THE
PEDIATRIC
ANESTHESIA
HANDBOOK

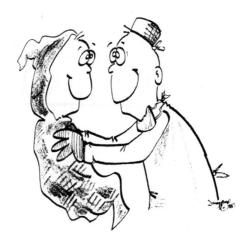

in your hands

now i lay me down to
sleep
all my trust in those who
seek
to ease my pain and my fears
to fix what's broken without my tears
and when I awake, I hope to be
on my way to
recovery

Adrienne Coleman

THE PEDIATRIC ANESTHESIA HANDBOOK

SECOND EDITION

Edited by

Charlotte Bell, M.D.
Associate Professor of Anesthesiology

Zeev N. Kain, M.D.
Assistant Professor of Anesthesiology and Pediatrics

Department of Anesthesiology
Yale University School of Medicine
New Haven, Connecticut

Visiting Editor
Cindy Hughes, M.D.

with poetry by Rivian Bell, Adrienne Coleman, and Mack T. McCoy
and cartoons by Jack Maypole, M.D.

 Mosby

An Affiliate of Elsevier Science

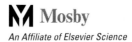
Mosby
An Affiliate of Elsevier Science

Vice President and Publisher: Anne S. Patterson
Editor: Laurel Craven
Developmental Editor: Wendy Buckwalter
Project Manager: Mark Spann
Production Editor: Steve Hetager
Book Design Manager: Judi Lang
Manufacturing Supervisor: Karen Boehme
Cover Art: Bob Messick

Great care has been used in compiling and checking the information in this book to ensure its accuracy. However, because of changing technology, recent discoveries, research, and individualization of prescriptions according to patient needs, the uses, effects, and dosages of drugs may vary from those given here. Neither the publisher nor the authors shall be responsible for such variations or other inaccuracies. We urge that before you administer any drug you check the manufacturer's dosage recommendations as given in the package insert provided with each product.

Printed in the United States of America

Mosby Inc.
11830 Westline Industrial Drive
St. Louis, Missouri 63146

ISBN 0-8151-0659-9

02 03 04 / 9 8 7 6 5

CONTRIBUTORS

The following people are recognized for their many contributions to this edition of *The Pediatric Anesthesia Handbook* in the areas of manuscript preparation, referencing, proofreading, and editing. The culmination of their efforts has made this book possible.

Lisa Caramico, M.D.
Kelly Colingo, M.D.
Cynthia Ferris, M.D.
Dorothy Gaal, M.D.
Antonio Hernandez Conte, M.D.
David Jaeger, M.D.
Boonsri Kosarussavadi, M.D.
Ben Lee, M.D.
Kathryn E. McGoldrick, M.D.
Gail Rasmussen, M.D.
Stephen Rimar, M.D.
Michelle Sanders, B.A.
Anne Savarese, M.D.
Martha Spieker, M.D.
Cephas Swamidoss, M.D.
Rachel Villaneuva, B.S.
Patricia Van der Mark, M.D.
Steven Weisman, M.D.
Shu Ming Wang, M.D.

FROM THE FIRST EDITION

Some material from the previous edition appears in this text. We would like to acknowledge the contributions of these authors:

Susan M. Chlebowski, M.D.; Richard A. DuBose, M.D.; Stephen A. Eige, M.D.; Jody Shapiro Gettleman, M.D.; Jonathan D. Halevy, M.D.; Roberta L. Hines, M.D.; Michael D. Ho, M.D.; Frederick C. Jacobson, M.D.; Karen M. Kabat, M.D.; Boonsri Kosarussavadi, M.D.; Kathryn E. McGoldrick, M.D.; Francis X. McGowan, M.D.; Kevin S. Morrison, M.D.; Tae Hee Oh, M.D.; Gail E. Rasmussen, M.D.; A. Pamela Reichheld, M.D.; Stephen Rimar, M.D.; Christine S. Rinder, M.D.; William H. Rosenblatt, M.D.; Anne M. Savarese, M.D.; Mary M. Stenger, M.D.; Harvey Stern, M.D.; Michael K. Urban, M.D.; Edward Weingarden, M.D.; Howard A. Zucker, M.D.

dedicated to
Tae Hee Oh, M.D.,
founder of the Section of Pediatric Anesthesia
at Yale,
colleague,
mentor,
and dear friend

PREFACE

The first edition of *The Pediatric Anesthesia Handbook* was a gamble. We took a huge amount of information and organized it to include pediatric physiology, drug dosing, equipment sizes, and treatment protocols. Such minutiae are difficult to remember, even for those of us who treat children every day, so we knew such a handbook would be valuable; it was just a matter of getting in all the detail. This second edition fine tunes the first, five years later. It expands areas from the first edition that proved to be most pertinent for readers, and refocuses other sections that had fewer clinical applications than we originally envisioned. We maintained the handbook's format, as accessibility, organization, simplification, and completeness were central to accomplishing our goal of making the *Handbook* a text that any health care provider could pick up and use at a moment's notice.

Specifically, information on physiology and anesthetic implications is more completely cross-referenced to supply the reader with more information without repetition. Whenever possible, the tabular format has been retained, especially for treatment protocols and drug dosing. Since this book is designed to be a handbook and brevity is essential, the reader may still desire more detail on certain topics. Therefore, we increased the number of referenced contemporary textbooks and journal articles in both the anesthetic and pediatric literature that provide further explications of such topics.

Some sections of the *Handbook* have been expanded to reflect contemporary pediatric anesthetic practice. For example, the chapter on congenital heart disease includes more physiologic explanations and illustrations of complex surgical repairs, as these children are commonly presenting for minor surgical procedures in locations away from tertiary care centers. We included more information on management of the difficult airway, in both urgent and elective situations, with emphasis on some of the new tools available (e.g., lightwand and laryngeal mask airway). The chapter on equipment and monitoring has been enlarged to reflect the importance of monitoring standards required by anesthesiology, pediatrics, hospitals, insurance companies, the legal profession, and most importantly, our patients and their families.

Since outpatient procedures are becoming the norm rather than the exception, we have eliminated the requisite chapter on anesthesia for ambulatory surgery. In its place you will find a chapter discussing the *unanticipated* pediatric admission, by Kathryn E. McGoldrick, M.D., director of the Yale Ambulatory Surgery Center and renowned expert. Drug lists and eponym lists have been updated. And finally, more emergency treatment protocols and information have been added to the appendixes for rapid location of information in urgent clinical situations. All other sections of the *Handbook* have been rewritten and newly referenced based on current anesthetic or pediatric practice.

It is a great pleasure for us to introduce the creative artists who have added a dimension to the *Handbook* which is singular among anesthesiology textbooks. We are pleased to precede each chapter with poetry as we did with the first edition. This time, however, all of the poetry is original and specifically written for the *Handbook*. Some of the poetry is humorous, some touching, but all reflecting the many emotions that are present when we care for these very special children. Rivian Bell and Adrienne Coleman have added a unique perspective to this book by sharing their literary gift. We are awed by their talent and grateful for their contributions.

By a stroke of luck, one of us (C.B.) happened to meet Mack McCoy in Washington, D.C., while traveling to give a lecture. From the driver's seat of his taxicab, he explained his self-expression through poetry, and his poem *no end* seemed the perfect way to bring the book to closure. It appears great things are sometimes found when you least expect them.

Jack Maypole, M.D., whose original cartoons are scattered throughout the book, has only recently graduated from Yale Medical School and is pursuing a career as a pediatrician. He is an accomplished student, an exceptionally talented artist, and a careful and caring physician. It has been an honor and a pleasure to have him join us in creating the *Handbook*.

Rachel Villanueva and Michelle Sanders, also Yale medical students, contributed to manuscript preparation. We thank them both for their hard work, infectious enthusiasm, and friendship.

We would like to express our gratitude to several others for their help and participation in completing this book. Our colleagues in the Section of Pediatric Anesthesia at the Children's Hospital at Yale have contributed material, references, photographs, and tables.

We are also indebted to Yale faculty in other sections and to a few Yale alumni who contributed their expertise on special topics. In particular, Rodrigio Nehgme, M.D., Section of Pediatric Cardiology at Yale, was kind enough to review and correct cardiac arrhythmia protocols.

We are especially grateful to Sarah Wheeler, Administrative and Editorial Assistant, for her expert management of all aspects of this *Handbook*'s evolution. Without her skill, quiet assurance, and sense of humor this book would have never reached conclusion.

And finally, we must thank the many readers of the first edition for your support, which encouraged us to undertake this mammoth effort once again.

The Editors

PERSONAL THANKS

I am truly indebted to my family for their constant support throughout the process of writing this book. My husband, John R. Loeffler, the only surgeon I've known to drive patients home from the hospital and deliver medication to those who can't get to his office, continues to be my model of the consummate physician and the ultimate source of my achievements and accomplishments. And to our three children, Caitlin, Zachary, and Burke, now too old to appear as photographic models in this edition, but whose love and acceptance have taught me the most important details about the care of children.

Charlotte Bell

The completion of this book is in no small measure due to the understanding, love, and continual support of my family. My wife, Tatiana Kain, a gifted radiologist, is my emotional center; without her I would not be who I am today. My children, Danielle and Alexandra, make me proud and make me laugh and remind me of the special needs of children everywhere. My mother and father, Samuel and Lea, have been my model for life and endurance. They survived the Holocaust and rebuilt their lives, providing a caring home for their children. I am grateful for all these people in my life.

Zeev Kain

CONTENTS

APPENDIXES

THE
PEDIATRIC
ANESTHESIA
HANDBOOK

I

PERIOPERATIVE GENERAL CONSIDERATIONS

PREOPERATIVE EVALUATION

as he sailed into
OR
seems the drugs had not gone
far
timothy tossed the gurney
round
nurse elaine had to calm him
down
no one understood—this was tim before
bed
until he had *Goodnight Moon*
read
all the strangers, all around
want to calm my screaming down
let my mom come in with me
read the story 'bout the sea
rub my head, sing lullabies
rock me 'till i close my eyes

Adrienne Coleman

GOALS

With the increase in ambulatory procedures and same-day surgery has come an inevitable decrease in time allotted for the preoperative interview, as well as preparation time for children and their families. However, obtaining a thorough medical history, performing a physical examination and successfully establishing rapport and trust with child and family still require a relaxed, unhurried interview, despite recent changes in medical economics.

Several techniques have been developed to successfully accomplish the preoperative interview within the resources of a given hospital. These include:

1. A complete preoperative program whereby patients and their families come to the operating room several days before an elective procedure. At this time the anesthesiologist can obtain the history and physical, any needed laboratory procedures are obtained, instructions are given, records are ordered, and play therapy and/or tours are provided.

2. Patients and families are interviewed the same day as scheduled surgery.
3. Telephone interviews with the parents are arranged to obtain needed information and relay instructions.[1]
4. A combination of 1, 2, and 3.

Regardless of the technique used, the preoperative interview should be designed to meet the following objectives:

1. To obtain essential details of the child's present illness and medical history
2. To assess potential anesthetic risk factors and discuss their likelihood and treatment with the patient and family
3. To initiate an anesthetic plan that is acceptable to the patient and family (including invasive procedures and monitoring) and secure informed consent
4. To discuss recovery, postoperative analgesia, and discharge planning and to answer questions
5. To allay anxiety and to establish trust and confidence with the patient and family
6. To offer play therapy and tours of operating, induction, and recovery rooms so that unfamiliar procedures become routine

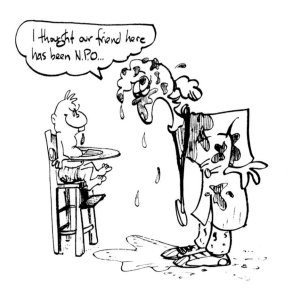

ANESTHETIC RISK

The preoperative interview should allow the anesthetist sufficient time to assess the problems listed below and to determine which intraoperative and postoperative problems are likely to occur and how they can best be managed.

Preoperative problems

Prematurity
Congenital malformations
Inherited disorders
Respiratory dysfunction
- Apnea
- RDS/BPD
- Asthma/bronchospasm
- Aspiration
- Infections (URI)

Intraoperative problems

Separation anxiety
Dental injury
Blood transfusions

Postoperative problems

Behavioral changes
Postoperative admission
Prolonged mechanical ventilation

Prematurity (see p. 409)

Chronic respiratory dysfunction with risk of *apnea* is the most common sequela to *prematurity*; it is seen even in compensated patients scheduled for minor elective procedures. Controversy persists regarding at what age former premature infants are no longer at risk for postoperative apnea, with ages ranging from 44 weeks postconceptional age (PCA) to 60 weeks PCA.[2,3] Several authors have also reported clinically significant apnea in full-term infants.[4-7] Regional procedures without sedation (spinal, caudal) seem to offer less risk of apnea, desaturation, and bradycardia for patients undergoing herniorrhaphy.[8-10] Other reported risk factors are listed on p. 6.

Author, year	Risk factors
Steward, 1982[11]	Apnea associated with prematurity in infants ‹3 kg and ‹10 wk postnatal age
Liu, 1983[12]	Apnea associated with PCA* ‹41 wk, history of apnea, and use of muscle relaxants
Mayhew, 1987[13]	Apnea associated with history of apnea and BPD
Kurth, 1987[3]	Apnea associated with PCA ‹60 wk, history of NEC, may occur as late as 12 hr
Welbourn, 1989[14]	Apnea found in patients *not* receiving caffeine pre-operatively
Kurth, 1991[15]	Mixed apnea (central and obstructive); leads to a lower SpO$_2$
Welborn, 1991[16]	Apnea associated with low hematocrit
Warner, 1992[17]	Apnea associated with age ‹49 wk, history of apnea, RDS, ventilator support, anemia
Gollin, 1993[18]	Apnea associated with history of RDS/BPD and PDA

*PCA, postconceptional age; *BPD,* bronchopulmonary dysplasia; *NEC,* necrotizing enterocolitis; *RDS,* respiratory distress syndrome; *PDA,* patent ductus arterious.

Congenital/Inherited Disorders

Congenital malformations and inherited disorders may be already diagnosed or suspected from the family history. Occasionally, previously undiagnosed disorders lead to anesthetic complications (see p. 486). In known disorders, the child may well have been seen and treated by multiple specialists. Acquiring old records and contacting the primary care physician become a necessity.

Respiratory Dysfunction

Respiratory disorders present such a wide range of disease processes that assigning risk preoperatively becomes difficult for even the experienced practitioner. Chronic lung disease as a result of prematurity may substantially increase the risk of respiratory complications after general anesthesia in young infants.[18] Conversely, there is little concrete data to predict morbidity after anesthesia in children with asthma (see p. 118). Children with chronic reflux/aspiration disorders are at increased risk because of the frequent simultaneous occurrence of pulmonary and neurologic disease.

UPPER RESPIRATORY INFECTIONS (URI)[19-21]

Most anesthesiologists agree that the presence of an acute purulent URI, fever, or any symptomatology of a lower respiratory infection would be sufficient grounds to postpone an elective surgical procedure. However, the child with the nonpurulent, nonacute URI nearly always presents a conundrum for even the most experienced anesthesiologist. Evidence exists to support the following statements:

1. Children with URI, particularly those less than 1 year of age, have an increased risk of respiratory-related adverse events intraoperatively and postoperatively.[22,23]
2. Symptomatic infants with URI have a decreased time to desaturation during apnea.[23]
3. Temperature regulation may be disrupted during URI.[23]
4. Endotracheal intubation seems to be a major risk factor for hypoxemia, bronchospasm, and atelectasis in children with URI.[20,22,23]
5. Inhalation agents may actually decrease the severity of viral URI in animals.[24]
6. Temporary airway hyperreactivity exists for 6 weeks after a viral infection.[25]
7. Most complications seen in older children (over 1 year of age) with mild, nonacute, nonpurulent URI after anesthesia are mild and easily treated.[20,23]

This evidence leads to the widely accepted recommendation that it is probably safe to proceed with minor procedures not requiring endotracheal intubation when a child over age 1 has a mild nonpurulent, nonacute URI. If it is deemed appropriate to postpone after considering the psychological, physiological, and economic implications, then waiting 4 to 6 weeks will minimize the chances of airway hyperreactivity.

Separation Anxiety

Information is becoming increasingly available on factors that may influence the occurrence of *separation anxiety,* including: (1) age ‹6, (2) lack of a preoperative visit, and (3) anxious behavior noted at the preoperative visit.[26] Conversely, recent evidence suggests that a preoperative visit designed to decrease anxiety may actually have the opposite effect in some children, perhaps because this population uses avoidance as a primary coping mechanism.[27] There is also evidence to suggest that prolonged behavior changes after surgery may be linked to preoperative anxiety.[28] A realistic discussion with parents, along with suggestions to minimize psychological trauma (e.g., premedication, play therapy, parental presence), will allow parents an opportunity to prepare for and assess potential psychological changes rather than regarding them as "complications."

Blood Transfusions

During the preoperative interview, the potential for transfusion of blood or blood products should be discussed. This discussion should include indications for transfusion, risk of any infection (according to local or state blood banks), and availability of directed donor or autologous transfusion.

Dental Trauma

The potential for damage to a child's nondeciduous teeth is minimal. However, the overwhelmingly negative response elicited from parents when this complication occurs is sufficient to warrant mentioning during the preoperative interview. It may be wise to plan removal of loose deciduous teeth just prior to intubation to prevent injury or aspiration. This should be agreed upon in advance with parents, child, and surgeon.

Admission to the Hospital

In this age of medical-economic crisis, many elective procedures are given outpatient standing regardless of the patient's preoperative medical condition. Parents and patients should be advised preoperatively of the likelihood of admission even if insurance carriers preclude the option of planned elective admission.

Postoperative Mechanical Ventilation/Intensive Care Admission

Likewise, a preoperative discussion of possible prolonged mechanical ventilation or ICU stay helps parents and patients to perceive these as anticipated sequelae and not complications.

HISTORY AND PHYSICAL

The preoperative history and physical for the pediatric patient consist of pertinent maternal history, birth and neonatal history, childhood history, review of systems, physical examination, and evaluation of height, weight, and vital signs. Because this process may be very brief in the healthy child, the use of preprinted admission forms is popular, particularly in busy output settings.

Maternal history with commonly associated neonatal problems

Maternal history	Anticipated neonatal sequelae
Rh-ABO incompatibility	Hemolytic anemia, hyperbilirubinemia, kernicterus
Toxemia	Small birth weight–associated problems (see p. 409), muscle relaxant interaction after magnesium therapy
Hypertension	Small birth weight
Infection	Sepsis, thrombocytopenia, viral infection
Hemorrhage	Anemia, shock
Diabetes	Hypoglycemia, birth trauma, macrosomia, or small birth weight
Polyhydramnios	Tracheoesophageal fistula, anencephaly, multiple anomalies
Oligohydramnios	Renal hypoplasia, pulmonary hypoplasia
Cephalopelvic disproportion	Birth trauma, hyperbilirubinemia, fractures
Alcoholism	Hypoglycemia, congenital malformation, fetal alcohol syndrome, small birth weight

Adapted from Coté CJ, Todres ID, Ryan JF: Preoperative evaluation of pediatric patients. In Coté CJ, Todres ID, Ryan JF, Goudsouzian NG, eds: *A practice of anesthesia for infants and children,* Philadelphia, 1993, WB Saunders, p 41.

Past medical history

Birth history	Maternal health, labor history, prematurity, condition at delivery

Neonatal history	Respiratory
	  RDS/BPD
	  Apnea
	  Congenital malformations
	Congenital cardiac anomalies
	Neurological problems
	  Congenital malformations/infections
	  Hemorrhage
	  Encephalopathy
	Metabolic/endocrine
	  Inborn errors of metabolism
	  Hypoglycemia
	  Hyperbilirubinemia
	Hematologic
	  Hemoglobinopathy
	  Rh or ABO incompatibility
	  Disseminated intravascular coagulation
	Renal
	Infections (STORCH)
	  Syphilis
	  Toxoplasmosis
	  Respiratory syncytial virus (RSV)
	  Cytomegalovirus (CMV)
	  Herpes
	Gastrointestinal
	  Congenital
	  Necrotizing enterocolitis

Childhood history	Chronic infections Croup Bronchospasm Review by systems (see table on p.11) Growth and development Previous surgery/anesthesia/hospitalizations Previous blood transfusions Medications Allergies and drug sensitivity Family history

Review by systems (acute and chronic conditions)

Respiratory

Asthma
Croup
Recent upper respiratory tract infection
Nasal congestion
Cough
History of apnea/bradycardia
Snoring, sleep apnea

Cardiovascular

Murmur
Easy fatigability
Dyspnea
Cyanosis

Neurologic

Seizures
Headache and vomiting
   (suggestive of elevated ICP)
Spasticity
Hypotonia
Developmental delay

Gastrointestinal

Reflux
Vomiting
Aspiration
Last oral intake

Renal

Time of last urination
   (urine specific gravity to assess
   hydration status)
Urinary tract infections

Metabolic/endocrine

Steroid medications
Growth failure
Last menstrual period of adolescent females

Hematologic

Easy bleeding/easily bruised
Anemia
Sickle cell trait/disease

Infectious

Recent upper respiratory
   infection
Fever
Otitis

Oral/dental

Loose or missing teeth
Caries
Conditions of soft and hard
   palates
Macroglossia
Micrognathia

Physical examination

Vital signs
General appearance
- Color
- Nutrition
- Hydration
- Mental status/activity

Head
- Fontanelle
- Craniofacial dysmorphisms, particularly of the nose, mouth, and jaw

Eyes/ears
- Strabismus
- Pupillary size and reactivity

Nose/mouth
- Oropharyngeal aperture
- Condition of soft and hard palates
- Dentition
- Size of tongue
- Adenotonsillar hypertrophy
- Dysmorphic mandible or maxilla

Neck
- Thyroid gland size
- Tracheal deviation

Chest
- Pattern and depth of spontaneous breathing
- Use of accessory muscles of respiration (e.g., neck muscles, intercostal retractions)
- Breath sounds (e.g., rales, stridor, wheezes, rhonchi, equality)

Cardiovascular
- Auscultation for S_1 and S_2, murmurs and their location
- Neck veins (distended, flat)
- Peripheral pulses and perfusion

Abdomen
- Size
- Contour (scaphoid, flat, protuberant, distended)
- Note tenderness and/or rigidity

Neurologic
- Mental status
- Development
- Gait, muscle strength
- If regional anesthetic planned, inspect back for vertebral landmarks, scoliosis/curvatures, flexibility, spina bifida, or sacral dimple

Growth characteristics: 50% for age values[29]

	Weight (kg)		Height (cm)		Head circumference (cm)	
	Male	Female	Male	Female	Male	Female
Full term	3.4	3.2	51	50	35	34
1 to 6 mo	4	4	54	54	37	36
6 mo to 1 yr	8	7	68	66	44	43
1 to 2 yr	10	10	76	74	47	46
2 to 3 yr	13	12	88	86	49	48
3 to 6 yr	15-19	14-18	95-110	94-108	50	50
6 to 9 yr	21-25	20-25	116-127	115-127	52	51
9 to 12 yr	28-40	28-42	132-149	132-151	53	52
12 to 16 yr	45-62	46-56	156-173	157-163	55	54

Vital signs[30-32]

Age	HR	Systolic BP	RR
Preterm infant	120-180	40-60	55-60
Newborn	95-145	50-70	35-40
6 mo	110-180	60-110	25-30
1 to 2 yr	100-160	65-115	20-24
2 to 3 yr	90-150	75-125	16-22
3 to 5 yr	65-135	80-120	14-20
5 to 8 yr	70-115	92-120	12-20
9 to 12 yr	55-110	92-130	12-20
12 to 14 yr	55-105	100-140	10-14

ANESTHETIC PLAN

Preoperative fasting guidelines
Preoperative laboratory data
Inpatient orders
Induction schemes
Choosing premedication
Recovery
Pstoperative pain management

During the preoperative evaluation, each topic listed above should be considered as part of the anesthetic plan and communicated to appropriate staff, surgical or pediatric colleagues, parents and child. One of the most important considerations when formulating the anesthetic plan is that all patients, including and perhaps especially children, need to have a sense of control and therefore should be included in the selection process at whatever level is appropriate. This may be as simple as a young child selecting a favorite toy for the operating room or as significant as an older child selecting an inhalation versus intravenous induction.

This section will cover all aspects of the plan except premedication, recovery, and pain management, which are discussed in Chapters 2, 5, and 20, respectively.

Preoperative Fasting Guidelines

Recent studies have favored the liberalization of fasting guidelines in children.[33-36] Although individual institutional guidelines may vary, the following data have helped to decrease controversy:

1. Aspiration pneumonitis in children is extremely rare. Of 40,000 cases involving use of anesthetics prospectively studied in France, the reported incidence of aspiration was 1:10,000 in children, with no reports of pneumonitis.[37]
2. Drinking clear liquids up to 2 hours prior to surgery has little effect on the gastric volume or pH.[33,36]
3. Drinking clear liquids may decrease irritability and thirst[33,38] and minimize dehydration and hypoglycemia.[34]
4. Emptying times of breast milk may be unpredictable. As such, it may be considered as a solid, especially in infants at risk for aspiration.[39]

Given the parameters above, many institutions now recommend a 4-hour fast for solids and/or milk (breast or formula) in infants and a 6- to 8-hour fast for older children, with *ad libitum* clear liquids for all patients until 2 hours preoperatively.

Preoperative Laboratory Data

The value of routine preoperative laboratory testing for healthy children undergoing minor procedures is questionable and has not been justified by recent studies.[40-42] However, most practitioners request a hemoglobin/hematocrit for infants, for patients with hemoglobinopathy or chronic disease and for procedures with anticipated blood loss. Other laboratory data are usually requested only when warranted by the preoperative medical evaluation or scheduled surgical procedure.

Common pediatric laboratory values*[43-45]

	Full term	Newborn	< 2 yr	2-15 yr
Electrolytes,[†] mEq/L (mmo/L)				
Sodium	130-140	135-145		
Potassium	3.5-6.0		3.5-5.0	
Chloride	96-109			
Bicarbonate	18-26	20-25	22-26	
Miscellaneous chemistries				
Total calcium, mg/dl (mmol/L)	6-10 (1.5-2.5)	7.0-12.0 (1.75-3.0)	8-10.5 (2-2.6)	
Glucose, mg/dl (mmol/L)	20-65 (1.1-3.6)	40-110 (2.2-6.4)	60-105 (3.3-5.8)	
Urea nitrogen, mg/dl (mmol/L)	5-25 (1.8-9.0)			
Creatinine, mg/dl (μmol/L)	0.3-1.0 (27-88)	Infant 0.2-0.4 (18-35)	Child 0.3-0.7 (27-62)	Adolescent 0.5-1.0 (44-88)
Magnesium, mEq/L (mmol/L)	1.5-2.3 (0.75-1.15)		1.4-2 (0.7-1)	

*Values expressed as mean or range. SI units and values are shown in parentheses.
[†]For electrolytes, mEq/L = mmol/L.

Common pediatric laboratory values*[43-45]

	Preterm	Full term	1-3 days	1 mo	2-6 mo	6 mo-2 yr	2-12 yr
Hematology							
Hgb, g/dl	13-15	13-19	14-24	11-17	10-14	11-15	12-15
Hct, %	41-47	51	55	35-50	30-40	37	37-40
White blood cells, $10^3/mm^3$	8-38			11.5-14	6-17	5-15.5	4.5-13.5
Platelets, $10^3/mm^3$	180-300	300	200	250	150-350		
Coagulation							
Prothrombin time (PT), sec	12-21	13-20		12-14			
Activated partial thromboplastin time (PTT), sec	70	45-65				30-45	
Fibrinogen, mg/dl (g/L)	200-400 (2-40)						

*Values expressed as mean or range. SI units and values are shown in parentheses.

Inpatient Orders

1. Specify fasting guidelines.
2. If a preoperative intravenous catheter should be placed, specify when, which fluid, and at what rate.
3. Clarify which routine medications should be given, at what time, and by which route. Consider also antibiotic prophylaxis and stress steroid coverage (see pp. 627 and 666).
4. Order premedications and specify dose, time, and route of administration.
5. Request that all current and old records and current inpatient day sheets be sent to the operating room with the patient.
6. Order transport monitoring and oxygen therapy during transport when appropriate.

Induction Schemes

Induction plans are usually selected on the basis of the child's preoperative medical condition, the presence or absence of an intravenous catheter, and, not insignificantly, the child's (or parent's) choice. Regardless of the method selected, the preoperative interview is the appropriate time to discuss the induction process with the child and parents. Allowing the child to actually practice the induction technique through play therapy is a useful technique to allay anxiety about new and unfamiliar procedures. Likewise, many practitioners have found the presence of a parent helpful in ensuring patient cooperation, allowing for a smoother induction. The success of each technique is dependent upon the anesthetist's skill and experience, representing the interface of art and science in pediatric anesthesiology. Parents and children should always be assured that more than one technique can be used and that a backup or alternative plan will be discussed.

References

1. Patel RI, Hannallah RS: Preoperative screening for pediatric ambulatory surgery: evaluation of a telephone questionnaire method, *Anesth Analg* 75:258-261, 1992.
2. Welborn LG, Ramirez N, Oh TH, et al: Postanesthetic apnea and periodic breathing in infants, *Anesthesiology* 65:658-661, 1986.
3. Kurth CD, Spitzer AR, Broennle AM, Downes JJ: Postoperative apnea in preterm infants, *Anesthesiology* 66:483-488, 1987.
4. Coté CJ, Kelly DH: Postoperative apnea in a full-term infant with a demonstrable respiratory pattern abnormality, *Anesthesiology* 72:559-561, 1990.
5. Tetzlaff JE, Annand DW, Pudimat MA, Nicodemus HF: Postoperative apnea in a full-term infant, *Anesthesiology* 69:426-428, 1988.
6. Karayan J, LaCoste L, Fusciardi J: Postoperative apnea in a full-term infant, *Anesthesiology* 75:375, 1991.
7. Noseworthy J, Duran C, Khine HH: Postoperative apnea in a full-term infant, *Anesthesiology* 70:879-880, 1989.
8. Welborn LG, Rice LJ, Hannallah RS, Broadman LM, Ruttiman UE, Fink R: Postoperative apnea in former preterm infants: prospective comparison of spinal and general anesthesia, *Anesthesiology* 72:838-842, 1990.
9. Krane EJ, Haberkern CM, Jacobson LE: Postoperative apnea, bradycardia, and oxygen desaturation in formerly premature infants: prospective comparison of spinal and general anesthesia, *Anesth Analg* 80:7-13, 1995.
10. Cox RG, Goresky GV: Life-threatening apnea following spinal anesthesia in former premature infants, *Anesthesiology* 73:345-347, 1990.
11. Steward DJ: Preterm infants are more prone to complications following minor surgery than are term infants, *Anesthesiology* 56:304-306, 1982.

12. Liu LMP, Coté CJ, Goudsouzian NG, et al: Life threatening apnea in infants recovering from anesthesia, *Anesthesiology* 59:506-510, 1983.

13. Mayhew JF, Bourke DL, Guinee WS: Evaluation of the premature infant at risk for postoperative complications, *Can J Anaesth* 34:627-631, 1987.

14. Welborn LG, Hannallah RS, Fink R, Ruttimann UE, Hicks JM: High-dose caffeine suppresses postoperative apnea in former preterm infants, *Anesthesiology* 71:347-349, 1989.

15. Kurth CD, LeBard SE: Association of postoperative apnea, airway obstruction, and hypoxemia in former premature infants, *Anesthesiology* 75:22-26, 1991.

16. Welborn LG, Hannallah RS, Luban NL, Fink R, Ruttiman UE: Anemia and postoperative apnea in former preterm infants, *Anesthesiology* 74:1003-1006, 1991.

17. Warner LO, Teitelbaum DH, Caniano DA, Vanik PE, Martino JD, Servick JD: Inguinal herniorrhaphy in young infants: perianesthetic complications and associated preanesthetic risk, *J Clin Anesth* 4:455-461, 1992.

18. Gollin G, Bell C, Dubose R, et al: Predictors of postoperative respiratory complications in premature infants after inguinal herniorrhaphy, *J Pediatr Surg* 28:244-247, 1993.

19. Kinouchi K, Tanigami H, Tashiro C, Nishimur M, Fukumitsu K, Takauchi Y: Duration of apnea in anesthetized infants and children required for desaturation of hemoglobin to 95%: the influence of upper respiratory infection, *Anesthesiology* 77:1105-1107, 1992.

20. Rolf N, Coté CJ: Frequency and severity of desaturation events during general anesthesia in children with and without upper respiratory infections, *J Clin Anesth* 4:200-203, 1992.

21. Martin LD: Anesthetic implications of an upper respiratory infection in children, *Pediatr Clin North Am* 41:121-130, 1994.

22. DeSoto H, Patel RI, Soliman IE, et al: Changes in oxygen saturation following general anesthesia in children with upper respiratory infection signs and symptoms undergoing otolaryngological procedures, *Anesthesiology* 68:276, 1988.

23. Cohen MM, Cameron CB: Should you cancel the operation when a child has an upper respiratory tract infection? *Anesth Analg* 72:282-288, 1991.

24. Tait AR, Davidson BA, Johnson KJ, et al: Halothane inhibits the intraalveolar recruitment of neutrophils, lymphocytes, and macrophages in the response to influenza virus infection in mice, *Anesth Analg* 76:1106, 1993.

25. Aquilina AT, Hall WJ, Douglas RG Jr, et al: Airway reactivity in subjects with viral upper respiratory tract infections: the effects of exercise and cold air, *Am Rev Respir Dis* 122:3, 1980.

26. Vetter TR: The epidemiology and selective identification of children at risk for preoperative anxiety reactions, *Anesth Analg* 77:96-99, 1993.

27. Kain ZN, Mayes L, Nygren MA, Spieker M, Brandiff C, Rimar S: Does a preparation program decrease preoperative anxiety in children and parents? *Anesthesiology* 81(3A):A1362, 1994.

28. Kain ZN, Mayes L, Nygren M, Rimar S: Behavioral disturbances in children following surgery, *Anesthesiology* 81(3A):A1382, 1994.
29. Hamill VV et al: Physical growth: National Center for Health Statistics percentiles, *Am J Clin Nutr* 32:607-629, 1979.
30. Ingelfinger JR, Powers L, Epstein MF: Blood pressure norms in low birthweight infants: birth through four weeks, *Pediatr Res* 17:319A, 1983.
31. Kendig EL, Chernick V, eds: *Disorders of the respiratory tract in children,* Philadelphia, 1983, WB Saunders.
32. Nelson WE, ed: *Textbook of pediatrics,* ed 13, Philadelphia, 1987, WB Saunders.
33. Schreiner MS, Triebwasser A, Keon TP: Ingestion of liquids compared with preoperative fasting in pediatric outpatients, *Anesthesiology* 72:593-597, 1990.
34. Nicolson SC, Dorsey AT, Schreiner MS: Shortened preanesthetic fasting interval in pediatric cardiac surgical patients, *Anesth Analg* 74:694-697, 1992.
35. Larsson LE, Nilsson K, Niklasson A, Andreasson S, Ekström-Jodal B: Influence of fluid regimens on perioperative blood glucose concentrations in neonates, *Br J Anaesth* 64:419-424, 1990.
36. Splinter WM, Steward JA, Muir JG: Large volumes of apple juice preoperatively do not affect gastric pH and volume in children, *Can J Anaesth* 37:36-39, 1990.
37. Tiret L, Nivoche Y, Hatton F, Desmonts JM, Vourc'h G: Complications related to anaesthesia in infants and children: a prospective survey of 40240 anaesthetics, *Br J Anaesth* 61:263-269, 1988.
38. Splinter WM, Schaefer JD: Ingestion of clear fluids is safe for adolescents up to 3 h before anaesthesia, *Br J Anaesth* 66:48-52, 1991.
39. Litman RS, Wu CL, Quinlivan JK: Gastric volume and pH in infants fed clear liquids and breast milk prior to surgery, *Anesth Analg* 70:482-485, 1994.
40. Roy WL, Lerman J, McIntyre BG: Is preoperative haemoglobin testing justified in children undergoing minor elective surgery? *Can J Anaesth* 38:700-703, 1991.
41. Hackmann T, Steward DJ, Sheps SB: Anemia in pediatric day-surgery patients: prevalence and detection, *Anesthesiology* 75:27-31, 1991.
42. O'Connor ME, Drasner K: preoperative laboratory testing of children undergoing elective surgery, *Anesth Analg* 70:176-180, 1990.
43. Johnson KB, ed: *The Harriet Lane Handbook,* ed 13, St. Louis, 1993, Mosby.
44. Wallach J, ed: *Interpretation of pediatric tests: a handbook synopsis of pediatric, fetal, and obstetric laboratory medicine,* Boston, 1983, Little, Brown.
45. Silver HK, Kempe CH, Bruyn HB, Fulginitti VA, eds: *Handbook of pediatrics,* East Norwalk, Conn, 1987, Appleton & Lange.

PREMEDICATION

2

rock a bye
the butterflies
shaky knees and
twitching eyes . . . .

take a breath
close your eyes
a little 'dazzler
is advised

Adrienne Coleman

GOALS OF PREMEDICATION

The primary goals of premedication in children are to facilitate a smooth separation from the parents and to ease the induction of anesthesia. Other effects that may be achieved by pharmacologic preparation of the patient include:

1. Amnesia
2. Anxiolysis
3. Prevention of physiologic stress (e.g., avoiding tachycardia in patients with cyanotic congenital heart disease)
4. Reduction of total anesthetic requirements
5. Decreased probability of aspiration of acidic stomach contents
6. Vagolysis
7. Decreased salivation and secretions
8. Antiemesis
9. Analgesia

CONSIDERATIONS FOR PREMEDICATION

1. Should the drug be given as a premedication, or would the drug effect be achieved more predictably by intravenous injection (e.g., atropine IM premedication versus IV preintubation)? Is sufficient time available for the drug to achieve the desired effect?

2. Does the patient have any contraindications to receiving a sedative, such as altered mental status, increased intracranial pressure, a difficult airway, compromised respiratory function, or hypovolemia?

3. Which route of administration (table on p. 23) will achieve the desired effect most effectively and be most acceptable to patient and parent?

4. Is the patient and/or parent able to participate in this decision (e.g., selecting IM or PO)?

5. Do the negative effects of the drug, such as respiratory or cardiovascular depression, tachycardia, or sedation lasting beyond the operation, outweigh the relative benefits of the premedication?

6. Has the child's age been considered? Infants less than 6 months of age can be separated easily from their parents by cuddling, keeping them warm, and allowing them to suck a pacifier. The more difficult airway and decreased respiratory reserve present in this age group add to the downside of using premedication. Conversely, patients who probably will benefit from premedication include:
   a. Toddlers and preschoolers, in whom separation anxiety is paramount
   b. Adolescents, who are particularly sensitive about body image and loss of control
   c. Patients with previous unpleasant hospital experiences
   d. Patients who are unable to communicate or cooperate (e.g., developmentally delayed)

7. Should the parents accompany the child into the operating room? Parental presence during induction of anesthesia has been suggested as a nonpharmacological intervention for reduction of preoperative anxiety.[1] The decision of applying this intervention should be individualized to the child, parent, and anesthesiologist. Although parental presence may be effective in some cases, it may lead to increased anxiety and decreased cooperation in others.[2]

8. EMLA (eutectic mixture of local anesthetics) cream supplies effective topical analgesia to intact skin if placed at least 1 hour prior to venipuncture and covered with an occlusive dressing. Parents (or older patients) can apply the EMLA cream. EMLA is

contraindicated in children with methemoglobinemia and should not be used in combination with drugs that induce methemoglobinemia. It is not recommended on mucous membranes and in children less than 1 month of age[3] (see p. 480).

Selecting a premedication by route of administration

PO (per os, orally)	Clonidine Diazepam Midazolam	Ketamine Pentobarbital Secobarbital
IN (intranasal)	Sufentanil Midazolam	Ketamine
PR (per rectum)	Pentobarbital Secobarbital Methohexital	Diazepam Midazolam Ketamine
OT (oral transmucosal)	Fentanyl lollipops	Midazolam
IM (intramuscular)	Pentobarbital Secobarbital Morphine Meperidine	Diazepam Midazolam Ketamine

ANXIOLYTICS
Benzodiazepines

Diazepam. Diazepam is given to allay anxiety and produce amnesia with minimal respiratory or cardiovascular depression. It rarely causes nausea or vomiting. Absorption from the gastrointestinal tract is more predictable than from the intramuscular route. Diazepam tends to precipitate and cause burning when given IV. It also can be administered rectally. Paradoxical excitement and lack of inhibition often occur, particularly at lower doses. Onset is slow and duration of action very long.

> Dose: diazepam   0.1 to 0.5 mg/kg PO, PR, IM

Midazolam. Midazolam is one of the most commonly used premedications. It has rapid onset and predictable effect without causing cardiorespiratory depression. Midazolam has short duration that does not delay emergence from general anesthesia or discharge from the PACU even for brief procedures.[4,5] It can be given by any route as dictated by the clinical setting. The intranasal route provides predictable effects within 10 minutes.[6] However, most children object strongly to the bitter taste and burning sensation. When mixed with fruit-flavored syrup and given orally, midazolam provides excellent sedation and anxiolysis in 30 to 45 minutes.[7] Sublingual, undiluted midazolam has been demonstrated to be as effective as nasal midazolam.[8] The tip of the syringe containing the midazolam can be dipped in candy flavor essence, then dipped in granulated sugar. The drug is then placed under the tongue and the child is instructed not to swallow the medication for 30 seconds. Sedation is obtained within 10 minutes after administration.[8] Unlike most other benzodiazepines, the intramuscular absorption of midazolam is reliable. It can be given per rectum, although this route may be objectionable to older children.

Dose: midazolam	0.2 to 0.3 mg/kg IN[5]
	0.5 mg/kg PO[4]
	0.08 to 0.5 mg/kg IM
	0.2 mg/kg OT[8]
	1 mg/kg PR[9]

Barbiturates

Pentobarbital or secobarbital. Pentobarbital or secobarbital produces sedation with minimal cardiovascular and respiratory depression and rarely causes nausea or vomiting. Each drug has a bitter taste when taken by mouth and can cause persistent pain at the injection site if given by intramuscular injection. Paradoxical responses (agitation and disorientation instead of sedation) are not uncommon, particularly in older children (>3 years of age).

Dose: pentobarbital or secobarbital	2 to 3 mg/kg PO
	2 to 4 mg/kg PR
	3 to 4 mg/kg IM

OPIOIDS

Morphine or meperidine.   Morphine or meperidine given intramuscularly produces both analgesia and sedation. However, opioids are potent respiratory depressants and can cause nausea, vomiting, pruritus, and dysphoria. In combination with barbiturates and/or scopolamine they produce excellent sedation and amnesia, particularly for patients with cyanotic congenital heart disease.

Dose: morphine   0.1 to 0.2 mg/kg IM
meperidine   1 to 2 mg/kg IM

Fentanyl. Fentanyl's lipid solubility makes it an ineffective premedication parenterally. However, oral transmucosal absorption in the form of the lollipop reportedly has produced effective preoperative sedation and facilitates inhalation induction of anesthesia.[10] At doses above those recommended by the manufacturers, transmucosal fentanyl causes pruritus of the nose and eyes in most patients; postoperative nausea and vomiting are common and are not significantly reduced by prophylactic droperidol.[10,11] To date, there are no outcome data based on use of the lower doses recommended by the manufacturers.

Dose: fentanyl   10 to 15 μg/kg OT

Sufentanil. Sufentanil has been given intranasally as a premedication.[12] Within 10 minutes of administration the patient should feel calm, cooperative, possibly euphoric, and easily separated from the parents. However the majority of patients will have an oxygen saturation of less than 95%.[13] There are also high incidences of apnea, laryngospasm, and chest wall rigidity.[14] When compared with nasal midazolam, sufentanil's risks outweigh the benefits.[15]

Dose: sufentanil   1.5 to 3 μg/kg IN

α-AGONIST

Clonidine. Clonidine is an α_2 agonist that when given in combination with atropine produces satisfactory preoperative sedation, easy separation from parents, and mask acceptance within 30 minutes.[16] Clonidine also attenuates the hemodynamic response to tracheal intubation. With the recommended dose, preoperative hypotension is not observed.[16] Premedication with oral clonidine also reduces the dose of intravenous thiamylal required for the induction of anesthesia.[17]

Dose: clonidine   4 μg/kg PO   *Administered together*
atropine   0.03 mg/kg PO

HYPNOTICS

Chloral hydrate and triclofos.   Chloral hydrate and triclofos are converted in the body to trichloroethanol, an active hypnotic agent. These agents are relatively safe, producing minimal respiratory depression, and are therefore used frequently by nonanesthesiologists. Chloral hydrate is the least palatable oral premedication and can cause gastric irritation. In contrast to older children and adults, neonates may manifest accumulation of chloral hydrate metabolites, leading to prolonged sedation.[18] In addition, administration of high doses to newborns may increase the serum direct bilirubin.[18]

Dose: chloral hydrate	25 to 75 mg/kg PO (max 1 g)
triclofos	70 mg/kg PO

ANTICHOLINERGICS

Current inhalation anesthetics do not stimulate salivary or tracheobronchial secretions. Therefore, premedication with anticholinergic drugs is not routinely indicated, and may cause fever, confusion, flushing, or an extremely dry mouth. Anticholinergics may be given during the operative procedure for their antisialagogue effect (e.g., oral surgery, airway manipulation), or vagolysis (e.g., traction on peritoneum, strabismus surgery, or preceding succinylcholine administration). Atropine is a better vagolytic agent than scopolamine; however, scopolamine produces amnesia and a better drying effect. Glycopyrrolate is the only agent that does not cross the blood-brain barrier, so it does not cause confusion. When compared to atropine, it is less effective in attenuating bradycardia during induction.[19] Preoperative administration of oral atropine or oral glycopyrrolate does not alter the incidence or degree of hypotension during induction of anesthesia.[19]

Dose: atropine	0.02 mg/kg IM, PO
	0.01 mg/kg IV
scopolamine	0.02 mg/kg IM
	0.01 mg/kg IV
glycopyrrolate	0.01 mg/kg IV, IM

ANTIHISTAMINE

Hydroxyzine. Hydroxyzine produces mild sedation with antiemetic, antihistaminic, and antispasmodic effects. When hydroxyzine is given in combination with narcotics, the sedative effects are additive.

> Dose: hydroxyzine   0.5 to 1 mg/kg PO, IM

H_2 antagonists/gastric motility stimulants. Seventy-five percent of fasting children have a gastric volume greater than 0.4 ml/kg and a pH less than 2.5, and are therefore at risk of developing acid aspiration syndrome following inhalation of gastric contents.[20] H_2 antagonists directly elevate gastric pH; metoclopramide decreases gastric fluid volume. This combination is effective when given by mouth 4 hours before operating.[21] These drugs usually are indicated in patients with gastrointestinal disorders.

H_2 antagonists	Dose: cimetidine ranitidine	7.5 mg/kg, PO, IV 2 mg/kg PO 0.5 to 1 mg/kg IV
Gastric stimulants	Dose: metoclopramide	0.1 mg/kg PO, IV

PREMEDICATION/INDUCTION

Methohexital. Methohexital can be used for premedication/induction when given rectally through a well-lubricated red rubber catheter. The child can be allowed to fall asleep in the parent's arms, which greatly reduces separation anxiety. Sedation occurs in 4 to 8 minutes and lasts 30 to 40 minutes. When compared with rectal pentobarbital, methohexital resulted in a significantly shorter awakening and recovery times.[22] A 10% solution may cause sufficient rectal irritation to precipitate defecation. For repeated administration (e.g., daily radiation therapy) a more dilute solution should be used to avoid proctitis.

> Dose: methohexital   1%-10% solution to
20-30 mg/kg PR

Thiopental and propofol. In patients who present to the operating room with established intravenous access, the use of small boluses of thiopental or propofol carries with it significant advantages. Patient cooperation with this technique is high. Patients will fall asleep rapidly in their parents' presence, avoiding separation anxiety. Caution should be taken not to administer high doses, which may lead to respiratory depression or arrest.

> Dose: thiopental   1 to 2 mg/kg IV
> propofol   0.5 to 1 mg/kg IV

Ketamine.   Ketamine is especially useful as a premedication/induction agent for uncooperative patients. Given intramuscularly it acts rapidly, usually causing loss of consciousness in less than 5 minutes. It stimulates the cardiovascular system (increasing heart rate and blood pressure). It preserves airway reflexes, but secretions, blood, or gastric regurgitant can trigger laryngospasm. An antisialagogue should be given simultaneously to minimize secretions. Parents should be apprised of the appearance of the dissociative state produced by ketamine. When mixed with cola-flavored soft drink and given orally, ketamine provides predictable sedation in 20 to 25 minutes.[23] The nasal route provides excellent sedation at similar doses.[24]

> Dose: ketamine   2 to 5 mg/kg IM
> 6 mg/kg PO[25]
> 3 mg/kg IN[14]
> 8 to 10 mg/kg PR

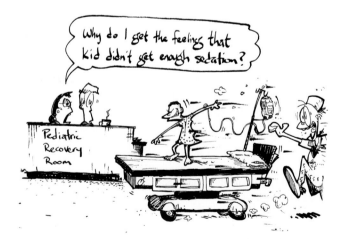

ANTIBIOTIC PROPHYLAXIS AGAINST BACTERIAL ENDOCARDITIS

See Appendix F, p. 666.

PREMEDICATION PHARMACOLOGY— SEDATIVES

Category/ medication	Dosage/route	Onset (T¹/₂)	Side effects/ contraindications
Barbiturates			
Pentobarbital or secobarbital	2-3 mg/kg PO 2-4 mg/kg PR 3-5 mg/kg IM	60-90 min 60-90 min 10-15 min (17-50 hr)	May cause paradoxical reaction Bitter taste when taken PO May cause persistent pain at IM injection site Contraindicated in porphyria
Methohexital	20-30 mg/kg PR	4-8 min (1.5-4 hr)	Unpredictable systemic bioavailability May cause rectal irritation or defecation Contraindicated in temporal lobe epilepsy or porphyria
Opioids			
Morphine	0.1-0.2 mg/kg IM	15-30 min (2-4 hr)	Potent respiratory depressant May cause pruritis, nausea, vomiting
Meperidine	1-2 mg/kg IM	15-30 min (3-4 hr)	As for morphine
Fentanyl lollipop	10-15 µg/kg OT	5-20 min (3-3.5 hr)	High incidence of itchy nose May cause respiratory depression, nausea, vomiting
Sufentanil	1.5-3 µg/kg IN	7.5 min (148 min)	Profound respiratory depression (resuscitative equipment and personnel must be present) Can cause poor chest compliance, apnea, laryngospasm

PREMEDICATION PHARMACOLOGY— SEDATIVES—cont'd

Category/ medication	Dosage/route	Onset (T$^1/_2$)	Side effects/ contraindications
Benzodiazepines			
Diazepam	0.1-0.5 mg/kg PO, PR, IM	30-90 min (21-37 hr)	Slow onset and prolonged action Insufficient doses may cause disinhibition and decrease patient cooperation
Midazolam	0.5 mg/kg PO 0.08-0.3 mg/kg IM 0.4-1 mg/kg PR 0.2-0.3 mg/kg IN 0.2 mg/kg OT	15-30 min 10 min 10 min 10 min 10 min (1-2 hr)	May cause respiratory depression, particularly in combination with narcotics
Dissociative anesthetics			
Ketamine	2-5 mg/kg IM 6 mg/kg PO 3 mg/kg IN 8-10 mg PR	30-40 sec 10 min <30 min 10 min (1-2 hr)	Contraindicated in patients with increased intracranial pressure Increases heart rate and blood pressure (not reported with oral routes) Accumulation of pharyngeal secretions may cause laryngospasm
Hypnotics			
Chloral hydrate	50-75 mg/kg PO (max 1 g)	1-2 hr (8 hr)	Gastric irritation
Triclofos	70 mg/kg PO	1-2 hr (8 hr)	Gastric irritation
α-Agonist			
Clonidine/ atropine	4 µg/kg PO 0.03 mg/kg PO	30-60 min (6-20 hr)	Perioperative hypotension has been demonstrated in adults
Antihistamines			
Hydroxyzine	0.5-1 mg/kg PO, IM	1 hr (3 hr)	Unpredictable level of sedation

PREMEDICATION PHARMACOLOGY—NONSEDATIVES

Category/medication	Dosage/route	Onset (T$^1/_2$)	Side effects/contraindications
Anticholinergics			
Atropine	0.02 mg/kg IM, PO 0.01 mg/kg IV	2-4 min 30 min (2-3 hr)	Can cause fever, extremely dry mouth, flushing, tachycardia
Scopolamine	0.02 mg/kg IM 0.01 mg/kg IV	30 min 5 min	May cause confusion Long duration
Glycopyrrolate	0.01 mg/kg IV 0.01 mg/kg IM	1 min 15 min	No CNS effects Long duration
H$_2$ Antagonists			
Cimetidine	7.5 mg/kg PO, IV	60-90 min (1.5-2 hr)	Decreases hepatic extraction of propranolol, phenytoin, diazepam Avoid use in patients with thrombocytopenia, neutropenia
Ranitidine	2 mg/kg PO (given 4 hr preop) 0.5-1 mg/kg IV	30-60 min (2-3 hr)	Does not alter hepatic extraction of drugs Fewer side effects than cimetidine
Gastric motility stimulants			
Metoclopramide	0.1 mg/kg PO (given 4 hr preop) 0.1 mg/kg IV	40-120 min 15-30 min (2-4 hr)	A single recommended dose does not cause extrapyramidal symptoms Contraindicated in gastrointestinal obstruction and pheochromocytoma

References

1. McGill WA, Hannallah RS: Parental presence during induction of anesthesia in children, *Semin Anesth* 11:259-264, 1992.
2. Kain ZN: Parental presence during induction of anesthesia (editorial), *Paediatr Anaesth* 5:209-212, 1995.
3. Gajraj NM, Pennant JH, Watcha MF: Eutectic mixture of local anesthetics (EMLA) cream, *Anesth Analg* 78:574-583, 1994.
4. McMillan CO, Spahr-Schopfer IA, Sikich N, Hartley E, Lerman J: Premedication of children with oral midazolam, *Can J Anaesth* 39(6):545-550, 1992.
5. Davis PJ, Tome JA, McGowan Jr. FX, Cohen T, Latta K, Felder H: Preanesthetic medication with intranasal midazolam for brief pediatric surgical procedures, *Anesthesiology* 82:2-5, 1995.
6. Wilton NCT, Leigh J, Rosen DR, Pandit UA: Preanesthetic sedation of preschool children using intranasal midazolam, *Anesthesiology* 69:972-975, 1988.

7. Weldon BC, Watcha MF, White PF: Oral midazolam in children: effect of time and adjunctive therapy, *Anesth Analg* 75:51-55, 1992.

8. Karl HW, Rosenberger JL, Larach MG, Ruffle JM: Transmucosal administration of midazolam for premedication of pediatric patients, *Anesthesiology* 78:885-891, 1993.

9. Spear RM, Yaster M, Berkowitz ID, Maxwell LG, Bender KS, Naclerio R, Manolio TA, Nichols DG: Preinduction of anesthesia in children with rectally administered midazolam, *Anesthesiology* 74:670-674, 1991.

10. Friesen RH, Lockhart CH: Oral transmucosal fentanyl citrate for preanesthetic medication of pediatric day surgery patients with and without droperidol as a prophylactic anti-emetic, *Anesthesiology* 76:46-51, 1992.

11. Nelson PS, Streisand JB, Mulder SM, Pace NL, Stanley TH: Comparison of oral transmucosal fentanyl citrate and an oral solution of meperidine, diazepam, and atropine for premedication in children, *Anesthesiology* 70:616-621, 1989.

12. Henderson JM, Brodsky DA, Fisher DM, Brett CM, Hertzka RE: Preinduction of anesthesia in pediatric patients with nasally administered sufentanil, *Anesthesiology* 68:671-675, 1988.

13. Karl HW et al: Nasal midazolam or sufentanil for preinduction of anesthesia in pediatric patients: implications for intraoperative management, *Anesthesiology* 71:A1169, 1989.

14. Tasi SK, Wei CF, Mok MS: Intranasal ketamine vs sufentanil as premedication in children, *Anesthesiology* 71:A1173, 1989.

15. Karl HW, Keifer AT, Rosenberger JL, Larach MG, Ruffle JM: Comparison of the safety and efficacy of intranasal midazolam or sufentanil for preinduction of anesthesia in pediatric patients, *Anesthesiology* 76:209-215, 1992.

16. Mikawa K, Maekawa N, Nishina K, Takao Y, Yaku H, Obara H: Efficacy of oral clonidine premedication in children, *Anesthesiology* 79:926-931, 1993.

17. Nishina K, Mikawa K, Maekawa N, Takao Y, Obara H: Clonidine decreases the dose of thiamylal required to induce anesthesia in children, *Anesth Analg* 79:766-768, 1994.

18. Steinberg AD: Should chloral hydrate be banned? *Pediatrics* 92:442-446, 1993.

19. Cartabuke RS, Davidson PJ, Warner LO: Is premedication with oral glycopyrrolate as effective as oral atropine in attenuating cardiovascular depression in infants receiving halothane for induction of anesthesia? *Anesth Analg* 73:271-274, 1991.

20. Coté CJ, Goudsouzian NG, Liu LMP, Dedrick DF, Szyfelbein SK: Assessment of risk factors related to the acid aspiration syndrome in pediatric patients: gastric pH and residual volume, *Anesthesiology* 56:70-72, 1982.

21. Lerman J, Christensen SK, Farrow-Gillespie AC: Effects of metoclopramide and ranitidine on gastric fluid pH and volume in children, *Anesthesiology* 69:A748, 1988.

22. Christensen PA, Balslev T, Hasselstrøm L: Comparison of methohexital and pentobarbital for premedication in children, *Acta Anaesthesiol Scand* 34:478-481, 1990.

23. Gutstein HB, Johnson KL, Heard MB, Gregory GA: Oral ketamine preanesthetic medication in children, *Anesthesiology* 76:28-33, 1992.

24. Weksler N, Ovadia L, Muati G, Stav A: Nasal ketamine for paediatric premedication, *Can J Anaesth* 40:119-121, 1993.

25. Gutstein HB et al: Oral ketamine premedication in children, *Anesthesiology* 71:A1176, 1989.

EQUIPMENT AND MONITORING

3

Martin knew monsters who crawled near his bed
They tickled his ankles and circled his head,
There were deep-throated dragons and silver snakes,
And they put him to sleep and kept him awake.

One day Martin listened and thought that he heard
In the monster's strange language a kind-hearted word.
They were there for his comfort and to help him to mend
And Martin's old monsters became Martin's new friends.

Rivian Bell

The success of a pediatric procedure depends not only on the skill and knowledge of the anesthesiologist, but also on the possession and utilization of the proper equipment. The same method of setup should be used each time, to avoid overlooking critical items and to ensure that all equipment is functioning properly.

AIRWAY EQUIPMENT
Circuits[1-4]

1. Circuits commonly used for children under 12 to 15 kg include Mapleson D, Bain, Jackson-Rees modification of Ayre's T-piece, and pediatric circle.
2. The circuits used for pediatrics were traditionally designed specifically to:
   a. Decrease the resistance to breathing by eliminating valves
   b. Decrease the amount of dead space in the circuit
   c. In the case of the Bain circuit, decrease the amount of heat loss by means of a coaxial circuit with warm exhaled gas surrounding the fresh gas inflow

However, resistance is only problematic in the small, spontaneously breathing patient. Furthermore, the narrow endotracheal tube offers more resistance than the circuit. In fact, all of these circuit types can be used effectively in infants and children, provided care is taken in control of ventilation, adequacy of fresh gas flows, and observation of capnography.

3. Semiopen systems (Mapleson) require high fresh gas flows to prevent rebreathing of exhaled gases. Several different methods of calculating required fresh gas flow (FGF) exist, as listed in the box on the next page. In the final analysis, capnometry

Circuit	Schematic	Advantages	Disadvantages
Mapleson D (semiopen)		Valveless (less work of breathing) Minimal dead space Short time constant for more rapid induction	Requires high fresh gas flows Increases heat and moisture loss Breath sounds may be obscured by water condensation in tubing
Bain (semiopen)		Valveless (less work of breathing) Minimal dead space Theoretically conserves heat because inspired gas tubing is surrounded by exhaled gas Short time constant	Requires high fresh gas flows Heat and moisture losses still occur Cracks in coaxial tubing lead to rebreathing of expired gases
Modified Ayre's T-piece (semiopen)		Simplicity Valveless (less work of breathing) Less dead space Short time constant	Bulky because the reservoir bag is close to the airway Requires high fresh gas flows Increased heat and moisture loss
Pediatric circle (semiclosed)		Simplicity Familiar system No need to disassemble anesthesia machine for setup	CO_2 absorber creates resistance Valves create resistance and can malfunction

helps to monitor rebreathing, allowing the anesthesiologist to adjust fresh gas flows accordingly.

a. FGF = 2½ to 3 times minute ventilation
   Minute ventilation = 150 ml × kg
   where minute ventilation is defined as tidal volume (V_T) × respiratory rate (RR)
b. FGF = 1000 ml + 100 ml/kg
c. FGF = minimum of 3 L/min for all children
d. FGF exceeds peak inspiratory flow.

4. The reservoir bag should contain a volume similar to that of the child's vital capacity. Children are more susceptible than adults to barotrauma that can occur with the higher pressures and volumes generated by an excessively large reservoir bag. Appropriate sizes, based on age, follow:

Age	Reservoir bag
Newborn	0.5 L
1-3 yr	1.0 L
3-5 yr	2.0 L
>5 yr	3.0 L

5. Humidification is helpful when a nonrebreathing circuit is used, to prevent excessive heat loss (high flows of cold gas can rapidly cool a small child), and to keep airway secretions moist. When a heated humidifier is used, airway temperatures should not exceed 32° C and condensed water should be drained periodically from the circuit. Fresh-water drowning can result from obstruction of the endotracheal tube and airway by water. A small pediatric humidivent offers humidification without an exogenous heat source and avoids the possibility of water overload.

Ventilators[1,4]

Ventilators that commonly accompany anesthesia machines in North America (North American Dräger, Telford, Pa; Ohmeda, Madison, Wisc.) are not designed specifically for infants and children. Like the larger adult ventilators, they are pneumatically driven, time-cycled, constant flow generators designed to deliver a specified inspiratory volume, respiratory rate, and I:E ratio. Ventilators can be adapted for children by changing to a pediatric bellows attachment. Several factors are noticeable:

1. The tidal volume delivered to the patient is significantly affected by the compressive volume of the pediatric circuit

and by the size of the leak around the endotracheal tube. Increasing fresh gas flow can augment tidal volume.

2. The respiratory rate and I:E ratio are set before attaching the ventilator and circuit with the volume and flow turned off. The tidal volume is then gradually increased until the desired chest movement and inspiratory pressures are obtained. This technique prevents the barotrauma that can occur from inadvertently connecting the child to a ventilator with preset high volume or flow.

3. Infants who require high inspiratory pressures or high levels of PEEP or CPAP are probably best managed with ventilators primarily designed for the intensive care unit. Unless these ventilators are specifically modified to use an anesthetic gas vaporizer, it is prudent to use a pure intravenous anesthetic technique.

4. Controversy continues regarding the relative advantages of manual versus mechanical ventilation. Although it has been documented that the overly compliant circuit makes it nearly impossible to appreciate changes in pulmonary compliance, even when ventilation is performed by an "educated hand,"[5] many anesthesiologists feel that manual ventilation offers significant information about the patient's respiratory state. Conversely, mechanical ventilation does free the anesthesiologist's hands for other tasks and provides consistent repetitive ventilation. Adequacy of ventilation is probably best ensured by a combination of factors, including mode of ventilation, auscultation, observation of the patient, and continuous monitors (especially capnography).

Oxygen[6]

Oxygen must be available from more than one source, and this availability must be checked before each procedure.

1. Wall oxygen delivered at 50 psi should be connected to the anesthesia machine and ventilator.

   a. Oxygen delivery by flow meters is delivered at low pressure because of reducing valves in the anesthesia machine.

   b. Oxygen from the fresh gas inlet will flow at a rate of 35 to 75 L/min, depending upon the machine. Flushing the pediatric circuit with these flows can result in pulmonary barotrauma in infants and young children.

2. A full oxygen reserve tank should be attached to every anesthesia machine and checked before each procedure. A free-standing oxygen source with separate circuit is recommended for backup (e.g., power failure) and for transport.

3. A green "E" cylinder contains compressed oxygen gas and is fitted with a gas regulator, serving both as a pressure-reducing valve and a flow meter. When filled, the "E" cylinder weighs approximately 7 kg and contains 625 L of oxygen pressurized to 2200 psi.

4. Its duration of use depends on two factors: the gas capacity of the cylinder (measured indirectly by cylinder pressure) and the rate of gas flow delivered. Approximate usable duration can be calculated by the following formula:

Duration of flow (min) for an E cylinder:

$$\frac{\text{Cylinder pressure (PSI)} \times 0.28}{\text{Flow rate (L/min)}}$$

For example, following are calculated durations of flow for two flow rates and three cylinder pressures:

Cylinder pressure

Flow rate	2200 PSI (full)	1200 PSI (½ full)	600 PSI (¼ full)
10 L/min	61 min	33 min	16 min
6 L/min	102 min	56 min	28 min

OXYGEN DELIVERY SYSTEMS

1. Any of the following can be used for oxygen delivery: nasal cannulae, oxygen hood, mask in the spontaneous breathing patient, or a positive-pressure delivery system connected to a mask, endotracheal tube, or tracheostomy tube.

2. An Ambu bag with nonrebreathing valve or a Jackson-Rees modification of Ayre's T-piece is useful for delivery of positive pressure. Important features include:

   a. Ability to use the system with either spontaneous or controlled ventilation. However, some Ambu bags contain valves that only allow inspiration of room air, not O_2 during spontaneous ventilation.

   b. High fresh gas flows (either 8 to 10 L/min or 2 times minute ventilation) are required to avoid CO_2 rebreathing and ensure delivery of FIO_2 greater than 90%.

   c. Pressure-limiting relief valves are needed to minimize the risk of barotrauma or overdistension of the lungs.

   d. The Ambu system may be fitted with a PEEP valve as well.

3. The type of oxygen delivery system selected for the unintubated patient depends on the age, size, and degree of cooperation of the patient and the goals of therapy (see next table).

Modes of oxygen therapy

Mode	Apparatus	Inspiratory reservoir	Ambient air entrainment	Rebreathing	Valves	O$_2$ flow delivery rate (set on flow meter)	Delivered Fio$_2$*	Comments	Disadvantages
Nasal cannulae	Nasal prongs	Yes (anatomic nasopharynx and oropharynx)	Possible	No	No	2-6 L/min	Variable: 0.27-0.39 (usually increases Fio$_2$ by 0.03 for each L/min of blood flow)	Ensure proper fit and positioning of prongs	Inability to measure Fio$_2$ Nasal irritation and drying
Oxygen hood	Plastic hood, which covers the head and neck	Yes (mixing of gases within the hood)	No	Yes	No	6-8 L/min	Pre-blended range of 0.28-0.60	Must provide adequate fresh gas flow to ensure mixing of delivered gases and flushing of exhaled gases	O$_2$ gradients can form from the top to the bottom of the hood Cold, humidified gases can contribute to thermal stress in small infants

Simple mask	Mask with exhalation side-ports	No	Yes (through side-ports)	No	No	6-10 L/min	Variable: 0.35-0.55	Limited concentration of delivered oxygen	Delivered FIO₂ varies with O₂ delivery, patient's inspiratory time, and peak inspiratory flow rate
Partial rebreathing mask	Mask with exhalation side-ports and a reservoir bag	Yes (bag)	Yes (through side-ports)	Yes	Yes	8-15 L/min	Variable: 0.60-0.80	Tight fit of mask is essential. Delivered flow must exceed peak inspiratory flow so reservoir does not collapse on inspiration	Requires high gas flows to maintain reservoir
Venturi, or entrainment, mask	Mask fitted with O₂ jet nozzle and entrainment ports	No	Yes (oxygen jet velocity is transferred to entrained air)	No	No	8-15 L/min	Variable: 0.24-0.60 (depends on jet velocity and size of entrainment ports)	Delivered flow must exceed peak inspiratory flow to ensure accurate FIO₂ delivery	If fresh gas flow fails, total rebreathing may occur (some are fitted with either non-valved perforations or a valve to allow ambient air to enter)

*For all the above modes, desired FIO₂ is delivered only if delivered fresh gas flow exceeds the patient's peak inspiratory flow rate (typically ≥6 L/min for an infant and 20-60 L/min for an adult).

Masks[7]

A child's face tends to be round and flat in comparison to the adult face, in which the chin and nose are more prominent. The original Rendell-Baker-Soucek mask was made to conform to the shape of a child's face and to reduce the amount of dead space in the mask. In addition, it is made of clear plastic, which allows for observation of the child's color, humidity from expired gases, and presence of secretions and vomitus.

Disposable plastic masks with inflatable rims are currently made in a variety of sizes. Some are even marketed with candy-flavor aromas and colors, although it is simple enough to add standard candy flavors or odorants to the side of the mask if it appears this will increase a child's compliance with induction. These masks offer all of the advantages of the Rendell-Baker-Soucek model and do not need to be washed or sterilized.

Rubber masks are rarely used in pediatric operating rooms because of the emerging problems with latex allergy (see p. 213).

Airways[7]

The smooth Guedel airway is most often selected for children. To fit properly, the tip of the oral airway should align just before the angle of the mandible when held against the side of a patient's face with the opening against the mouth. An airway that is too large can push the epiglottis down. One that is too small can push the tongue against the posterior oropharynx.

Care must be taken in placing a nasal trumpet to avoid injuring the hypertrophied adenoids and causing bleeding. The presence of either the nasal or oral airway near the glottis can precipitate laryngospasm in the lightly anesthetized patient or in the early phases of an inhalation induction.

Oral airway sizes for children

Age	Size	cm
Preterm	000 or 00	3.5 or 4.5
Neonate to 3 mo	0	5.5
3-12 mo	1	6.0
1-5 yr	2	7.0
>5 yr	3	8.0

Laryngoscopes

1. The use of a small pediatric handle is recommended. It is less bulky, allowing laryngoscopy to be performed while cricoid pressure is applied with the fifth finger of the same hand.

2. In general, straight blades (Miller) are used in infants to facilitate picking up the elongated epiglottis and exposing the vocal cords. The wider-phlanged Wis-Hippel or Robert-Shaw blades are sometimes preferred for ease of exposure.

Laryngoscope blades	Age
Miller 0	Preterm, neonate
Miller 1	Neonate to age 2
Miller 2	Age 3 and older
Wis-Hippel 1.5	Age 2-5
Macintosh 2	Age 3-6

3. The oxyscope has a separate port to which oxygen tubing can be attached. It is useful for passive insufflation of oxygen during intubation, particularly if respiratory compromise is present or a difficult intubation is anticipated.
4. The light wand (a rigid stylet with a light at the tip) facilitates blind intubation of the trachea by providing external visualization of light in the neck rather than requiring direct visualization of the larynx.[8-10] It is particularly useful in children with oral aperture limitations and micrognathia (e.g., Pierre Robin). It is available in sizes small enough to accommodate infant endotracheal tubes and requires minimal technical expertise (see Fig. 8-2, p. 183).

BULLARD LARYNGOSCOPE

The Bullard laryngoscope (Circon ACMI, Stamford, Conn.) consists of a rigid blade with a fixed fiberoptic bundle. It is manufactured in adult and pediatric sizes and can facilitate difficult intubation.[11,12]

Uses

1. The Bullard allows direct visualization of the larynx in a patient whose larynx cannot be seen by standard direct laryngoscopy (mandibulofacial abnormalities).
2. It is also recommended when the oral aperture is inadequate for a standard laryngoscope (e.g., burns) or when the head and neck cannot be repositioned, as with head or cervical trauma.
3. The superior optics provide enhanced depth and width of field.
4. Its use is noninvasive and requires minimal technical expertise.

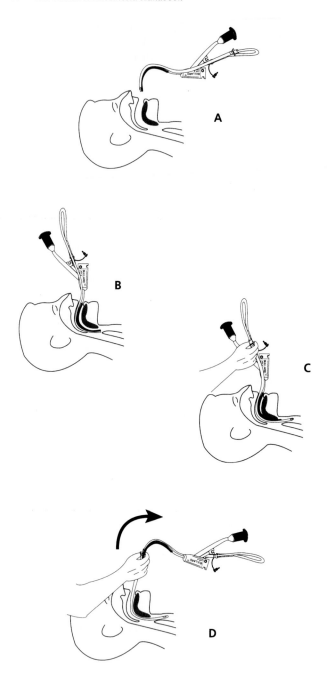

FIG. 3-1

Technique for endotracheal intubation
1. The laryngoscope is inserted in the mouth with the handle parallel to the body (Fig. 3-1, *A*).
2. The blade is rotated around the tongue until the handle is turned 90 degrees (vertical to the body) (Fig. 3-1, *B*).
3. The glottic aperture is visualized by elevating the blade against the tongue's surface (Fig. 3-1, *C*).
4. The endotracheal tube is positioned and the blade removed in the reverse process (Fig. 3-1, *D*).
5. To facilitate intubation:
   a. A stylet can be attached to the laryngoscope, over which the endotracheal tube is advanced.
   b. Grasping forceps can be inserted through a side channel to grasp the Murphy eye and direct the endotracheal tube through the larynx.
   c. A jet ventilation catheter may also be passed through the side-port.

Endotracheal Tubes
1. Small-diameter endotracheal tubes increase airway resistance and work of breathing. An oversized endotracheal tube can injure the narrow cricoid area and predispose to postintubation croup. The anesthesiologist should calculate ideal tube size from the table below and then prepare (or have available) endotracheal tubes one size larger and one size smaller.

Age	Endotracheal tube size (inner diameter in mm)
Premature <2kg	2.5
>2kg	3.0
Neonate	3.0-3.5
0-6 mo	3.5
6-12 mo	4.0
12-18 mo	4.0-4.5
2 yr	4.5
2-3 yr	4.5-5.0
>4 yr	(Age [yr]+16) ÷ 4 or (wt [kg] + 35) ÷ 10

2. Cuffed tubes increase pressure and the potential for damage in the narrow subglotic area. The cuff also reduces the maximum tube size allowable. Cuffed tubes are generally not used for patients under age 8.
3. Ultimately, the proper tube size is confirmed by the ability to generate positive pressure greater than 30 cm H_2O and by the presence of a leak at less than 20 cm H_2O.

4. A stylet should be placed in the endotracheal tube or be readily available to facilitate tracheal intubation.
5. The tube should be secured so that the second mark at the tip just passes through the cords. Recommended tube-to-lip taping distances are listed below. The correct taping distance can be estimated by adding 10 to the child's years of age.
6. Extending the neck decreases tube depth; flexing the neck (chin down) deepens the tube position within the trachea.[13] In the infant, neck flexion may result in endobronchial placement. Placing a small roll under the shoulder and thus extending the neck will reposition the tube in midtrachea without retaping, which can cause inadvertent extubation.

Methods of verification of endotracheal tube depth

Method	Comment
X-ray	Impractical in the operating room Useful in the ICU, but assumes child's head and neck position will remain constant
Tube markings	Requires controlled intubation by experienced individual The average distance from cords to carina in a neonate is 5 cm; placement of the tube with the first single line at the cords will put the tube midway in the trachea
1,2,3,4,7,8,9,10 rule for premature infants	The weight of the child is used as a guide: <table><tr><td>kg</td><td>cm at lip</td></tr><tr><td>1</td><td>7</td></tr><tr><td>2</td><td>8</td></tr><tr><td>3</td><td>9</td></tr><tr><td>4</td><td>10</td></tr></table>
Age + 10 rule	The centimeter mark at the lip should equal the age (in years) + 10

COMMON SEQUELAE OF INTUBATION IN CHILDREN[14,15]

Endobronchial intubation occurs typically into the right mainstem bronchus. It may be difficult to detect in neonates, because breath sounds are transmitted well throughout the chest. A decrease in SpO_2, unequal breath sounds, or wheezing may indicate that the endotracheal tube should be repositioned in midtreachea. Pulling up on the chin before retaping is a simple technique to see if repositioning will correct the problem.

The incidence of postintubation croup in children is 1% to 6%. Risk factors include age (6 months to 4 years), length of intubation, lack of leak around the tube, and increased head movement. Treatment includes inhaled cold oxygenated mist and nebulized 2.25% racemic epinephrine (0.05 ml/kg/dose in 3 ml of normal saline). Use of steroids to reduce edema is controversial (see also p. 507).

Complications of intubation based on time of occurrence

Laryngoscopy

Cardiovascular changes (hypertension, tachycardia)
Dental and soft tissue damage
Aspiration
Laryngospasm

Tube In situ

Obstruction or kinking of tube
Endotracheal intubation
Inadvertent extubation
Increased resistance to breathing
Bronchospasm
Tracheal mucosal ischemia

PostIntubation

Laryngospasm
Laryngitis
Granuloma formation
Tracheitis
Tracheal stenosis
Vocal cord paralysis
Arytenoid cartilage dislocation

Laryngospasm is defined as approximation of true vocal cords or both true and false cords. It is caused most often by inadequate depth of anesthesia with sensory stimulation (secretions, manipulation of airway, surgical stimulation). Treatment includes removal of stimulus, 100% oxygen, continuous positive pressure by mask, and muscle relaxants if necessary.

Laryngeal Mask Airway (LMA)
DESCRIPTION[16,17]

1. The latex-free LMA consists of a silicone tube fused to a spoon-shaped mask with an inflatable cuff. The cuff is inflated similarly to an ETT by means of an attached valved pilot balloon.
2. The LMA is reusable and may withstand multiple sterilizations when cleaned with mild detergent and sterilized at temperatures not exceeding 134° C (with cuff deflated) for 4 to 5 minutes.
3. It is currently manufactured in five sizes.

Descriptions of different sizes of laryngeal mask airways

Mask size	Patient weight (kg)	Internal diameter (ID, mm)	Cuff volume (ml)	Largest ETT (ID, mm)	Fiberoptic bronchoscope size (mm)
1	<6.5	5.25	2-5	3.5	2.7
2	6.5-20	7.0	7-10	4.5	3.5
2½	20-30	8.4	14	5.0	4.0
3	30-70	10	15-20	6.0 cuffed	5.0
4	>70	10	25-30	6.5 cuffed	5.0

From Pennant JH, White PF: *Anesthesiology* 79:144-163, 1993.

USES/INDICATIONS

1. The LMA is indicated in patients who are candidates for inhalation anesthesia with spontaneous ventilation who do not require intubation.
2. It has also proved useful to maintain airways in children whose tracheae are difficult to intubate (e.g., congenital dysmorphism, burns)[18,19] or to facilitate fiberoptic intubation (see Fig. 8-3, p. 183).[20]
3. Although not usually recommended for positive-pressure ventilation because of potential gastric distension, the LMA has proved effective and easy to use for neonatal resuscitation.[21] Adequate positive pressure can be generated without the occurrence of audible leak when the LMA is held in place with continuous forward pressure.
4. The LMA is useful for anesthesia outside of the operating room, particularly for the following procedures when the sedation necessary for endotracheal intubation exceeds that necessary for the procedure:
   a. Radiation therapy (RT)
   b. Computerized tomography (CT)
   c. Magnetic resonance imaging (MRI)
5. The LMA is contraindicated in patients at risk for aspiration, as the airway is not protected.
6. The LMA offers the following advantages:
   a. Less pressure on the face/eyes than a mask
   b. Anesthetist's hands are free
   c. Less cardiovascular response than with endotracheal intubation
   d. Less sore throat than with endotracheal intubation

INSERTION

1. A plane of anesthesia sufficient for placement of an oral airway is achieved either by inhalation or by intravenous agents. In children, greater anesthetic depth may be required than for adults. When propofol is used, doses greater than those recommended for adults may be required for children (pediatric dose, 3 mg/kg).
2. The child is placed in classic "sniff" position with the head extended and neck flexed.
3. Insertion for adults is described with the cuff fully deflated and laryngeal aperture inserted against the tongue and away from the palate. However, in children, partial cuff inflation and "upside-down" insertion with rotation in the posterior pharynx (like a Guedel airway) decreases the time required and improves the rate of successful insertion.
4. Airway irritability during insertion (coughing, gagging) is best remedied by deepening the anesthetic rather than removing the LMA.

5. The black midline indicator on the silicone tube should be in the midline when the tube is secured with tape to prevent dislodgement. A bite-block is recommended; rolled gauze covered with tape is usually sufficient.
6. Successful placement is confirmed by synchronous movement of the chest, abdomen, and circuit reservoir bag, as well as by capnography and bilateral lung auscultation.
7. The use of 2% lidocaine gel for insertion is as effective as morphine at reducing cough on emergence when the LMA is not removed until protective airway reflexes have returned.[22] Conversely, removing the LMA while the patient remains anesthetized also facilitates a smooth emergence.

COMPLICATIONS/PROBLEMS OF THE LMA[16,17,23]

1. Unsuccessful insertion/positioning/maintenance
2. Laryngospasm/bronchospasm
3. Coughing
4. Breath holding/apnea
5. Vomiting/aspiration
6. Excessive salivation
7. Desaturation
8. Airway obstruction
9. Gastric distension (from air swallowing or positive-pressure ventilation)
10. Airway trauma
11. Cuff overinflation due to expansion when using nitrous oxide
12. Sore throat

MONITORING CARDIAC FUNCTION
Electrocardiography (ECG)[24-26]

Continuous monitoring of the pediatric ECG provides a determination of heart rate and rhythm abnormalities and of alterations in configuration of the complex. Because the rate and complex configuration are different from adults, some modifications in monitoring are helpful to improve detection of abnormalities.

HEART RATE

1. The rapid heart rate of children (up to 3 or 4 Hz or 180 to 240 beats/min) requires that the ECG have a digital rate meter with adjustable gain to eliminate artifacts.
2. The T waves in infants are much larger, because the electrodes are situated much closer to the heart, and may be of the same amplitude as the QRS. This can lead to erroneous counting of heart rates or double counting. The ability to remove this artifact is helpful.

RHYTHM ABNORMALITIES

1. Monitoring lead II provides the best P wave configuration to help with dysrhythmia detection.
2. A variable sweep rate controls the speed at which the ECG is recorded. The standard speed for adults is 25 mm/sec, but faster rates may be necessary for the rhythm analysis of children. Rates of 50 mm/sec or 100 mm/sec will enable P-R and Q-T interval interpretation and facilitate arrhythmia detection.

ECG COMPLEX CONFIGURATION

1. The most prominent P wave in infants is seen in lead III, because of R axis shift.
2. Changes in the P wave or QRS configuration are usually the result of dysrhythmias.
3. Use of the monitor mode implies the presence of a narrow band width, which minimizes motion and respiratory artifact, high-frequency noise, baseline drift, and 60 Hz interference. It also distorts the S-T segment away from the baseline.
4. To accurately determine if S-T segment changes are present, the diagnostic mode must be used, which utilizes a wider band width filter.
5. S-T changes may indicate electrolyte imbalance (potassium and calcium), ischemia, pericarditis, or myocarditis, or may represent nonpathologic early repolarization (J point elevation). Automated S-T segment trending can be modified for use with rapid infant heart rates by manually resetting the J point.[25]

LEAD PLACEMENT

1. Leads placed on extremities (shoulders, thighs) will result in less movement artifact from breathing.
2. Smaller leads generate a higher current density in the presence of electrosurgical units (cautery), which can result in burns, particularly in older-model ECG units with grounded reference electrodes.
3. Leads should not be placed on bony protuberances, to avoid pressure necrosis.
4. To avoid trauma to fragile ribs, snap-on electrodes should be snapped to the lead before being stuck to the chest.
5. Leads for preterm infants should be changed as infrequently as possible, to avoid skin trauma.
6. Leads placed on the nipple bud of preterm infants may cause permanent damage on removal.

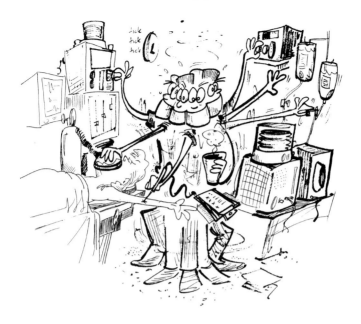

Echocardiography[27-34]

Transesophageal echocardiography (TEE) is becoming an important tool for intraoperative assessment of cardiac function, flow defects, cardiac morphology, and adequacy of repair during and after surgical procedures for congenital heart disease. Placement of the probe in the intubated and anesthetized infant is usually the responsibility of the anesthesiologist. However, it is generally advocated that interpretation of the echocardiogram and any subsequent decision making which arises from that interpretation result from a collaboration between the involved teams: surgery, anesthesiology, pediatric cardiology and echocardiographic imaging.

1. Small color flow probes (6.8 mm diameter) are available for infants as small as 3 kg.
2. Esophageal damage is reportedly minimal, although susceptibility to injury may increase with extreme probe flexion for greater periods of time.
3. Epicardial techniques offer better visualization of the right ventricular outflow tract than TEE and also offer continuous-wave Doppler capability for analysis of higher flow velocities. However, epicardial imaging necessitates interrupting the surgical procedure and carries the risks of arrhythmias and hypotension because of direct contact with the heart.

4. Transient bacteremia after TEE is common, and cardiac prophylaxis is therefore recommended.

5. Particularly in small infants or children, there is a risk of dislodging the endotracheal tube during insertion or removal of the TEE probe.

6. Compression of the left mainstem bronchus has been reported, with resultant cardiorespiratory compromise (simultaneous decrease in end-tidal CO_2 and SpO_2). Compression of the descending aorta with posterior rotation and flexion of the probe has also been described and can be diagnosed by changes in pulse oximeter plethysmography or the lower extremity intraarterial waveform.

MONITORING OF CENTRAL CIRCULATION

Percutaneous insertion of catheters into the central circulation allows for both continuous monitoring of central pressure and access to the central circulation through large-bore catheters for volume replacement or drug administration.

1. The internal jugular is a common site of insertion because it is easily accessible to the anesthesiologist during the surgical procedure. (For technique, see Appendix C, Fig. C-3, p. 659). Percutaneous insertion is more difficult in very young (less than 3 months) or very small infants (less than 4 kg).[35] Complications include arterial puncture, catheter malposition, hematoma formation, and pneumothorax.

2. The external jugular vein is a superficial vessel in the neck that allows catheter placement under direct vision. However, accessing the central circulation with a guide wire from the external jugular is often difficult in very young children.

3. In neonates, the umbilical vein may be easily cannulated. Position above the liver and ductus venosus must be confirmed by radiographs. Complications may include thrombosis, sepsis, hypertension, necrotizing enterocolitis, and hemorrhage.

4. The femoral vein may be easily accessible for percutaneous cannulation. Large-bore catheters can usually be placed into this vessel. However, the area may be predisposed to infection and is not always available to the anesthesiologist during surgical procedures. This site may be particularly useful for monitoring and venous access during craniotomy, as the area is located in proximity to the anesthesiologist and away from the surgical site. (See Appendix C, Fig. C-4, p. 660.)

5. Pulmonary artery catheters are rarely placed in pediatric patients. They are most useful for patients with congenital heart disease during and after cardiac surgery to provide information about chamber pressure and vascular resistance. Placement is often complicated by unusual anatomy and aberrant flow across shunts or stenotic areas so that fluoroscopic guidance is required. Complications include arrhythmias, catheter migration, thrombocytopenia, and thrombosis.[36]

6. Surgically placed indwelling central venous catheters are commonly used for children with chronic illness or difficult percutaneous venous access, or those requiring prolonged parenteral nutrition or chemotherapy. Although these catheters are usually available to the anesthesiologist for central monitoring and venous access, they are sometimes dedicated for specific infusions and cannot be violated. Strict aseptic technique must be followed before accessing these catheters, and a heparin flush (usually 100 μg/ml) must be administered when discontinuing catheter use. Protocols for accessing and anticoagulation may vary from institution to institution; however, these protocols should be well known and carefully followed by every anesthesiologist who elects to access the port.

BLOOD PRESSURE MONITORING[37-40]
Cuff Size

A blood pressure cuff with too narrow a bladder is the most common cause of hypertension in children. Too large a cuff may underestimate blood pressure. Accurate cuff size can be determined using the following criteria:

1. Cuff bladder width should be keyed to arm circumference, not to upper arm length.
2. The cuff bladder width should be approximately 40% of the arm circumference for closest approximation to intra-arterial readings.
3. Bladder length should be 90 to 100% of the arm circumference (in contrast to 80% for adults) to avoid overestimating blood pressure.

Noninvasive Monitoring

1. *Auscultation.* A blood pressure cuff and stethoscope are secured to the child's arm. The cuff is manually inflated, and Korotkoff's sounds are auscultated as the cuff is deflated 2 to 3 mm Hg at a time.

2. *Doppler.* An ultrasound transducer is placed over an artery, distal to the blood pressure cuff. Systolic pressure is recorded when the sound of pulsatile flow is first appreciated.
3. *Distal flow detection.* Similar in use to the Doppler, several other detectors of blood flow may be placed distal to the blood pressure cuff. Palpation, a plethysmograph, and an oximeter probe are some of the more common techniques used.
4. *Oscillation:* Manual oscillation describes the systolic blood pressure as the pressure at which oscillations, or "bounces," of the needle occur on the manometer after the cuff is deflated. Automated oscillometric devices measure the beginning oscillation as the systolic pressure and maximum oscillation as the mean pressure (DINAMAP: Device for Indirect Noninvasive Automated Mean Arterial Pressure, Critikon, Inc., Tampa, Fla.). Systolic, diastolic, and mean pressure and heart rate are digitally displayed. Given that the appropriate cuff size is selected, this type of noninvasive pressure monitoring is very accurate on upper and lower extremities and requires little user training. Automated oscillometric readings in very low birth weight infants must be carefully verified, as overestimation has been reported when the mean arterial pressure is below 40 mm Hg.

Invasive Monitoring[41-44]

1. Placement of an intraarterial catheter is requisite for invasive monitoring of blood pressure. Nontapered Teflon catheters are commonly used. Catheters made of an elastomeric hydrogel polymer blend (Streamline, Menlo Care, Menlo Park, Calif.) that expands intravascularly may be useful in patients with minimal access, but they are expensive and require special care in placement.
2. Smaller catheters provide greater accuracy in monitoring, but larger catheters are more practical for blood sampling. However, larger catheters may also predispose to distal ischemia, as the incidence of arterial occlusion increases linearly with an increase in the ratio of cannula outer diameter to vessel diameter.[45] General sizing recommendations for intraarterial catheter placement are as follows:

Size	Child
24 g	Neonates, infants
22 g	Less than 5 years old
20 g	More than 5 years old

3. Preductal catheter placement is optimal for:
   a. Infants with patent ductus arteriosis (PDA)
   b. Coarctation repair
   c. Diaphragmatic hernia repair
4. The right radial artery is used for preductal monitoring. Use of

the temporal arteries is not advised because of the possibility of cerebral hemispheric infarct if ischemia occurs as a result of spasm or clot formation. Although the brachial artery is avoided because it has no collateral blood flow, axillary artery monitoring has proven accuracy in an intensive care setting and carries few complications.[45] The ulnar artery is another alternative to radial artery insertion, but should probably be avoided when radial artery cannulation on the same wrist has already been attempted.[42] The umbilical artery, a postductal site, may be accessible for monitoring during the first 2 to 3 days of life, but carries a high complication rate for lower extremity ischemia, necrotizing enterocolitis, and renovascular thrombosis.[47] Femoral arteries are easily cannulated, but are exposed to infection from fecal and urine contamination and may cause lower extremity ischemia.

Complications of intraarterial catheters

Complications	Comments
Hematoma	More common if vessel is transfixed during cannulation.
Infection	Common when catheters are left in place for more than 4 days.
Ischemia	50% of all children will have distal ischemia after percutaneous placement; the vessel usually recannulizes within 7 to 14 days.
Embolization	Retrograde embolization into the central circulation has occurred with aggressive flushing. Gentle flushing of the catheter by hand with a syringe is advised.
Necrotizing enterocolitis Renovascular hypertension Leg ischemia	95% of all umbilical artery catheters demonstrate clot formation.

TEMPERATURE MONITORING[48-51]

The ability to maintain normothermia for pediatric patients (particularly infants) is challenging, as the higher body surface area–to–weight ratio increases susceptibility to heat loss by radiation, convection, evaporation, and conduction. The consequences of thermal stress include cerebral and cardiac depression, increased oxygen demand, acidosis, hypoxia, and intracardiac shunt reversal.

Types of Temperature Monitors

1. Thermistors are temperature-sensitive resistors placed in soft plastic tubing (e.g., esophageal stethoscope).
2. Thermocouples are used for tympanic membrane monitoring.

3. Liquid crystal thermometers are placed on self-adhesive strips, which can easily be attached to the forehead to measure skin temperature. Temperature readings are usually about 3° C below core, but trends can be followed and these monitors are easily transported to sites away from the operating suite.

Preferred Sites for Temperature Monitoring

1. Esophageal temperatures will more accurately represent core if the thermistor is located in the distal third of the esophagus. More proximal placement close to the tip of the endotracheal tube may underestimate temperature if anesthetic gases are unheated.[52] The ideal location for core temperature monitoring may not correspond to the best anatomic location for monitoring heart and breath sounds with the esophageal stethoscope.

2. Rectal temperatures are not recommended for very small infants because of the possibility of trauma to rectal mucosa. Furthermore, rectal temperatures do not reflect rapid core temperature changes (as seen with cardiopulmonary bypass).

3. Tympanic membrane temperatures correlate well with core temperatures. Equipment specific for this site should be used, to avoid trauma to the external canal and tympanic membrane.

4. Nasopharyngeal temperatures also show good correlation with core temperatures, but epistaxis is a frequent complication.

5. Skin temperature monitors pose little risk of trauma, but show great variability in their correlation with core temperatures. Wide discrepancies between skin and core temperatures may provide information about peripheral resistance, but the exact clinical interpretation of this information remains controversial.

Equipment for Maintaining Normothermia

1. Covering the patient with clear plastic wrap or warm blankets helps to decrease losses by convection, conduction, and radiation.

2. Radiant heat lamps are useful for the small patient, whose entire body falls within the path of heat from the bulbs. The child must be uncovered; heat is reflected off white blankets. Placing the heat lamps too close to the patient may result in burns.

3. Warm-water mattresses with temperature and thermostatic control help to prevent heat loss by transferring heat across the skin surface.

4. Warmed washing solutions and sterile drapes help to decrease heat losses.

5. Rapid infusions of cold blood or crystalloid will drop core temperature. This can be prevented by warming all intravenous fluids.

6. Heated humidifiers add heat and moisture to inhaled gases to

prevent evaporative losses. However, accumulation of water within the circuit and endotracheal tube can lead to fresh-water drowning. Filters that prevent evaporative loss without adding humidification are manufactured in sizes that do not add significant dead space to the circuit. These are probably as effective and pose less danger for infants than humidifiers or nebulizers, but may increase work of breathing during spontaneous ventilation.

7. Forced-air warming devices have been shown to be most effective at warming during anesthesia, even when they are only applied to part of the body.

8. It is sometimes necessary to increase the operating room temperature in order to maintain normothermia.

OXIMETRY[53-62]

Indications

Use of the oximeter is particularly important in pediatrics because of the greater tendency of the infant to develop rapid desaturation and hypoxemia (because of low functional residual capacity, high closing capacity, and greater O_2 consumption). Care of critical infants requires the ability to closely follow arterial saturation in order to treat respiratory distress syndrome and congenital heart disease with minimal complications from oxygen usage (e.g., retinopathy of prematurity oxygen toxicity). However, just as it has been recognized for nearly half a century that visual observation of cyanosis is an inaccurate indicator of hypoxemia,[53,63] the principles and limitations of oximetry must also be understood to accurately interpret the SpO_2 display.

Principles

1. Pulse oximetry only *measures* functional hemoglobin:

$$\text{Functional hemoglobin} = \frac{\text{Oxyhemoglobin (oxyHgb)}}{\text{oxyHgb} + \text{deoxyHgb}}$$

2. No oximeter can measure fractional hemoglobin:

$$\text{Fractional hemoglobin} = \frac{\text{oxyHgb}}{\text{oxyHgb} + \text{deoxyHgb} + \text{dysHgb}}$$

3. Since most people have some percentage of dyshemoglobin (COHgb, metHgb, sulfHgb, etc.), some oximeters *calculate in* a small percentage of dyshemoglobin to more closely approximate fractional hemoglobin.

4. Oxygen saturation in patients with large amounts of dyshemoglobin (e.g., burn patients with large percentages of carboxyhemoglobin, sickle cell patients) should be determined by hemoximetry.

5. The presence of fetal hemoglobin (HgbF) does not seem to interfere with the accuracy of pulse oximetry. The goal of neonatal oxygen monitoring is to maintain saturation in the low 90s to minimize risks of oxygen toxicity. The pulse oximeter is a poor monitor of hyperoxia in that it cannot reflect changes in PO_2 greater than 100 mm Hg (correlating with $SpO_2 = 100\%$), at which point the oxyHgb dissociation curve becomes completely flat.

6. Response time to desaturation and resaturation varies with the anatomic site of sensor placement. Delay times of 30 to 60 seconds are reported with hand/finger monitoring and 60 to 80 seconds with toe /foot monitoring.[64] Ear sensors show the shortest lag time (5 to 10 seconds) but are difficult to affix to children.

7. Many common clinical situations affect oximeter accuracy. As with all monitoring devices, the observer must interpret information projected in light of the clinical situation. For example, desaturation to 85% during crying may be due to monitor artifact if the child is moving the arm or leg where the sensor is attached.

Sources of inaccurate saturations obtained from pulse oximetry

Type of interference	Cause	Solution
Excessive ambient light*	Operating room lights Bilirubin treatment lights Bright fluorescent lighting Infrared heating Sunlight Xenon surgical lamps	Cover sensor with opaque material (e.g., blanket, foil).
Optical shunt*	Too large a sensor, which allows light to reach the sensor without passing through a pulsatile bed	Sensor must completely adhere to skin and be of the appropriate size so that the light-emitting device and photodiode are opposed. Disposable adhesive band sensors or reusable adult-sized clips are equally accurate for children. Infant sensors are best placed across the foot or palm to keep the light source detector opposed.

*Many sources of interference allow the oximeter to inaccurately calculate an SpO_2 of 85%, falsely elevating the saturation in the cyanotic child and falsely lowering the saturation in the normoxic child. Please see reference 57 for a more complete explanation.

Sources of inaccurate saturations obtained from pulse oximetry

Type of interference	Cause	Solution
Optical cross talk	Multiple sensors too close to one another	Cover sensors with opaque material or separate sensors (one per extremity).
Movement artifact*	Shivering Motion of the extremity in the awake patient is interpreted as heart rate by the oximeter	Actual heart rate must correlate with rate displayed by oximeter before credence can be given to oximeter reading. Moving the probe to a more central location (ear vs. finger). Change the oximeter to a longer averaging time. Use new-technology filters.
Absorption of light by non-Hgb sources	Intravenous dyes Nail polish Bilirubin	Remove nail polish. Verify readings with hemoximetry.
Electrical interference*	Usually caused by cautery; can be affected by 60-Hz interference	60-cycle interference may be improved by moving the plug to another outlet. Some machines have built-in mechanisms to decrease interference by cautery.
Low perfusion	Cold extremities Decreased cardiac output Peripheral vasoconstriction	Warm extremities. Use inotropic agents or vasodilators. Use a more central location for probe site (tongue or ear).
Active venous bed	Right heart failure Tricuspid regurgitation	Using an oximeter with visual display of plethysmograph waveform may help interpretation.
Altered hemoglobin	HgbF: oximeter remains in the range of acceptable accuracy. HgbS: possibly accurate if oxygenated; probably very inaccurate in a sickle crisis Methemoglobin*: SpO_2 85% Carboxyhemoglobin: falsely elevated SpO_2	Verify readings with laboratory hemoximetry.

GAS MONITORING

Capnometry[65-70]

The measurement of CO_2 is mandated by law in some states (e.g., New York) for all patients under general anesthesia. The ASA lists capnometry as a monitoring standard.

Capnography provides additional information on airway dynamics, cardiac output, amount of rebreathing, patency of the endotracheal tube, and state of neuromuscular relaxation (see table at right).

1. Techniques of measuring CO_2 include the following:
   a. Infrared analysis
   b. Mass spectrometry
   c. Raman scattering
2. Adult flow-through devices for measurement are bulky, can increase dead space, and can cause circuit disconnections. Pediatric sampling chambers are smaller, have minimal dead space, and are reuseable.
3. Side-stream or aspirated gas samples are affected by several factors:
   a. The size of the patient. The most accurate sampling of gas in children under 12 kg is thought to be from a distal port on the endotracheal tube.
   b. Dilution of expired gas by high fresh gas flows needed with nonrebreathing circuits.
   c. Amount of gas aspirated for sampling.
4. Patient pathophysiology may contribute to an increased gradient between end-tidal and arterial CO_2 measurements, usually by increasing shunt ($\dot{V}/\dot{Q}$ mismatch) and increasing dead space (V_D/V_T).
   a. In children with cyanotic heart disease, end-tidal underestimates arterial CO_2, since venous blood passes directly into the arterial circulation without going through the lungs.
   b. Low tidal volumes, rapid respiratory rates, and changing intrapulmonary shunts make $ETCO_2$ accuracy variable for infants with respiratory distress syndrome (RDS).
   c. Pulmonary edema may cause $ETCO_2$ to overestimate arterial CO_2 as alveolar CO_2 approximates venous values.
   d. $\dot{V}/\dot{Q}$ mismatch may change in normal children as a result of changes in body position, muscle relaxation, body temperature, and depth of anesthesia. Techniques to improve accuracy of capnography are listed in the table at right.

Examples of capnographs

Capnograph	Figure	Explanation
Normal		Rapid increase P to Q End-tidal CO_2 is equivalent to alveolar CO_2 *only* when the plateau Q to R is nearly horizontal End-tidal = R Rapid decrease from R to zero during inspiration
Pediatric		Moderate rebreathing Absence of plateau Rapid rate
Obstruction • Kinked tube • Asthma		Slowed expiratory phase Poor plateau Elevated CO_2
Curare cleft		Caused by lack of coordination between diaphragm and intercostal muscles with waning muscle relaxation Cleft occurs in last third of plateau Depth of cleft ∝ degree of muscle relaxation
Camel capnogram		Seen in patients in lateral position or if there is asymmetric pressure on one side of the chest Differential lung emptying with spontaneous or positive-pressure ventilation
Patient breathing against ventilator		Interrupts regular pattern of capnography Capnography of ventilator and of spontaneous ventilation are merged
Cardiac oscillation		Commonly seen during inspiration in children Does not indicate pathology
Decreased height of capnogram		Hyperventilation Decreased cardiac output Air embolism

Techniques to improve accuracy of P_{ETCO_2} in infants and children

Technique	Advantage	Disadvantage
Distal sampling	Decreases dilution by fresh gas flows (FGF)	Requires special sampling port
Cuffed tube (absence of leak)	Decreases dilution by ambient air in oropharynx	Increases incidence of subglottic stenosis
Circle system	Valves isolate FGF to minimize dilution of sample	Valves increase work of breathing in infants who are spontaneously ventilating
Low fresh gas flows	Decrease dilution of expired sample	May increase rebreathing in a Mapelson D or Bain system
Lower sampling rates	Minimize dilution by FGF	Decrease accuracy by increasing lag time and reducing response time, especially at rapid respiratory rates and low tidal volumes (does not record true CO_2 peak)
Long I:E ratios (1:3.5)	Prevent rebreathing	Probably not significant
Controlled ventilation	Increases tidal volume relative to FGF	Prevents weaning from mechanical ventilation
Discontinuation of FGF during sampling	Prevents dilution of sample	Interrupts normal ventilation
Mainstream capnometer	Prevents plugging of the sample line with secretions or humidity. Decreases response time. Minimally affected by fresh gas flow	Adds dead space and weight. Patient must be intubated

Adapted from Bell C, Hughes C, Gaal D: Monitoring for pediatric anesthesia. In Saidman LJ, Smith NT, eds: ed 3, *Monitoring in anesthesia*, Boston, 1993, Butterworth.

Halogenated Agents

Measuring the concentration of halogenated agents in inspired and expired gases serves to monitor the accuracy of a vaporizor and can help prevent accidental overdose from volatile agents.

Methods used to measure halogenated agents include the following:

1. Mass spectrometry
2. Raman scattering
3. Silicon rubber relaxation
4. Crystal oscillation

MONITORING OF NEUROMUSCULAR BLOCKADE[70-72]

Although muscle relaxation is a common ingredient of most pediatric anesthetics, clinical indices of recovery may be more elusive than for the adult patient.

1. Infants will not display head lift or respond to commands, even with full return of neuromuscular function.
2. Lifting both legs (for neonates) may indicate a likelihood that the patient can generate adequate negative inspiratory force, but tells little about gag, cough, or ability to maintain a patent airway.
3. Stimulation of peripheral nerves offers objective evidence about return of neuromuscular function but does not guarantee adequacy or completeness of return. Nerve stimulation does help to guide re-dosing. Furthermore, it is recommended that eliciting three (3) responses to a train-of-four stimulus prior to anticholinesterase reversal helps to ensure rapid antagonism.
4. Nerve stimulation is recommended at the following locations:
   a. Superficial ulnar nerve: the negative lead is placed about 1 cm proximal to the wrist crease, slightly radial to the flexor carpi ulnaris tendon. The positive electrode is positioned slightly more proximally along the volar forearm.
   b. Posterior tibial nerve: the electrodes are placed posterior to the medial malleolus, just above and below. Stimulation produces plantar flexion of the big toe.
5. The facial nerve is not recommended, as the orbicularis oculi muscle is more resistant to neuromuscular blockade and twitch depression at this site, which may underestimate the degree of motor depression elsewhere.

INTRAVENOUS EQUIPMENT

Precise measurement of intravenous fluids for premature infants, neonates, and small children is crucial.

1. Small-gauge nontapered Teflon catheters are available for venous cannulation and are preferable to metal butterflies, which can easily perforate the vessel wall. Use of a 22-gauge catheter is suitable from neonate to 3 or 4 years. A 24-gauge catheter is reserved for use in small infants, and a 25- or 27-gauge catheter for very small premature infants.

2. Use of a T-piece connector directly attached to the venous catheter limits the amount of dead space in tubing during drug administration and provides almost instant access into the vasculature. Use of the T-piece connector is recommended for all children under 1 year of age.

3. Because of the possibility of an intracardiac shunt, all IVs in infants and children should have air bubbles scrupulously removed. Air filters in the IV tubing will assist in keeping the lines bubble-free. Air should also be aspirated from the needle or injection site before injection into any IV tubing.

4. To prevent volume overload, a burette (150-ml capacity) should be used for fluid administration. Also useful is a minidrop (60 gtt/ml) to control the infusion rate over time.

5. Positive-pressure infusion pumps are especially helpful with pediatric patients to control the small amount of fluid given and avoid inadvertent IV boluses, which can cause hemodilution and pulmonary edema. Accuracy at low flow rates is ±1% to 5%, even with the minor occlusions not uncommon with small pediatric catheters. However, low-flow delivery may persist when significant occlusions exist, worsening the severity of infiltrations. Furthermore, bolus delivery may occur after release of the occlusion. Syringe pumps carry these same advantages and disadvantages, but use a smaller reservoir, decreasing medication waste for infants.

   "Smart" pumps calculate and deliver accurate dosages when a patient's weight and drug concentration are entered into the program. Computer-assisted continuous-infusion systems use known pharmacokinetic data and a drug redistribution model to maintain accurate drug plasma concentrations. This infusion technique may provide for improved intraoperative hemodynamics and earlier wakeup.[73-75]

References

1. Hillier SC, McNiece WL: Pediatric anesthesia systems and equipment. In Ehrenwerth J, Eisenkraft J, eds: *Anesthesia equipment: principles and applications,* St Louis, 1993, Mosby.

2. Rose DK, Byrick RJ, Froese AB: Carbon dioxide elimination during spontaneous ventilation with a modified Mapleson D system: studies in a lung model, *Can Anaesth Soc J* 25:353-365, 1978.

3. Conterato JP, Lindahl SGE, Meyer DM, Bires JA: Assessment of spontaneous ventilation in anesthetized children with use of a pediatric circle or a Jackson-Rees system, *Anesth Analg* 69:484-490, 1989.

4. Coté CJ: Pediatric breathing circuits and anesthesia machines, *Int Anesthesiol Clin* 30:51-61, 1992.

5. Spears RS, Yeh A, Fisher DM, Zwass MS: The "educated hand": can anesthesiologists assess changes in neonatal compliance manually? *Anesthesiology* 75:693-696, 1991.

6. Dorsch JA, Dorsch SE: Medical gas cylinders and containers. In Dorsch JA, Dorsch SE, eds: *Understanding anesthesia equipment: construction, care, and complications,* ed 3, Baltimore, 1994, Williams & Wilkins.

7. Pullerits J: Routine and special pediatric airway equipment, *Int Anesthesiol Clin* 30:109-130, 1992.

8. Holzman RS, Nargozian CD, Florence B: Lightwand intubation in children with abnormal upper airways, *Anesthesiology* 69:784-787, 1988.

9. Krucylak CP, Schreiner MS: Orotracheal intubation of an infant with hemifacial microsomia using a modified lighted stylet, *Anesthesiology* 4:826-827, 1992.

10. Fox DJ, Matson MD: Management of the difficult pediatric airway in an austere environment using the lightwand, *J Clin Anesth* 2:123-125, 1990.

11. Borland LM, Casselbrant M: The Bullard laryngoscope: a new indirect oral laryngoscope (pediatric version), *Anesth Analg* 70:105-108, 1990.

12. Brown RE, Vollers JM, Rader GR, Schmitz ML: Nasotracheal intubation in a child with Treacher Collins syndrome using the Bullard intubating laryngoscope, *J Clin Anesth* 5:492-493, 1993.

13. Sugiyama K, Yokoyama K: Displacement of the endotracheal tube caused by change of head position in pediatric anesthesia: evaluation by fiberoptic bronchoscopy, *Anesth Analg* 82:251-253, 1996.

14. Koka BV, Jeon IS, Andre JM, MacKay I, Smith RM. Postintubation croup in children, *Anesth Analg* 56:501-505, 1977.

15. Leicht P, Wisborg T, Chraemmer-Jorgensen B. Does intravenous lidocaine prevent laryngospasm after extubation in children? *Anesth Analg* 64:1193-1196, 1985.

16. Pennant JH, White PF. The laryngeal mask airway, *Anesthesiology* 79:144-163, 1993.

17. Haynes SR, Morton NS. The laryngeal mask airway: a review of its use in paediatric anaesthesia, *Pediatr Anaesth* 3:65-73, 1993.

18. Markakis DA, Sayson SC, Schreiner MS: Insertion of the laryngeal mask airway in awake infants with the Robin sequence, *Anesth Analg* 75:822-824, 1992.

19. Chadd GD, Crane DL, Phillips RM, Tunell WP: Extubation and reintubation guided by the laryngeal mask airway in a child with the Pierre Robin syndrome, *Anesthesiology* 76:640-641, 1992.

20. Reynolds PI, O'Kelly SW: Fiberoptic intubation and the laryngeal mask airway, *Anesthesiology* 79:1144, 1993.

21. Paterson SJ, Byrne PJ, Molesky MG, Seal RF, Finucane BT: Neonatal resuscitation using the laryngeal mask airway, *Anesthesiology* 80:1248-1253, 1994.

22. O'Neill B, Templeton JJ, Caramico L, Schreiner MS: The laryngeal mask airway in pediatric patients: factors affecting ease of use during insertion and emergence, *Anesth Analg* 78:659-662, 1994.

23. Dubreuil M, Laffon M, Plaud B, Penon C, Ecoffey C: Complications and fiberoptic assessment of size 1 laryngeal mask airway, *Anesth Analg* 76:527-529, 1993.

24. Lake CL: Monitoring of the pediatric cardiac patient. In Lake CL, ed: *Pediatric cardiac anesthesia,* ed 2, Norwalk, Conn, 1993. Appleton & Lange.

25. Bell C, Rimar S, Barash P: Intraoperative ST-segment changes consistent with myocardial ischemia in the neonate: a report of three cases, *Anesthesiology* 71:601-604, 1989.

26. Yemen TA: Noninvasive monitoring in the pediatric patient, *Int Anesthesiol Clin* 30:77-90, 1992.

27. Muhuideen IA, Roberson DA, Silverman NH, Haas GS, Turley K, Cahalan MK: Intraopertive echocardiography for evaluation of congenital heart defects in infants and children, *Anesthesiology* 76:165-172, 1992.

28. Hickey PR: Transesophageal echocardiography in pediatric cardiac surgery, *Anesthesiology* 77:610-611, 1992.

29. Muhuideen IA, Silverman NH: Response to "Transesophageal echocardiography in pediatric cardiac surgery," *Anesthesiology* 77:610-611, 1992.

30. Gilbert TB, Panico FG, McGill WA, Martin GR, Halley DG, Sell JE: Bronchial obstruction by transesophageal echocardiography probe in a pediatric cardiac patient, *Anesth Analg* 74:156-158, 1992.

31. Görge G, Erbel R, Henrichs KJ, Wenchel HM, Werner HP, Meyer J: Positive blood cultures during transesophageal echocardiography, *Am J Cardio* 65:1404-1405, 1990.

32. Shah PM, Stewart S III, Calalang CC, Alexson C: Transesophageal echocardiography and the intraoperative management of pediatric congenital heart disease: initial experience with a pediatric esophageal 2D color flow echocardiographic probe, *J Cardiothorac Vasc Anesth* 6:8-14, 1992.

33. Urbanowicz JH, Kernoff RS, Oppenheim G, Parnagian E, Billingham ME, Popp RL: Transesophageal echocardiography and its potential for esophageal damage, *Anesthesiology* 72:40-43, 1990.

34. Lunn RJ, Oliver WC, Hagler DJ, Danielson GK: Aortic compression by transesophageal echocardiographic probe in infants and children undergoing cardiac surgery, *Anesthesiology* 77:587-590, 1990.

35. Hayashi Y, Uchida O, Takaki O, Ohnishi Y, Nakajima T, Kataoka H, Kuro M: Internal jugular vein catheterization in infants undergoing cardiovascular surgery: an analysis of the factors influencing successful catheterization, *Anesth Analg* 74:688-693, 1992.

36. Introna RPS, Martin DC, Pruett JK, Philpot TE, Johnston JF: Percutaneous pulmonary artery catheterization in pediatric cardiovascular anesthesia: insertion techniques and use, *Anesth Analg* 70:562-566, 1990.

37. Gillman MW, Cook NR: Blood pressure measurement in childhood epidemiological studies, *Circulation* 92:1049-1057, 1995.

38. Friesen RH, Lichtor JL: Indirect measurement of blood pressure in neonates and infants utilizing an automatic noninvasive oscillometric monitor, *Anesth Analg* 60:72, 1981.

39. Diprose GK, Evens DH, Archer LN, Levene MI: Dinamap fails to detect hypotension in very low birthweight infants, *Arch Dis Child* 61:771-773, 1986.

40. Wareham JA, Haugh LD, Yeager SB, Hombar JD: Prediction of arterial blood pressure in the premature neonate using the oscillometric method, *Am J Dis Child* 141:1108-1110, 1987.

41. Soderstrom CA, Wasserman DH, Dunham CM, Caplan ES, Cowley RA: Superiority of the femoral artery for monitoring: a prospective study, *Am J Surg* 144:309-312, 1988.

42. Miyasaka K, Edmonds J, Corm A: Complications of radial artery lines in the paediatric patient, *Can J Anaesth* 23:9-14, 1976.

43. Lowenstein E, Little JW, Lott H: Prevention of cerebral embolization from flushing radial artery cannulas, *N Engl J Med* 285:414-415, 1971.

44. Neal WA, Reynolds JW, Jarvis CW, Williams HJ: Umbilical artery catheterization: demonstration of arterial thrombosis by aortography, *Pediatrics* 50:6-13, 1972.

45. Bedford RF: Radial artery function following percutaneous cannulation with 18 and 20 gauge catheters, *Anesthesiology* 47:37-39, 1977.

46. Lawless S, Orr R: Axillary arterial monitoring of pediatric patients, *Pediatrics* 84:273-275, 1989.

47. Goodwin SR, Graves SA, VanDer Aa J: Umbilical catheters and arterial blood pressure monitoring, *J Clin Monit* 1:227-231, 1985.

48. Freed GL, Fraley JK: Lack of agreement of tympanic membrane temperature assessments with conventional methods in a private practice setting, *Pediatrics* 89:384-386, 1992.

49. Nilsson K: Maintenance and monitoring of body temperature in infants and children, *Pediatr Anaesth* 1:13-20, 1991.

50. Hynson JM, Sessler DI: Intraoperative warming therapies: a comparison of three devices, *J Clin Anesth* 4:194-199, 1992.

51. Bissonnette B, Sessler DI, LaFlamme P: Passive and active inspired gas humidification in infants and children, *Anesthesiology* 71:350-354, 1989.

52. Bloch EC, Ginsberg B, Binner RA Jr: The esophageal temperature gradient in anesthetized children, *J Clin Monit* 9:73-77, 1993.

53. Coté CJ, Goldstein EA, Coté MA, Hoaglin DC, Ryan JF: A single-blind study of pulse oximetry in children, *Anesthesiology* 68:184-188, 1988.

54. Bell C, Hughes C, Gaal D: Monitoring for pediatric anesthesia. In Saidman LJ, Smith NT, eds: *Monitoring in anesthesia,* ed 3, Boston, 1993, Butterworth, pp. 255-289.

55. Kurki TS, Smith NT, Sanford TJ Jr, Head N: Pulse oximetry and finger blood pressure measurement during open-heart surgery, *J Clin Monit* 5:221-228, 1989.

56. Severinghaus JW, Naifeh KH: Accuracy of response of six pulse oximeters to profound hypoxia, *Anesthesiology* 67:551-558, 1987.

57. Barker SJ, Hyatt J, Shah NK, Kao J: The effect of sensor malpositioning on pulse oximeter accuracy during hypoxemia, *Anesthesiology* 79:248-254, 1993.

58. Barker SJ, Tremper KK: Pulse oximetry. In Ehrenwerth J, Eisenkraft Jr, eds: *Anesthesia equipment: principles and practice,* St Louis, 1993, Mosby, pp. 24-63.

59. Macnab AJ, Baker-Brown G, Anderson EE: Oximetry in children recovering from deep hypothermia for cardiac surgery, *Crit Care Med* 18:1066-1069, 1990.

60. Bell C, Nicholson J, Luther M, Fox C, Hirsh J., O'Connor T: The effect of probe design on accuracy and efficacy of pulse oximetry in pediatric patients, *Anesthesiology* 79:A257, 1993.

61. Brooks TD, Gravenstein N: Pulse oximetry for early detection of hypoxemia in anesthetized infants, *J Clin Monit* 1:135-137, 1985.

62. Schmitt HJ, Schuetz WH, Proeschel PA, Jaklin C: Accuracy of pulse oximetry in children with cyanotic congenital heart disease, *J Cardiothorac Vasc Anesth* 7:61-65, 1993.

63. Comroe JH Jr, Botelho S: The unreliability of cyanosis in the recognition of arterial anoxemia, *Am J Med Sci* 214:1-6, 1947.

64. Reynolds LM, Nicolson SC, Steven JM, et al: Influence of sensor site location on pulse oximetry kinetics in children, *Anesth Analg* 76:751-754, 1993.

65. Badgwell JM, Heavner JE: End-tidal carbon dioxide pressure in neonates and infants measured by aspiration and flow-through capnography, *J Clin Monit* 7:285-288, 1991.

66. Coté CJ, Rolf N, Liu LMP, et al: A single-blind study of combined pusle oximetry and capnography in children, *Anesthesiology.* 74:980-987, 1991.

67. Rich GF, Sullivan MP, Adams JM: Is distal sampling of end-tidal CO_2 necessary in small subjects? *Anesthesiology* 73:265-268, 1990.

68. Isserles SA, Breen PH: Can changes in end-tidal PCO_2 measure changes in cardiac output? *Anesth Analg* 73:808-814, 1991.

69. Badgwell JM, Kleinman SE, Heavner JE: Respiratory frequency and artifact affect the capnographic baseline in infants, *Anesth Analg* 77:708-712, 1993.

70. Badgwell JM: Respiratory gas monitoring in the pediatric patient, *Int Anesthesiol Clin* 30:131-146, 1992.

71. Meistelman C, Debaene B, D'Hollander A, Donati F, Saint-Maurice, C: Importance of the level of recovery for a rapid antagonism of vecuronium with neostigmine in children during halothane anesthesia, *Anesthesiology* 69;97-99, 1988.

72. Law CS, Brandom BW: Monitoring neuromuscular function in the pediatric patient, *Int Anesthesiol Clin* 30:147-162, 1992.

73. Zarmsky RF, Parker AJ, Sinatra RS: Infusion pumps. In Ehrenwerth J, Eisenkraft J, eds: *Anesthesia equipment: principles and applications,* St Louis, 1993, Mosby.

74. Kern FH, Ungerleider Rm, Jacobs JR, et al: Computerized continuous infusion of intravenous anesthetic drugs during pediatric cardiac surgery, *Anesth Analg* 72:487-492, 1989.
75. Holzman RS: Intravenous infusion equipment, *Int Anesthesiol Clin* 30:35-50, 1992.

FLUIDS, ELECTROLYTES, AND TRANSFUSION THERAPY

4

Water, water everywhere
Flows in rivers, suspends in air
Ships in trains across the map
Moves through pipes and out the tap
Freezing in snowflakes,
Ice cubes or hail
Makes a home for the fishes,
A home for the whales

Water to cool us
When we're at play
Water for baths
At the end of the day
Water for paints so that
Artists we'll be
Water for new life
In flowers and trees

You think that the world
Must depend upon land
And rock solid places
On which you can stand
But you're bound to admit
When the days become hotter
That no one could live
In a world without water.

Rivian Bell

PRINCIPLES OF FLUID MANAGEMENT

Fluid requirements in children must be carefully calculated pre-operatively and repeatedly evaluated intraoperatively by the anesthesiologist. Persistent vigilance is mandatory, as the pediatric patient's smaller blood volume is more sensitive to overhydration or underhydration.

Fluid, electrolyte, and transfusion therapy is based upon the patient's weight. The use of body surface area or caloric expenditure yields large variations in dosing of parenteral fluid therapy. A system based on body weight is preferable, as it is far easier and faster for the anesthesiologist to obtain a consistent, accurate measurement of weight in the preoperative assessment.

Parenteral fluid therapy is administered in the operating room with the following goals in mind:

1. To preserve hydration
2. To compensate for fluid and electrolyte deficits caused by patient disease or enforced preoperative fasting
3. To replace ongoing losses resulting from evaporation, insensible losses, or surgical bleeding
4. To compensate for acute changes in autonomic function that occur during anesthesia. Alterations in sympathetic and parasympathetic tone can markedly alter preload and afterload, with subsequent decreases in cardiac output and perfusion.

Effects of anesthetics on fluid and electrolyte balance

- Enforced preoperative fasting increases fluid deficit.
- Surgical trauma to tissues causes capillary leaks and tissue edema, decreasing intravascular volume.
- Decreased sympathetic tone caused by general or regional anesthetics increases venous capacitance with a resultant decrease in cardiac output.
- Baroreflexes are blunted.
- Cardiac output is depressed by halothane, enflurane, isoflurane, sevoflurane, desflurane, thiopental, and propofol.
- Decreased cardiac output decreases glomerular filtration rate and renal blood flow.
- Total peripheral resistance is decreased by isoflurane, enflurane, sevoflurane, desflurane, and morphine.
- Hyperventilation causes a relative hypokalemia.
- Mechanical ventilation and CPAP cause an increased secretion of atrial natriuretic factor (ANF), which increases sodium and water excretion.
- Decreased energy expenditures during anesthesia decrease requirements for fluid, sodium, and potassium.
- ADH secretion is increased by the sympathoadrenal axis (decreased excretion of sodium and water).
- Hyperglycemia commonly results from the "stress response" (increased sympathoadrenal activity).
- Effectiveness of insulin is impaired and glucose tolerance is decreased.
- Hypothermia increases oxygen consumption, thereby increasing caloric and water requirements.

FLUID REQUIREMENTS

1. Water is necessary to replace evaporative and fecal losses, to excrete renal solute, and for metabolic processes.
2. Preterm and small infants have a relatively high percentage of total body water (85% in a preterm and 75% in a full-term infant).
3. The minimum amount of water required to meet ongoing insensible losses is 60 to 100 ml/kg/day.
4. Preoperative assessment of the child's fluid status is important to determine intraoperative needs. The anesthesiologist should consider the duration of fasting, urine output, and amount of diarrhea or vomiting. Also, cardiopulmonary status and underlying systemic diseases may influence the fluid balance.
5. The relative percentages of the various fluid compartments are different for infants, children, and adults.

	Infant	Child	Adult
Fat	16%	23%	30%
Total body water (TBW)	75%	70%	55%-60%
Extracellular fluid (ECF)	40%	30%	20%
Intracellular fluid (ICF)	35%	40%	40%

Dehydration

The severity of dehydration (described as a percent change in body weight secondary to dehydration) should be estimated on the basis of patient history and clinical observations, as laboratory data are not useful in predicting severity. Dehydration is classified by its tonicity according to the concentration of serum sodium. To differentiate among isotonic, hypotonic, and hypertonic dehydration, serum osmolarity can be calculated by the following formula:

$$\text{Serum osmolarity} = 2(Na^+ + K^+) + \frac{BUN}{2.8} + \frac{Glucose}{18}$$

If BUN and glucose are within normal ranges, then:

$$\text{Serum osmolarity} = 2(Na^+)$$

Classification of dehydration by tonicity

Type	Serum osmolarity	Serum sodium	Etiology
Isotonic	270-300	130-150 mmol/L	Hypotonic losses (fasting, thirsting, diarrhea, vomiting), with replacement by hypotonic fluids
Hypotonic	<270	<130 mmol/L	Ongoing Na^+ loss with replacement by Na^+-poor beverages
Hypertonic	>310	>150 mmol/L	Inadequate replacement of free water

Severity of dehydration

Percent of body weight lost	Signs and symptoms	Amount of body fluid lost, ml/kg (%)	
		Infants	Older children and adults
Mild 1%-5%	History of 12-14 hours of vomiting and diarrhea Dry mouth Decreased urination	50 (5%)	30 (3%)
Moderate 6%-10%	Skin tenting Sunken eyes Depressed fontanelles Oliguria Lethargy	100 (10%)	60 (6%)
Severe 11%-15%	Cardiovascular instability: Mottling Hypotension Tachycardia Anuria Sensorium changes	150 (15%)	90 (9%)
20%	Coma Shock		

Replacement of Fluid Deficits

1. Selection of fluid
   a. Generally either lactated Ringer's or normal saline is used for routine intraoperative fluid administration, because they closely resemble the intravascular fluids lost during surgery.
   b. Half-normal saline is often used preoperatively for gradual (8- to 24-hour) replacement of dehydration deficits, with frequent clinical and laboratory reassessment.
   c. Crystalloid (lactated Ringer's or normal saline) or colloid (hetastarch or albumin) can be used in cases of acute vol-

ume loss. While crystalloid is considerably less expensive, hetastarch may be more effective in acutely expanding the intravascular space.

2. Insensible losses generally result from evaporation, either from the incision site and viscus exposure or from respiration. These losses increase with a larger incision and with higher respiratory rates.

3. Adequacy of replacement can be determined by the following:
   a. Routine noninvasive hemodynamic monitoring: heart rate may be a more sensitive guide of fluid changes than blood pressure. It is important to note that a child will compensate for hypovolemia and maintain cardiac output and blood pressure by increasing the systemic vascular resistance and increasing heart rate.
   b. Urine output (> 0.5 ml/kg/hr)
   c. Urine specific gravity (1.010 or less if no proteinuria or glucosuria)
   d. Urine osmolality
   e. Central venous pressure monitoring

4. When acute intravascular volume loss has occurred, the rapid administration of 10 to 20 ml/kg of lactated Ringer's or normal saline may be warranted to restore cardiovascular stability and renal perfusion. If losses are ongoing, invasive monitoring will be necessary.

5. The effects of anesthetics on autonomic tone, reflexes, and cardiac output may also increase fluid needs, even though an absolute fluid deficit does not exist. Fluids necessary to compensate for a relatively decreased preload resulting from autonomic effects should be given on a dose-response basis. The decrease in systemic vascular resistance that occurs with the induction of general anesthesia may be reversed at emergence, when pain and agitation increase catecholamines. This process should be considered when fluid boluses are administered, to avoid postoperative hypervolemia.

Intraoperative fluid requirements

1. Estimated fluid requirement (EFR) per hour (maintenance fluids)	0-10 kg = 4 ml/kg/hr + 10-20 kg = 2 ml/kg/hr + > 20 kg = 1 ml/kg/hr
2. Estimated preoperative fluid deficit (EFD)	Number of hours fasting × EFR 1st hr, infuse $\frac{1}{2}$ EFD + EFR 2nd hr, infuse $\frac{1}{4}$ EFD + EFR 3rd hr, infuse $\frac{1}{4}$ EFD + EFR

3. Insensible losses (IL)	Minimal incision 3-5 ml/kg/hr
	Moderate incision
	  with viscus exposure 5-10 ml/kg/hr
	Large incision
	  with bowel exposure 8-20 ml/kg/hr

4. Estimated blood loss (EBL)	Replace maximum allowable
	  blood loss (ABL) with crystalloid 3:1.
	  (See transfusion therapy section, p 83.)

5. Total intraoperative fluid replacement	EFR + EFD + IL + EBL

Liberalization of fasting criteria prior to surgery has decreased the severity of preoperative fluid deficits. Normal children who have fasted minimally and who are expected to resume oral intake in the immediate postoperative period (e.g., myringotomy, nevus excision, etc.) do not usually require calculated replacement of fluid deficits. However, attention should be paid to the length of fast before the time of surgery, especially in neonates and infants.

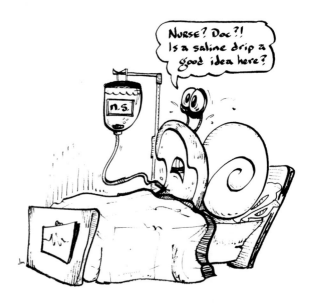

Composition of intravenous crystalloid solutions

Solution (pH, osmolarity)	Glucose (mg/dl)	Na$^+$ (mmol/L)	K$^+$ (mmol/L)	Cl$^-$ (mmol/L)	Lactate (mmol/L)	Ca^{++} (mmol/L)
5% Dextrose (5.0, 253)	500	—	—	—	—	—
Ringer's (6.0, 309)	—	147	4	155	—	4
Lactated Ringer's (6.7, 273)	—	130	4	109	28	3
D$_5$ lactated Ringer's (5.3, 527)	500	130	4	109	28	3
D$_5$ 0.22% NSS* (4.4, 330)	500	38.5	—	38.5	—	—
D$_5$ 0.45% NSS (4.2, 407)	500	77	—	77	—	—
0.9% NSS (5.7, 308)	—	154	—	154	—	—
Normosol R (7.4, 295)	—	140	5	98	Acetate 27 Gluconate 23	—

Adapted from Stoelting RK: *Pharmacology and physiology in anesthetic practice*, ed 2, Philadelphia 1991, JB Lippincott.
*NSS, Normal saline solution.

Composition of intravenous colloid solutions

Solution	Composition	Comments
Dextran: D_{40} = low molecular weight D_{70} = high molecular weight	Branched-chain polysaccharides	• Remains in intravascular compartment longer than crystalloid. • Interferes with platelet function, stimulates fibrinolysis, and may cause renal failure. • May cause anaphylactic reactions, fever, and rash. • Use of a filter is not necessary.
Hydroxyethyl starch (HES): 6% solution in normal saline solution	Starch composed of amylopectin ethoxylated to retard degradation by amylase	• Fewer side effects than dextran. • May cause pruritus. • May cause coagulation defects. • Use of a filter is not necessary.
Albumin: 5% solution 25% solution	Donor plasma derived from blood by plasmapheresis. Contains: 96% albumin 4% globulin Na^+ = 145 mmol/L	• Used for hypovolemia with hypoproteinemia. • 5% solution is osmotically equivalent to plasma. • No ABO testing or blood filter is required. • Heat process prevents viral transmission.

Glucose Requirements[4-8]

Glycogen stores in the neonatal liver are limited and are rapidly depleted within the first few hours of life. Neonates tolerate fasting poorly because of their high metabolic demands and limited energy stores. The routine intravenous replacement solution for normal neonates contains 10% dextrose. At 100 ml/kg/day, this solution will provide only 40 kcal/kg/day, or one third of the infant's basal metabolic requirements. Without further nutritional support, the infant will have a negative nitrogen and caloric balance.

Caloric requirements for children are as follows:

Age (yr)	kcal/kg/day
Preterm	120
0-1	90-100
1-7	75-90
7-12	60-75

The intraoperative use of glucose-containing solutions for children must be individualized on the basis of fasting and caloric requirements. When intraoperative parenteral glucose is administered to infants and children, an attempt must be made to balance the risk of hypoglycemia against the detrimental effects of hyperglycemia.

Children at increased risk for hypoglycemia

Those in the lower percentiles of weight
Those with chronic debilitating illness
Those whose preoperative fast has been extensive
Those who have been receiving total parenteral nutrition
All term neonates
Preterm infants
Infants of diabetic mothers
Infants small for gestational age
Infants with erythroblastosis fetalis
A small percentage of normal, healthy infants and children will exhibit mild hypoglycemia preoperatively or intraoperatively even without an extended fast.

Intraoperative *hyperglycemia* in children seems to occur frequently when solutions containing glucose are given. Hyperglycemia is usually a result of the "stress response" to surgery. Increased sympathoadrenal activity results in decreased glucose tolerance, decreased glucose utilization, and increased gluconeogenesis. The increased osmotic load caused by hyperglycemia may result in osmotic diuresis when the renal threshold is exceeded, which may impair the determination of adequate cardiac output and cause intraventricular hemorrhage in preterm infants.

Recommendations for intraoperative glucose administration include:

1. Consideration of the length of fast before surgery. Most centers have liberalized the fasting period prior to surgery; therefore, preoperative hypoglycemia may occur less often.
2. Dextrose-containing solutions should be avoided in patients at risk for complete cerebral ischemia (craniotomy, cardiac bypass). In these patients, dextrose infusions prior to ischemia have been shown to correlate with worsened neurologic outcome. During hypothermic cardiopulmonary bypass, gluconeogenesis continues despite a dearth of insulin production, posing a threat of extreme hyperglycemia. Patients having craniotomy or cardiac surgery will have intraarterial access, so that it becomes simple to check glucose levels frequently.
3. Infants and chronically ill patients at greatest risk of hypoglycemia (or of adverse effects from hypoglycemia) should

have frequent intraoperative blood glucose measurements.
4. Use of dextrose concentrations of less than 5% (2.5% recommended) is probably sufficient to prevent hypoglycemia and decreases the likelihood of hyperglycemia.

TOTAL PARENTERAL NUTRITION[9]

Infants and children who fast briefly in the perioperative period do not require parenteral protein. However, the anesthesiologist may encounter patients who are chronically unable to tolerate enteral feeding and are therefore maintained on total parenteral nutrition.

Perioperative Management of Total Parenteral Nutrition (TPN)

1. Peripheral TPN can provide up to 80 kcal/kg/day. The maximum allowable dextrose concentration by this route is 10%, and amino acids should not exceed 2%.
2. Central-vein TPN is indicated when high caloric requirements are present (burns, sepsis, major surgery) or the bowel cannot be used for feeding. The maximum allowable concentration of dextrose given by central vein is 25%; the maximum for amino acids, 3%. Lipid emulsions can be administered as a source of fatty acids and calories. A 25% dextrose solution allows for a small volume relative to the amount of calories to be infused. Lipids should make up no more than 60% of the total daily caloric intake.
3. An additional peripheral intravenous catheter may be placed if the TPN infusion catheter provides the only intravenous access. Third-space losses and blood should be replaced through the peripheral catheter in order to avoid introducing infection into the TPN infusion. Drugs should be administered through the peripheral catheter because of possible drug incompatibilities.
4. The key to intraoperative management of TPN, regardless of the dextrose concentration being used, is frequent glucose monitoring. The stress of surgery alone is likely to cause hyperglycemia, and the concomitant administration of a concentrated glucose solution could induce severe hyperglycemia, glycosuria, osmotic diuresis, and associated fluid and electrolyte derangements. A sudden withdrawal of TPN, on the other hand, could result in rebound hypoglycemia. An infusion of 10% dextrose should be started if TPN is to be discontinued intraoperatively. If TPN is continued, the rate may be decreased by half to avoid hyperglycemia. In either case, blood glucose should be assessed at frequent and regular intervals.

ELECTROLYTE MANAGEMENT

The principles behind electrolyte management in children are similar to those in adults. Replacement needs to be administered on a mg/kg or mmol/kg basis.

**Daily electrolyte requirements
(1 mEq = 1 mmol)**

Na^+	0.5-2.0 mmol/kg/day
K^+	0.5-2.0 mmol/kg/day
Cl^-	0.5-2.0 mmol/kg/day
Ca^+	20-100 mg/kg/day

Management of Electrolyte Imbalances

Repetition of laboratory results is often indicated, as hemolysis secondary to difficult venipuncture may result in a falsely elevated K^+. ECG monitoring for arrhythmias is also required.

Imbalance	Treatment
Hyperkalemia, acute (K^+ > 6.5 mmol/L)	1. Hyperventilation 2. Sodium bicarbonate 1-2 mmol/kg (bolus not to exceed 0.5 mmol/kg) 3. Calcium chloride 5-10 mg/kg IV 4. Glucose (0.5g/kg) and regular insulin (0.3 unit/g glucose) IV
Hyperkalemia, chronic (K^+ > 6.5 mmol/L)	Administration of perioperative sodium poly-styrene sulfonate (Kayexalate), 1-2 g/kg/day orally or rectally in divided doses
Hypokalemia (K^+ < 3.5 mmol/L)	Urine output should be at least 0.5 ml/kg/hr before potassium replacement is started. 1. Total amount of K^+ to be replaced may be calculated as follows: Weight × ($C_D - C_M$) × 0.3 = mmol required C_D = Serum concentration desired C_M = Serum concentration measured 2. Infusion should proceed at rates ≤ 0.5 mmol/kg/hr
Hypernatremia (Na^+ > 160 mmol/L)	Gradual hydration over 48 hours with isotonic solutions; rapid fall in intracellular sodium can cause cerebral edema
Hyponatremia (Na^+ < 130 mmol/L)	1. Can usually be treated with isotonic solutions 2. Although administration of hypertonic saline may be hazardous, it has been used for children with severe hyponatremia (Na < 120 mmol/L) and symptoms of cerebral edema (seizures, coma).
Hyperchloremia (Cl^- > 109 mmol/L)	Excess will usually self-correct when offending problem is resolved (often caused by large infusions of saline).
Hypochloremia (Cl^- < 95 mmol/L)	1. Commonly seen in pyloric stenosis accompanied by metabolic alkalosis and hypokalemia 2. Infusion of isotonic saline and potassium will correct Cl^- and K^+ deficits and therefore alkalosis.

TRANSFUSION THERAPY[10-12]

Transfusion of blood components is indicated to increase oxygen-carrying capacity (red cells) or to improve coagulation (fresh frozen plasma, platelets). Rapid blood loss in the infant can lead to significant hemodynamic compromise more rapidly than in the larger adult, and therefore transfusion is often required sooner. If rapid or massive blood loss is anticipated, invasive monitoring (particularly the arterial pressure tracing) will be needed to see rapid changes in hemodynamics. The following guidelines should assist the anesthesiologist in managing intraoperative blood loss:

1. The maximum allowable blood loss (ABL) before transfusion should be calculated preoperatively for any operation in which blood loss is anticipated (see table on p. 83).
2. Blood losses less than the ABL can be replaced by crystalloid or colloid. Either 2 to 3 ml of balanced salt solution or 1 ml of 5% albumin can be used to replace each ml of blood lost. No conclusive studies have been done supporting the preferential use of either crystalloid or colloid solution in children.
3. Specific techniques to quantitate blood loss, such as small traps in suction circuits and weighing bloody sponges, will help to estimate the amount of blood loss intraoperatively.

Normal and Acceptable Hematocrit in Pediatric Patients[13] (See also Anemia, p. 281)

The risk of transmitting blood-borne pathogens, such as the hepatitis virus and HIV, has led to the development of some arbitrary guidelines concerning recommended threshold hematocrit values. The concepts of an acceptable hematocrit and a normal hematocrit will assist the physician in determining when transfusion should occur. A normal hematocrit is often defined as a hematocrit within two standard deviations. If the hematocrit is below two standard deviations, then an attempt should be made to delineate the etiology of the anemia. An acceptable hematocrit is defined as a hematocrit tolerated by infants and children without the need for blood transfusion. The term "acceptable hematocrit" has not been clearly delineated for different age groups and will likely vary from patient to patient according to underlying disease, ability to compensate for lowered red cell mass, and the proposed surgery. Children with normal cardiac physiology can compensate for a lower hematocrit by increasing cardiac output. Increasing FIO_2 is also useful to improve oxygen delivery.

Calculating allowable blood loss and transfusion requirements

Several different techniques/formulas are given to assist the anesthesiologist in determining transfusion requirements.

1. Calculate the estimated blood volume (EBV).	Premature infant 90-100 ml/kg Full-term infant 80-90 ml/kg 3 mo-1 yr 75-80 ml/kg > 1 yr 70-75 ml/kg
2. Calculate allowable blood loss by simple proportion. ABL = Allowable blood loss EBV = Estimated blood volume Hct_{pt} = Patient hematocrit (decimal) Hct_{LA} = Lowest allowable hematocrit (decimal)	$ABL = \dfrac{EBV \times (Hct_{pt} - Hct_{LA})}{Hct_{pt}}$
3. Calculate by estimating red cell mass loss (RCML). EBV = Estimated blood volume Hct_{pt} = Patient hematocrit (decimal) $ERCM_{pt}$ = Estimated red cell mass (patient) Hct_{LA} = Lowest allowable hematocrit (decimal) $ERCM_{LA}$ = Estimated red cell mass (lowest allowable) ARCML = Allowable red cell mass loss (maximum) ABL = Allowable blood loss (maximum)	$EBV \times Hct_{pt} = ERCM_{pt}$ $EBV \times Hct_{LA} = ERCM_{LA}$ $ERCM_{pt} - ERCM_{LA} = ARCML$ $ARCML \times 3 = ABL$
4. Calculate the volume of whole blood to be transfused. RBV = Blood volume to be replaced AcBL = Actual measured (or estimated) blood loss ABL = Calculated allowable blood loss	$RBV = AcBL - ABL$
5. Convert the volume of whole blood to the volume of packed red blood cell transfusion necessary to increase the hematocrit to the desired level. RBV = Blood volume to be replaced Hct_{LA} = Lowest allowable hematocrit $Hct_{prbc}\%$ = Hematocrit of packed red blood cells to be transfused (ADSOL blood: hematocrit 55%; CPDA blood: hematocrit 70%)	$\dfrac{RBV \times Hct_{LA}\%}{Hct_{prbc}\%}$ = ml necessary to achieve lowest allowable hematocrit (Hct_{LA})

Blood Components[10]

WHOLE BLOOD

A unit of whole blood contains approximately 450 ml of blood and 60 ml of anticoagulant preservative. It is obtained from a single donor and is not separated into components; its hematocrit is usually 36% to 44%. If used within 24 hours of donation, whole blood also contains viable platelets. However, using it within the first 24 hours of donation is virtually impossible because of donated blood testing requirements.

Whole blood is used for actively bleeding patients who require an increased oxygen-carrying capacity and expansion of blood volume. Fresh whole blood may also be chosen for trauma patients, transplant patients, or infants needing exchange transfusion or having open heart surgery. It is rarely available, however, because of the widespread use of component therapy.

The components of whole blood are susceptible to aging. Few viable platelets or granulocytes exist after the first 24 hours. 2,3-DPG levels decrease significantly after the first 7 days. Factor V and VIII levels decrease according to storage time but are probably sufficient for normal clotting (> 20% to 30%).

RED BLOOD CELLS[10,14]

Indications

1. Red cell transfusions increase oxygen-carrying capacity of blood in anemic normovolemic patients (abnormally low red cell mass or poorly fucntioning red blood cells).
2. Pediatric patients who are anemic and hypovolemic from acute blood loss during surgery may require transfusion and hydration if losses exceed ABL calculations.
3. Coexistent disease (dyshemoglobinemia, chronic pulmonary or cardiac disease) that impairs oxygen-carrying capacity may necessitate transfusion in the presence of surgical losses.
4. Additional considerations exist for the full-term or preterm neonate, based on the presence of Hgb F and concurrent medical problems.

Administration of red cells

1. The use of a standard 170-μm filter is requisite to trap debris.
2. For pediatric patients, red cells are generally not diluted to ease administration, because of the risk of hypervolemia.
3. Clinically significant hemolysis does not occur with infusions through 25- or 26-g intravenous catheters if the driving pressure is less than 300 mm Hg.
4. Blood used for neonatal transfusion should be frozen, deglycerolized, or less than 7 days old in order to preserve 2,3-DPG levels. It may also be irradiated to prevent graft-versus-host disease.
5. It may be preferable to intraoperatively transfuse slightly more blood than required rather than expose the child to a second unit of blood in the postoperative period, especially when ongoing losses are anticipated.

Categories of red blood cell transfusion preparations[10]

Type	Preparation	Indications for use	Comments
RBC/CPDA* preservative	Preserved with adenine to increase ATP, which results in a shelf life[†] of 35 days	Treatment of anemia; improves oxygen-carrying capacity	Potassium content, 15-25 mmol/L Decreases factors V, VIII Absent platelets Decreased 2,3-DPG Hct approx. 70% (10 ml/kg raises Hct about 10%
RBC/ADSOL preservative (adenine saline solution)	Preservative contains mannitol, dextrose, and adenine in a 100-ml volume (extends shelf life to 42 days)	As above	As above except Hct approx. 55% (10 ml/kg raises Hct about 7%)
Frozen thawed deglycerolized RBC	Glycerol added to blood < 6 days old and frozen	Depleted of leukocytes; safe for infants < 1200 g at risk for CMV (decreases risk of seroconversion)	Low potassium Nearly normal 2,3-DPG No fibrinogen Less red cell mass and almost no citrate
Irradiated RBC	Blood irradiated with cesium-137 (1-5 min with 1500 rads) to eradicate lymphocytes	To prevent graft-versus-host disease in immunocompromised patients or for exchange transfusion in infants	Functional components other than lymphocytes are not affected.
Leukocyte-poor (saline-washed) RBC	Blood centrifuged and filtered to remove "buffy coat" (leukocytes and platelets)	Used in patients with recurrent or severe febrile nonhemolytic reactions due to alloimmunization to leukocyte antigens or plasma proteins	After washing, shelf life is decreased to 24 hours because of possible bacterial contamination. 30% of red cells may be lost during washing.

*Citrate phosphate dextrose adenine preservative.
[†]Shelf life: number of days during which blood cells maintain 75% viability 24 hours after infusion.

All red blood cell categories listed in the table above are prepared by removing 200 to 250 ml of plasma from whole blood and then storing it in various preservatives and anticoagulants at 1° to 6°C.

Alternatives to homologous red cell transfusion[15,16]

1. *Autologous transfusion:* Patients scheduled for nonemergent procedures may donate blood several weeks prior to surgery for availability when needed. Autologous donations minimize the risk of transmission of infectious disease in blood. Some patients (i.e., those who are severely anemic or have a coexisting disease) may not be suitable candidates for donation. Contraindications include anemia, bacteremia, HIV-positive antibodies, hepatitis B surface antigen, and syphilis. Increased cost is associated with autologous transfusion.

2. *Directed donor:* Similar to the autologous transfusion, except an individual is selected by the patient to serve as the blood donor. Directed donor blood may present less risk; however, this increase in safety is controversial.

3. *Hetastarch:* This may be used for acute blood loss, as it remains in the intravascular space longer than crystalloid. It can prolong the protime and partial thromboplastin time (PT/PTT) and should not be used if coagulation abnormalities are present or anticipated.

4. *Acute perioperative phlebotomy/isovolemic hemodilution:* The purpose of this technique is to lower the hematocrit but not the vascular volume prior to surgical blood loss, with the ability to transfuse autologous blood if necessary. Advantages include lower cost and less planning than for preoperative autologous donation. Disadvantages include causing acute anemia. It is contraindicated in patients unable to tolerate rapid blood loss or lowered hematocrit.

5. *Controlled hypotension:* This method has the twofold benefit of decreasing blood loss and producing a drier surgical field. Hypotension is induced by pharmacologic agents such as trimethaphan, sodium nitroprusside, or nitroglycerin. Invasive arterial monitoring is recommended (see p. 264).

6. *Cell salvage:* This procedure requires the use of an intraoperative device to scavenge lost red blood cells. Not usually used in pediatric procedures, it may be useful in large-blood-loss operations. It is useful when transfusion therapy is contraindicated or not possible (e.g., Jehovah's Witness, hemolytic reactions) but is contraindicted in the presence of bacteremia or evidence of malignancy.

Pharmacologic alternatives to blood transfusion[17-22]

Drug	Mechanism of action	Patient population	Dose
Erythropoietin	Stimulates production of red blood cells by acting at the kidney or liver	Patients with chronic renal disease Jehovah's Witnesses	100 units 2-3 times/wk
Aprotinin	Protease inhibitor that inhibits kallikrein and plasmin, thus inhibiting fibrinolysis	Prophylactic use to reduce perioperative blood loss, especially in patients undergoing cardiopulmonary bypass	Adult dose: 1 ml test followed by 100 ml loading dose over 20-30 min; then, 100 ml into pump prime; then 25 ml/hr infusion*
Desmopressin	Synthetic analogue of antidiuretic hormone Increases factor VIII	Von Willebrand's disesase Hemophilia A Patients with post-bypass bleeding	0.3-0.5 mg/kg

*Extrapolation to pediatric dosing on a mg/kg basis has not been verified.

Jehovah's Witnesses[18,23]

The treatment of the children of Jehovah's Witnesses often presents a moral and ethical dilemma to the physician in the operating room when transfusion must be considered. Alternatives to homologous transfusion, such as hetastarch infusion, hemodilution, preoperative erythropoietin therapy, blood scavenging systems, and cardiopulmonary bypass (any system where the patient's blood is in a continuous circuit with the patient) may be acceptable to Jehovah's Witnesses.

Legal and ethical concerns arise when parents refuse blood transfusion for their children. It should be noted that the courts have consistently supported physicians who transfuse the child of a Jehovah's Witness as a life-saving measure. In nonemergent situations, the need for transfusion must be weighed against the parental decision. A preoperative conference that includes the family, primary care physician, surgeon, and anesthesiologist is recommended prior to elective surgery. Finally, when transfusion is unavoidable, judicial support (court order) should be obtained before transfusing whenever possible.

FRESH FROZEN PLASMA (FFP)[23]

FFP is the supernatant component of a single unit of blood, consisting of water, protein, carbohydrates, and lipids. It is separated from the red cells and frozen within 6 hours of phlebotomy. All clotting factors are present, and 1 ml of FFP contains 1 unit of coagulation factor activity. FFP should be given through a filter in a dose of 10 to 20 ml/kg if bleeding is acute.

Indications

1. For patients with active bleeding, and a PT or PTT patient:control ratio of at least 1.5, as a result of:
   a. Factor deficiency secondary to liver disease
   b. Disseminated intravascular coagulation (DIC)
2. For patients with congenital factor deficiencies for which no coagulation concentrate is available
3. To reverse the effects of warfarin or coumarin in actively bleeding patients who cannot wait for reversal by vitamin K or when emergent surgery is necessary
4. For infants with immunodeficiency as a result of protein-losing enteropathy
5. May be useful for the treatment of thrombotic thrombocytopenic purpura and hemolytic-uremic syndrome

CRYOPRECIPITATE

Cryoprecipitate is derived from the cold-insoluble precipitate remaining after FFP is thawed and refrozen. Each 20- to 40-ml bag contains 80 to 100 units of factor VIII activity and 100 to 350 mg of fibrinogen.

Indications

1. Cryoprecipitate was previously used in the treatment of a congenital deficiency of factor VIII. It has now been replaced by the development of an ultrapure commercial concentrate prepared by immunoaffinity chromatography using monoclonal antibodies (see p. 293 for dose).
2. Useful in treating a quantitative or qualitative deficiency of fibrinogen
3. Useful in treating hemophilia A and von Willebrand's disease (congenital or acquired)

ALBUMIN[25,26]

Albumin is a plasma component containing 96% albumin and 4% globulin heated to 60°C for 10 hours. It is available in a 5% solution ($Na^+ = 145$ mEq/L), which is osmotically equivalent to plasma, or in a 25% solution.

Plasma protein fraction (PPF) contains approximately 83% albumin and 17% globulins because it goes through less purification than albumin. Like albumin, it is also available in a 5% solution.

The presence of sodium acetate and Hageman factor may produce hypotension during rapid infusion.

Albumin cannot transmit viral disease because of the heating process. ABO antigens and antibodies are absent, so blood typing is unnecessary. It can be stored for up to 5 years at 2° to 10°C, and administration through a filter is not necessary.

Indications

1. Hemolytic disease of the newborn (binds indirect bilirubin during exchange transfusion)
2. To support blood pressure in patients who are hypovolemic and hypoproteinemic (usual dose: 10 ml/kg of the 5% solution)
3. Albumin will not correct chronic hypoalbuminemia, and it should not be used for long-term therapy.
4. Dose: 1 ml per 1 ml fluid deficit (or per 1 ml blood loss) to restore intravascular volume.

PLATELETS[27]

One unit of platelets is obtained by centrifuging a single unit of whole blood. Each unit contains at least 5.5×10^{10} platelets in 50 to 70 ml of plasma. Platelet concentrates are usually stored at 20° to 24°C for up to 5 days with constant gentle agitation to preserve cell survival; refrigeration kills platelets. The usual dose is 1 unit/10 kg or 20 ml/kg. Administration through a filter is necessary. Red cell compatibility testing is not necessary.

Indications

1. Active bleeding with either a platelet count of less than 50,000/μl or abnormal platelet function with template bleeding time greater than twice normal
2. Prophylaxis against bleeding in patients with platelets less than 20,000/μl. Children with accelerated platelet destruction who are scheduled for splenectomy can be given platelet transfusions after the spleen is removed.
3. Dilutional thrombocytopenia associated with massive transfusion when active bleeding and documented thrombocytopenia are present
4. *Not* indicated for routine prophylaxis after cardiac surgery[28]

Risks of platelet transfusion[29]

1. Alloimmunization to platelets or leukocytes may occur in patients receiving repeated transfusions (e.g., oncology patients). Antibodies to subsequent platelet transfusion may result in platelet destruction, and further platelet transfusion must be HLA matched.
2. Infection:
   a. Viral risk increases exponentially with each transfusion, because of pooling of concentrates from multiple donors.
   b. Bacterial risk is increased by storage at 20° to 24°C.

3. Graft-versus-host disease can be prevented by irradiation of platelets for immunocompromised patients.
4. Large-pore filters must be used, since micropore filters adsorb platelets.
5. Platelets contain large amounts of histamine, and rapid infusion may result in vasodilation and hypotension.

GRANULOCYTES[30,31]

Granulocytes are usually prepared by centrifugation electrophoresis of a single donor and must be infused within 24 hours of collection. Neonatal granulocyte transfusions use "buffy coat" preparations. Irradiation will help to decrease the incidence of graft-versus-host disease.

Indications

1. Neonatal sepsis-induced neutropenia, especially if the sepsis is unresponsive to antibiotic therapy
2. Pediatric patients with qualitative and/or quantitative neutrophil defects
3. Patients with hypoplastic bone marrow with a reasonable chance of recovery

PLASMA DERIVATIVES TO REPLACE CONGENITAL DEFICIENCIES (SEE P. 293)

Derivative	Preparation and indications
Cryoprecipitated antihemophilic factor (AHF)	• Contains concentrated factor VIII:C, factor VIII:vWF (von Willebrand factor), fibrinogen, factor XIII • Useful for hemophilia A, von Willebrand's disease, congenital or acquired fibrinogen deficiency, factor XIII deficiency, and consumptive coagulopathy
Factor VIII concentrate	• Indicated for the treatment of hemophilia A • Prepared from pooled plasma with techniques that reduce (*not* eliminate) viral transmission
Factor IX concentrate	• Factor IX complex (prothrombin complex) contains factors IX (1%-5%), II, VII, X • Coagulation Factor IX contains Factor IX (20%-30%), trace II, VII, X • Useful for patients with Christmas disease (factor IX deficiency, or hemophilia B) • Heat treated to reduce (*not* eliminate) viral transmission
Antithrombin III concentrate[32]	• Fraction of pooled plasma used to treat congenital deficiency of antithrombin III with associated thrombosis and to restore response to heparin • Heat treated to reduce (*not* eliminate) viral transmission
Alpha$_1$-proteinase inhibition concentrate (alpha$_1$-antitrypsin)[33]	• Fraction of pooled plasma used for patients with severe alpha$_1$-antitrypsin deficiency and demonstrable emphysema • Heat treated to reduce (*not* eliminate) viral transmission

Transfusion Reactions[10]

ACUTE HEMOLYTIC REACTIONS

ABO incompatibility (intravascular hemolysis).   This reaction is usually the result of clinical errors. It is caused by activation of complement to C_9 by anti-A or anti-B with resultant intravascular hemolysis. Clinical symptoms include:

1. Chest and back pain
2. Fever
3. Hemodynamic instability and cardiorespiratory failure
4. Disseminated intravascular coagulation (DIC)
5. Renal damage from renovascular thrombosis, prolonged hypotension, or vasoconstriction of renal microcirculation. Renal dysfunction is probably not due to inspissation of hemoglobin in renal tubules.

Treatment is as follows:

1. Transfusion is immediately stopped.
2. Blood bank is notified and samples of patient blood are sent for Coombs test to verify transfusion reaction.
3. Crystalloid is infused; furosemide can be used to maintain urine output and increase renal cortical blood flow.
4. Low-dose dopamine also increases renal circulation and supports systemic blood pressure (3 to 5 µg/kg/min).
5. An anticoagulated blood sample should be centrifuged and assessed for hemolysis.
6. Baseline coagulation profile, BUN, and creatinine should be obtained.

Extravascular hemolysis.   This reaction is usually seen when antibodies other than ABO (e.g., Kell, Duffy, Kidd) are present. No activation of C_9 occurs. Clinical symptoms include fever, anemia, increased bilirubin, and positive direct antiglobulin test. These reactions may occur up to 14 days after transfusion and usually require only supportive care.

Nonimmune hemolysis.   Nonimmune hemolysis is caused by mechanical or osmotic factors. These include exposure to hypotonic solutions, exposure to dextrose, warming of blood products to more than 45°C, cardiopulmonary bypass, and prosthetic valves. When possible, the offending agent should be discontinued to stop further hemolysis.

FEBRILE REACTIONS

Antibodies against leukocytes or platelets usually precipitate the reaction. Symptomatology includes chills and a rise in temperature without other signs of transfusion reaction. Repeat reactions are uncommon but can be prevented by using leukocyte-poor red cells. Fever can be treated with acetaminophen. Meperidine may be used to stop shaking chills in older children.

ALLERGIC REACTIONS

1. Urticaria is caused by antibodies to plasma proteins. Once it is determined that an intravascular hemolytic reaction is not occurring, the transfusion may continue with antihistamine administration to alleviate symptoms.
2. Anaphylaxis is seen in patients with IgA deficiency who have anti-IgA antibodies as a result of a previous transfusion. No fever is present. The blood is discontinued and epinephrine is administered. The diagnosis is confirmed by measuring patient IgA levels.

PULMONARY EDEMA

1. Transfusion-related acute lung injury (TRALI) with noncardiogenic pulmonary edema and hypoxemia can occur minutes to hours after transfusion.[34,35] Caused by an antigen-antibody reaction with resultant increased microvascular lung permeability (plasma and cells), the pulmonary edema usually responds to positive-pressure ventilation.
2. Hypervolemia occurs when normovolemic patients receive rapid blood transfusion. Pulmonary edema and hypertension may develop, necessitating diuresis and ventilatory support.

SEPSIS

Bacterial sepsis is caused by transfusion of a contaminated unit of blood component and consists of fever, chills, and cardiovascular collapse. The diagnosis is differentiated from hemolytic reaction by negative Coombs test and the absence of hemolysis. The transfusion should be discontinued. Hemodynamic support and antibiotics are needed.

Complications of Massive Transfusion[11,12,36]

PLATELET DEPLETION

A significant decrease in platelet count occurs in pediatric patients when two blood volumes are lost. Platelet administration is indicated, at a dose of 1 unit/10 kg or 20 ml/kg, if the platelet count is less than 50,000 μl or abnormal bleeding time is present.

DEPLETION OF FACTORS V AND VIII

Fresh frozen plasma is routinely given in a dosage of 20% to 30% of each blood volume lost (or 10 to 20 ml/kg) to compensate for anticipated factor depletion.

HYPERKALEMIA

1. As blood ages, the K^+ concentration can increase by 17 to 27 mmol/L, although it usually averages 3 to 6 mmol/L. However, K^+ in transfused blood moves into the intracellular compartment and is not usually a problem unless active hemolysis is occurring.
2. Frozen red blood cells have a low K^+ content and may cause hypokalemia.
3. Serum K^+ should be monitored frequently and hyperkalemia treated if necessary (see table on p. 81).

HYPOCALCEMIA

1. Hypocalcemia occurs when citrate in FFP or blood chelates calcium, lowering serum ionized calcium.
2. No treatment is indicated unless hemodynamic deterioration is present and consistent with ECG changes (prolonged Q-T, decreased S-T segment, flattened T waves), or ionized serum calcium levels are lowered.
3. Treatment: calcium chloride 2.5 mg/kg (should be given centrally) or calcium gluconate 7.5 mg/kg (may be given peripherally). Dosages may be repeated as necessary.

ACID-BASE CHANGES

Alkalosis caused by the conversion of citrate to bicarbonate in the liver may occur with massive transfusion.

PULMONARY INJURY

Embolization may occur as a result of microaggregates of non-viable cells or debris. Although microaggregate filters are available (20- to 40-μm pores), they have not been shown to be beneficial on a routine basis.[37] Noncardiogenic pulmonary edema may occur from an inflammatory reaction (probably caused by leukocyte antibodies) in the pulmonary microvasculature.[34,35]

INFECTIONS[36,38,39]

Hepatitis. The incidence of postranfusion hepatitis is 3% to 15%. The incidence increases as the number units of blood transfused increases. The frequency of transfusion-transmitted infection of hepatitis B is 1:50,000 per recipient or 1:200,000 per unit. Current estimates suggest the risk of hepatitis C may be 0.15 cases per 1000 units transfused.

Human immunodeficiency virus (HIV)[40]. HIV is known to be transmitted by transfusion of whole blood, red blood cells, platelets, and plasma. Overall risk of infection is 1:450,000 to 1:660,000 per unit. However, reported ranges for risk of infection vary widely.

Cytomegalovirus (CMV). The risk of CMV transmission is 2% to 12%. Morbidity is significant only in immunocompromised patients or preterm infants of CMV-negative mothers. The use of leukocyte-depleted blood lowers the incidence of CMV infection.

HYPOTHERMIA

1. Blood products have a temperature of 4° to 6°C. Massive transfusion without warming can easily result in hypothermia or even cardiac arrest.[41]
2. Energy must be expended by the infant or child to warm the infused blood. This process greatly increases oxygen consumption.
3. Warming blood to more than 45°C may result in hemolysis.

OXYHEMOGLOBIN DISSOCIATION

Shifting the oxyhemoglobin dissociation curve to the left decreases hemoglobin's capacity to release oxygen to tissue. The following factors are responsible for the leftward shift:

1. Hypothermia caused by unwarmed blood products
2. Alkalosis caused by conversion of citrate to bicarbonate in the liver
3. Decreased 2,3-DPG, which is minimally present in CPDA- or ADSOL-preserved cells.

Frozen red cells contain no citrate and normal amounts of 2,3-DPG and should cause a minimal shift in oxyhemoglobin dissociation.

References

1. Lattanzi WE, Siegel NJ: A practical guide to fluid and electrolyte therapy, *Curr Probl Pediatr* 16:1-43, 1986.
2. Lindahl SGE: Energy expenditure and fluid and electrolyte requirements in anesthestized infants and children, *Anesthesiology* 69:377-382, 1988.
3. Dabbagh S, Ellis D, Gruskin AB: Regulation of fluids and electrolytes in infants and children. In Motoyama EK, Davis PJ, eds: *Smith's anesthesia for infants and children,* ed 6, St Louis, 1996, Mosby.
4. Lanier WL, Stangland KJ, Scheithauer BW, Milde JH, Michenfelder JD: The effects of dextrose infusion and head position on neurologic outcome after complete cerebral ischemia in primates: examination of a model, *Anesthesiology* 66:39-48, 1987.
5. Payne K, Ireland P: Plasma glucose levels in the perioperative period in children. *Anaesthesia* 39:868-872, 1984.
6. Sieber FE, Smith DS, Traytsman RJ, Wollman H: Glucose: a reevaluation of its intraoperative use, *Anesthesiology* 67:72-81, 1987.

7. Welborn LG, McGill WA, Hannallah RS, Nisselson CL, Ruttimann UE, Hicks JM: Perioperative blood glucose concentrations in pediatric outpatients, *Anesthesiology* 65:543-547, 1986.

8. Bell C, Hughes CW, Oh TH, Donielson DW, O'Connor T: The effects of intravenous dextrose infusion on postbypass hyperglycemia in pediatric patients undergoing cardiac operations, *J Clin Anesth* 5:381-385, 1993.

9. Lipsky CL, Spear ML: Recent advances in parenteral nutrition, *Clin Perinatol* 22:141-155, 1995.

10. Pisciotto PT, ed: *Blood transfusion therapy: a physician's handbook,* ed 4, Arlington, Va, 1989, American Association of Blood Banks.

11. DePalma L, Luban NLC: Blood component therapy in the perinatal period: guidelines and recommendations, *Semin Perinatol* 14:403-415, 1990.

12. Coté CJ: Strategies for blood product management and blood salvage. In Coté CJ, Ryan JF, et al, eds: *A practice of anesthesia for infants and children,* ed 2, Philadelphia, 1993, WB Saunders.

13. Welch HG. Meehan KR, Goodnough LT: Prudent strategies for elective red blood cell transfusion, *Ann Intern Med* 116:393-402, 1992.

14. NIH Consensus Development Conference: Perioperative red cell transfusion, *JAMA* 7:2700-2703, 1988.

15. Adzick NS, deLorimier AA, Harrison MR, Glick PL, Fisher DM: Major childhood tumor resection using normovolemic hemodilution anesthesia and hetastarch, *J Pediatr Surg* 20:372-375, 1985.

16. Milligan NS, Edwards JC, Monro JL, Atwell JD. Excision of giant haemangioma in the newborn using hypothermia and cardiopulmonary bypass, *Anaesthesia* 40:875-878, 1985.

17. Levine EA, Rosen AL, Gould SA, et al: Recombinant human erythropoietin and autologous blood donation, *Surgery* 104:365-369, 1988.

18. Rothstein P, Roye D, Verdisco L, Stern L: Preoperative use of erythropoietin in an adolescent Jehovah's Witness, *Anesthesiology* 73:568-570, 1990.

19. Gallagher P, Ehrenkranz R: Erythropoietin therapy for anemia of prematurity, *Clin Perinatol* 20:169-191, 1993.

20. Guay J, Reinberg C, Poitras B, et al: A trial of desmopressin to reduce blood loss in patients undergoing spinal fusion for idiopathic scoliosis, *Anesth Analg* 75:405-410, 1992.

21. Davis R, Whittington R: Aprotinin: a review of its pharmacological and therapeutic efficacy in reducing blood loss associated with cardiac surgery, *Drugs* 49:954-983, 1995.

22. Royston D: Blood-sparing drugs: aprotinin, tranexamic acid, and epsilonaminocaproic acid, *Int Anesthesiol Clin* 33:155-179, 1995.

23. Layon AJ, D'Amico R, Caton D, Mollet CJ: And the patient chose: medical ethics and the case of the Jehovah's Witness, *Anesthesiology* 73:1258-1262, 1990.

24. NIH Consensus Development Conference: Fresh frozen plasma—indications and risks, JAMA 253:551-553, 1985.

25. Tullis JL: Albumin 2: guidelines for clinical use, *JAMA* 237:460-463, 1977.

26. Erstad BL, Gales BJ, Rappaport WD: The use of albumin in clinical practice, *Arch Intern Med* 151:901-911, 1991.

27. NIH consensus development conference: platelet transfusion therapy, *JAMA* 257:1777-1780, 1987.
28. Mannucci PM. Federici AB, Sirchia G: Hemostasis testing during massive blood replacement: a study of 172 cases, *Vox Sang* 42:113-123, 1982.
29. Kickler TS: The challenge of platelet alloimmunization: management and prevention, *Transfus Med Rev* 4:8-18, 1990.
30. Christensen RD et al: Granulocyte transfusions in neonates with bacterial infection, neutropenia, and depletion and mature marrow neutrophils, *Pediatrics* 70:1-6, 1982.
31. Dutcher JP: Granulocyte transfusion therapy, *Am J Med Sci* 287:11-17, 1984.
32. Menache D, Grossman BJ, Jackson CM: Antithrombin III: physiology, deficiency, and replacement therapy, *Transfusion* 32:580-588, 1992.
33. Wewars MD, Casolaro MA, Sellers SE, et al: Replacement therapy for $alpha_1$-antitrypsin deficiency associated with emphysema, *N Engl J Med* 316:1055-1062, 1987.
34. Popovsky MA, Moore SB: Diagnostic and pathogenic considerations in transfusion-related acute lung injury, *Transfusion* 5:573-577, 1985.
35. Lane TA, Anderson KC, Goodnough LT, et al: Leukocyte reduction in blood component therapy, *Ann Intern Med* 117:151-162, 1992.
36. Sloand EM, Pitt E, Klein HG: Safety of the blood supply, *JAMA* 274:1368-1373, 1995.
37. Snyder El, Hezzey A, Barash G, Palermo G: Microaggregate blood filtration in patients with compromised pulmonary function, *Transfusion* 22:21-25, 1982.
38. Dodd RY: The risk of transfusion-transmitted infection (editorial), *N Engl J Med* 327:419-421, 1992.
39. Badon SJ, Cable RG: Diseases transmissible by transfusion: changing risks and new surveillance recommendations, *Conn Med* 58:541-543, 1994.
40. Lackritz EM, Satten GA, Aberle-Grasse J, et al: Estimated risk of transmission of the human immunodeficiency virus by screened blood in the United States, *N Engl J Med* 26:1721-1725, 1995.
41. Boyan CP, Howland WS: Cardiac arrest and temperature of bank blood, *JAMA* 183:58-60, 1963.

EMERGENCE AND RECOVERY

5

Jeremy dreamt of rocket ships
Of satellites and stars,
And creatures with a thousand hands
Who traveled here from Mars.

They showed him lands of sparkling lights
And oceans made of clay,
The cloudlike homes and sunless worlds
Beyond the Milky Way

Jeremy dreamt but wasn't sure
About the dream he'd made up,
And wondered if he'd get back home
Or if he'd even wake up.

Rivian Bell

PRIMARY GOALS OF RECOVERY

The primary goal of the postanesthesia care unit (PACU) is to provide a safe environment (with presence of skilled nurses, appropriate monitoring, and resuscitative equipment), where patients can return to their preanesthetic homeostasis. The specific anatomic and physiologic differences in children as compared with adult patients often necessitate increased observation and vigilance during the recovery period.

In a recent 5-year study of pediatric PACU events,[1] the highest rate of adverse events (38%) was noted among neonates less than 1 month of age, with respiratory system problems having the most frequent occurrence. Also, the incidence of postoperative nausea and vomiting approached 33% in children over 1 year of age. These data represent a greater incidence of adverse postoperative events in children than adults.

Goals of recovery

Goals	Indicators
Primary goals	
Ventilation	Patent airway Clear breath sounds by auscultation Good chest excursion No stridor, retractions, or nasal flaring No wheezing Normal respiratory patterns without apnea or periodic breathing
Oxygenation	$SpO_2 > 90\%$ on room air
Consciousness	Response to verbal stimuli Return of reflexes: • Ability to maintain patent airway • Ability to cough • Presence of baroreceptor and chemoreceptor reflexes
Normothermia	Temperature of 36° to 37.5° C
Reversal of neuromuscular blockade	Return of muscle strength; assess by peripheral nerve stimulation or clinical indices: • Inspiratory force > –20 cm H_2O • Vital capacity > 15 ml/kg • Ability to protrude tongue and lift head for more than 5 seconds • Knee flexion in infants
Secondary goals	
Relief from pain	In preverbal children, absence of physiologic responses that may indicate presence of pain (i.e., tachycardia, hypertension, nausea, vomiting, agitation)
Relief from nausea and vomiting	In the absence of raised intracranial pressure, acute intraabdominal process or severe gastric distention, treatment should allow for oral consumption of fluids
Reduction of psychologic and physiologic stress	Normal hemodynamic parameters Calm, cooperative behavior

Ventilation

Upon the patient's arrival in the recovery room, attention should be focused on patency of the airway and adequacy of ventilation. The chest should always be auscultated by the nurse as well as the physician. If there is any doubt about the adequacy of ventilation, the airway should be supported. Cyanosis, poor chest excursion, grunting, retractions, nasal flaring, stridor, and wheezing should be noted and treated.

Oxygenation

Children recovering from general anesthesia are at greater risk for hypoxia than adults because of higher minute ventilation/ functional residual capacity (FRC) ratio, higher closing volumes, and greater oxygen consumption. The pulse oximeter is now the standard for monitoring oxygenation during recovery. In adults, significant cost savings have been achieved by administering supplemental oxygen only when the SpO_2 falls below 94%.[2] However, the continuous administration of oxygen during monitoring of SpO_2 has been advocated for children[3] because of the unreliability of pulse oximetry in wriggling infants and toddlers. It is equally important to administer oxygen and monitor SpO_2 in the transfer from operating room to PACU when infants and children are at increased risk for hypoxia.[4]

Awakening

The most important aspect of awakening is the return of cardiorespiratory reflexes: the ability to gag and cough to protect the airway, the return of baroreceptor reflexes to support perfusion, and the return of chemoreceptor responses to hypercapnia and hypoxia. The presence of a safe airway in children may be predicted by spontaneous eye opening in the immediate postanesthetic period.[5] The child also needs to achieve a level of consciousness sufficient to allow the assessment of level of comfort.

The practice of extubating the trachea during deep anesthesia or in the awake state is based on the patient's history, NPO status, difficulty in airway management, surgical procedure, and the anesthesiologist's preference and experience. Emergence through Stage II can be complicated by laryngospasm and vomiting.[6] Patel and colleagues reported no difference in hemoglobin desaturation among deeply anesthetized and awake children after tracheal extubation.[7] No increase in airway reactivity was noted in children anesthetized with isoflurane as compared to those anesthetized with halothane when extubation occurred during deep anesthesia.[8] When tracheal extubation was performed awake, patients receiving isoflurane had significantly more coughing, airway obstruction, and adverse respiratory events. Nevertheless, deeply anesthetized children should be closely observed until they have regained consciousness and control of airway reflexes. The skills and capabilities of the PACU personnel must be considered before a decision is made to have a deeply anesthetized child recover outside of the operating room. Personnel skilled in airway management need to be readily available.

Normothermia

Both hypothermia and hyperthermia are common intraoperative problems, particulary in infants. The inability to regulate body temperature under general anesthesia, cold operating rooms, and continued heat loss are major reasons for hypothermia.[9] Although minor hypothermia (34° to 36°C) has not been found to influence the recovery period (no impact upon time to awakening, incidence of apnea, or episodes of desaturation to < 90%),[10] it is best to restore normothermia prior to discharge from the PACU to avoid increased oxygen consumption, cardiovascular manifestations of hypothermia (increased heart rate and blood pressure),[11] and prolonged metabolism and excretion of anesthetic drugs. In comparing warmed cotton blankets to forced-air systems for rewarming, a study has found the forced-air systems more efficient in raising patients' temperatures to normothermic levels, decreasing the incidence of shivering, and decreasing the length of stay in the PACU.[12]

Similarly, hyperthermia may be seen as a result of dehydration, atropine administration, or overaggressive attempts to warm the child. On rare occasions malignant hyperthermia may be present (see Chapter 21). The etiology of the aberrancy in body temperature must be sought and corrected.

Reversal of Neuromuscular Blockade (NMB)

NMB in toddlers and school-age children can be assessed by the same clinical indices as in adults: full train-of-four and sustained tetany on NMB monitor, inspiratory force greater than −20 cm H_2O, and a vital capacity of at least 15 ml/kg. Brisk flexion of the hips and knees is an indication of return of adequate peripheral muscle strength in infants.[13] However, because of poorly developed musculature around the neck and glottic region, clinical judgment is required to assess the infant's motor ability to maintain airway patency.

Infants are at increased risk of upper airway obstruction when even minimal residual blockade exists, because of poorly developed airway musculature. As the infant attempts to breathe against the closed glottis, increased venous return to the right heart and pulmonary capillary leak can cause acute negative-pressure pulmonary edema. Recent evidence indicates that the acute hypoxia from airway obstruction (causing increased sympathetic tone and increased afterload) may be more responsible for the subsequent pulmonary edema than the negative intrathoracic pressure.[14]

If glottic weakness is noted after tracheal extubation, placing the infant in the lateral position or applying continuous positive airway pressure by face mask can help to prevent the development of pulmonary edema while motor strength is returning. If negative-pressure pulmonary edema develops, treatment includes reintubation and positive-pressure ventilation. Symptoms frequently resolve within 12 to 24 hours.

SECONDARY GOALS OF RECOVERY
Analgesia (see also Chapter 20)

Preverbal children cannot convey their perceptions of pain. However, prompt treatment of pain is urged, for both physiologic and psychologic well-being. Crying is not always an indicator of pain, but may represent other sources of discomfort such as anxiety, hunger, thirst, or nausea. Physiologic responses such as tachycardia, hypertension, nausea, vomiting, and agitation may be important indicators of analgesic needs in the preverbal child.

Intravenous opiates are used most commonly to treat moderate to severe pain. The intravenous route allows quicker onset and a more predictable and earlier peak effect than intramuscular injections, and facilitates titrating dose to response. Carefully titrated intravenous narcotics present few untoward effects.

Treatment of pain in the PACU

Mild to moderate

Ketorolac	0.75-1.0 mg/kg IV
Ibuprofen	10 mg/kg PO
Acetaminophen	10-15 mg/kg PO/PR

Moderate to severe (usually begin with $1/2$ dose and titrate to effect)

Morphine	0.1 mg/kg IV
Demerol	1.0 mg/kg IV
Fentanyl	1.0 µg/kg IV
Codeine	1.0 mg/kg PO

Control of Nausea and Vomiting

Nausea and vomiting occur frequently after eye or ear surgery but can occur after any procedure or anesthetic. Some recent studies quote an overall incidence of 20% to 30%,[15] while others have found that the problem is even more widespread (39% to 73%).[16] The physiologic mechanisms for postoperative nausea include central causes (opiates), gastrointestinal malfunction (ileus or gastric distention), the surgical procedure itself (eye and ear, most commonly), fear, anxiety, and postoperative pain. More serious causes, such as raised intracranial pressure (ICP), should be considered before any antiemetic is given.

Control of nausea and vomiting no longer remains purely within the domain of the PACU, but begins in the selection of agents/techniques used for anesthesia. For example, induction and maintenance of anesthesia with propofol-air-oxygen is associated with only a 23% incidence of nausea and vomiting, as compared to a 50% incidence using halothane-N_2O-droperidol for strabismus surgery.[17] Other studies have suggested that even a single dose of morphine can increase the incidence of nausea and vomiting.[18] Similarly, other authors advocate avoiding nitrous oxide to reduce postoperative emesis.[19]

Pretreatment with ondansetron 0.15 mg/kg,[20] droperidol 0.075 mg/kg,[21,22] or metoclopramide 0.15 mg/kg[23,24] has been very successful in reducing nausea and vomiting for patients at higher risk, such as those undergoing tonsillectomy, strabismus repair, or chemotherapy.

Ondansetron, a selective serotonin antagonist, is particularly effective in reducing postoperative nausea and vomiting when used prophylactically.[25,26] Although it is more expensive than other antiemetics, its significant efficacy makes it cost effective when used for procedures with a high incidence of nausea and vomiting (e.g., stabismus repair, tonsillectomy). Benzodiazepines are useful in patients with chemotherapy-induced nausea[27] (for adolescents or older children: lorazepam 1-2 mg IV or midazolam 1-2 mg IV or SL).

Treatment of postoperative nausea and vomiting	
Droperidol	10-20 µg/kg IV
Diphenhydramine	0.75-1.0 mg/kg IV
Promethazine	0.25-0.5 mg/kg IV
Metaclopramide	0.10-0.15 mg/kg IV
Ondansetron	0.05-0.10 mg/kg IV

Psychological Stress

Many children are terrified in the recovery room. They awaken in a strange place with unfamiliar people and may be disoriented from residual effects of the anesthesia. Some children may experience nightmares, develop enuresis, or have behavioral problems after a surgical procedure.[28] Delirium has been reported after sedation or induction with ketamine,[29] which may be more problematic when ketamine is used for short procedures. Measures taken to calm and comfort the child may reduce the incidence of these sequelae and aid in the overall recovery.

An agitated child will not return to physiologic baseline as quickly as a calm child. Increased catecholamines can result in poor perfusion and increased shunting. In the presence of intracardiac shunts, crying may increase pulmonary vascular resistance, causing right-to-left shunting and cyanosis. Comforting the child with warm blankets, rocking him, and having a familiar toy available can be reassuring. Many institutions have found that allowing parents to soothe the child during recovery is beneficial.

PACU SCORING SYSTEM AND CRITERIA FOR DISCHARGE

A variety of criteria for discharge from the PACU have been developed; however, discharge ultimately must be based on clinical judgment. Discharge criteria for outpatients tend to be more strict, as these patients do not have immediate access to skilled medical personnel, intravenous hydration, and analgesics.

In 1970, Aldrete developed a scoring system to help quantitate recovery from anesthesia.[30] He modified and updated this scoring system in 1995 to reflect current technological standards (pulse oximetry) and contemporary standards for ambulatory patients.[31] A score of 18 is considered the minimal requirement for discharge of outpatients.

Modified Postanesthetic Recovery (PAR) Score

For all patients

Activity	
Able to move four extremities voluntarily on command	2
Able to move two extremities voluntarily on command	1
Able to move no extremities voluntarily on command	0
Respiration	
Able to breathe deeply and cough freely	2
Dyspnea, limited breathing, or tachypnea	1
Apneic or on mechanical ventilator	0
Circulation	
Blood pressure ±20% of preanesthetic level	2
Blood pressure ±29% to 49% of preanesthetic level	1
Blood pressure ±50% of preanesthetic level	0
Consciousness	
Fully awake	2
Arousable on calling	1
Not responding	0
Oxygen saturation	
Able to maintain O_2 saturation >92% on room air	2
Needs O_2 inhalation to maintain O_2 saturation >90%	1
O_2 saturation <90% even with O_2 supplement	0

For ambulatory patients

Dressing	
Dry and clean	2
Wet but stationary or marked	1
Growing area of wetness	0
Pain	
Pain free	2
Mild pain handled by oral medication	1
Severe pain requiring parenteral medication	0
Ambulation	
Able to stand up and walk straight*	2
Vertigo when erect	1
Dizziness when supine	0
Fasting-feeding	
Able to drink fluids	2
Nauseated	1
Nausea and vomiting	0
Urine output	
Has voided	2
Unable to void but comfortable	1
Unable to void and uncomfortable	0

From Aldrete JA: The postanesthesia recovery score revisited, *J Clin Anesth* 7:89–91, 1995.
*Romberg's test, or picking up 12 clips in one hand, may be substituted.

PACU emergencies

Problem/predisposing factors	Diagnosis/therapy
Hypoxia Decreased FRC, with increased closing volume causing atelectasis and intrapulmonary shunt High metabolic requirements Increased right-to-left intracardiac shunting All factors leading to hypercapnia can also lead to hypoxia: airway obstruction, central hypoventilation, splinting from pain or tight dressings	• Pulse oximetry for early recognition of hypoxia • Oxygen therapy after general anesthesia • Correction of predisposing factors • Assisted ventilation with bag and mask • Reintubation if necessary
Hypercapnia Hypoventilation caused by: Residual anesthetic and narcotics Airway obstruction Incomplete reversal of neuromuscular blockade Atelectasis Splinting secondary to pain Tight dressings Malignant hyperthermia	• Suspect hypercapnia in the restless, agitated, or overly narcotized patient • Stimulate child • Analgesics when indicated • Reversal of neuromuscular blockade if indicated • Assist ventilation with bag and mask • Reintubation if necessary
Bradycardia Hypoxia Vagal response Drugs (fentanyl, neostigmine, edrophonium) Increased intracranial pressure (ICP)	• Assist ventilation and oxygenation • Atropine • Lower ICP with hyperventilation, pharmacotherapy
Laryngospasm During emergence: Secretions Stimulation Positive-pressure ventilation	• Continuous positive pressure with oxygen • Suction of secretions • Atropine (0.010-0.020 mg/kg) and succinylcholine (2 mg/kg IV or 4 mg/kg IM)
Bronchospasm Preexisting reactive airway disease (asthma) Allergy/anaphylaxis Histamine release Mucous plugging Aspiration Pulmonary edema/cardiogenic asthma Foreign body	• Oxygen • Inhaled bronchodilators: nebulized albuterol or metoproterenol 0.5 ml + 2.5 ml saline • Terbutaline (MDI or SC) • Epinephrine 0.010 mg/kg IV bolus (may repeat) • Antihistamine (diphenhydramine 1 mg/kg IV) • Dexamethasone • Suction of secretions; removal of foreign body • Support ventilation; reintubation

PACU emergencies—cont'd

Problem/predisposing factors	Diagnosis/therapy
Tachycardia Hypoxia and/or hypercapnia Hypovolemia Sepsis Hyperthermia Heart failure Pain Drugs (atropine/epinephrine) Psychologic stress	• Administer oxygen • Assist ventilation • Evaluate fluid and cardiac status • Use analgesics and/or sedatives • Lower temperature
Hypotension Cuff of inappropriate size (too large) Hypovolemia Cardiac failure	• Cuff of appropriate size ($^2/_3$ length of upper arm) • Fluid resuscitation (10 ml/kg isotonic crystalloid) • Inotropic agents or vasopressors
Hypertension Cuff of inappropriate size (too small) Pain, stress Hypercarbia Drugs (epinephrine, ketamine) Bladder distension	• Cuff of appropriate size • Assist ventilation • Analgesics and sedatives • Foley catheter • Vasodilator therapy
Subglottic edema (postintubation croup)[32] Age 1-4 yr Traumatic intubation Tight fit of endotracheal tube (air leak > 25 cm H_2O) Coughing with the endotracheal tube in place Change in position of patient while intubated Surgery of head and neck Duration of surgery >1 hr	• Humidified oxygen (cold steam) • Nebulized racemic epinephrine (0.05 ml/kg/dose diluted to 3 ml with saline), not more frequently than every 2 hr (maximum dose 0.5 ml) • Helium/oxygen mixture (70%/30%)[33] • Dexamethasone 0.1-0.2 mg/kg • Calm the child with judicious use of narcotics or parental presence • Consider overnight admission for outpatients; edema may rebound after racemic epinephrine • Reintubation if airway is severely compromised

Edematous upper airway, macroglossia[34]
Surgery around the airway
Prone position intraoperatively
Craniofacial abnormalities
Trauma from clamps/retractors in the mouth
Common procedures:
  Cleft palate repair
  Resection of cystic hygroma
  Tonsillectomy
  Adenoidectomy
  Tongue resection
	• Stimulate patient
	• Support airway by head tilt and jaw displacement
	• Nasal/oral airway
	• Early reintubation if severe compromise of airway
	• Emergency cricothyroidotomy if failed reintubation
	• Upper airway obstruction may rarely result in pulmonary edema (see next page)

Continued.

PACU emergencies—cont'd

Problem/predisposing factors	Diagnosis/therapy
Negative-pressure pulmonary edema[14] Upper airway obstruction Laryngospasm Incomplete reversal of neuro- muscular blockade Significant period of hypoxia	• Reintubation • Ventilator support • Oxygen therapy • Diuretics • Hemodynamic support as neces- sary if transient cardiomyopathy develops
Bleeding tonsil[35] Inadequate surgical hemostasis Severe coughing Bleeding diathesis Rarely occurs postoperatively; most common presentation is at 7 to 10 days with separation of eschar	• Blood available in OR • No premedication • Intravenous placement and hy- dration are desirable but not al- ways possible; treatment consists of swift surgical ligation • Rapid-sequence induction after intravenous catheter placement and hydration is ideal. However, when bleeding is life threatening, treatment consists of swift surgi- cal ligation. Awake intubation or inhalation induction (head-down, lateral position) may be life-sav- ing while an assistant obtains emergency intravenous access (cutdown or intraosseous). See also Appendix C, Fig. C-5, p. 661.

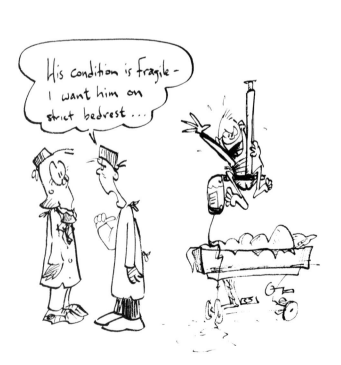

His condition is fragile—
I want him on
strict bedrest...

References

1. Cohen MM, Cameron CB, Duncan PG: Pediatric anesthesia morbidity and mortality in the perioperative period, *Anesth Analg* 70:160-167, 1990.

2. Motoyama EK, Glazener CH: Hypoxemia after general anesthesia in children, *Anesth Analg* 65:267-272, 1986.

3. DiBenedetto RJ, Graves SA, Gravenstein N, Konicek C: Pulse oximetry monitoring can change routine oxygen supplementation practices in the postanesthesia care unit, *Anesth Analg* 78:365-368, 1994.

4. Kataria BK, Harnik EV, Mitchard R, Kim Y, Admed S: Postoperative arterial oxygen saturation in the pediatric population during transportation, *Anesth Analg* 67:280-282, 1988.

5. Berde CB, Todres ID: Recovery from anesthesia and the postanesthesia care unit. In Coté CJ, Ryan JF, Todres ID, Goudsouzian NG, eds: *A practice of anesthesia for infants and children,* ed 2, Philadelphia, 1993, WB Saunders.

6. Miller KA, Harkin CP, Bailey PL: Postoperative tracheal extubation, *Anesth Analg* 80:149-172, 1995.

7. Patel RI, Hannallah RS, Norden J, Casey WF, Verghese ST: Emergence airway complications in children: a comparison of tracheal extubation in awake and deeply anesthetized patients, *Anesth Analg* 73:266-270, 1991.

8. Pounder DR, Blackstock D, Steward DJ: Tracheal extubation in children: halothane versus isoflurane, anesthetized versus awake, *Anesthesiology* 74:653-655, 1991.

9. Imrie MM, Hall GM: Body temperature and anesthesia, *Br J Anaesth* 64:346-354, 1990.

10. Bissonnette B, Sessler DI: Mild hypothermia does not impair postanesthetic recovery in infants and children, *Anesth Analg* 76:168-172, 1993.

11. Frank SM, Higgins MS, Breslow MJ, et al: The catecholamine, cortisol, and hemodynamic responses to mild perioperative hypothermia: a randomized clinical trial, *Anesthesiology* 82:83-93, 1995.

12. Lennon RL, Hosking MP, Conover MA, Perkins WJ: Evaluation of a forced-air system for warming hypothermic postoperative patients, *Anesth Analg* 70:424-427, 1990.

13. Mason LJ, Betts EK: Leg lift and maximum inspiratory force: clinical signs of neuromuscular blockade reversal in neonates and infants, *Anesthesiology* 52:441-442, 1980.

14. Ruffle J, Gleason M, Domino KB, Gersony WM, Zucker HA: Pulmonary edema and transient cardiomyopathy in a previously healthy adolescent after general anesthesia, *J Cardiothorac Vasc Anesth* 8:463-470, 1994.

15. Watcha MF, Simeon RM, White PF, Stevens JL: Effect of propofol on the incidence of postoperative vomiting after strabismus surgery in pediatric outpatients, *Anesthesiology* 75:204-209, 1991.

16. Cohen MM, Duncan PG, DeBoer DP, Tweed WA: The postoperative interview: assessing risk factors for nausea and vomiting, *Anesth Analg* 78:7-16, 1994.

17. Watcha MF, Bras PJ, Cieslak GD, Pennant JH: The dose-response relationship of ondansetron in preventing postoperative emesis in pediatric patients undergoing ambulatory surgery, *Anesthesiology* 82:47-52, 1995.

18. Weinstein MS, Nicholson SC, Schreiner MS: A single dose of morphine sulfate increases the incidence of vomiting after outpatient inguinal surgery in children, *Anesthesiology* 81: 572-577, 1994.

19. Wetchler BV: Control of nausea and vomiting in the postanesthesia care unit, *Anesthesiology Rev* 8:19-22, 1991.

20. Litman RS, Wu CL, Catanzaro FA: Ondansetron decreases emesis after tonsillectomy in children, *Anesth Analg* 78:478-481, 1994.

21. Lerman J, Eustis S, Smith DR: Effect of droperidol pretreatment on postanesthetic vomiting in children undergoing strabismus surgery, *Anesthesiology* 65:322-325, 1986.

22. Abramowitz MD, Oh TH, Epstein BS, Ruttiman UE, Friendly DS: The antiemetic effect of droperidol following outpatient strabismus surgery in children, *Anesthesiology* 59:579-583, 1983.

23. Ferrari LR, Donlon JV: Metoclopramide reduces the incidence of vomiting after tonsillectomy in children, *Anesth Analg* 75:351-354, 1992.

24. Broadman LM, Ceruzzi W, Patane PS, Hannallah RS, Ruttimann U, Friendly D: Metoclopramide reduces the incidence of vomiting following strabismus surgery in children, *Anesthesiology* 72:245-248, 1990.

25. Ummenhofer W, Frei FJ, Urwyler A, Kern C, Drewe J: Effects of ondansetron in the prevention of postoperative nausea and vomiting in children, *Anesthesiology* 81:804-810, 1994.

26. Furst SR, Rodarte A: Prophylactic antiemetic treatment with ondansetron in children undergoing tonsillectomy, *Anesthesiology* 81:799-803, 1994.

27. Grunberg SM, Hesketh PJ: Control of chemotherapy-induced emesis, *N Engl J Med* 329:1790-1796, 1993.

28. Kain ZN, Mayes L, Nygen MA, Rimar S: Behavioral disturbances in children following surgery, 81:A1382, 1994.

29. Donahue PJ, Dineed PS: Emergence delirium following oral ketamine, *Anesthesiology* 77:604-605, 1992.

30. Aldrete JA, Kroulik D: A postanesthetic recovery score, *Anesth Analg* 49:924-934, 1970.

31. Aldrete JA: The postanesthesia recovery score revisited, *J Clin Anesth* 7:89-91, 1995.

32. Koka BV, Jean IS, Andre JM, MacKay I, Smith RM: Postintubation croup in children, *Anesth Analg* 56:501-505, 1977.

33. Kemper KJ, Ritz RH, Benson MS, Bishop MS: Helium-oxygen mixture in the treatment of postextubation stridor in pediatric trauma patients, *Crit Care Med* 19:356-359, 1991.

34. Bell C, Oh TH, Loeffler JR: Massive macroglossia and airway obstruction after cleft palate repair, *Anesth Analg* 67:71-74, 1988.

35. Motoyama EK: Anesthesia for ear, nose, and throat surgery. In Motoyama EK, Davis PF, eds: *Smith's anesthesia for infants and children,* St. Louis, 1990, Mosby, pp 649-674.

II

CLINICAL MANAGEMENT

RESPIRATORY PHYSIOLOGY AND DISEASE PROCESSES

6

shake, rattle and roll
breath . . .
in and out real slow
hold it now, then let go
shake, rattle and roll

Adrienne Coleman

ANATOMY AND PHYSIOLOGY[1]

Anatomy of the Upper Airway: Differences Between Children and Adults

See also Chapters 3 and 8.

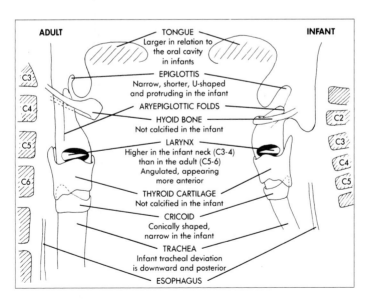

FIG. 6-1. Anatomic differences between the infant airway and the adult airway. (Adapted from Coté CJ, Todres ID: The pediatric airway. In Ryan JF et al, eds: *A practice of anesthesia for infants and children,* Orlando, 1986, Grune & Stratton.)

Tongue.   The infant tongue is large in relation to the oral cavity, predisposing to airway obstruction.

Larynx.   The infant larynx is higher in the neck (C3 to C4) than in the adult (C5 to C6).

1. This high position allows swallowing to occur simultaneously with nasal breathing but also places the tongue against the soft palate during quiet respirations, causing oral airway obstruction.
2. Infants are obligate nasal breathers until the age of 3 to 5 months.
3. The acute angulation of the infant larynx at the base of the tongue makes intubation difficult by creating the impression of an anterior larynx. The larynx is not anatomically more anterior but is anterior to the line of view of the laryngoscope.
4. External laryngeal pressure during intubation helps push the larynx into view. A straight laryngoscope blade also makes it easier to lift the base of the tongue and epiglottis to visualize the larynx.

Epiglottis.   The infant epiglottis is narrow, short, and U-shaped and protrudes posteriorly over the larynx at a 45-degree angle.

Vocal cords.   The anterior attachment of the vocal cords is more caudal in infants. This slant in the vocal cords predisposes toward catching the tip of the endotracheal tube in the anterior commissure during intubation. Turning the endotracheal tube 90 degrees during intubation improves the angle of entry into the trachea.

Cricoid cartilage.   The narrowest part of the upper airway in the infant is at the conically shaped cricoid cartilage.

1. Rather than an endotracheal tube (ETT) size being selected to fit between the cords, the pediatric ETT must fit through the cricoid cartilage.
2. This narrowing assumes special importance because the resistance to laminar air flow is proportional to the fourth power of the radius. For example, 1 mm of circumferential edema in a 4-mm infant airway will reduce cross-sectional area by 75% and increase the resistance 16 times. The same amount of edema in an 8-mm adult airway will decrease the cross-sectional area by 44% and increase the resistance 3 times.
3. The cricoid narrowing and angulation of the cords generally disappear by 10 to 12 years of age.

Tonsils.   The tonsils and adenoids are small in a neonate but grow during childhood to achieve their maximal size by 4 to 7 years of age, after which they gradually recede.

Large occiput.   The relatively large size of the infant head and the short cords-to-carina distance (4 to 5 cm) can cause the tip of the endotracheal tube to move down the trachea with head flexion and up with head extension by as much as 2 cm. A small rolled towel beneath the neck when the infant is lying supine will prevent neck flexion caused by the large occiput.

Angulation of trachea.   In the infant, tracheal deviation is downward and posterior. In the adult, it is straight downward. Cricoid pressure is thus more effective in aiding endotracheal intubation in infants.

Respiratory Physiology: Basic Pulmonary Mechanics
MECHANICS OF BREATHING

Quiet tidal breathing occurs when there is active inspiratory contraction of the diaphragm and intercostal muscles, followed by relaxation and passive expiration resulting from elastic recoil of the lungs and chest wall. Contraction of the accessory muscles of respiration (strap muscles of the neck, sternocleidomastoid, anterior serratus, and external intercostals) augments forced inspiration. This effect, however, is diminished in the neonate, who has a "floppy," highly compliant chest wall and poorly developed musculature. Consequently, attempts at forceful inspiration in neonates appear as chest and sternal retractions with tracheal "tugging." Forceful expiration is equally difficult for neonates because of their poorly developed abdominal and internal intercostal musculature. These features illustrate why the only significant means for enhancing alveolar minute ventilation in neonates is by increasing respiratory frequency. The cost of enhanced minute ventilation includes increased work of breathing, increased oxygen consumption, increased dead space ventilation, ventilation/perfusion ($\dot{V}/\dot{Q}$) mismatching, and susceptibility to fatigue and respiratory failure.

At about 6 months of age, the chest wall begins to stiffen, the elastic recoil of the lungs increases, overall compliance decreases, and the ventilatory musculature develops. These developments allow for increased tidal volume (V_T), decreased respiratory frequency, and improved performance of forced inspiratory and expiratory maneuvers (e.g., sigh and cough).

Pulmonary function: normal values [2]

Components of pulmonary function	Neonate 0-3 days	Infant 1 year	Child to adult
Resting oxygen consumption ($\dot{V}O_2$)(ml/kg/min)	5-8	5	3-4
Minute ventilation (V_E)(ml/kg/min)	200-260	175-185	80-100
Respiratory frequency (rpm)	30-50	20-30	12-16
Tidal volume (V_T)(ml/kg)	6-8	6-8	7-8
Dead space (V_D)(ml/kg)	2-2.5	2-2.2	2-2.2
V_D/V_T ratio	0.3	0.3	0.3
Vital capacity (VC) (ml/kg)	35-40	45-50	50-60
Functional residual capacity (FRC) (ml/kg)	22-25	25-30	30-45
Lung compliance (C_L)(ml/cm H_2O)	5-6	15-20	130-150
Airway resistance (R_{aw})(cm H_2O/L/sec)	25-30	10-15	1.5-2
Peak flow rate (L/min)	10		350-450

LUNG VOLUMES AND CAPACITIES

1. *Functional residual capacity* (FRC) as it relates to overall respiratory reserve is critical to the anesthetic management of the pediatric patient. FRC is the volume of gas in the lung at the end of tidal expiration, when there is zero gas flow and alveolar pressure equals ambient pressure. Preserving or restoring FRC is a major goal of clinical interventions such as chest physiotherapy, diuretic and bronchodilator therapy, PEEP/CPAP, and positive-pressure mechanical ventilation, as well as adequate postoperative analgesia and early ambulation following major thoracic or abdominal surgery.

2. FRC *decreases* under the following conditions:
   - General anesthesia with either spontaneous or controlled ventilation; increasing depth of anesthesia changes compliance as the outward recoil of the thorax decreases with muscle relaxation:

   $$\downarrow \text{Compliance} \rightarrow \text{Airway closure} \rightarrow \downarrow \text{FRC}$$

   - Neuromuscular blockade, from loss of residual end-expiratory muscle tone
   - Pulmonary edema
   - Pulmonary fibrosis
   - Neonatal respiratory distress
   - Kyphoscoliosis
   - Restrictive lung disease
   - Obesity
   - Pregnancy
   - Lateral decubitus or Trendelenburg position
   - The first 24 hours of the newborn period

3. FRC *increases* with the following:
   - Increasing height (a linear relationship)
   - Male sex
   - Erect body position (versus supine)
   - Positive end-expiratory pressure (PEEP) or continuous positive airway pressure (CPAP)
   - Chronic obstructive pulmonary disease (COPD), because of decreased elastic recoil of the lungs (this has a salutary effect because at higher lung volumes airway resistance decreases and gas flow increases)
4. The adverse consequences of diminished FRC include:
   - Small airway closure
   - Uneven distribution of ventilation
   - $\dot{V}/\dot{Q}$ mismatching
   - Hypoxemia
5. The *dynamic* FRC in spontaneously breathing infants is maintained at about 40% of total lung capacity (as in the supine adult) by three mechanisms:
   - Premature cessation of the expiratory phase by glottic closure; also referred to as "laryngeal braking"
   - Forced expiration against a partially closed glottis; also referred to as "grunting" or "auto-PEEP"
   - Maintenance of continuous, tonic inspiratory muscle tone in the diaphragm and intercostals, thereby stiffening the chest wall to oppose the elastic recoil of the lungs, which improves compliance and diminishes airway closure

AIRWAY CLOSURE

Airway collapse may be either *volume related* or *flow related*. Except at total lung capacity, airways and alveoli are smaller in dependent lung regions than in the top regions. The *closing capacity* (CC) is the lung volume above the residual volume at which airways in dependent lung zones begin to close. In most patients, closing capacity is less than FRC. Closing capacity approaches FRC with aging, in the supine position, and under general anesthesia. When tidal breathing occurs within the closing capacity range of lung volume, then pulmonary blood flow is directed to areas of low ventilation, leading to increased shunt and hypoxemia.

In infants, closing capacity approaches tidal breathing, especially during spontaneous ventilation under general anesthesia. The application of CPAP during spontaneous ventilation with a face mask will help to maintain patency of the upper and lower airways (alveoli).

The Effects of Anesthesia on Pulmonary Physiology

In the normal infant or child, general anesthetics depress respiration by the mechanisms listed below.

Effects of anesthesia and surgery on respiration[3]

Respiratory variable	Effects of anesthesia
↓ VC	A restrictive pattern with diminished lung volumes VC is reduced as little as 25% with lower abdominal procedures and up to 70% with thoracic.
↓ FRC	25% decrease with general anesthesia, supine position Persists up to 5 to 7 days postoperatively
↓ V_T	Decreases 20% with inhalation anesthesia
↑ V_D/V_T ratio	0.3 awake 0.5 anesthetized with an ETT 0.7 anesthetized with a mask
↑ RR	Increases 25% with inhalation anesthesia Hyperventilation postoperatively reflects a compensatory response for the decreased FRC. May also be associated with pain
↑ $\dot{V}/\dot{Q}$ mismatching	Secondary to alveolar hypoventilation and increased closing capacity Absent "sigh" Increased airway resistance leads to loss of lung volume.
Pulmonary toilet	A decrease in cough, mucociliary transport, and "sigh" occurs because of pain, splinting, inhalation anesthetics, narcotics, mechanical ventilation, and immobilization.
Inspiratory muscle tone	Impaired diaphragmatic function is thought to be centrally mediated by increased descending inhibitory input. Decreased genioglossus and pharyngeal/laryngeal abductor motor tone contributes to upper airway obstruction. The genioglossus is most sensitive as depth of anesthesia increases, followed by the intercostal muscles, and finally by the diaphragm.
Respiratory depression and CO_2/O_2 ventilation response curves	All inhalation anesthetics produce respiratory depression in a dose-related fashion, mostly by decreasing tidal volume. Minute ventilation is preserved by increasing respiratory rate. All inhalation anesthetics depress hypoxic ventilatory drive, even at low concentrations. All inhalation anesthetics depress the ventilatory response to CO_2 in a dose-dependent manner. At 1 MAC, in spontaneously breathing patients, Pa_{CO_2} is highest with enflurane, followed in descending order by isoflurane, halothane, and nitrous oxide. Respiratory depression is potentiated by systemic narcotics and sedative/hypnotic drugs.

The neonate is particulary susceptible to respiratory depression because of increased O_2 requirements (higher metabolic rate). Although the FRC approaches adult levels within days, the persistently high closing capacity increases the likelihood of alveolar collapse and intrapulmonary shunt.

Neonatal respiratory characteristics that increase anesthetic risk

- Decreased FRC until about 24 hours old; after which FRC approaches normal infant/adult levels.
- Closing volume and closing capacity encroach upon FRC and tidal breathing.
- Chest wall compliance is high, secondary to poorly developed musculature and nonossified ribs. Lung compliance is low, contributing to increased work of breathing to maintain lung volume and airway caliber.
- $\dot{V}O_2$ is twice that of the adult and increases with hypothermia.
- Increased CO_2 production is a result of a high metabolic rate.
- Increased respiratory rate is required to maintain alveolar minute ventilation, which increases susceptibility to fatigue.
- Work of breathing increases because of high-resistance, small-caliber airways.
- Reduced Type I sustained-twitch muscle fibers in the diaphragm increases susceptibility to fatigue.
- Immature central nervous system predisposes to periodic breathing and apnea.
- Residual left-to-right shunt (through the patent ductus) worsens intrapulmonary shunt.

The oxyhemoglobin dissociation curve for neonates is shifted to the left. This shift represents the increased affinity for oxygen of fetal hemoglobin (HbF), indicated by a P_{50} of 19 mm Hg as compared to a P_{50} of 27 for adult hemoglobin ($P_{50} = PaO_2$ of whole blood at 50% saturation). A relatively low concentration of 2,3-DPG in fetal hemoglobin is responsible for the increased oxygen affinity. In contrast, children between the ages of 3 months and 10 years have a P_{50} of approximately 30, which is probably related to accelerated growth and development. As a result of the leftward shift of the curve, neonates require a higher hemoglobin level to maintain adequate O_2 delivery to the tissue. Alkalosis, hypocapnia, and hypothermia will also cause a leftward shift of the curve. See Fig. 6-2.

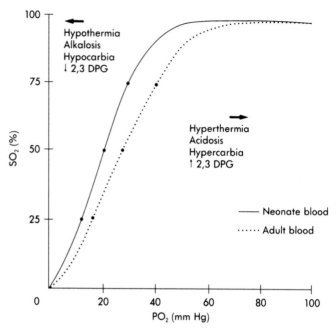

FIG. 6-2. Oxyhemoglobin curve. The oxyhemoglobin dissociation curve for fetal hemoglobin is shifted leftward ($P_{50} = 19$ mm Hg) compared to adult hemoglobin ($P_{50} = 27$ mm Hg), indicating an increased affinity of hemoglobin for oxygen. Alkalosis, hypocarbia, and hypothermia will also result in a leftward shift. Conversely, acidosis, hypercarbia, and hyperthermia shift the curve to the right, increasing the unloading of oxygen at the tissue level.

ANESTHETIC IMPLICATIONS OF PULMONARY DISEASES IN CHILDREN

Upper Respiratory Infections

One of the more confusing and common issues presented to the anesthesiologist is the child with symptoms consistent with an upper respiratory infection (URI), especially since the average child will have multiple respiratory infections per year.

It is important to distinguish between an upper respiratory illness and an allergic response. Many children have seasonal allergies, and a thorough history must be obtained from the parents to determine whether the child's rhinorrhea, cough, and infected mucosa are a chronic problem or represent an acute change. For a more detailed discussion regarding anesthetic implications of upper respiratory infections, please refer to p. 7.

Asthma[4-8]

Asthma is a common disease in the pediatric population, with increasing prevalence.[9] Fifty percent of children with asthma have symptoms by 3 years of age and 80% by 5 years of age.[10] Asthmatic patients are reportedly at increased risk for operative and postoperative complications. [11-13]

PATHOPHYSIOLOGY

Many factors contribute to increased airway reactivity and inflammation causing acute bronchospasm and airway obstruction. [14]

Asthma: triggering factors

Respiratory infections (especially viral)
Aeroallergens (dust, animal danders, etc.)
Air pollutants (including cigarette smoke)
Temperature changes
Exercise
Emotion and anxiety

Recent data have indicated that chronic airway inflammation is seen in asthmatic patients, and greater focus is now being given to the role of the inflammatory process rather than the acute bronchospastic aspect of the disease. [14]

Pathological features of asthma[10]	Clinical signs of asthma[15]
Airway inflammation	Dyspnea
Plasma exudation	Wheezing
Edema	Cough
Smooth muscle hypertrophy	Chest tightness
Mucous plugging	
Shedding of epithelium	

PHARMACOTHERAPY

Based on the history and physical examination, asthmatic patients will usually fall into one of three groups.

Group 1   Patients who have a history of asthma but have been asymptomatic and are on no routine medications currently

Group 2   Patients who have recurrent attacks of asthma and are on prophylactic medications but are not actively symptomatic

Group 3   Patients who are symptomatic or who have deteriorated from their normal condition

1. β-*adrenergic agents* are widely used in the treatment of asthma to provide rapid relief of acute bronchospasm. This class of medication leads to smooth muscle relaxation and increased mucociliary clearance by activating adenylate cyclase to increase cAMP levels. β-adrenergic agents may be administered

by metered dose inhalers (MDI), nebulizer, or oral or intravenous routes. Inhalation administration provides faster peak bronchodilation and fewer systemic side effects than other routes of drug delivery.[16]

2. *Cromolyn sodium* is used prophylactically to reduce the incidence of asthmatic attacks. Although the precise mechanism of action is unknown, it is believed to inhibit release of mediators from mast cells. It is usually administered by MDI or nebulizer and causes few adverse effects.

3. *Corticosteroids* are now initiated much earlier in the treatment of asthma, because of their potent antiinflammatory properties. Inhaled corticosteroids are efficacious and have reduced systemic side effects at low doses. Oral steroids are used during acute episodes of asthma resistant to inhaled agents, and intravenous corticosteroids may be given in cases of severe asthma.

4. *Anticholinergics* produce bronchodilation by inhibiting mucus hypersecretion and cholinergic activation of airway smooth muscle. Ipratropium bromide may be administered by MDI.

5. *Methylxanthines.* Theophylline and related drugs offer a narrow therapeutic margin and the potential for serious toxicity.[17] The side effects of methylxanthines include nausea, vomiting, headache, seizures, cardiac arrhythmias, and behavioral disturbances. Since the risks of toxicity and side effects outnumber the benefits, these drugs are rarely used in the acute management of bronchospasm.

Treatment of asthma

Severity of asthma	Symptoms	Treatment
Mild	Infrequent, brief Good exercise tolerance Asymptomatic between exacerbations Infrequent nocturnal symptoms	Inhaled β-agonist Oral β-agonist for infants and young children
Moderate	Symptoms > 2 per week Diminished exercise tolerance Emergency room visits Exacerbations last several days Symptoms at night 2 or 3 times/week	Cromolyn sodium and inhaled corticosteroids for prophylaxis β-agonists as needed for acute episodes
Severe	Continuous symptoms Limited activity Frequent exacerbations Nocturnal symptoms every night Hospitalization	Oral corticosteroids plus inhaled corticosteroids and β-agonist as needed

ANESTHETIC MANAGEMENT OF ASTHMATIC PATIENTS

Preoperative evaluation.   Usually patients in groups 1 and 2 (mild to moderate symptoms) do not require further workup prior to anesthesia. Patients in group 3 who are actively symptomatic should have any elective surgery postponed and their conditions optimized prior to elective surgery. Further workup may entail blood count with differential, chest radiograph, blood gases, electrocardiogram, and pulmonary function testing. Patient medications (dose, type, and frequency) should be reviewed and optimized in consultation with the primary physician.

1. A *complete history* should focus on the following points:
    - Age of onset
    - Nature and severity of symptoms
    - Triggering events
    - Management of acute episodes
    - Allergies
    - Interference with sleep
    - Cough, sputum, change in sputum color
    - Previous anesthetic history
    - Hospital visits (clinic, emergency department, ward, intensive care)
    - Aggressive therapy (intubation, intravenous infusions)
    - Medication regimen
    - Activity level
2. *Physical examination* should include documentation of:
    - Vital signs
    - Use of accessory muscles
    - Wheezing
    - Cough
    - Nature and symmetry of breath sounds
    - Cyanosis
    - Altered mental status
    - Hydration

Preoperative pharmacotherapy

Premedications.   The advantages or disadvantages of premedication for asthmatic patients have not been confirmed in controlled investigations. Opioids should be used cautiously, since they may lead to respiratory depression.[13,18] Conversely, anxiety may precipitate acute bronchospasm.

Preoperative bronchodilators.   Prophylactic inhaled β-agonists prior to anesthetic induction may improve air flow and decrease the risk of bronchospasm.

Stress-dose steroid coverage.   Patients who have received steroid therapy within 6 months may be at risk for adrenal suppression and should receive stress-dose steroid coverage.

Anesthetic technique. Regional anesthesia avoids airway manipulation but may not be feasible in pediatric patients or appropriate for the site of surgery. With general anesthesia, endotracheal intubation is the most important risk factor for bronchospasm.[12] Avoiding intubation by using a face mask or laryngeal mask airway may be useful. Ensuring a deep plane of anesthesia prior to intubation, by either intravenous or inhalation induction, helps to decrease risk of bronchospasm.

Effects of induction agents on the asthmatic patient

Technique or drug	Advantages	Disadvantages
Intravenous		
Thiopental	Rapid onset; blunts airway reflexes	Histamine release may precipitate bronchospasm
Ketamine	Bronchodilation	Increased secretions and airway irritability
Inhalation		
Halothane	Bronchodilation	May precipitate dysrhythmias when used with adrenergic agents or methylxanthines
Enflurane	Bronchodilation	Respiratory depression; elevated $PaCO_2$ with spontaneous ventilation
Isoflurane	Bronchodilation	Increased incidence of breath-holding and laryngospasm

Intraoperative management
1. Intraoperatively, all gases should be humidified to prevent inspissation of dried secretions.
2. Suction of the trachea should be performed only while the patient is deeply anesthetized.
3. Mechanical ventilation should be instituted with low inflating pressures and a prolonged expiratory time.
4. Deep extubation of the trachea avoids the risk of bronchospasm from coughing on the endotracheal tube during emergence but adds the risk of aspiration.

Postoperative course
1. Humidified oxygen should be delivered during recovery.
2. Bronchodilator therapy is instituted if needed.

3. Aggressive pain management increases the likelihood of adequate pulmonary toilet.

Anesthesia for the symptomatic asthmatic child

1. Preoperative therapy with inhaled and intravenous bronchodilators and steroids should be continued intraoperatively.
2. Preoperative laboratory studies include CBC, CXR, bedside pulmonary function tests, arterial blood gas determinations, and theophylline levels.
3. Premedication is usually avoided to prevent further respiratory depression.
4. Regional anesthesia, if appropriate for patient age and level of cooperation, will avoid intubation. However, loss of accessory muscles of respiration can diminish vital capacity.
5. Atropine may help to dry secretions and prevent reflex bradycardia but may also cause inspissated mucus that will exacerbate wheezing.
6. Intravenous lidocaine or fentanyl preintubation helps to decrease airway reactivity.
7. Agents that release histamine are avoided if possible (e.g., thiopental, propofol, succinylcholine, d-tubocurarine, morphine, atracurium).
8. Intraoperative management includes inhalation agents for bronchodilatory effect, humidified gases, aggressive hydration, and mechanical ventilation with long expiratory times and low inflation pressures.
9. Deep extubation is usually not useful in emergency situations because of aspiration risks. Intravenous lidocaine may attenuate airway reactivity on emergence. Severely symptomatic patients may require prolonged intubation and intensive care admission.

Pharmacologic therapy for acute intraoperative bronchospasm

The following treatments should be initiated after eliminating other causes of intraoperative wheezing or airway obstruction:

1. Deepen anesthesia with inhalational agents or opioids.
2. β-agonist bronchodilators (albuterol, metaproterenol) using metered dose inhalers through the endotracheal tube.
3. Adrenergic agents:
   a. Epinephrine 0.1-1.0 μg/kg IV bolus, may repeat
   b. Epinephrine infusion 0.01 - 0.1 μg /kg/min
   c. Isoproterenol infusion 0.01 - 0.1 μg /kg/min
4. Methylxanthines: aminophylline 5-7 mg/kg IV load over 30 min; infusion: 0.6 - 1 mg /kg/hr (therapeutic level: 10-20 μg/ml)
5. Corticosteroids:
   a. Hydrocortisone 5 mg/kg IV q6h
   b. Methylprednisolone 1 mg/kg IV load, then 0.8 mg/kg q4-6h

Cystic Fibrosis

Cystic fibrosis (CF) is most common in Caucasians, with an incidence of approximately 1:2500.[19] The management of CF patients has greatly improved over the years, leading to longer life expectancy; 50% of patients live to be older than 27 years.[20] Many cystic fibrosis patients require surgical procedures related to complications of their disease.

PATHOPHYSIOLOGY[19,21]

CF is a disease of the exocrine glands involving the respiratory, digestive, and reproductive systems and sweat glands. It is inherited as an autosomal recessive gene located on chromosome 7. Mutations in this gene lead to defects in the chloride resorptive mechanism, resulting in increased loss of chloride and sodium. Patients with CF produce abnormal secretions, by alterations in electrolyte content, water deficit, and abnormal mucus glycoprotein. Exocrine gland duct obstruction often occurs.

CLINICAL MANIFESTATIONS[21,22]

The pulmonary system is typically affected in CF patients, and over 90% of the mortality and most of the morbidity are related to involvement of this system. The combination of viscous secretions and abnormal mucociliary clearance seen in CF patients leads to airway obstruction, which in turn leads to chronic pulmonary infections (*Pseudomonas aeruginosa* and *Staphylococcus aureus*) and ultimately tissue destruction. Chronic hypoxemia from advanced pulmonary disease can lead to cor pulmonale.

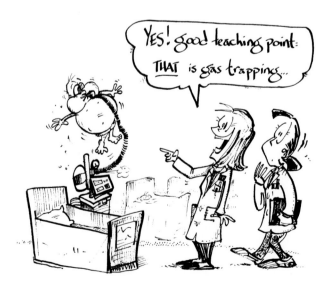

The gastrointestinal manifestations of CF may also have some important anesthetic considerations. CF patients may have intestinal malabsorption, which leads to deficiencies of fat-soluble vitamins. Vitamin K deficiency can lead to reduced levels of clotting factors II, VII, IX, and X. Pancreatic insufficiency may also contribute to the malabsorption. Patients with CF are also at increased risk for diabetes mellitus.

Clinical manifestations and complications of cystic fibrosis[23]

Respiratory tract	
Upper airway	Increased mucoid secretions
	Chronic polypoid sinusitis
Lungs	Cough, wheezing
	Atelectasis
	Bronchitis
	Bronchiectasis
	Recurrent pneumonia/lung abscesses
	Hemoptysis
	Pneumothorax, pneumomediastinum
	Abnormal pulmonary function: increased airway resistance; gas trapping; increased FRC, decreased FEV_1, decreased VC, decreased PaO_2, increased $PaCO_2$, $\dot{V}/\dot{Q}$ mismatch, hypoxemia
Cardiac	Right ventricular hypertrophy
	Cor pulmonale
Gastrointestinal tract	
Pancreas	Pancreatic insufficiency
	Hyperglycemia
	Recurrent acute pancreatitis
Biliary tract	Cholelithiasis, obstructive jaundice
	Focal biliary cirrhosis
	Portal hypertension
Bowel	Malabsorption—deficiency of vitamins A, D, E, K
	Intestinal intussusception
	Fecal impaction
	Rectal prolapse
	Meconium ileus
	Steatorrhea
	Esophageal varices

OPERATIVE MANAGEMENT

Preoperative considerations. Vigorous chest physiotherapy can maximize pulmonary function in the immediate preoperative period. A complete history and physical examination should detail the following:

1. Any acute pulmonary changes
2. Nutritional status
3. Clotting abnormality
4. Adequacy of control of blood glucose levels
5. Cardiac function

Maintenance therapy for cystic fibrosis patients
Chest physical therapy
Antibiotics
Oral
Inhalational
Intravenous
Bronchodilators
Aerosolized
Oral
Antiinflammatory agents [24]
Corticosteroids[25]
Ibuprofen
Pancreatic enzyme replacement
Vitamin and mineral replacement
Vitamins A, D, E, and K

Premedication

1. Narcotic premedication or anxiolysis should be used with caution because of the risks of respiratory depression.
2. All current medications are continued (for pancreatic insufficiency, antifibrosis, bronchodilation, etc.).
3. Vitamin K should be considered if clotting abnormalities exist (48 to 72 hours are needed for effective treatment).

Laboratory data.   Recent pulmonary function tests, electrolytes, chest roentgenograms, arterial blood gas values, and echocardiograms (right heart function) should be reviewed.

Anesthetic technique

1. If coagulation is normal, regional techniques may be used with older children. Regional anesthesia avoids the need for intubation but may cause decompensation if accessory muscles of respiration are blocked. Many children with CF must also sit up to spontaneously ventilate, which may make the use of regional techniques for certain operative procedures less favorable.
2. For general anesthesia, endotracheal intubation is usually required to facilitate airway control and to allow suction of secretions. Most intraoperative difficulties arise as a result of copious secretions, airway irritability, and inability to oxygenate.

Intraoperative management

1. Nitrous oxide is avoided if cystic lesions are present by x-ray.
2. Opioids should be titrated to effect to prevent further respiratory depression.
3. Lower pressure settings are used for mechanical ventilation to avoid pneumothorax.
4. Aggressive hydration helps to prevent inspissation of mucus. Frequent endotracheal suction of mucus plugs is required.

Postoperative management

1. CF patients are at risk for respiratory failure, atelectasis, pneumonia, pneumothorax, and airway obstruction; prolonged mechanical ventilation is often required. Humidified oxygen, intravenous hydration, chest physiotherapy, and antibiotics should be continued in the postoperative period.

2. Regional pain management techniques and neuroaxial opioids allow for vigorous chest physiotherapy, earlier extubation, and less respiratory depression than intravenous opioids.

3. All preoperative medications should be resumed as soon as possible.

Common surgical procedures related to cystic fibrosis[22,26]

Endoscopic sinus surgery (polypectomy)
Central venous catheter placement
Bronchoscopy
Lobectomy
Pneumonectomy
Pleurodesis
Abdominal exploration for meconium ileus intestinal obstruction
Colostomy

Respiratory Distress Syndrome
(see also p. 409)

Respiratory distress syndrome (RDS) is largely a disease of premature infants who require mechanical ventilation within the first 12 hours of life. The disease is caused by a deficiency in pulmonary surfactant, produced by type II pneumocytes. The recent ability to treat premature infant lungs by delivering surfactant has greatly reduced the incidence and morbidity of RDS.

An intraarterial catheter (often umbilical) is useful for infants with RDS requiring surgery, to assess oxygenation, avoid hyperoxia, and prevent respiratory and metabolic acidosis. Positive end-expiratory pressure and prolonged mechanical ventilation may also be needed to prevent respiratory insufficiency. Pneumothorax is a common complication secondary to barotrauma. In patients who tolerate early tracheal extubation, postoperative cardiopulmonary monitoring for apnea and bradycardia is warranted.

Bronchopulmonary Dysplasia[27-31]

Bronchopulmonary dysplasia (BPD) is a chronic pulmonary disease first described in 1967 in premature infants with RDS who were treated with oxygen and mechanical ventilation. Pulmonary air leak, pulmonary edema, and pulmonary infection can also contribute to the pathogenesis of BPD. In addition, meconium aspiration pneumonia, neonatal pneumonia, congestive heart failure, and Wilson-Mikity syndrome can all lead to BPD.

DIAGNOSTIC CRITERIA FOR BPD[27]

1. Positive-pressure ventilation during the first 2 weeks of life for a minimum of 3 days
2. Respiratory compromise persisting past 28 days of age
3. Supplemental O_2 requirements greater than 28 days of life (to maintain $PaO_2 > 50$ mm Hg)
4. Chest x-ray findings of increased interstitial markings and peribronchial cuffing.

CLINICAL COURSE

1. Etiology: Many factors contribute to the development of BPD, including lung immaturity, high oxygen requirements, barotrauma, and inflammation. Also, immature lungs do not have adequate antioxidant defense mechanisms.
2. Pathophysiology includes:
   - Pulmonary edema
   - Bronchoconstriction and airway hyperactivity
   - Airway inflammation
   - Chronic lung injury and repair
3. Complications of BPD include:
   - Pulmonary hypertension
   - Cor pulmonale
   - Right or biventricular hypertrophy
   - Systemic hypertension
   - Tracheomalacia
   - Recurrent respiratory infections
   - Altered growth, nutrition, and metabolism
   - Hypertrophy of systemic to pulmonary collateral vessels

TREATMENT OF BPD[32]

1. Oxygen therapy optimally maintains a $PaO_2 > 55$ mm Hg and an SpO_2 of 92% to 96%.
2. Treating hypoxemia prevents increased pulmonary vascular resistance and optimizes growth.
3. In mechanically ventilated patients, inspiratory pressures are limited to minimize barotrauma.
4. Bronchodilators (methylxanthines, beta-adrenergic agents, and anticholinergic agents) are used to improve air flow and minimize reactivity.
5. Diuretics (spironolactone, thiazides, and furosemide) decrease pulmonary edema.
6. Corticosteroids decrease airway inflammation.

ANESTHETIC CONSIDERATIONS FOR PATIENTS WITH BPD

Preoperative assessment

1. Coexisting problems of prematurity are noted (intracranial hemorrhage, retinopathy of prematurity, developmental delay, poor musculature, apnea).

2. Pulmonary status is evaluated, including current oxygen requirements, pulmonary function tests, and blood gases. Pulmonary function is optimized with vigorous pulmonary toilet and, when indicated, preoperative bronchodilators, diuretics, and/or steroid therapy.
3. Long-term medication should be continued throughout the perioperative period. Stress steroid coverage may be indicated.
4. Cardiovascular status, including presence of right ventricular hypertrophy, cor pulmonale, or systemic hypertension, should be evaluated and treated.

Intraoperative considerations
1. Bronchospasm may occur, particularly during placement of the endotracheal tube. Prophylactic bronchodilators and deep anesthetic planes prior to intubation help to minimize this risk.
2. High inflating pressures may cause pneumothorax.
3. Pulmonary hypertension is worsened by acidosis, hypercapnia, hypothermia, and hypoxia.
4. An adequate FIO_2 should be delivered to maintain a PaO_2 of 50 to 70 mm Hg
5. Fluid administration is restricted to minimize risks of pulmonary edema.

Postoperative complications
1. Prolonged mechanical ventilation is often required, necessitating adequate sedation. Tracheostomy may be needed if ventilatory support is long-term.
2. Pneumonia, atelectasis, pneumothorax, and bronchospasm are common postoperative pulmonary complications.
3. Acute congestive heart failure may occur in susceptible patients (history of right ventricular hypertrophy or cor pulmonale).

References

1. McGoldrick KG: The larynx: normal and congenital anomalies. In McGoldrick KG, ed: *Anesthesia for ophthalmologic and otolarygologic surgery,* Philadelphia, 1992, WB Saunders.
2. Motoyama EK: Respiratory physiology in infants and children. In Motoyama EK, Davis PJ, eds: *Smith's anesthesia for infants and children,* ed 6, St. Louis, 1995, Mosby.
3. Stevens WC, Kingston HGG: Inhalation anesthesia. In Barash PG, Cullen BF, Stoelting RK, eds: *Clinical anesthesia,* ed.2, Philadelphia, 1992.
4. Rachelefsky GS, Warner JO: International concensus on the management of pediatric asthma: a summary statement, *Pediatr Pulmonol* 15:125-127, 1993.
5. Stempel DA, Szefler SJ: Management of chronic asthma, *Pediatr Clin North Am* 39: 1293-1310, 1992.
6. Stempel DA, Redding GT: Management of acute asthma, *Pediatr Clin North Am* 39: 1311-1325, 1992.
7. Powell CV: Asthma in childhood, *Br J Hosp Med* 49:127-130, 1993.

8. Larsen GL: Review article: asthma in children, *N Engl J Med* 526:1540-1545, 1992.

9. Shapiro GG: Childhood asthma: update, *Pediatrics in Review* 13:403-412, 1992.

10. Woodhead M: Guidelines on the management of asthma, *Thorax* 48:S1-24, 1993.

11. Gold MI, Helrich M: A study of the complications related to anesthesia in asthmatic patients, *Anesth Analg* 42:283-293, 1963.

12. Shnider SM, Papper EM: Anesthesia for the asthmatic patient, *Anesthesiology* 22:886-92, 1961.

13. Kingston HGG, Hirshman CA: Perioperative management of the patient with asthma, *Anesth Analg* 63:844-855, 1984.

14. Hill M, Szefler SJ, Larsen GL: Asthma pathogenesis and the implications for therapy in children, *Pediatr Clin North Am* 39:1205-1224, 1992.

15. Murphy S, Kelly HW: Asthma, inflammation, and airway hyperresponsiveness in children, *Cur Opin Pediatr* 5:255-265, 1993.

16. Wolfe JD, Shapiro GG, Ratner PH: Comparison of albuterol and metaproterenol syrup in the treatment of childhood asthma, *Pediatrics* 88:312-318, 1991.

17. Strauss RE, Wertheim DL, Bonagura VR, Valacer DJ: Aminophylline therapy does not improve outcome and increases adverse effects in children hospitalized with acute asthmatic exacerbations, *Pediatrics* 93:205-210, 1994.

18. Morray JP, Krane EJ, Geiduschek JM, Pearl-O'Rourke P: Anesthesia for thoracic surgery. In Gregory GA, ed: *Pediatric anesthesia,* ed 3, New York, 1994, Churchill Livingstone.

19. Wilmott RW, Fiedler MA: Recent advances in the treatment of cystic fibrosis, *Pediatr Clin North Am* 41:431-451, 1994.

20. Cole RR, Cotton RT: Preventing postoperative complications in the adult cystic fibrosis patient, *Int J Pediatr Otorhinolaryyngol* 18:263-269, 1990.

21. Doershuk CF, Reyes AL, Regan AG, Matthews LW: Anesthesia and surgery in cystic fibrosis, *Anesth Analg* 51; 413-421, 1972.

22. Lamberty JM, Rubin BK: The management of anaesthesia for patients with cystic fibrosis, *Anaesthesia* 40:448-459, 1985.

23. Boat TF: The respiratory system: acquired disease. In Behrman RE, ed: *Nelson textbook of pediatrics,* ed 14, Philadelphia, 1992, WB Saunders.

24. Konstan MW, Hoppel Cl, Chai BL, Davis PB: Ibuprofen in children with cystic fibrosis: pharmacokinetics and adverse effects, *J Pediatr* 118:956-964, 1991.

25. Auerbach HS, Williams M, Kirkpatrick JA, Colten HR: Alternate-day prednisone reduces morbidity and improves pulmonary function in cystic fibrosis, *Lancet* 2:686-688, 1985.

26. Olsen MM, Gauderer MWL, Girz MK, Izant Jr RJ: Surgery in patients with cystic fibrosis, *J Pediatr Surg* 22:613-618, 1987.

27. Northway WH: Commentary: bronchopulmonary dysplasia twenty-five years later, *Pediatrics* 89:969-973, 1992.

28. Northway WH: Bronchopulmonary dysplasia: then and now, *Arch Dis Child* 65:1076-1081, 1990.

29. Northway WH: An introduction to bronchopulmonary dysplasia, *Clin Perinatol* 19:489-495, 1992.
30. Rush MG, Hazinski TA: Current therapy of bronchopulmonary dysplasia, *Clin Perinatol* 19:563-590, 1992.
31. Abman SH, Groothius JR: Pathophysiology and treatment of bronchopulmonary dysplasia, *Pediatr Clin North Am* 41:277-315, 1994.
32. Tnog WE, Jackson JC: Alternative modes of ventilation in the prevention and treatment of bronchopulmonary dysplasia, *Clin Perinatol* 19:621-647, 1992.

ANESTHESIA FOR CHILDREN WITH CONGENITAL HEART DISEASE

7

You hear it in the dead of night
You feel it when you're jumpy
It races when you're scared or sick
And pounds when you get grumpy.

It swells with pride and stirs at tales
Of beauty, truth and spirit
It sings of love and warms the soul
For those prepared to hear it.

It forms our ballast, anchors us
And makes life stop and start
No, nothing in the universe
Can match the human heart.

Rivian Bell, 1995

The incidence of congenital heart disease (CHD) is approximately 6 to 8 per 1000 births. Premature infants have a 2 to 3 times higher incidence. Associated anomalies are not uncommon in infants with congenital heart disease, particularly those of the genitourinary tract.[1]

Several techniques exist for the detection and confirmation of congenital heart disease in children:

1. History and physical examination may identify the presence of heart murmurs, rales, cyanosis, tachypnea, hypertension, or failure to thrive.
2. The electrocardiogram may give evidence of chamber enlargement, axis deviation, or conduction defects.
3. The chest radiograph may note heart size and shape and the prominence of pulmonary vascularity.
4. Transthoracic echocardiography is useful to define anatomically the presence of a defect, and color flow imaging with echocardiography can reveal directionality of flow through the defect or valvular lesions.[2]
5. Finally, cardiac catheterization is the ultimate technique by which the size and location of defects are determined, as well as the degree of stenosis or shunt.

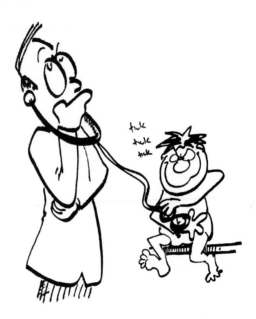

CARDIAC CATHETERIZATION

The objective of cardiac catheterization is to obtain hemodynamic data about suspected cardiac anomalies by measuring pressures and oxygen saturations in each chamber and great vessel. The mixed venous oxygen saturation is usually obtained in the superior vena cava or proximal to the area where the shunt occurs. For example, an increase in saturation at the level of the right atrium would indicate the presence of left-to-right shunting at the atrial level. Similarly, a step-up in saturation in the right ventricle would indicate a left-to-right shunt at the ventricular level. Normally a slight step-down in saturation occurs between the right atrium and the right ventricle because of the addition of coronary sinus blood. Low saturations obtained in the left atrium or ventricle are usually indicative of a right-to-left shunt.

Determination of Shunt Direction: Ratio of Pulmonary to Systemic Blood Flow

Measured oxygen saturation can be used to calculate *oxygen content (O_2C):*

$$O_2C = (1.34 \times \text{hemoglobin} \times \text{saturation}) + (.0031 \times \text{PaO}_2)$$
Normal O_2C = 15-20 ml O_2/100 ml blood

Oxygen saturation or oxygen content can be used to calculate the amount of shunt present by determining the Q_p/Q_s, or ratio of pulmonary blood flow to systemic blood flow. A Q_p/Q_s ratio > 1 is indicative of a left-to-right shunt. A Q_p/Q_s ratio < 1 is indicative of a right-to-left shunt.

Determination of Q_p/Q_s

Equation	Variables
$Q_p \text{ (L/min)} = \dfrac{\dot{V}o_2}{Spvo_2 - Spao_2}$ $Q_s \text{ (L/min)} = \dfrac{\dot{V}o_2}{Sao_2 - Smvo_2}$ $Q_p/Q_s = \dfrac{Sao_2 - Smvo_2}{Spvo_2 - Spao_2}$	$\dot{V}o_2$ = Oxygen consumption Sao_2 = Systemic arterial oxygen saturation* $Smvo_2$ = Mixed venous oxygen saturation (SVC) $Spvo_2$ = Pulmonary venous oxygen saturation $Spao_2$ = Pulmonary artery oxygen saturation

*O_2 content may replace O_2 saturation (Cao_2, $Cmvo_2$, $Cpvo_2$, $Cpao_2$).

Clinical findings with variations in Q_p/Q_s

Q_p/Q_s	Interpretation	Physical findings
< 1.0	Right-to-left shunt	Cyanosis
1.0-1.5	Minimal left-to-right shunt	Asymptomatic Loud murmur Normal ECG
1.5-3.0	Moderate left-to-right shunt	+/–symptomatic Signs of failure on chest x-ray
3.0-5.0	Large left-to-right shunt	Very symptomatic: • Failure to thrive • Congestive heart failure • Repeated respiratory infections • Cyanosis ECG: biventricular enlargement Chest x-ray: failure

Pressures and Gradients

Pressures and gradients are determined during cardiac catheterization by the percutaneous placement of catheters directly into the vessel or chamber to be measured. This information can describe the amount of stenosis across a valvular lesion or express the amount of shunt present. For example, in a large ventricular septal defect, the left and right ventricular pressures may be equal. Vascular resistance can be calculated if both pressure and flow are known (see table, pp. 136-139).

Angiography

Angiography utilizing intravenous contrast techniques gives a definitive radiographic image of the congenital lesions. Simultaneous transesophageal echocardiography helps to improve accuracy in size, shape, and directionality of flow in these defects.

Cardiac catheterization data

	How derived	Normal values	Comments
Q_s Systemic blood flow	$$\dfrac{\dot{V}O_2}{SaO_2 - SmvO_2}$$	2.5-4.5 L/min/m²	Cardiac output decreases with age and decreases 10% from the supine to the sitting position.
Q_p Pulmonary blood flow	$$\dfrac{\dot{V}O_2}{SpvO_2 - SpaO_2}$$	2.5-4.5 L/min/m²	$Q_p = Q_s$ if no shunting is present.
$\dot{V}O_2$ Oxygen consumption	Calculated by using a Douglas bag to collect and measure O_2 and CO_2 in expired gas and comparing these values to those of the ambient air	5-8 ml/kg/min	$\dot{V}O_2$ is heart rate and age dependent. For calculations, FEO_2 and FIO_2 must be room air or 100% O_2 and be carried to four decimal places.
Q_p/Q_s Ratio of pulmonic to systemic blood flow	$$\dfrac{SaO_2 - SmvO_2}{SpvO_2 - SpaO_2}$$ *or* $$\dfrac{CaO_2 - CmvO_2}{CpvO_2 - CpaO_2}$$	1/1	$Q_p>Q_s$ if left-to-right shunts are present. $Q_p<Q_s$ if right-to-left shunts are present.
CaO_2 Systemic arterial oxygen content	Calculated from PaO_2, SaO_2, and Hgb	15-20 ml/L	This value may be 1%-2% less than $CpvO_2$ secondary to drainage of the coronary venous blood through the thebesian veins.
$CmvO_2$ Mixed venous oxygen content	Calculated from $PmvO_2$, $SmvO_2$, and Hgb	14-15 ml/L	In absence of intracardiac shunts, this equals $CpaO_2$. In the presence of intracardiac shunts, it could be measured from the right atrium or SVC.

Cpvo$_2$ Pulmonary venous oxygen content	Calculated from Ppvo$_2$, Spvo$_2$, and Hgb	20-21 ml/L	High pulmonary blood flows, as with ASD, VSD, will decrease the value. Since it depends on V/Q, lung disease can affect the value depending on where sampling occurs.
Cpao$_2$ Pulmonary artery oxygen content	Calculated from Ppao$_2$, Spao$_2$, and Hgb	14-15 ml/L	The value should be the same as that taken in the RV. A 3% step-up or more between the PA and RV is significant. In DORV or VSD, a step-up is seen in the PA secondary to their subpulmonic nature.
PAP Pulmonary artery pressure	Measured	Newborn: $\dfrac{65\text{-}80}{35\text{-}50 \text{ mm Hg}}$ Child: $\dfrac{15\text{-}25}{10\text{-}16 \text{ mm Hg}}$	Increases with left-to-right shunting, cor pulmonale.
LAP Mean left atrial pressure	Measured	Newborn: 3-6 mm Hg Child: 5-10 mm Hg	A dominant V wave is related to increased pulmonary blood flow.

Continued.

Cardiac catheterization data—cont'd

	How derived	Normal values	Comments
PCWP Pulmonary capillary wedge pressure	Measured	Newborn: 6-9 mm Hg Child: 8-11 mm Hg	PCWP shows damping of the a and v waves and has a mean level of 2-3 mm Hg higher than the pulmonary venous pressure.
SVR Systemic vascular resistance	$\dfrac{MAP - CVP*}{Q_s}$	Neonate: 10-15 Woods units (mm Hg/L/min/m^2) Infancy to adulthood: 20 Woods units or 800-1500 $\dfrac{dynes \times sec}{cm^5}$ (equation multiplied by 80)	SVR is lower in the newborn; at 12-18 months, SVR gradually rises to adult levels.
PVR Pulmonary vascular resistance	$\dfrac{PAP - LAP\ (PCWP)}{Q_p}$	Older children and adults: 1-3 Woods units (mm Hg/L/min/m^2) or 150-250 $\dfrac{dynes \times sec}{cm^5}$ (equation multiplied by 80)	The value is considerably higher in the neonate up to 2 months of age.

*MAP = Mean arterial pressure; CVP = Mean central venous pressure (measured in right atrium).

		2.6-3.5 cm² in adults	Neonatal aortic stenosis determined by the presence of a critical gradient across the valve, rather than determination of the valve area (critical gradient = ≥ 50 mm Hg). Treatment is seldom required before the fourth decade (adult valves). 44.5 is also used for calculation of the pulmonic valve.
AVA Aortic valve area	$\dfrac{Q\ (ml/sec)}{44.5 \times \sqrt{\Delta P}}$		
MVA Mitral valve area	$\dfrac{Q\ (ml/sec)}{31.5 \times \sqrt{\Delta P}}$	4.6 cm² in adults	≤1 cm² usually leads to symptoms. 1.5-2.5 cm² will precipitate symptoms with moderate to severe exercise.
F Flow	CO ml/min $\dfrac{}{\text{Diastolic filling pressure (sec/min)}}$ or systolic ejection period (sec/min)	Variable, depending upon preload, afterload, and contractility	For the mitral valve, flow is calculated during diastole. For the aortic valve, flow is calculated during systole.
ΔP Mean pressure gradient across the valvular orifice	Difference between simultaneously measured pressures in two chambers	Minimal gradients should be present across normal valves	Critical stenosis is implied by the following gradients: Aortic: > 40 mm Hg justifies operative intervention Pulmonic: 10-15 mm Hg

CLASSIFICATION OF CONGENITAL HEART DISEASE

Congenital lesions of the heart are generally classified according to the physiologic problems produced by a given lesion or defect.

1. *Left-to-right:* The term simple shunt generally describes a single connection (or hole) between the venous and arterial systems. Blood flows unidirectionally from the area of higher pressure to lower pressure (left to right). These children usually display right-sided failure because of the increased pulmonary blood flow.

2. *Right-to-left:* A connection between the venous and arterial systems with obstruction to outflow on the right side will preferentially shunt blood in the other direction (right to left). Venous blood is therefore ejected systemically by the left ventricle, and these children are cyanotic.

3. *Complex:* Complex shunts or mixing lesions generally are cardiac defects where all venous and arterial blood is mixed before being ejected from the heart. There may or may not be obstruction to flow. Because the venous and arterial circulation cannot be separated, all blood ejected from the heart has a "mixed" saturation (70% to 80%).

4. *Obstructive:* Obstructive lesions, such as valvular stenosis or coarctation of the aorta, can prevent ventricular outflow from either side of the heart, diminishing cardiac output into the pulmonary or systemic vasculature and causing ventricular failure.

Common congenital cardiac defects classified by physiology

Left-to-right shunts Lesions with increased pulmonary blood flow (failure)	Atrial septal defect Ventricular septal defect Patent ductus arteriosus Endocardial cushion defect Aortopulmonary window
Right-to-left shunts Lesions with decreased pulmonary blood flow (cyanotic)	Tetralogy of Fallot Pulmonary atresia Tricuspid atresia Ebstein's anomaly
Complex shunts Mixing of pulmonary and systemic circulation	Truncus arteriosus Transposition of the great vessels Total anomalous pulmonary venous return Double outlet right ventricle Hypoplastic left heart syndrome
Obstructive lesions	Aortic stenosis Mitral stenosis Pulmonic stenosis Coarctation of the aorta Cor triatriatum Interrupted aortic arch

General Principles of Anesthetic Management for Patients with CHD

The relationship of flow, pressure, and resistance in the cardio-vascular system is crucial to understanding the pathophysiology of congenital heart disease:

$$Q = \frac{P}{R}$$

Where:

Q = Blood flow (cardiac output)
P = Pressure within a chamber or vessel
R = Vascular resistance of the pulmonary or systemic bed

Thus the cardiac output from the left ventricle is dependent upon the pressure generated by the ventricle and the resistance to outflow from the aorta and systemic vasculature. A similar situation exists on the right side of the heart between the right ventricle and the pulmonary vascular system. If a shunt exists between the right and left sides of the heart, then the flow across the shunt is likewise determined by the pressure generated across the shunt and the resistance to flow. A shunt across the ventricular septum will have left-to-right directionality as relatively high left ventricular pressures increase flow against the relatively lower pulmonary vascular resistance. Conversely, a shunt occurring within the ventricular septum could have right-to-left flow if pulmonary resistance becomes higher than systemic, as occurs in children with concurrent VSD and pulmonic stenosis.

The ability to alter the relationship of flow, pressure, and resistance is the basic tenet of anesthetic management for children with congenital heart disease. Although pressure (P) within a given intracardiac chamber can be manipulated with positive and negative inotropic agents and flow (Q) can be directly improved by maximizing hydration and preload, the anesthesiologist's principal focus is an attempt to manipulate resistance (R) by the use of various dilators and constrictors.

Left-To-Right Shunts

Simple left-to-right shunts include the defects which connect the arterial and venous circulation, resulting in increased pulmonary blood flow. These include:

Atrial septal defect
Ventricular septal defect
Patent ductus arteriosus
Atrioventricular canal
Aortopulmonic window

PATHOPHYSIOLOGY

Initially, patients with left-to-right shunts exhibit pulmonary congestion and heart failure from the increased pulmonary blood flow. Because there is no anatomic impedance to pulmonary blood flow, oxygenated blood is ejected from the left heart. Therefore, these children are often described as "pink." However, in severe failure, pulmonary edema may inhibit oxygen diffusion, resulting in hypoxemia and cyanosis. Therefore, it would be more physiologically correct to describe children with left-to-right shunts as "wet" without attempting to predict the adequacy of oxygenation or presence of cyanosis.

Long-standing left-to-right shunts with significant increases in pulmonary blood flow can eventually cause pulmonary hypertension in response to the increased pressure and volume in the pulmonary vasculature. If pulmonary hypertension becomes severe, pulmonary vascular resistance may exceed systemic vascular resistance, resulting in shunt reversal. A right-to-left shunt with cyanosis in a patient with a history of uncorrected left-to-right shunt and pulmonary hypertension is called *Eisenmenger's syndrome*.

PREOPERATIVE TREATMENT[3]

Preoperative therapeutic maneuvers that have been used in infants with left-to-right shunts include indomethacin (to close the patent ductus) and a digoxin/diuretic regimen to control congestive heart failure. If a satisfactory therapeutic response is not seen with medical therapy, a band can be surgically placed around the main pulmonary artery to increase resistance to blood flow and reduce the magnitude of the left-to-right shunt. Ideally, the band should decrease distal pulmonary artery pressures to one third to one half of aortic pressures, resulting in a slight decrease in central venous pressure and a rise in aortic or systemic pressure. Placement of a pulmonary artery band is considered a temporizing technique until the infant is large enough or well enough to undergo open-heart surgery and definitive repair. If the band is left in place over months to years, resistance to flow may increase significantly, since the band does not grow with the child. Initiation of positive-pressure ventilation with the induction of anesthesia in a child with an unrepaired shunt and a long-standing band may increase pulmonary resistance sufficiently to reverse shunt flow. This iatrogenic "Eisenmenger's syndrome" causes rapid desaturation and cyanosis.

ANESTHETIC TECHNIQUES

1. Premedication should be used judiciously in patients with severe heart failure.
2. All patients should receive endocarditis prophylaxis (see Appendix F, p. 666).
3. Meticulous removal of all air bubbles from intravenous tubing will help to prevent venous air emboli from crossing the shunt and entering the systemic circulation.
4. If myocardial function is preserved, induction of anesthesia may include either intravenous or inhalation techniques. Dosages should be appropriately modified for the patient with severe failure.
5. Continuous dilution in the pulmonary circulation may slow the onset time of intravenous agents. Speed of induction with inhalation agents is usually not affected in a left-to-right shunt unless cardiac output is significantly reduced.
6. Induction techniques:
   a. *Positive-pressure ventilation:* increases pulmonary vascular resistance and decreases flow through the pulmonary vessels
   b. *Low inspired oxygen concentration (FIO_2):* limits pulmonary blood flow, as oxygen is a direct pulmonary vasodilator
   c. *Nitrous oxide:* helps to limit the amount of inspired oxygen but probably has little direct effect on the pulmonary vasculature in children[4]
   d. *Inhalation agents:* reduce systemic resistance, improving systemic flow[5]
   e. *Opiates:* In the failing heart, high-dose fentanyl techniques probably have the least effect on myocardial performance and help to block the stress response[5,6]
   f. *Ketamine:* increases both pulmonary and systemic vascular resistance, which may increase left-to-right shunting[7]
7. The degree of right ventricular overload and/or failure is often underappreciated in children with left-to-right shunting. Marked increases in preload or afterload and negative inotropy (e.g., high concentrations of halothane) may initiate an irreversible decline in right ventricular performance, with disastrous consequences.

POSTOPERATIVE PROBLEMS

The following problems may be anticipated after surgical closure of septal defects:

1. Supraventricular tachycardia (SVT) and atrioventricular (AV) conduction disturbances are common in the early postoperative period. Conduction delays may persist indefinitely and necessitate pacing.

2. If PVR was elevated before surgery, the increase in RV afterload after closure may not be tolerated and maneuvers to decrease PVR may be necessary (e.g., high FIO_2, vasodilators, isoproterenol, nitric oxide).[8,9]

3. Postoperative valvular incompetence is most common after repair of canal defects.

4. Prolonged postoperative mechanical ventilation is usually not necessary for simple asymptomatic ASD secundum closures. Patients with signs or symptoms of congestive failure usually require continued ventilatory assistance.

Septal defects

Atrial

Primum	Defect is usually associated with a mitral cleft and possibly mitral regurgitation.
Secundum	Patients are usually asymptomatic and tolerate early extubation (before leaving the OR).
Sinus venosus	The defect includes RA, SVC, and partial anomalous pulmonary venous return.

Ventricular

Supracristal	Defect lies just below the aortic annulus and above the crista supraventricularis so that the right coronary cusp of the valve may lack support.
Infracristal (membranous)	The most common form (80%); the defect is found beneath the crista supraventricularis in the membranous septum.
Canal type	Defect lies very high in the septum and is associated with an AV canal.
Muscular	The defect may contain multiple small holes ("swiss cheese") and is located lower in the muscular septum.

Right-To-Left Shunts[10,11]

Lesions that produce a right-to-left shunt contain not only a connection between the right and left heart, but also must offer increased resistance to blood flow through the pulmonary vasculature. Children with these defects have marked hypoxemia and cyanosis. These lesions include:

Tetralogy of Fallot
Tricuspid atresia
Pulmonary atresia
Ebstein's anomaly (downward displacement of the tricuspid valve
   with hypoplastic right ventricle)

The goal of preoperative and intraoperative management is to increase pulmonary blood flow to improve oxygenation.

1. In the neonate, infusions of prostaglandin E_1 (0.03 to 0.10 μg/kg/min) will help to maintain patency of the ductus arteriosus to increase pulmonary blood flow. Complications related to PGE_1 use include vasodilation, hypotension, bradycardia, arrhythmias, apnea or hypoventilation, seizure-like activity, and hyperthermia.[10,12]

2. Palliative shunts are usually placed to provide additional pulmonary blood flow until definitive repair is undertaken. Shunt placement both improves hypoxemia and stimulates growth in the pulmonary artery to aid the technical feasibility of future repair. The eponyms for various surgical shunts are listed below. Selection of a particular shunt is dependent upon the patient's diagnosis and the specific anatomy of the lesion.

Eponyms of surgical shunts to improve pulmonary blood flow

Procedure	Most common indication	Description
Rashkind-Miller	Transposition of great vessels	Balloon atrial septostomy
Blalock-Hanlon	Transposition of great vessels	Open atrial septostomy
Blalock-Taussig	Tetralogy of Fallot Pulmonary atresia Tricuspid atresia	Anastomosis between subclavian artery and pulmonary artery
Potts	Tetralogy of Fallot Pulmonary atresia Tricuspid atresia	Anastomosis between descending aorta and left pulmonary artery
Waterston	Tetralogy of Fallot Pulmonary atresia Tricuspid atresia	Anastomosis between descending aorta and right pulmonary artery
Central	Any cyanotic lesions	A gortex graft is placed between ascending aorta and main pulmonary artery
Glenn	Tetralogy of Fallot Ebstein's anomaly Pulmonary atresia Tricuspid atresia	End-to-end anastomosis between SVC and distal end of transected right pulmonary artery
Bidirectional (modified) Glenn	Tetralogy of Fallot Ebstein's anomaly Pulmonary atresia Tricuspid atresia	End-to-side anastomosis between transected SVC and distal intact RPA to decrease ventricular volume burden and increase flow to the RPA and LPA

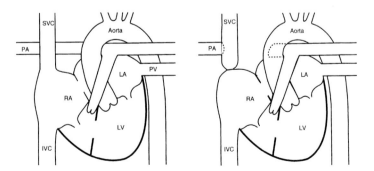

FIG. 7-1. Classic Glenn shunt to increase pulmonary blood flow: end-to-end anastomosis between superior vena cava and distal end of transected right pulmonary artery.

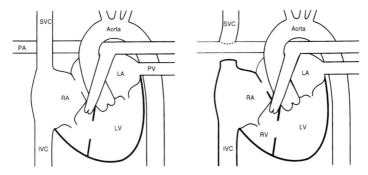

FIG. 7-2. Bidirectional (modified) Glenn shunt: end-to-side anastomosis between transected superior vena cava and distal intact right pulmonary artery to decrease ventricular volume burden and increase flow to the right and left pulmonary arteries.

ANESTHETIC MANAGEMENT

The goal of anesthetic management for right-to-left shunts is to selectively improve pulmonary blood flow by maintaining or increasing systemic vascular resistance and lowering pulmonic vascular resistance.

Preoperative management

1. Premedication is recommended to prevent crying and agitation, which can increase pulmonary vascular resistance and worsen right-to-left shunting.
2. The meticulous removal of all air bubbles from intravenous lines is critical, since venous air emboli can pass directly into the systemic or cerebral circulation.
3. Prostaglandin infusions should be maintained into the intraoperative period.
4. Endocarditis prophylaxis is recommended (see Appendix F, p. 666).
5. Altered pharmacokinetics should be anticipated. Inhalation induction is prolonged by limited pulmonary blood flow. Intravenous induction times are more rapid because dilution in the pulmonary circulation is bypassed and drugs are distributed directly to the systemic and cerebral circulation through the shunt.

Induction techniques.   The goal of induction is to improve pulmonary blood flow to reduce hypoxemia and cyanosis.

1. *Oxygen* is the cornerstone of intraoperative management, as the only readily available drug (pending use of nitric oxide) that specifically dilates the pulmonary vascular bed. High levels of inspired oxygen along with low peak inspiratory pressure can maximize pulmonary blood flow.

2. *Hydration* helps to maintain adequate right-sided filling pressures needed to overcome obstruction to pulmonary outflow. Adequate hydration is also necessary in the child with polycythemia secondary to long-standing hypoxemia. Dehydration increases the risk of cerebral vascular accidents and other sequelae of thrombotic events. Intravenous fluids should be started if a prolonged preoperative fast is anticipated.

3. *Spontaneous ventilation* or gentle assisted ventilation is recommended during induction. Positive-pressure ventilation increases intrathoracic pressure and thereby increases PVR. A trial of positive pressure is recommended before instituting muscle relaxation.

4. *Ketamine* raises both SVR and PVR and is therefore ideal for lesions where pulmonary flow is determined more by fixed obstruction than by dynamic pulmonary vascular resistance.[13,14] Its analgesic and sedative effects are also useful to calm a crying child while maintaining spontaneous ventilation.

5. *Morphine* is also useful for sedation and analgesia, although it theoretically lowers both SVR and PVR.

6. *Fentanyl* in doses sufficient to block the stress response (50 μg/kg) has been suggested to decrease morbidity and mortality in infants undergoing open-heart procedures.[6]

7. *Beta blockade* has been used in children over the age of 6 months to relax infundibular spasm (dynamic outflow obstruction) and slow the heart rate.[10,11] The short duration of action of esmolol makes it a more attractive choice in the operating room than propranolol, whose negative inotropic effects can persist for hours.

8. *Halothane* offers similar attributes to beta blockade therapy (slow heart rate and negative inotropy to relax infundibular spasm) and can be rapidly turned on and off.

9. *Enflurane* and *isoflurane,* which increase heart rate and decrease systemic vascular resistance, are less attractive choices.[5]

10. *Nitrous oxide* lowers the concentration of oxygen administered. It may also constrict the pulmonary vasculature.[4]

11. *Slower heart rates* are recommended to maximize the flow time across obstructed valvular lesions; vagolytic agents should be avoided.

TETRALOGY OF FALLOT[11,15]

This disease complex comprises about 10% of all CHD and is the most common right-to-left shunt. It is particularly challenging to the anesthesiologist because of the wide range and severity of symptoms. The four anomalies that make up the tetrad include:

1. Right ventricular outflow tract obstruction (infundibular stenosis, pulmonic stenosis, or supravalvular stenosis)

2. Subaortic VSD
3. Overriding aorta
4. Right ventricular hypertrophy

Traditionally, palliative shunts were placed to improve pulmonary blood flow. Primary pulmonary artery reconstruction with complete repair at any earlier age is now more common.

Hypercyanotic ("tet") spells occur because of infundibular spasm, low pH, or low PaO_2. Episodes in the awake patient manifest as acute cyanosis and hyperventilation and may occur with feeding, crying, defecation, or stress. Hypercyanosis may also occur during anesthesia, usually as a result of acute dynamic infundibular spasm. Recommended treatment is listed below.

Treatment of hypercyanotic spells

Treatment	Effect
High FIO_2 (1.0)	Acts as a specific pulmonary vasodilator, decreasing pulmonary vascular resistance (PVR)
Hydration (volume bolus)	Opens the right ventricular outflow tract
Morphine	Sedation, decreases PVR
Ketamine	Maintains systemic vascular resistance (SVR); provides sedation and analgesia, improving pulmonary blood flow
Phenylephrine	Increases SVR
Propranolol	Decreases heart rate (HR), improving flow time across an obstructed valve; decreases infundibular spasm (negative inotropy)
Halothane	Negative inotropy; decreases HR
Thiopental	Negative inotropy
Squatting Abdominal compression	Increases SVR

Anesthetic agents contraindicated or not useful for hypercyanotic spells

Atropine	Increases HR, resulting in decreased blood flow across the stenotic pulmonary valve
N_2O	Decreases FIO_2; may increase PVR
Isoflurane/enflurane	Decreases SVR, increases HR
Epinephrine	May cause spasm of right ventricular outflow tract; increases heart rate
Dopamine	May cause spasm of right ventricular outflow tract; increases heart rate; increases PVR at $\propto$ doses
Halothane in extreme right ventricular failure	Negative inotropy

Complex Congenital Heart Disease[16-18]

Complex lesions include the "mixing lesions" and bidirectional shunts, which produce both cyanosis and congestive heart failure. These include:

Transposition of the great vessels
Truncus arteriosus
Total anomalous pulmonary venous return
Double-outlet right ventricle
Hypoplastic left heart syndrome

PATHOPHYSIOLOGY

Continuous mixing of venous and arterial blood results in cyanosis. Since there is no obstruction to pulmonary flow, high-pressure left-to-right shunting results in simultaneous pulmonary edema. In severe left-to-right shunts, the placement of a PA band may protect the lungs from progressive (and irreversible) pulmonary hypertension.

Preoperative review of recent cardiac catheterization data is critical to determine degree and direction of shunting and therefore direct anesthetic management. Because these children are chronically cyanotic, these lesions are often included with right-to-left shunts. However, an overzealous approach to improve pulmonary blood flow may actually "steal" blood from the aorta. This situation may result in systemic hypotension and coronary insufficiency. As a result, ischemic changes on ECG may be seen even in infants or children. A susceptibility to severe right heart failure unresponsive to inotropic agents (as exists for left-to-right shunts) may also be present.

ANESTHETIC MANAGEMENT

1. Since all of the venous and arterial blood is pooled before ejection from the heart, it is not possible to improve oxygenation by increasing pulmonary blood flow.
2. Manipulating pulmonary or systemic vascular resistance will not improve oxygenation and may acutely worsen biventricular failure.
3. Attempting to improve pulmonary blood flow (by increasing FIO_2 or SVR) will steal circulation from the aorta and may cause coronary ischemia.
4. Generally, maintaining "status quo" with high-dose opiates (fentanyl or sufentanil) that do not significantly affect heart rate, contractility, or resistance is recommended.
5. For short, noncardiac procedures, a slow and gradual induction with halothane (at low doses) will have the least positive chronotropic effect and the least effect on peripheral resistance.

The use of nitrous oxide will limit FIO_2 and help to prevent coronary steal while decreasing halothane requirements.

TYPES OF MIXING LESIONS

Transposition of the great arteries.   The aorta originates from the RV and the pulmonary artery arises from the LV, creating two parallel circulations. In the "D" type the aorta is to the right of the pulmonary artery; the "L" type bases the aorta to the left of the PA. As mixing of pulmonary and systemic circulation is necessary to maintain life, many of these patients also have a VSD (50%). In the absence of a septal defect, ductal patency for mixing may be maintained by prostaglandin infusion. If mixing is inadequate, a Rashkind balloon septostomy of the atrial septum is performed emergently in the neonatal period.

Historically, the Mustard and Senning procedures created an atrial baffle to divert pulmonary venous return to the right side of the heart and aorta. These procedures carried significant complications and left the right ventricle as the systemic pumping chamber. The Jatene switch procedure is now the recommended surgical correction[19] (see p. 152).

Truncus arteriosus.   The truncus is one large rudimentary vessel arising from both ventricles and overriding a large VSD. It represents a failure of separation between the systemic and pulmonary circulations. Three types are identified: (1) the truncus divides into an aorta and main pulmonary artery; (2) the pulmonary arteries arise posteriorly from the truncus; (3) the pulmonary arteries arise laterally from the truncus. Because of the large VSD without obstruction to flow, pulmonary overperfusion and cardiac failure are common. Mortality is very high if complete repair is not performed within the first year of life. Placement of a pulmonary artery band will temporize on the development of pulmonary hypertension, but will not improve RV failure.

Anomalous pulmonary venous return.   In total anomalous pulmonary venous return, an ASD must be present in order for oxygenated blood from the lungs to reach the left side of the heart. Pulmonary congestion and hypertension are common. A partial anomaly is recognized by a step-up in saturation in the right atrium and is treated like an ASD. Four sites of drainage are described:

1. Supracardiac—pulmonary veins drain into the SVC, creating a left-to-right shunt (pulmonary recirculation)
2. Infracardiac—pulmonary veins drain into the portal or hepatic system
3. Cardiac—pulmonary veins drain into the right atrium or coronary sinus
4. Mixed

Double-outlet right ventricle.   Both great arteries arise from the RV, and a VSD is always present. There may also be pulmonic stenosis. Anesthetic management depends on the amount of pulmonary blood flow. If the Q_p/Q_s ratio is high, the anesthetic management is similar to VSD. The defect is corrected by a baffled closure of the VSD so that the PA remains on the right and the aorta arises from the left. If significant right ventricular outflow tract obstruction is present, the anesthetic management resembles tetralogy of Fallot.

Hypoplastic left heart syndrome.   In this complex syndrome, the LV is hypoplastic or atretic, as are the proximal aorta, aortic valve, and mitral valve. The neonate's survival is dependent upon ductal patency, as mixed blood in the RV is ejected out the single great vessel (PA) to both the lungs and (through the PDA) the systemic circulation. Severe congestive failure is present, and mortality is usually anticipated within the first month of life without either transplant or the palliative Norwood procedure (see p. 155).

SURGICAL CORRECTION OF COMPLEX MIXING LESIONS

Many different procedures have been developed to palliate or attempt correction of complex heart lesions. The eponyms these techniques have been given often represent a series of procedures, which are confusing to most practitioners unless encountered routinely in practice. The Fontan, Jatene, and Norwood procedures are now most commonly encountered, because they attempt to aggressively correct severe lesions rather than only palliate. These three surgical techniques are discussed below, followed by a table briefly describing more historical procedures. Older children and young adults who have had these earlier corrections may be admitted for noncardiac surgery or obstetric care.

Jatene.[19]   This procedure provides anatomic correction of transposition of the great arteries by division of both great vessels and reattachment to their correct ventricular outflow. The coronary arteries are reimplanted into the "new" aorta. The technique has been successfully performed in neonates with large VSDs and therefore high LV and pulmonary pressures and also in neonates with intact ventricular septa. Delaying the procedure in the latter group predisposes the unprepared LV to failure when it becomes the systemic pumping chamber. Prior to surgical correction, adequate mixing must be maintained through the patent ductus or atrial or ventricular septal defects.

Advantages (over the Mustard, Senning, Rastelli)
1. Fewer arrhythmias
2. Less frequent obstruction of the systemic or pulmonary venous return
3. The RV is not required to be the systemic pumping chamber

Complications
1. Pulmonary outflow tract obstruction
2. Supravalvular aortic stenosis
3. Coronary insufficiency with myocardial ischemia and ventricular dysfunction
4. Myocardial infarction
5. LV failure if it is not adequately prepared to pump systemic pressures

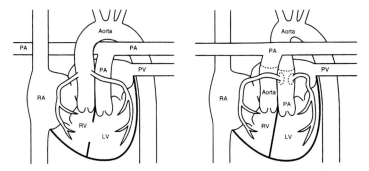

FIG. 7-3. Jatene procedure for transposition of the great arteries: this procedure provides anatomic correction by division of both great vessels and reattachment to their correct ventricular outflow. The coronary arteries are reimplanted into the "new" aorta.

Fontan.[20,21] This surgical technique was originally developed over 20 years ago as a definitive treatment for tricuspid atresia, based on the concept that venous pressure is sufficient to drive blood through the pulmonary circulation if pulmonary hypertension is not present. The procedure not only delivers venous blood to the pulmonary vasculature, but effectively separates the circulation. It is now used not only for tricuspid atresia but also for pulmonic atresia and single ventricle and as part of the Norwood procedure for hypoplastic left heart (see p. 155).

The technique is an extension of the Glenn shunt (SVC to PA) and generally consists of a (homograft) right atrial to pulmonary artery connection with closure of the ASD. Although valved conduits were initially described, the valve may actually predispose to later obstruction and does not necessarily contribute to the delivery of blood to the pulmonary vasculature. At a later procedure (to avoid volume overload), the inferior vena cava is connected to the pulmonary artery by formation of a lateral tunnel through the right atrium. A small window in the tunnel into the atrium serves as a pop-off to prevent overload and ventricular failure at the price of a small right-to-left shunt and decrease in oxygenation. The window is closed later with either an umbrella device placed during cardiac catheterization or a slip suture.

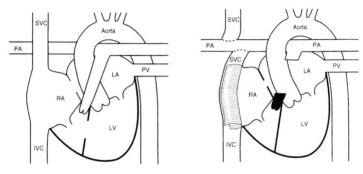

FIG. 7-4. Fontan procedure.

Selection criteria for the Fontan procedure
_____

Over 4 years of age
Normal sinus rhythm
Normal vena caval drainage
Right atrium of normal volume
Mean PA pressure up to 15 mm Hg
Pulmonary resistance below 4 units/m^2
Diameter of PA at least 75% of diameter of aorta
Normal ventricular function (ejection fraction at least 0.6)
No AV valve incompetence
No impairment due to previous shunt

From Choussat A, Fontan F, Besse P, et al: Selection criteria for Fontan's procedure. In Anderson RH, Shinebourne EA, eds: *Pediatric cardiology*, Edinburgh, 1978, Churchill Livingstone.

Anesthetic management.[22,23]   The induction technique is dependent upon the anatomy and physiology of the original lesion (see relevant sections above in this chapter). The postbypass and recovery phases demand a relatively high central venous pressure (driving force) and a relatively low pulmonary vascular resistance. These criteria necessitate maintaining normocapnia and avoiding acidosis while maintaining preload. Inotropic support that decreases PVR is desirable. High doses ($\propto$ range) of dopamine have been shown to markedly increase PVR. Dobutamine has less effect on the pulmonary vasculature; amrinone has also been used successfully to support the ventricle without increasing pulmonary resistance.[24]

Complications of Fontan procedure
1. Pleural effusion
2. Ascites
3. Chylothorax
4. Renal failure
5. Low cardiac output
6. Obstruction or deterioration of conduits or valves
7. Cirrhosis
8. AV valve insufficiency
9. Cardiomyopathy

Norwood.[25] The three-stage Norwood procedure was initially developed over 15 years ago as palliative treatment for hypoplastic left heart syndrome (HLHS). Because the three procedures are undertaken over a period of months to years, these infants often come to the operating room for noncardiac surgery at different stages of palliation/repair.

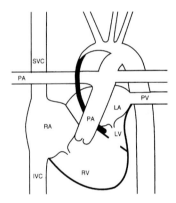

FIG. 7-5. Hypoplastic left heart: before Norwood procedure.

Stage I (neonate)
1. A large atrial septectomy is formed to prevent pulmonary venous hypertension.
2. The main pulmonary artery is transected and separated from the RV.
3. The ascending aorta is augmented with a patch of pulmonary artery and attached to the RV to ensure systemic flow from the single ventricle.

4. The ductus is ligated and replaced with a synthetic graft either from aorta to PA (central shunt) or from subclavian to PA (Blalock-Taussig shunt), which helps ensure growth of the pulmonary arteries.

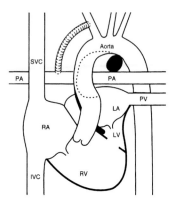

FIG. 7-6. Hypoplastic left heart syndrome: after Norwood repair stage I.

Stage II (1 to 2 yr)
1. A hemi-Fontan or bidirectional Glenn shunt (SVC to PA) directs about one third of the systemic venous return directly to the pulmonary vasculature. Completion of the Fontan at this stage (i.e., including the IVC) can significantly drop ventricular end-diastolic volume and result in severe ventricular dysfunction with fall in cardiac output. Staging the Fontan decreases the chance of ventricular failure.
2. The central or Blalock-Taussig shunt is ligated.
3. Any atrial restriction is relieved.

Stage III (6 to 12 mo after Stage II)
1. The Fontan is completed by connecting the inferior vena cava to the PA.
2. Any intraatrial obstruction is relieved.

Regardless of the stage of completion at which these children are seen, the morphologic right ventricle continues to be the chamber responsible for maintaining systemic cardiac output. As such it may be exquisitely sensitive to marked increases in preload, afterload, or negative inotropy. Induction even for simple procedures should strive to maintain a relatively low pulmonary vascular resistance, with a very gradual titration of anesthetic agents to assess ventricular tolerance. A slow and careful inhalation induction with halothane and oxygen is often recommended because of the minimal changes in resistance and because it offers the ability to control the speed of induction, allowing the anesthesiologist the opportunity to respond to gradual hemodynamic changes. Because the ventricle has little reserve, it is likewise sensitive to small hemodynamic changes in the postoperative period, and clinicians should be observant for signs of failure. Even those children who appear well compensated before surgery are unlikely candidates for ambulatory procedures.

Eponyms of surgical procedures for correction of congenital heart disease

Eponyms of procedure	Disease	Technique
Blalock-Hanlon	Transposition of great vessels (TOGV)	1. Open atrial septectomy 2. Clamping of the right pulmonary veins during septal excision
Damus-Kaye-Stansel	TOGV with poor coronary anatomy for the Jatene procedure Double-outlet right ventricle (DORV)	1. The PA is cut with its proximal end anastomosed to the side of the aorta, establishing left ventricle to aorta flow. 2. A valved conduit from the RV to the distal PA establishes pulmonary flow.
Danielson	Ebstein's anomaly	Plication of atrialized portion of the RV, bringing the anterior and posterior leaflets of the tricuspid valves back to the normal annulus.
Mustard	TOGV	1. After excision of the interatrial septum, an interatrial baffle using pericardium or synthetic material is created. 2. The baffle directs pulmonary venous blood across the tricuspid valve into the RV, with systemic venous blood passing below the baffle through the mitral valve.
Rastelli	TOGV Left ventricular outflow obstruction with VSD	1. Oversewing of the main PA 2. Conduit from the RV to the distal main PA 3. Closure of the VSD such that the LV outflow is directed to the aorta
Senning	TOGV	As for the Mustard procedure except autologous atrial tissue is used, with the theoretical advantage that it can grow with the heart

Obstructive Lesions
PATHOPHYSIOLOGY

Obstructive lesions may be either valvular stenosis or vascular bands (such as coarctation of the aorta), which cause decreased perfusion and pressure overload of the corresponding ventricle. Congestive failure is a consistent finding in this group of anomalies. Obstruction to left ventricular outflow in the infant is often more devastating than in adults because of the severity of obstruction, poor myocardial tolerance, and difficulty of repair.

ANESTHETIC MANAGEMENT

The pressure gradient across an obstructive lesion will direct anesthetic management.

- Lesions with a large pressure gradient (>50 mm Hg) and congestive failure are best managed with an opiate technique (fentanyl or sufentanil), which maintains a slow heart rate and minimally affects ventricular performance or vascular resistance. Tachycardia increases myocardial demand and decreases flow across the obstruction.
- Preload is maximized to improve flow beyond the lesion. Central pressure monitoring will help to prevent ventricular overload while maintaining preload.
- In patients with critical gradients, inhalation agents may cause negative inotropy and decrease vascular resistance, worsening the gradient and thereby flow past the obstruction.
- Patients with smaller pressure gradients (< 40 mm Hg) and good perfusion beyond the obstruction will likely tolerate a variety of induction techniques, including the use of inhalation agents.

COARCTATION OF THE AORTA[26]

Description. *Preductal* coarction is a narrowing of the aortic isthmus, which coexists with other anomalies in 90% of patients. As a patent ductus is necessary to perfuse the lower body, PGE infusions are used to maintain ductal patency. *Postductal* patients are usually asymptomatic until ductal closure. Extensive collaterals often develop from the intercostal or mammary arteries to feed the lower body.

Pathophysiology. Congestive failure in infancy and hypertension in the upper extremities are classic physical findings. Surgery is indicated when the pressure gradient exceeds 40 mm Hg or systolic blood pressure is greater than 180 mm Hg. The risk of cerebral aneurysm is greater for these children.

Anesthetic considerations

- Endocarditis prophylaxis is recommended (Appendix F, p. 666)
- Preductal placement of intraarterial catheters is most accurate. If possible, placement of arterial catheters preductally (right ra-

dial) and postductally (umbilical or lower extremity) is ideal for blood pressure management and assessment of perfusion to upper and lower extremities. Central pressure monitoring helps to maximize preload. Preductal and postductal oximetry is recommended, although the presence of functional oximetry distal to the obstruction does not guarantee adequacy of perfusion (see also p. 57).

- Lowering blood pressure can be accomplished by using inhalation agents or vasodilator therapy.
- Intraoperative cooling to 33° C aids in preservation of spinal cord function if aortic cross-clamping is necessary during repair. Evoked potentials may also be used to monitor spinal cord function.
- Postoperatively, hypertension is common and usually necessitates both vasodilator therapy and beta blockade. Mesenteric enteritis with abdominal pain and even bowel ischemia is also seen, as a result of increased sympathetic tone. Regional pain management techniques (e.g., epidural opiates/local anesthetics) for the lateral thoracotomy incision are useful for blocking sympathetic response and thereby help to decrease hypertension and abdominal symptoms.

INTERRUPTED AORTIC ARCH

This lesion results from failure of the fourth to sixth aortic arches to fuse. The pathophysiology and anesthetic management are similar to those for a preductal aortic coarctation, and repair is necessary during the neonatal period. The lower body is dependent upon ductal patency for perfusion, and, therefore, prostaglandin infusion is maintained. Commonly associated anomalies include VSD, aortopulmonic window, and truncus arteriosus.

Three types of interrupted arch are commonly described:

1. Type A—interruption distal to the left subclavian
2. Type B—interruption between left carotid and left subclavian (most common)
3. Type C—interruption between the innominate artery and the left carotid

AORTIC STENOSIS

Description.   Three types of congenital aortic stenosis are described. All may have symptoms of left ventricular hypertrophy, syncope, angina, and congestive failure.

1. Valvular—stiff, thickened bicuspid valve fused at the commissures (80%)
2. Subvalvular—eventually turbulence develops beyond the initial obstruction, causing thickening of valve leaflets and incompetence (10%)
3. Supravalvular—associated with Williams syndrome; tortu-

ous coronary arteries with a predilection for early athero-
sclerosis evolve because of proximal location to the obstruction and subjection to high pressures

Anesthetic considerations

- Endocarditis prophylaxis is recommended (Appendix F, p. 666)
- Patients with valvular and supravalvular obstruction do not tolerate myocardial depressants or tachycardia. Hypotension can
  be catastrophic because coronary perfusion will markedly decrease. Therefore, an opiate technique (fentanyl or sufentanil) is
  recommended.
- Subvalvular stenosis can behave like idiopathic hypertrophic
  subaortic stenosis (IHSS). Hypovolemia, hypotension, tachycardia, and vasodilation augment the obstruction and worsen perfusion. Negative inotropy and slow heart rate (with beta blockade
  or halothane) while maintaining preload and afterload will relax
  outflow obstruction and maximize flow (see also IHSS, p. 166).

MITRAL STENOSIS

Description.   Mitral stenosis is an uncommon congenital lesion,
seen more often in males. Chronic ischemia and fibrosis in severe
obstruction lead to left ventricular dysfunction. Elevated left atrial
pressures cause pulmonary hypertension and cor pulmonale.

Anesthetic considerations

- Endocarditis prophylaxis is recommended (Appendix F, p. 666).
- Left ventricular filling is optimized by slower heart rates and
  sinus rhythm.
- Maximized preload is monitored with central or pulmonary
  artery pressure monitoring.
- Opiate techniques (fentanyl or sufentanil) are recommended for
  patients with ventricular failure.
- Postoperatively, reduction of pulmonary and systemic vascular
  resistance with vasodilator therapy is often needed.

COR TRIATRIATUM

Description.   The left atrium is partitioned into a superior chamber, which receives pulmonary venous return, and an inferior
chamber, which communicates with the mitral valve. The chambers are connected by a fenestrated membrane. Pathophysiology
resembles mitral stenosis, with pulmonary hypertension and cor
pulmonale developing within the first year of life.

Anesthetic considerations.   Similar to those for mitral stenosis.

CARDIOPULMONARY BYPASS[27]
Goals

1. Adequate perfusion of the patient's organs without using the
   heart as a pump

2. Maintenance of CVP for effective drainage into the extracorporeal circuit
3. Maintenance of normal PaO_2, pH, and $PaCO_2$

Cannulation

Venous.   Usually two separate cannulas are placed, one in the SVC and one in the IVC. Any major vein can be used, the femoral vein being the most common alternative to central vein cannulation

Arterial.   Usually a single cannula in the anterior aspect of the ascending aorta is placed. If an interrupted aortic arch is present, cannulation of both the proximal and distal ends of the aorta is performed. The femoral artery can be used if necessary.

Oxygenators

1. Membrane oxygenators permit gas exchange through a synthetic membrane. They offer the advantage over bubble oxygenators of improved platelet survival and fewer microemboli.
2. Bubble oxygenators permit gas exchange by bubbling the gas flow through the blood, defoaming and filtering the blood, then transfusing it back to the patient. Advantages include simplicity in the setup and the prime, and the capacity to oxygenate a large volume of blood. Disadvantages include hemolysis, thrombocytopenia, and platelet dysfunction, especially when perfusion is necessary for more than 2 hours.

Prime[27]

Each circuit has its own obligatory prime volume: that volume of solution necessary to fill the circuit and ensure that no air is pumped. The Cobe Variable Prime Membrane Lung allows different amounts of priming volumes depending on the size of the child (220 ml, 290 ml, and 375 ml).

Hemodilution results from a volume of priming solutions considerably greater than the patient's blood volume. In addition, most primes are hyponatremic, hypocalcemic, hypomagnesemic, hypocapnic, acidotic, and hypoosmolar. Common sequelae of bypass therefore include hypoproteinemia, thrombocytopenia, anemia, hypocoagulability, and hypothermia. To avoid extreme hemodilution in small children, a combination of blood and plasma is frequently used. Mannitol is also added to promote an osmotic diuresis and to scavenge oxygen-free radicals.

Flow

Flow is measured by an electromagnetic flowmeter on the arterial side of the circuit. Optimal rates are dependent upon body mass and the ability to maintain organ perfusion as determined by blood gases, pH, and urine output. The rate is higher in pediatric cases because of higher metabolic demands (albeit reduced by hypothermia) and the compliance of the vascular tree. Flows as high as 150 to 175 ml/kg/min are common.

If perfusion pressure seems too low for the age and perfusion rate, the possibility of substantial aortopulmonary communication should be considered (undiagnosed shunt). All known shunts should be ligated before bypass.

Anticoagulation

Anticoagulation is accomplished with 3 to 4 mg/kg of IV heparin. An activated clotting time (ACT) of 300 to 400 seconds is adequate to assume CPB, but values greater than 400 are necessary to ensure no microscopic evidence of aggregates. The ACT should be checked every 30 minutes while the patient is on CPB.

Heparin reversal is accomplished with protamine, 1 mg for every mg of heparin administered. Hemostatis may be more problematic in infants and children because of the increased hemodilution, platelet inhibition by prostaglandin, and secondary fibrinolysis.

Hypothermia

Moderate hypothermia provides temperatures between 25° and 30° C. Profound hypothermia provides temperatures between 15° and 20° C. A combination of this temperature and circulatory arrest has the advantage of providing a bloodless field, decreased trauma to blood cells, and enhanced myocardial protection. Circulatory arrest can be maintained for up to 1 hour; however, neuropsychologic dysfunction (both transient and permanent) has been reported in 25% to 45% of infants after deep hypothermic circulatory arrest.[28-30] Trickle flow (very low pump flows) is more commonly used than complete circulatory arrest. Surface cooling can be accomplished with the room temperature reduced to 22° C, a cooling blanket at 15° C, and ice packed around the head. The effects of hypothermia are as follows:

1. Myocardial ATP stores are maintained at low temperatures.
2. It decreases the cerebral metabolic rate as well as total body oxygen consumption.
3. It leads to arrhythmias, bradycardia, and decreased contractility and compliance.
4. Increased blood glucose occurs secondary to decreases in insulin levels and increases in ACTH, cortisol, epinephrine, and norepinephrine. Gluconeogenesis in the liver usually persists during moderate hypothermia.
5. Hypothermia leads to intense vasoconstriction and poor rheologic characteristics because of the increased viscosity of blood; thus the need for hemodilution and systemic heparinization.

Anesthesia and CPB

1. Hypothermia decreases anesthetic requirements.
2. Priming solutions cause marked dilution of drugs, which necessitates the administration of additional doses in the postbypass period.
3. A volatile anesthetic vaporizer can be inserted into the gas delivery system. Isoflurane is an attractive choice because of its effect on cerebral EEG activity and reduction of peripheral vasomotor tone.

Rewarming

1. Ice bags are removed.
2. The operating room is warmed.
3. The heating blanket is warmed to 37° C.
4. The use of nitroprusside or droperidol (75 to 100 µg/kg) helps to ensure even warming by vasodilation.
5. Upon completion of rewarming, differences between core and peripheral blood temperatures (esophageal and rectal) should be no greater than 1° or 2°. Otherwise, increased organ damage and coagulopathies may result.
6. Sinus rhythm should be established. Cardioversion or pacing may be required.

Discontinuation of CPB

1. Monitors are recalibrated.
2. Adequate hematocrit level, ABGs, and electrolyte balance are ensured.
3. Ventilation with 100% oxygen is resumed.
4. Inotropic and vasodilator drugs in bolus and infusion doses are made available.
5. Difficulties in discontinuation from bypass may be due to inadequacy of the repair, a lengthy bypass period, electrolyte imbalance, or preexisting myocardial damage.

ANESTHETIC MANAGEMENT OF NONCARDIAC SURGERY IN CHILDREN WITH CONGENITAL HEART DISEASE[31,32]

As survival and quality of life for patients with congenital heart disease continue to improve, more patients are encountered in the operating room for noncardiac procedures.[33] These children may even be scheduled for ambulatory procedures, based on the principle that the surgery is "minor" and without regard for the effects of general anesthesia on shunt direction or ventricular decompensation. Many of these patients are adolescents or adults who have had palliative procedures many years prior to admission. The pregnant patient with palliated or uncorrected congenital heart disease is a particularly challenging clinical problem.

A current cardiac physiology profile is critical for determining shunt direction and therefore anesthetic management. The patient, surgeon, and pediatrician should also be apprised of complications anticipated from the anesthetic or surgery. It is important to remember that postoperative pain with increased catecholamines can affect vascular resistance and therefore shunt direction. Most of these patients are not candidates for outpatient surgery, although this consideration should be made on an individual basis.

1. Obtain history and physical, including:
   a. Presence of cyanosis or failure
   b. Growth percentiles
   c. Exercise tolerance
   d. Medications, laboratory data, ECG, chest x-ray
2. Review most recent echocardiographic and cardiac catheterization data.
   a. Q_p/Q_s (type and degree of shunt)
   b. Pressure gradients across obstruction
   c. Myocardial contractility
   d. Function of palliative shunts
   e. Anatomy
3. Order premedication based on age, presence of failure or cyanosis, degree of respiratory dysfunction.
4. Order antibiotic prophylaxis (see Appendix F, p. 666).
5. Use all standard monitors, especially oximetry. Quantitative capnometry may not be useful with right-to-left shunting. Consider need for invasive monitoring.
6. Plan induction based upon primary shunt flow (right-to-left or left-to-right). Avoid high-dose fentanyl techniques except when postoperative ventilation is anticipated. Low-dose halothane, which has little effect on heart rate or vascular resistance, may be tolerated well for brief procedures.
7. Anticipate severe conduction disturbances even after complete repair, and particularly in patients with previous or current septal defects.
8. Plan postoperative ICU stay based upon need for prolonged ventilatory or inotropic support or need for prolonged monitoring (anticipation of cardiac or respiratory dysfunction).

ACQUIRED HEART DISEASE

RHEUMATIC HEART DISEASE[34]
Description
- RHD is associated with group A β-hemolytic streptococcal infections of the upper airway and affects young children more commonly in the winter and spring.

- Clinical manifestations include carditis, polyarthritis, chorea, subcutaneous nodules, and erythema marginatum. In 76% of the cases, carditis appears within the first week of onset of the disease and may be treated with corticosteroids.
- Patients with recurrent infections or those with severe carditis may go on to develop rheumatic heart disease. The mitral valve is involved 85% of the time, the aortic valve 54%, and the tricuspid and pulmonary valves less than 5% of the time. Patients are predisposed to endocarditis.

Anesthetic considerations.   Anesthetic considerations are based on the specific cardiac involvement. Patients rarely require valvular replacement before adulthood.

KAWASAKI SYNDROME[35]

Description

- Mucocutaneous lymph node syndrome is an acute febrile exanthem of children, manifested by fever, conjunctival injection, oral erythema with crusting of the lips, induration of the hands and feet followed by erythema and desquamation of the soles and palms, a diffuse erythematous rash, and lymphadenopathy.
- Cardiac involvement occurs 20% of the time, manifested by pericarditis during the first and second weeks and coronary aneurysms between the second and sixth weeks. The majority of the aneurysms involve the coronary arteries, and most are detected by echocardiography.
- Sequelae include pericardial effusion with decreased ventricular function and failure, aneurysmal thrombosis or rupture leading to infarction, and arrhythmias.

Anesthetic considerations

- Children requiring anesthesia should be managed like adults with coronary artery disease.
- Tachycardia and myocardial depression may precipitate ischemia.
- A calibrated ECG or ST segment trending is indicated to monitor for ischemia.

TAKAYASU DISEASE[36]

Description

- Takayasu is a rare form of arteritis, primarily of females, involving the aorta and proximal branches and leading to occlusion.
- The disease can begin in childhood with symptoms of hypertension, cardiomegaly, dyspnea, ocular disturbances, and marked weakening of the pulses in upper extremities.
- Slow progression occurs even with treatment (steroids and cytotoxic drugs). Survival ranges between 1 and 20 years from the onset.

Anesthetic considerations.   Anesthetic considerations include control of hypertension and monitoring and treatment of myocardial ischemia.

CARDIOMYOPATHIES[37]

IDIOPATHIC HYPERTROPHIC SUBAORTIC STENOSIS (IHSS)

Description
- IHSS results from muscular growth of the left ventricular (LV) outflow tract.
- Symptoms of dyspnea, angina on exertion, and orthopnea are most consistently present. Sudden death occurs in 3% to 4% of cases.
- Patients often have some degree of mitral valve incompetence, resulting in a decrease in LV compliance.
- Surgical repair is indicated if the gradient between the LV and the aorta is over 40 mm Hg.

Anesthetic considerations
- The mainstays of treatment are beta blockade (negative inotropy to reduce outflow stenosis and slow heart rate) and maintenance of adequate preload and afterload. Filling volumes must be monitored so that hypovolemia, hypotension, reflex tachycardia, and vasodilation can be avoided.
- Preoperative anxiety should be tempered by premedication.
- Sinus rhythm should be maintained
- Regional anesthesia is not usually advocated, because of the decreased afterload and preload.
- Primary fentanyl techniques help to maintain a slow heart rate with few hemodynamic changes.
- Halothane helps to relax dynamic ventricular outflow and maintain a slow rate. It should be used cautiously with the failing ventricle because of its negative inotropic properties.

CARNITINE DEFICIENCY[38]

Description
- Carnitine is important in the transport of long-chain fatty acids into mitochondria. If it is deficient, cardiac enlargement and failure result.
- The deficiency responds well to L-carnitine therapy, which may improve ventricular function.

Anesthetic considerations
- Fentanyl, which has little effect on myocardial contractility, is usually recommended.
- Inhalation agents are best avoided when significant ventricular failure is present.
- Volume replacement must be sufficient to maintain cardiac output without resulting in pulmonary edema.

ARRHYTHMIAS

Common pediatric arrhythmias

Arrhythmia	Causes	Criteria	Treatment
Asystole	Hypoxia Ischemia Direct myocardial injury Severe electrolyte disturbances Succinylcholine	Isoelectric ECG without complexes	Adequate oxygenation Epinephrine (IV/ETT/intracardiac) Atropine Isoproterenol
Sinus bradycardia	Hypoxia Direct injury to sinus node Increased ICP Acidosis Vagal stimulation	Heart rate: <100 first year of life <80 ages 1-5 <60 over 5 years of age	Adequate oxygenation is first ensured If needed, drug therapy as in asystole Pacing, if needed
Sick sinus	Direct injury Cardiomyopathy Ischemia Myocarditis Digitalis toxicity Congenital anomalies ASD (sinus venosus) • Left atrial isomerism • TGA s/p Senning or Mustard procedures • s/p Fontan procedures	Sinus bradycardia or sinus arrest with modal or ventricular escape rhythms giving rise to tachyarrhythmias Stokes-Adams attacks	Permanent pacemaker, if symptomatic

Continued.

Common pediatric arrhythmias—cont'd

Arrhythmia	Causes	Criteria	Treatment
First-degree A-V block	Digitalis Inferior-wall infarction Hyperkalemia Acute rheumatic fever Calcium channel blocker toxicity	PR—age dependent	Rarely requires treatment
Second-degree heart block Mobitz I	Normal variant Inferior-wall infarction Digoxin excess	Progressive lengthening of PR interval until one P wave is not conducted	Rarely requires treatment
Mobitz II	Conduction pathology distal to bundle of His Anterior-wall infarction	PR intervals are constant before a dropped beat occurs	Permanent pacemaker may be required because progression to complete AV block is frequent
Complete heart block	Digitalis toxicity Connective tissue disease in mother Cardiac tumors Myocarditis L-TGA Left atrial isomerism Encocardial fibroelastosis	Atria and ventricles beat independently Rate of atria is faster than that of ventricle PR interval constantly changes	Isoproterenol Temporary pacemaker Permanent pacemaker
Atrial fibrillation	Wolff-Parkinson-White S/P cardiac surgery (Fontan, Senning) Rheumatic heart disease Mitral valve prolapse Ebstein's anomaly Cardiomyopathy	Rapid irregular ventricular rate; absent P waves	Synchronized cardioversion Anticoagulation required Digoxin Propranolol Verapamil*

Atrial flutter	S/P cardiac surgery (Fontan, Senning) Rheumatic heart disease Mitral valve prolapse Pericarditis Wolff-Parkinson-White	Sawtooth pattern between normal QRS	Digoxin Overdrive pacing (TE or IC) β-blockers (esmolol, propranolol) Cardioversion (synchronized) Ca^{++} channel blockers (verapamil,* diltiazem)
Paroxysmal atrial tachycardia	Often seen in healthy individuals	Three or more consecutive premature atrial contractions	Vagal maneuvers β-blockers (esmolol, propranolol) Ca channel blockers (verapamil,* diltiazem) Edrophonium
Supraventricular tachycardia	Reentry phenomenon through the A-V node or accessory pathways	Regular RR interval Narrow QRS Rate 200-300 in infants, 150-250 in older children	Vagal maneuvers Adenosine β-blockers (esmolol, propranolol) Ca channel blockers (verapamil,* diltiazem)
Frequent premature ventricular contractions and ventricular tachycardia	Ischemia Electrolyte disturbances Cardia tumors Idiopathic hypertrophic subaortic stenosis (IHSS) Long QT Cardiomyopathy	Wide QRS (depending on age) T wave and QRS usually point in opposite directions Often followed by a compensatory pause	Lidocaine Bretylium Phenytoin Procainamide Synchronized cardioversion .5-2 Joules/kg (if hypotensive) Amiodarone

*Contraindicated in children < 1 yr old.

Continued.

Common pediatric arrhythmias—cont'd

Arrhythmia	Causes	Criteria	Treatment
Long QT syndrome	Congenital form: associated with deafness and sudden death Familial tachycardia: QT prolongation occurs only with excessive exercise and not at rest Acquired causes: • Infarction • Myocarditis • Mitral valve prolapse • Head injury • Cervical injury • Adrenal insufficiency • Amyloidosis • Hypothermia • Hypocalcemia • Hypokalemia • Hypomagnesemia • Antiarrhythmic drugs	Depends on heart rate; normally, QT prolongation does not exceed half the PR interval if HR < 80	β-blockers Dilantin Bretylium Pacing Automatic implantable cardiac difibrillation (AICD) Left stellate ganglion block Acquired cases are treated with isoproterenol, correction of disturbance
Torsades de pointes	Electrolyte disturbances Drug toxicity • Quinidine • Disopyramide • Amiodarone	QRS twists and turns in opposite directions	Overdrive atrial pacing Bretylium Electrolyte correction

---

Anesthesia pearls for patients with congenital heart disease

- All air bubbles should be meticulously removed from intravenous tubing to prevent paradoxical air emboli from entering the systemic circulation.
- In general, hyperoxia, hypocapnia, alkalemia, and spontaneous ventilation (or low peak inspiratory pressure) decrease pulmonary vascular resistance and improve pulmonary blood flow.
- In general, a low FIO_2, hypercapnia, acidosis, and positive-pressure ventilation will increase pulmonary vascular resistance and decrease pulmonary blood flow.
- In general, opiate techniques (fentanyl) have the least effect on vascular resistance and myocardial contractility.
- Conduction disturbances are common in children with septal defects, even after repair.
- Although infants and children usually tolerate very rapid heart rates, patients with CHD favor slower heart rates to improve flow across stenotic valves or through narrow shunts.
- The following pharmacokinetic changes can be anticipated with intracardiac shunts:
    1. Intravenous agents may have slower onset times in patients with left-to-right shunts because of continuous dilution in the pulmonary circulation.
    2. Intravenous agents may have more rapid onset times with right-to-left shunts (decreased "vein-to-brain" time).
    3. Although a right-to-left shunt may result in a slower induction with inhalation agents (decreased pulmonary circulation), a left-to-right shunt probably has no effect on induction time if cardiac output is normal. Decreased cardiac output may speed induction with inhalation agents.

References

1. Fixler DE, Talner NS: Epidemiology of congenital heart disease. In Oski FA, ed: *Principles and practice of pediatrics,* Philadelphia, 1990, JB Lippincott, pp 349-352.
2. Daniel WG, Mügge A: Transesophageal echocardiography, *N Engl J Med* 332;1268-1279, 1995.
3. Mahoney LT: Acyanotic congenital heart disease: atrial and ventricular septal defects, atrioventricular canal, patent ductus arteriosus, pulmonic stenosis, *Cardiol Clin* 11:603-616, 1993.
4. Hickey PR, Hansen DD, Strafford M, Thompson JE, Jonas RE, Mayer JE: Pulmonary and systemic hemodynamic effects of nitrous oxide in infants with normal and elevated pulmonary vascular resistance, *Anesthesiology* 65:374-378, 1986.
5. Glenski JA, Friesen RH, Berglund NL, Hassanein RS, Henry DB: Comparison of the hemodynamic and echocardiographic effects of sufentanil, fentanyl, isoflurane, and halothane for pediatric cardiovascular surgery, *J Cardiothorac Anesth* 2:147-155, 1988.
6. Anand KJ, Hickey PR: Halothane-morphine compared with high-dose sufentanil for anesthesia and postoperative analgesia in neonatal cardiac surgery, *N Engl J Med* 329:1-9, 1992.
7. Morray JP, Lynn AM, Stamm SJ, Herndon PS, Kawabori I, Stevenson JG: Hemodynamic effects of ketamine in children with congenital heart disease, *Anesth Analg* 63:895-899, 1984.

8. Rich GF, Murphy Jr GD, Roos CM, Johns RA: Inhaled nitric oxide: selective pulmonary vasodilation in cardiac surgical patients, *Anesthesiology* 78:1028-1035, 1993.

9. Lawson CA, Smerling AJ, Naka Y, et al: Selective reduction of PVR by inhalation of a cGMP analogue in a porcine model of pulmonary hypertension, *Am J Physiol* 268:H2056-H2062, 1995.

10. Armstrong BE: Congenital cardiovascular disease and cardiac surgery in childhood. I: Cyanotic congenital heart defects, *Curr Opin Cardiol* 10:58-67, 1995.

11. Warnes CA: Tetralogy of Fallot and pulmonary atresia/ventricular septal defect, *Cardiol Clin* 11:643-650, 1993.

12. Silove ED: Prostaglandins in paediatric cardiology, *Br J Hosp Med* 45:309-310, 1991.

13. Hickey PR, Hansen DD, Cramolini GM, Vincent RN, Lang P: Pulmonary and systemic hemodynamic responses to ketamine in infants with normal and elevated pulmonary vascular resistance, *Anesthesiology* 62:287-293, 1985.

14. Berman Jr W, Fripp RR, Rubler M, Alderete L: Hemodynamic effects of ketamine in children undergoing cardiac catheterization, *Pediatr Cardiol* 11:72-76, 1990.

15. Pinsky WW, Arciniegas E: Tetralogy of Fallot, *Pediatr Clin North Am* 37:179-192, 1990.

16. Hickey PR, Hansen DD: High-dose fentanyl reduces intraoperative ventricular fibrillation in neonates with hypoplastic left heart syndrome, *J Clin Anesth* 3:295-300, 1991.

17. Hansen DD, Hickey PR: Anesthesia for hypoplastic left heart syndrome, *Anesth Analg* 65:127-132, 1986.

18. Nicolson SC, Jobes DR: Hypoplastic left heart syndrome. In Lake CL, ed: *Pediatric cardiac anesthesia,* Norwalk, Conn, 1993, Appleton & Lange, pp 271-280.

19. Jatene AD, Fontes VF, Sauza LCB, et al: Anatomic correction of transposition of the great vessels, *J Thorac Cardiovasc Surg* 83:20-26, 1982.

20. Kopf GS: Tricuspid atresia. In Mavroudis C, Backer CL, eds: *Pediatric cardiac surgery,* St Louis, 1994, Mosby, pp 379-400.

21. Kopf GS, Kleinman CS, Hijazi ZM, Fahey JT, Dewar ML, Hellenbrand WE: Fenestrated Fontan operation with delayed transcatheter closure of atrial septal defect, *J Thorac Cardiovasc Surg* 103; 1039-1048, 1992.

22. Hosking MP, Raimundo HS, Warner MA, Ensing GJ: Anesthetic management of the modified Fontan operation using an intra-atrial conduit for a single ventricle with anomalous systemic venous return, *J Cardiothorac Anesth* 3:601-606, 1989.

23. Hosking MP, Beynen FM: The modified Fontan procedure: physiology and anesthetic implications, *J Cardiothorac Vasc Anesth* 6:465-475, 1992.

24. Booker PD, Evans C, Franks R: Comparison of the haemodynamic effects of dopamine and dobutamine in young children undergoing cardiac surgery, *Br J Anaesth* 74:419-423, 1995.

25. Norwood WI, Lang P, Hansen DD: Physiologic repair of aortic atresia –hypoplastic left heart syndrome, *N Engl J Med* 308:23-26, 1983.

26. Gersony WM: Ventricular septal defects and left sided obstructive lesions in infants, *Curr Opin Pediatr* 6:596-599, 1994.
27. Kern FH, Gieser WG, Farrell DM: Extracorporeal circulation and circulatory assist devices in the pediatric patient. In Lake CL, ed: *Pediatric cardiac anesthesia,* ed 2, Norwalk, Conn, 1993, Appleton & Lange, pp 151-179.
28. Ferry PC: Neurologic sequelae of open-heart surgery in children: an irritating question, *Am J Dis Child* 144:369-373, 1990.
29. Bellinger DC, Jonas RA, Rappaport LA, et al: Developmental and neurologic status of children after heart surgery with hypothermic circulatory arrest or low-flow cardiopulmonary bypass, *N Engl J Med* 332:549-555, 1995.
30. Bellinger DC, Wernovsky G, Rappaport LA, et al: Cognitive development of children following early repair of transposition of the great arteries using deep hypothermic circulatory arrest, *Pediatrics* 87:701-707, 1991.
31. Karl HW, Hensley Jr. FA, Cyran SE, Frankel CA, Myers JL: Hypoplastic left heart syndrome: anesthesia for elective noncardiac surgery, *Anesthesiology* 72:753-757, 1990.
32. Hickey PR: The patient with congenital heart disease for noncardiac surgery: anesthesia for the reconstructed and unreconstructed heart, *Anesth Analg* 74 (suppl):551-554, 1992.
33. Morris CD, Menashe VD: 25-year mortality after surgical repair of congenital heart defect in childhood: a population-based cohort study, *JAMA* 266:3447-3452, 1991.
34. Burge DJ, DeHoratius RJ: Acute rheumatic fever, *Cardiovasc Clin* 23:3-23, 1993.
35. Kato H, Akagi T, Sugimura T: Kawasaki disease, *Coron Art Dis* 6:194-206, 1995.
36. Hall S, Buchbinder R: Takayasu's arteritis, *Rheum Dis Clin North Am* 16:411-422, 1990.
37. Kelly DP, Strauss AW: Inherited cardiomyopathies, *N Engl J Med* 330:913-919, 1993.
38. Martin A, Haller RG, Barohn R: Metabolic myopathies, *Curr Opin Rheumatol* 6:552-558, 1994.

ANESTHESIA FOR OTOLARYNGOLOGIC SURGERY

8

Brave little Bucky
Tired of being plucky
Wondered how it happened that
He was so unlucky.

Hurt to talk about it,
Brought him close to tears
Pain inside his throat and chest
Pain inside his ears.

Couldn't play in little league
Couldn't splash in water
Angry that he couldn't live
In the way he oughter.

Bucky was frustrated
And he felt degraded
But everything turned right-side up
Once they operated.

Rivian Bell

Otolaryngological procedures are often the most commonly performed operations in children in pediatric medical centers, community hospitals, and free-standing outpatient units. It is easy to classify these operations as "routine" and underestimate their anesthetic difficulty because of their frequent occurrence, short procedure length, and outpatient status. However, these procedures continue to be challenging even to the experienced anesthetist, as the airway is often included in the operative site and many patients present with preexistent airway problems.

DIAGNOSTIC PROCEDURES

Diagnoses of pediatric airway disorders are confirmed by procedures that visualize the anatomic pathology. Radiographs, computerized tomography, and magnetic resonance imaging are sometimes helpful to elucidate airway narrowing, masses, deviation, or presence of a foreign body. Transnasal flexible fiberoptic bronchoscopes may be used with local anesthesia and/or conscious sedation for laryngeal examination in older cooperative children or infants. Usually, general anesthesia is required for direct laryngoscopy and rigid bronchoscopy.

Direct Laryngoscopy/Rigid Bronchoscopy

This typically brief diagnostic procedure is always challenging to the anesthetist. Airway patency must be maintained in the absence of an endotracheal tube, and the airway must be relinquished to the operating surgeon. Usually, spontaneous ventilation is preferred to assure visualization of vocal cord mobility. The size of the bronchoscope refers to its internal lumen, with the smallest having a 4-mm external diameter and a 3.2-mm internal diameter (e.g., Storz).

PROCEDURE

1. Premedication is avoided when there are concerns about compromising spontaneous ventilation.
2. A gentle inhalation induction is preferred, halothane offering the least airway irritability. An FIO_2 of 1.0 is used if respiratory insufficiency or airway compromise is present. An intravenous induction with incremental doses of propofol will also maintain spontaneous ventilation.
3. Intravenous atropine (10 to 20 µg/kg) is given to infants to prevent the bradycardia that accompanies laryngeal stimulation. Glycopyrrolate (10 to 20 µg/kg) may be useful as an antisialogue in older children.
4. It is difficult to maintain general anesthesia at a depth sufficient for laryngeal stimulation and still maintain spontaneous ventilation. Topical lidocaine spray to the vocal cords will help to minimize reactivity. Because nebulized drugs are rapidly absorbed through the lungs, lidocaine doses should be the same as for intravenous use (1.0 to 1.5 mg/kg).
5. The rigid bronchoscope is placed under direct vision by the operating surgeon, using a laryngoscope. An oxyscope (laryngoscope that delivers oxygen through a side port) may be useful. Primary intubation of the trachea before bronchoscopy may be important when the airway must be rapidly secured because of obstruction or respiratory compromise. Avoiding pre-bronchoscopy intubation in the healthy patient will minimize subglottic trauma and subsequent edema.
6. The anesthesia circuit can be connected to the rigid bronchoscope from a proximal side port (see Figure 8-1). The increase in dead space caused by the bronchoscope makes it difficult to maintain anesthetic depth using inhalation agents alone. As an adjunct, incremental boluses or an infusion of intravenous

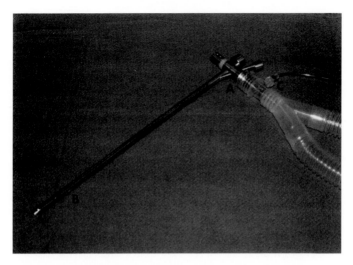

FIG. 8-1.   The anesthesia circuit can be connected to the rigid broncho-scope from the proximal side port (**A**). With the telescope removed, venti-lation is easily accomplished when all of the distal holes are placed below the level of the vocal cords (**B**). Although capnography can be monitored at the proximal port (**C**), the increased dead space caused by the broncho-scope may increase the alveolar–end tidal CO_2 difference.

> propofol allows tolerance of the bronchoscope, spontaneous ventilation, and rapid drug clearance.

7. Use of 100% oxygen while the bronchoscope is in the trachea offers a margin of reserve against possible hypoxia. Higher concentrations of halogenated agents may be needed both during instrumentation of the airway and while the patient is receiving 100% oxygen. Using higher concentrations of in-halation agents demands careful monitoring of exhaled gas concentrations to avoid administering toxic doses.

8. Hypercapnia frequently occurs because passive ventilation is difficult with the high airway resistance caused by the narrow bronchoscope. Capnography can be obtained at the side port, although the increased dead space caused by the broncho-scope will affect the accuracy of the capnogram.

9. Insertion of the telescope into the bronchoscope worsens air-way resistance. Resultant air trapping can lead to pneumotho-rax or impede venous return. The surgeon may need to remove the telescope at intermittent intervals so that the pa-tient can be adequately ventilated.

10. An *open bronchoscope* delivers oxygen through a high-pressure source. Room air is entrained by the Venturi effect. The actual delivered FIO_2 depends on the amount of entrained room air. The amount of gas delivered will decrease in less

compliant lungs. For children, spontaneous or assisted ventilation through a ventilating bronchoscope is preferred to jet
ventilation through an open bronchoscope because of the risk
of barotrauma, air trapping, and hypoxia.

11. Upon removal of the bronchoscope, an anesthesia mask can
be used to assist ventilation and deliver oxygen during emergence. Some anesthetists will prefer to intubate the trachea
with an endotracheal tube prior to emergence. Intubation
would be preferred if airway compromise, edema, blood, or
secretions are present.

12. Laser excision of lesions in the lower airway is usually accomplished with laryngoscopy under direct vision using the
carbon dioxide laser. Bronchial lesions are less common in
children but can be excised using the fiberoptic-directed YAG
laser. The YAG laser and other types of lasers are listed in the
box below.

Types of laser[1,2,3]

Type	Properties and uses
CO_2	Continuous emission of invisible infrared energy absorbed by water; therefore damages all surface tissue.
Helium-neon	Emits a visible beam of low energy, which does not affect tissue. Used to direct invisible laser beams (CO_2) and to focus x-rays.
Neodymium: yttrium-aluminum-garnett (Nd:YAG)	Pulsed emission preferentially absorbed by hemoglobin or melanin (not water), which can be directed via fiberoptics to tracheobronchial lesions. Primarily used for lower airway tumor debulking.
Pulsed dye	Pulsed emission absorbed by hemoglobin more than melanin; used primarily to target intravascular hemoglobin (port-wine stains).
Argon	Continuous emmision of visible radiation highly absorbed by hemoglobin or pigment and poorly absorbed by water; used on the retina or to photocoagulate large areas and for otologic procedures. May be transmitted fiberoptically.
Ruby	Pulsed emission absorbed by hemoglobin or melanin; also used primarily for ophthalmologic photocoagulation. May be transmitted via fiberoptics.

Anesthetic Techniques for Laser Microsurgery of the Airway

1. An ETT smaller than the calculated size is used.
2. If a cuffed tube is used, the cuff is filled with water, not air. Methylene blue may be added to the water so a leak can be easily detected.
3. A red rubber endotracheal tube is spirally wrapped with aluminum or copper foil tape, or manufactured tubes of stainless steel can be used. Laser-specific silicone tubes have been found to be combustible and should be avoided. Polyvinylchloride (PVC) tubes are not recommended, as they burn easily and release hydrochloric acid.[4,5]
4. Muscle relaxants are used to ensure an immobile surgical field.
5. The patient's eyes are protected with moist pads.
6. The use of O_2 and N_2O is minimized; they are replaced with air to decrease fire hazards.
7. 2.5 to 5.0 cm H_2O PEEP should be added to the breathing circuit during CO_2 laser operations in which wrapped PVC endotracheal tubes are used to reduce the risk of airway fires.[6]
8. The use of highly reflective instruments and mirrors is avoided in the surgical field
9. If a fire occurs, the flow of O_2 is discontinued, the ETT removed, the fire extinguished with saline, and tissue damage assessed with bronchoscopy.

Advantages of laser use

Precision
Lack of bleeding
Complete sterility
Reduced tissue reactions (edema)

Hazards of laser use

Operating room personnel are susceptible to eye injury and must wear protective goggles designed to absorb energy of the wavelength emitted by the laser in use.
Fire is an ever-present hazard even with dye-absorbing lasers. This risk increases in children because of the leak present around the endotracheal tube or the use of mask-assisted ventilation.
Direct laser ignition of the endotracheal tube with resultant airway fire, thermal burns, and smoke inhalation is possible.
Normal tissue can be damaged by reflected or misdirected laser beams.

GENERAL PRINCIPLES OF ANESTHETIC MANAGEMENT FOR AIRWAY PROCEDURES

Anatomic Location of Procedure

1. When providing anesthesia for ENT (ear/nose/throat) procedures, the anesthesiologist must assume that the airway will be shared with the surgical team. The responsibility for maintaining an adequate airway requires vigilance on the part of both teams.
2. The technique selected for airway control (face mask, endotracheal tube, laryngeal mask airway) must protect the airway from blood and obstruction and not hamper surgical visualization or technique, using the least invasive manner so as to minimize further trauma to the surgical field.
3. Securing the airway may also involve a cooperative effort between the surgeon and the anesthesiologist. In some cases the endotracheal tube may be sutured directly to a part of the airway by the surgeon or may be secured by the surgical retractors (e.g., the use of the Dingman gag for tonsillectomy, cleft palate repair).
4. The *anatomic location* of the surgical procedure has direct anesthetic implications:
   a. Lesions in the nose are easily anesthetized topically, allowing for decreased anesthetic requirements and hemostasis. For nasal procedures the airway can be secured orally without interfering with the surgical procedure.
   b. Oropharyngeal lesions may increase the difficulties of intubation or maintaining mask ventilation. Endotracheal tube security may be breached during the surgical procedure. Throat packs may help to decrease aspiration of blood, tissue, or secretions, particularly in young children, in whom a leak around the endotracheal tube is desirable. Delivered oxygen concentration should be kept as low as possible when electrocautery is being used in the oropharynx, to avoid fires.
   c. Procedures of the larynx, trachea, and bronchi necessitate the greatest anesthetic depth to prevent airway hyperreactivity. The ability to maintain anesthetic depth is complicated by the fact that spontaneous ventilation may also be required. These procedures carry significant risk of pulmonary compromise.

Induction Techniques

1. Inhalation inductions are commonly used in children undergoing otolaryngologic procedures in the situations listed below.

Halothane is selected most frequently because it causes the least amount of airway reactivity.

    a. Simple, brief procedures such as myringotomy and tube placement often can be completed safely with inhalation anesthesia without placing an intravenous catheter.

    b. In children with airway edema or foreign body, inhalation agents may improve bronchodilation and decrease airway reactivity.

    c. In children with airway emergencies, an inhalation induction allows for continuous maintenance of spontaneous ventilation and delivery of high concentrations of oxygen.

2. An intravenous induction may be more appropriate in the following situations:

    a. Removal of esophageal foreign bodies or lesions without airway compromise, but with risk of aspiration.

    b. In upper airway obstruction (e.g., large adenoids) when mask ventilation may be very difficult, but uneventful intubation is anticipated.

    c. As an adjunct to inhalation agents when it is difficult to reach desired anesthetic depth either because of delivery dead space (bronchoscopy) or because airway obstruction limits gas delivery. The judicious use of propofol in these scenarios may allow increased anesthetic depth and preserve spontaneous ventilation.

Commonly Anticipated Complications

Recognition and treatment of sequelae that occur after ENT procedures must also be shared by the anesthesiologist and surgeon. These include:

1. *Airway edema or obstruction:* The airway may be marginal because of postintubation subglottic edema (see also p. 105), the surgical procedure (e.g., cleft palate repair), surgical packing to the nose, or persistence of the preoperative disorder. Steroids rarely have any immediate effect on airway edema. Positioning children in a lateral or prone position may relieve some airway obstruction. Humidified oxygen should always be administered to help decrease edema and assist oxygenation.

2. *Bleeding:* Intraoperative aspiration of blood into the lungs is a particular risk in the young child with an uncuffed endotracheal tube. Throat packs help to minimize this possibility. Postoperatively, blood loss from the nose, mouth, or pharynx is often insidious, and blood may be swallowed without complaint by the drowsy child. Positioning in the prone or lateral position during recovery will allow recognition of bleeding.

3. *Nausea and vomiting:* Children undergoing tonsillectomy or otologic procedures are particularly vulnerable to postoperative nausea and vomiting, persisting after discharge from the postanesthesia care unit (see p. 101).

The Difficult Airway

Children with craniofacial deformities are often seen repeatedly for corrective procedures. The difficult airway in children differs from that in adults in that the upper airway is usually involved (micrognathia, small oral aperture, macroglossia, etc.). Furthermore, most children are not cooperative for awake fiberoptic intubations, even with sedation.

1. Awake intubation after administration of atropine is used most commonly for neonates with complicated airways. An oxyscope, which administers oxygen during laryngoscopy, is useful. The lightwand or laryngeal mask airway may assist in blind or fiberoptic tube placement if direct laryngoscopy is not successful. (See also pp. 43, 47, and 383.)

2. In older children, an inhalation induction with maintenance of spontaneous ventilation is usually advocated. Because the structural abnormalities are usually in the upper airway, mask ventilation may not be problematic. Preoperative placement of an intravenous catheter may be advisable. Halothane is usually selected as the agent least likely to cause airway irritability. Because of its high solubility, a lengthy induction is often required to reach anesthetic depth sufficient for laryngoscopy (either direct or fiberoptic). Topical anesthesia may help to decrease anesthetic requirements during laryngoscopy. Because of rapid absorption from the bronchial tree, lidocaine doses should be equivalent to intravenous to avoid toxicity (1.0 to 1.5 mg/kg).

3. The light wand (lighted stylet) is useful for blind intubations in children, as the relative sparsity of tissue anterior to the larynx makes accurately locating the light easier (see also p. 43) (see Fig. 8-2).

4. The laryngeal mask airway has also been advocated for use in children whose tracheas may be difficult to intubate. A blindly placed LMA serves as an easy guide for the fiberoptic bronchoscope. Two endotracheal tubes are placed in tandem over the fiberoptic scope, as the LMA tube is too long to remove over a single endotracheal tube (see Fig. 8-3). Pediatric flexible bronchoscopes are available with outside diameters as small as 2.7 mm to pass through endotracheal tubes with 3.0-mm internal diameters.

5. Cricothyrotomy is the technique of choice in emergent situations with an acutely obstructed airway when ventilation by other techniques has failed. This procedure may be quite

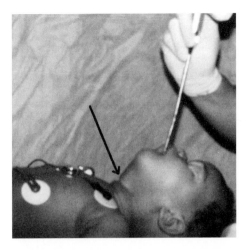

FIG. 8-2. The light wand can be passed blindly into the trachea of a child whose larynx is difficult to visualize with direct laryngoscopy. The light source is easily visualized in the anterior neck *(arrow)* when the light wand is correctly positioned.

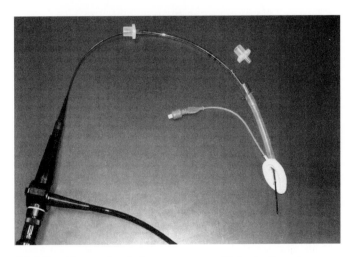

FIG. 8-3. A laryngeal mask airway serves as a guide for the fiberoptic bronchoscope when the larynx is poorly visualized. Two endotracheal tubes will be needed for intubation, in tandem over the fiberoptic scope and through the LMA. After successful tracheal intubation the LMA is removed, the two endotracheal tubes are separated, and the hub is replaced for connection to the anesthetic circuit.

difficult in the infant, whose trachea is small, pliable, and obscured by the soft tissue of the anterior neck. The hub of a 14-g intravenous catheter will attach directly to a 3.5-mm endotracheal tube adapter and connect directly to the anesthetic circuit (see Fig. 8-4). A small skin nick with a no. 15 surgical blade will eliminate skin resistance and facilitate placement of the IV catheter within the tracheal lumen. Tracheostomy is an elective surgical procedure not indicated in emergent situations.

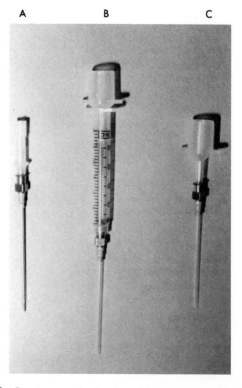

FIG. 8-4. Percutaneous cricothyrotomy. In an emergency, a 14-g intravenous catheter (**A**) can be converted for tracheal ventilation. A 3-ml syringe attached to the catheter allows for confirmation of placement in the trachea by aspiration of air. An anesthesia circuit or jet ventilator can be attached to the syringe by removing the plunger and adding an 8-mm ETT adapter (**B**). A 3.5-mm ETT adapter can be attached directly to the 14-g catheter (after the needle is removed) (**C**). Elimination of the 3-ml syringe decreases dead space and makes it easier to hold the catheter securely with one hand without kinking or dislodging.

6. Percutaneous transtracheal jet ventilation consisting of a jet injector and wall oxygen source at 50 psi is frequently advocated as the system of choice for rapidly establishing ventilation emergently.[7] These systems require that the natural airway be patent for passive exhalation, which is often not the case in children with airway obstruction (e.g., papillomas of the larynx). The rapid delivery of high-pressure oxygen to the lungs of an infant or small child (particularly without a source of egress) could result in barotrauma and pneumothoraces. In many cases it may be safer to ventilate more gradually using the anesthesia circuit, even though hypercapnia may result, until the percutaneous airway is converted to a tracheostomy.

Tracheostomy[8,9]

The indications for tracheostomy in children include:
1. Chronic airway obstruction, such as in laryngomalacia or bilateral vocal cord palsy
2. Pulmonary toilet when chronic ventilator support is required
3. As part of major head and neck surgery (e.g., cystic hygroma)
4. To urgently secure the airway when a temporary emergent airway has been obtained (e.g., after cricothyrotomy)
5. Rarely for prolonged ventilation, as nasotracheal intubation is well tolerated in children for long periods

ANESTHETIC TECHNIQUE
FOR TRACHEOSTOMY

1. The preferred surgical position is supine with the neck hyperextended. As the innominate vessels cross the trachea higher in children, the incision is often made lower in the neck than for adults.[8]
2. In this position, it may be possible to maintain general inhalation anesthesia by mask with spontaneous ventilation. Use of local anesthesia to the surgical site and the larynx decreases anesthetic requirements.
3. In children with pliable tracheas, tracheostomy is facilitated if the trachea is stented by an endotracheal tube. It is easier to intubate the trachea prior to positioning for tracheostomy.
4. Alternative methods of airway management should be available, including cricothyrotomy, jet ventilation, rigid bronchoscopy, light wand, and laryngeal mask airway.

Comparison of tracheostomy and endotracheal tubes

Approximate age of child	Tracheostomy tube (Shiley) size (ID mm)	Endotracheal tube size (mm)
Preterm	00(3.1)	3.0
Newborn to 3 mo	0(3.4)	3.5
3-10 mo	1(3.7)	4.0
10-12 mo	2(4.1)	4.5
13-24 mo	3(4.8)	5.0
2-9 yr	4(5.5)	5.5-6.5
>10 yr	6(7.0)	7.0-8.0

Adapted from Stool SE, Eavey RD: Tracheotomy. In Bluestone CD, Stool SE, Scheetz MD, eds: *Pediatric otolaryngology,* ed 2, Philadelphia, 1990, WB Saunders, pp 1226-1243.

CONGENITAL DISORDERS OF THE AIRWAY
Choanal Atresia[10,11]

1. Choanal atresia usually is not associated with other anomalies. It occurs in approximately 1 in 8000 births, when the bony or membranous portions of the nasopharynx fail to perforate during development. Because of the neonate's dependence upon nasal breathing, the child is cyanotic at rest and pink with crying.
2. Choanal atresia may occasionally be associated with Apert's or Crouzan's syndrome and is part of the CHARGE syndrome (*C*oloboma, *H*eart disease, *A*tresia choanae, *R*etarded growth, *G*enital abnormalities, *E*ar abnormalities).
3. Functional choanal obstruction can occur following traumatic suctioning and is managed conservatively with cool mist and topical vasoconstrictors such as phenylephrine.
4. Unilateral obstruction may be unrecognized.
5. The diagnosis usually is made shortly after birth, when a catheter fails to pass into the nasopharynx.
6. Early surgical repair is necessary to prevent respiratory distress. If respiratory distress develops, the airway should be secured by an oral airway or awake endotracheal intubation.

Cystic Hygroma[12]

Cystic hygroma is a congenital dysplasia of the lymphatics, consisting of multiple cavernous cysts that contain serous, serosanguinous, or bloody fluid. Hygromas are usually located in the posterior triangle of the neck (60% to 70%) or in communication with the axilla (20% to 30%). They can also be found, although rarely, in the anterior triangle of the neck with intraoral involvement. Present at birth, these hygromas can rapidly enlarge as a result of bleeding, infection, or fluid accumulation. The extent of the lesion and the existence of any mediastinal or oral involvement are determined during the preoperative evaluation.

If possible, surgery is delayed until age 18 to 24 months because spontaneous regression can occur in the interim. Surgery is necessary at an earlier age if the airway is obstructed either directly by the mass or by compression of surrounding tissues.

Neonates with large hygromas undergo awake tracheal intubation after administration of atropine. Older children may undergo inhalation induction, spontaneous ventilation being maintained until intubation is accomplished. The prognosis is poor for neonates with massive hygromas, as fluid usually reaccumulates in cystic areas after initial resection, necessitating long-term tracheostomy.

Laryngomalacia[13]

Laryngomalacia results from flaccid supraglottic laryngeal cartilage (epiglottic and aryepiglottic), which infolds with inspiration. It occurs as a result of retardation of tissue development and involves no underlying tissue pathology. High-pitched inspiratory stridor usually appears within the first few days or weeks of life. Crying aggravates symptoms; a prone position alleviates them. Rigid laryngo-bronchoscopy may be performed if severe stridor is present, to rule out other treatable causes (see p. 176 for anesthetic management). The condition usually resolves spontaneously between 12 and 24 months. Tracheostomy may be required if severe neonatal obstruction is present.

Head extension, jaw thrust, and continuous positive airway pressure can help alleviate acute episodes of obstruction. The flexible fiberoptic nasopharyngoscope may be used for diagnostic purposes, in which case general anesthesia is not usually needed.

Tracheomalacia[14]

Tracheomalacia is an uncommon anomaly, leading to collapse of the trachea during expiration and stridor. Rarely found as a primary deficit, it is more commonly associated with tracheoesophageal fistulas, extrinsic compression by vascular anomalies or mediastinal masses, Ehlers-Danlos syndrome, or Hunter's syndrome, or following prolonged tracheal intubation. The trachea stiffens with age, obviating the need for surgery in most children. Occasionally tracheostomy, vascular suspension of the aorta or innominate arteries, or implantation of a splint is necessary.

Laryngeal Web, or Laryngeal Atresia[15]

Complete laryngeal atresia requires immediate tracheostomy or bronchoscopy and may be an unrecognized cause of stillbirths. Diagnosis is made by direct laryngoscopy. A weak cry or aphonia at birth may be indicative of partial obstruction. Simple membranous webs can be treated by surgical endoscopic division. Thicker webs tend to recur and may require tracheostomy or laryngofissure with insertion of a prosthetic implant.

Cleft Lip and Palate[16-18]

1. The presence of isolated cleft palate may be associated with umbilical hernia, club feet, ear defects, and syndromes such as Pierre Robin and Klippel-Feil. Cleft lips are repaired surgically in early infancy. The repair of cleft palates is delayed until age 1 or later, preferably before children learn language skills.

2. An inhalation induction is typically selected. Because the nasopharynx forms a large continuous cavity, mask ventilation and intubation are not usually difficult with isolated cleft palate lesions. Difficulty may be encountered in the presence of micrognathia or associated dysmorphic syndromes. Careful stabilization of the endotracheal tube is particularly important because the tube is present in the operative site and subject to dislodgment during surgical repair.

3. The surgical site is commonly infiltrated with local anesthetic with epinephrine to provide hemostasis. The arrhythmogenic dose of epinephrine in children receiving halothane has yet to be determined, but at least 10 µg/kg of epinephrine may be safely used in normocapnic or hypocapnic pediatric patients who have no history of congenital heart disease. Tachycardia and premature atrial contractions have been reported with the use of halothane and epinephrine, without significant consequence.[19] Blood loss is usually not excessive, but may increase when a velopharyngeal flap is used to close palatal defects.

4. All pharyngeal packs are removed before extubation. Awake tracheal extubation reduces the chances of postextubation airway collapse, which may necessitate nasal airway placement and damage the repair. Some degree of upper airway obstruction is anticipated after palatal closure. Obstruction may be worsened by residual neuromuscular blockade or residual inhalation anesthetics, which relax the glossopharyngeus muscle causing the tongue to obstruct the posterior pharynx.[20] A strong suture is often placed in the tongue at the end of the operative procedure so that the tongue can be manually retracted if airway obstruction occurs in the postoperative period. Placing the child in the lateral or prone position may also decrease obstruction. Usually obstruction improves during the first 24 hours after repair as the swelling decreases and the child adapts to a smaller nasopharyngeal airway. Macroglossia and progressive airway obstruction have been reported after lengthy use of oral tongue retractors and necessitate prolonged postoperative intubation.[21]

Subglottic Hemangiomas[22,23]

Congenital hemangiomas occur in the laryngeal and subglottic regions of young infants. This diagnosis is suspected in those with a fluctuating pattern of respiratory obstruction, inspiratory stridor, and cutaneous hemangiomas. Spontaneous regression by the age of 2 years is typical. Resection with a CO_2 laser or cryoprobe, with concurrent use of systemic steroids, may become necessary. An inhalation induction, with gentle placement of the endotracheal tube to avoid bleeding, is indicated.

Cysts

Cysts (supraglottic, subglottic, or laryngocele) are not uncommon in premature infants who have had a long history of prolonged intubation. Induction of anesthesia and airway management are as for other airway lesions.

Subglottic Stenosis[24] (see also p. 190)

Congenital subglottic stenosis may cause neonatal respiratory distress that usually is less acute than with a web. The severity of stenosis usually is determined by bronchoscopy, requiring general anesthesia. Mask inhalation induction with gentle assisted ventilation helps to keep the airway from further soft-tissue obstruction. Lidocaine aerosol or spray can be applied directly to the trachea during laryngoscopy to minimize airway reactivity. A 3-ml syringe with an IV catheter attached can be used for lidocaine spray (maximum dosage: 1.0 to 1.5 ml/kg).

The surgical management of subglottic stenosis includes tracheostomy, with a series of tracheal dilations or initial tracheostomy followed by a laryngotracheoplasty with costal cartilage grafting when the child is older. An anterior cricoid cartilage split is sometimes performed in a larger neonate (>1500 g) who fails extubation attempts and does not have stenosis significant enough to warrant a tracheostomy. Complications of tracheal dilation are life threatening and include tracheal rupture, pneumothorax, and pneumomediastinum.

ACQUIRED AIRWAY DISORDERS

Macroglossia[25]

CAUSES

1. The term macroglossia broadly describes a tongue too large for the oral cavity. Primary macroglossia is a benign condition, generally not requiring surgical correction until later in childhood for orthodontic or speech problems. Secondary macroglossia arises from several causes, the most common of which is congenital lymphangioma (cystic hygroma, see p. 186).

2. A lingual thyroid may also cause macroglossia and occurs as an incomplete migration of thyroid tissue from its original po-

sition at the base of the tongue. More common in females, the mass may cause dysphagia and bleeding, although small tumors can be asymptomatic. Following thyroid function tests and radionuclide scanning, thyroid supplementation usually shrinks the gland.

3. Sublingual salivary, dermoid, and epidermal cysts may also cause macroglossia. They are either treated with marsupialization or excised.

4. Solid glossal tumors including hemangiomas, fibromatosis, and fibrolipomatous dysplasia are rare in children, as are childhood malignant tumors such as lingual carcinoma and rhabdomyosarcoma.

ANESTHETIC MANAGEMENT

1. Awake intubation is the safest approach to airway management. Occasionally, primary tracheostomy with local anesthesia is necessary. Lesions involving the neck make preoperative tracheostomy difficult if not impossible to perform.

2. Intraoperative blood loss may be significant. Pharyngeal packing during surgery may obstruct the airway or kink the endotracheal tube.

3. Postoperative edema and swelling, particularly if the operation involves the posterior tongue, require prolonged intubation or tracheostomy.

Subglottic Stenosis[24] (see also p. 189)

Although subglottic stenosis may be congenital, it is most often iatrogenic, usually due to prolonged intubation. Acquired subglottic stenosis is generally more severe and more difficult to treat than congenital. Infants often present at 2 to 3 months of age, when an upper respiratory infection causes sufficient airway edema to make the croupy cough or stridor become very noticeable. Diagnosis is confirmed in the presence of normal laryngoscopy, with stenosis seen on bronchoscopy.

Mild stenosis usually resolves with growth. Symptomatic stenosis is treated with tracheostomy below the area of stenosis. Antibiotics and steroids are usually administered for several weeks in an effort to resolve chronic scarring. These children often undergo multiple surgical procedures for visualization of the stenosis and eventual repair or decannulation.

ANESTHETIC MANAGEMENT

1. Patients with severe stenosis generally come to the operating room with tracheostomy in situ and therefore a secure airway.

2. The anesthesia circuit can be directly connected to the tracheostomy, or a gooseneck adapter can be used for inhalation induction. If the surgical procedure so dictates, the tracheostomy tube can be changed to an endotracheal tube after induction.

3. Direct endolaryngoscopy to visualize the stenotic area and remove any resectable granulation tissue is usually accomplished first. If the lesion is not repairable by this route, an external incision is made superior to the tracheostomy site through the cricoid cartilage (cricoid split).
4. The internal laryngo-tracheal surface is cored and denuded of scar tissue. It may be resurfaced with epithelium to prevent reformation of scar. Silastic stents or rib cartilage may be used to widen the narrowed cricoid area. Repeat procedures are needed to remove the stent.
5. The tracheostomy is left in place at the termination of the procedure. Because the airway is secure, the patient can be allowed to emerge in the recovery or intensive care area.
6. Decannulation is accomplished by changing to progressively smaller tracheostomy tubes over time.
7. Perioperative stress steroid coverage may be needed for patients who have received courses of steroids preoperatively.

Vocal Cord Paralysis[26]

Unilateral paralysis is more frequent than bilateral and suggests peripheral nerve injury. It is more common on the left because of the long course of the recurrent laryngeal nerve under the aortic arch. Left-sided paralysis may be indicative of cardiac, pulmonary, or esophageal anomalies. The occurrence of right-sided vocal cord paralysis after right-sided carotid artery cannulation for extracorporeal membrane oxygenation has also been described.

Bilateral paralysis is associated with central nervous system disease such as hydrocephalus, Arnold-Chiari malformation, intracerebral hemorrhage, encephalocele, and dysgenesis of the nucleus ambiguus.

Symptoms of unilateral paralysis include a weak cry, occasional choking, stridor, and coughing. Marked stridor, cyanosis with feeding, and intermittent aspiration are more common with bilateral paralysis. The diagnosis is made by direct laryngoscopy. If obstruction or aspiration is persistent, tracheostomy may be necessary.

Tumors
PAPILLOMATOSIS[3]

1. Juvenile papillomatoses are multiple tumorous growths with viral etiology found in the larynx, pharynx, trachea, and occasionally the lung tissue of children.
2. Although classified as benign entities, the nature of these tumors is aggressive and recurrent. The disease is self-limited, and most cases enter remission in puberty.
3. Hoarseness is usually the first symptom, and progressive respiratory obstruction often occurs.

4. Frequent endoscopic removal is required, often by laser excision (see p. 178 for types and principles of lasers). Spontaneous ventilation should be maintained to avoid pushing polypoid lesions into an already compromised airway.
5. A protected endotracheal tube for use with laser equipment should be selected, often several sizes smaller than age-predicted because of laryngeal narrowing by papillomas.
6. Tracheostomy may be required for severe obstruction but involves the risk of papilloma virus seeding the trachea.

ANGIOFIBROMAS[27]

Angiofibromas are the most common benign tumor of the nasopharynx in children, often presenting with episodic epistaxis in adolescent males. Controlled hypotension with nitroprusside is a useful technique to minimize bleeding during excision of this tumor. Intraoperative monitoring of the central venous pressure, arterial pressure, and hematocrit is essential during controlled hypotension (see p. 264). Surgery is usually staged, with initial devascularization followed later by transpalatal excision. Since the tumor is thought to be androgen dependent, preoperative estrogens have also been used.

Tonsillar Hypertrophy

Airway obstruction and recurrent infection are indications for tonsillectomy. Patients with chronic tonsillitis do not necessarily exhibit signs of sleep apnea and airway obstruction.

OBSTRUCTIVE SLEEP APNEA[28,29]

1. During rapid-eye-movement (REM) sleep, brief periods of apnea lasting less than 10 seconds are frequently seen in normal children. Pathologic apnea, however, is of longer duration and occurs frequently throughout the sleep cycle.
2. The definition of obstructive sleep apnea syndrome may vary from institution to institution, but is is usually defined as multiple apneic periods, each occurring for more than 10 seconds, during several consecutive hours of sleep. Other symptoms of the syndrome include excessive daytime sleepiness, enuresis, hyperactivity, declining school performance, and behavioral changes.
3. Sleep apnea can be classified as central, obstructive, or mixed. The majority of apneic events in children (excluding premature neonates) are of an obstructive nature. Although causes include enlarged tonsils and adenoids, choanal atresia or stenosis, nasal hamartomas or tumors, enlarged tongue, cleft palates, temporomandibular joint (TMJ) dysfunction, and facial anomalies, two thirds of children with obstructive sleep apnea respond to tonsillectomy and adenoidectomy.

4. Cor pulmonale can occur secondary to upper airway obstruction as a result of hypoxic pulmonary vasoconstriction during periods of apnea. With repeated episodes, the increased pulmonary vascular resistance can become chronic, with resultant dilatation and hypertrophy of the right side of the heart.

5. Changes in respiratory physiology are often seen in patients with obstructive sleep apnea. It is not uncommon to see a decreased CO_2 ventilatory response with CO_2 retention and dependence on hypoxic ventilatory drive. These changes involve a central component in the pathogenesis of obstructive apnea, perhaps implying mixed etiologies.

6. It is not uncommon for children with Down syndrome to have sleep apnea. It should not be assumed that tonsillectomy and adenoidectomy will relieve these symptoms. A central component or macroglossia can be part of the etiology.

TONSILLECTOMY/ADENOIDECTOMY

As indications for this previously routine procedure have become more stringent, anesthetic risks have also increased proportionately.

Preoperative evaluation.   Children undergoing tonsillectomy for recurrent infections (chronic tonsillitis) must be distinguished from those with a history of obstruction. Patients with a history of extreme obstructive symptoms and sleep apnea may benefit from a preoperative sleep study to document hypoxia, hypercapnia, incidence and duration of apnea, and central versus obstructive components. Echocardiography may also be indicated to determine presence of right heart dilatation or failure from chronic obstruction. Children with right heart failure are particularly susceptible to postobstructive (negative-pressure) pulmonary edema (see p. 106) and to volume overload. Judgment is required in managing the child with mild obstructive symptoms (such as snoring) in whom a preoperative sleep study has not been obtained.

Procedure/anesthetic management

Premedication.   Premedication should be used judiciously, if at all, in children with sleep apnea.

Induction.   A mask inhalation induction before intravenous (IV) cannulation is usually preferred by most children and parents. In extreme adeno-tonsillar hypertrophy, the nose may be completely obstructed and the mouth must be kept open during induction. Early placement of an oral airway during Stage I or II may induce coughing or laryngospasm. Airway obstruction during spontaneous ventilation may precipitate negative-pressure pulmonary edema. In these cases, an IV induction might be less hazardous, as visualization of the vocal cords and intubation are rarely difficult even with severe hypertrophy.

Maintenance.   A primary opioid anesthetic technique helps to provide postoperative analgesia. However, in patients with sleep apnea, intraoperative opioids should probably be avoided.

Emergence.   In healthy patients, tracheal extubation while they are deeply anesthetized may minimize trauma to the open surgical wound (tonsillar bed) that can result from coughing or "bucking" on the tube. However, most anesthesiologists feel the patient should have reflexes intact before extubation, because of the presence of blood and secretions in the airway. A history of sleep apnea demands a full emergence with intact reflexes and normal ventilatory pattern before tracheal extubation. In either case, it is best to minimize airway trauma that may be caused by vigorous suction or airway placement.[30] Emergence and extubation in the lateral position help to visualize secretions and bleeding and prevent aspiration. In this position, pooled secretions can be removed by suction of the buccal sulcus (cheek) rather than along the tonsil beds.

Postoperative problems

Vomiting.   The incidence of vomiting after tonsillectomy has been reported to exceed 50%[31] and may necessitate postoperative admission. The incidence and frequency of emesis may increase after discharge from the PACU. Metoclopramide (0.15 mg/kg) and ondansetron (50 to 100 µg/kg) have been shown to decrease vomiting,[32,33] whereas droperidol and pre-emergence gastric emptying have not been as effective.[31] Opioid administration even in small doses may increase vomiting, but the use of N_2O appears to have no effect.[34] Admission is necessary if vomiting prevents adequate oral hydration.

Pain.   Severity of post-tonsillectomy pain depends on several factors, including chronicity of infection and surgical technique. In one series, preincisional infiltration of bupivacaine into the fascia prior to tonsillectomy and adenoidectomy reduced pain acutely and for several days, as compared with controls.[35] Intraoperative nonsteroidal antiinflammatory drugs are not recommended, as they may increase bleeding.[36] Opioids may increase vomiting.[31] Usually pain is resolved by 7 to 10 days with sloughing of the eschar. Admission may be necessary if pain prevents adequate oral hydration.

Bleeding.   Post-tonsillectomy bleeding usually occurs either in the first 8 hours postoperatively or approximately 1 week later, when the eschar retracts (see also p. 106).[37,38]

Airway obstruction.   Overnight observation with apnea monitoring and oximetry is recommended for patients with tonsillectomy and/or adenoidectomy who have documented obstructive sleep apnea or meet any of the following high-risk criteria[39]:

1. Less than 2 years old
2. Craniofacial abnormalities affecting the pharyngeal airway
3. Failure to thrive
4. Hypotonia
5. Cor pulmonale

6. Morbid obesity
7. Previous airway trauma or an SaO_2 nadir <70%
8. Undergoing a uvulopalatopharyngoplasty, in addition to tonsillectomy and adenoidectomy
9. Respiratory disturbance index $\geq$ 40 (no. of apneic events and breathing related arousals/total hours of sleep)

FOREIGN BODY ASPIRATION[40-42]

1. Foreign body aspiration is common in children between 1 and 4 years of age. Any recent aspiration of a foreign body is considered urgent because of the possibility of obstruction, edema, or dislodgment. Emergent removal is indicated when a sharp object has been aspirated or in the presence of hemoptysis, dyspnea, or cyanosis. A peanut, because it releases inflammatory mediators, frequently causes pneumonitis and should also be urgently removed.
2. Most foreign bodies (95%) lodge in the right mainstem bronchus. The obstruction can be partial, producing wheezing that is unresponsive to bronchodilators. A greater degree of obstruction can result in a ball-valve phenomenon, leading to gas trapping and hyperinflation. Atelectasis results from more complete distal obstruction.
3. Most foreign bodies (90%) are radiolucent. Fluoroscopy or chest radiographs during exhalation, to look for air trapping on the obstructed side, are useful in making the diagnosis. Chronic cough and recurrent pneumonia are often the manifestations of a foreign body when there is no known history of aspiration.
4. The remaining 5% of foreign bodies lodge in the trachea, and are usually prevented from further passage through the trachea by their large size. Cough, voice change, drooling due to painful swallowing, and partial or complete obstruction can result.
5. Esophageal foreign bodies can produce obstruction at the level of the aortic arch or cricopharyngeus, producing drooling and dysphagia.
6. Foreign bodies are generally removed by direct laryngoscopy/ rigid bronchoscopy (see p. 176). Inhalation induction with maintenance of spontaneous ventilation may be prolonged, depending on the degree of airway obstruction. Avoidance of nitrous oxide is advised to prevent expansion of trapped gas. Intravenous atropine (10 to 20 $\mu g/kg$) helps to minimize secretions and prevent reflex bradycardia. Lidocaine spray provides additional topical anesthesia. Intravenous propofol also helps to maintain anesthetic depth.
7. The use of muscle relaxants during removal of a foreign body from the airway is controversial. Positive-pressure ventilation

can lodge the foreign body more distally or result in obstruction of a previously patent airway. Conversely, an ill-timed cough when grasping a fragile foreign body in the distal bronchus may cause it to fragment and shower particles throughout lung tissue. The surgeon and the anesthetist should discuss the planned technique and contingencies before starting the procedure.

INFECTIOUS AND IMMUNE DISORDERS

Epiglottitis[43,44]

1. Epiglottitis is an acute, life-threatening infection of the supraglottic area, usually due to *Haemophilus influenzae.* The region becomes edematous and inflamed, leading to the sudden onset of sore throat, fever, inspiratory stridor, and respiratory distress. Typically, the child will be leaning forward to breathe, drooling, and appearing quite toxic. The age of onset is usually 2 to 8 years. There is no seasonal predilection.

2. The patient should be kept calm and comforted by the parents. Radiographic studies and physical examination, including attempts to visualize the epiglottis, should be deferred because of the potential for laryngospasm and irrevocable loss of the airway.

3. A physician with the ability to perform emergent cricothyrotomy/tracheostomy in children should always be in attendance.

4. The patient is brought into the operating room under the supervision of an experienced anesthesiologist and surgeon.

5. The induction may be performed with the child sitting upright, possibly on a parent's lap to decrease anxiety. Forcing the child into a supine position may precipitate acute airway obstruction.

6. Inhalation anesthesia is induced with halothane and oxygen; spontaneous ventilation is continually maintained regardless of the patient's oral intake. Yankauer suction should be readily available. Airway obstruction will increase the amount of time necessary to produce deep anesthesia using an inhalation induction and may necessitate increasing gas concentration. Capnography with exhaled gas analysis will help to determine anesthetic depth and avoid toxicity from inhalation agents delivered at high concentrations. After deep plane of anesthesia is obtained, an intravenous cannula is placed and atropine administered.

7. Direct laryngoscopy and oral endotracheal intubation are performed using an endotracheal tube one size smaller than normal with a stylet in place. Spontaneous ventilation should always be maintained and muscle relaxants avoided. A rigid bronchoscope may be used for initial intubation.

8. Replacement of the oral tube with a nasal one is recommended when prolonged intubation is anticipated and if the change can be accomplished easily. If initial intubation is very difficult, the tube should be well secured and no further airway instrumentation should be attempted.

9. The patient is transferred to the intensive care unit. Intravenous sedation should ideally allow spontaneous ventilation by T-tube until defervescence and the presence of an air leak indicate improvement (usually 36 to 48 hours). "Second look" direct laryngoscopy with deep sedation or general anesthesia is performed to evaluate readiness for extubation.

Laryngotracheobronchitis (Croup)[44]

1. A common wintertime viral illness of the subglottic area in children, croup usually occurs between 6 months and 6 years of age.

2. Symptoms include an insidious onset of low-grade fever, a croupy or seal-bark cough, inspiratory stridor, retractions, and, if severe, cyanosis.

3. Differentiation from epiglottitis may be difficult, since the development of respiratory distress and stridor can be the final common pathway of both. Pathologic conditions that can have similar presentations include bacterial tracheitis, laryngeal foreign body, retropharyngeal abscess, and diphtheria. Radiographs help to differentiate croup from other disease entities. Classically subglottic edema appears as a "steeple" sign in the AP projection (whereas the swollen epiglottis of epiglottitis is seen in the latter view). Pharyngeal masses may also be seen in the lateral projection. Radiography should not be attempted with any child in respiratory distress. For these children, rapidly securing the airway should be of paramount concern, with attendance by both an experienced anesthesiologist and a surgeon capable of rapidly performing a cricothyrotomy if necessary.

4. Basic guidelines for care include keeping the patient calm and administering oxygen in cold steam (croup tent).

5. The use of aerosolized racemic epinephrine may temporarily improve symptoms, but rebound hyperemic obstruction may result after its use.

6. The use of steroids as a treatment option remains controversial, although positive results have been reported with nebulized glucocorticoids (budesonide and dexamethasone).[45,46]

7. The need for intubation or tracheostomy is unusual, but may be necessary in cases of severe respiratory compromise. The duration of usual intubation is longer than for epiglottitis (3 to 5 days), because of lack of specific antibiotic treatment for the viral pathogens.

Differential diagnosis of epiglottitis and croup

	Epiglottitis	Croup
Etiology	Bacterial	Viral
Age	2-8 yr	6 mo to 6 yr
Onset	Sudden	Slow, insidious
Season	No seasonal predilection	Wintertime

Signs and symptoms*	Sore throat
	Fever
	Inspiratory stridor and
	  respiratory distress
	Child may be leaning
	  forward and drooling
	Dysphagia
		Low-grade fever
		Croupy or seal-bark
		  cough
		Inspiratory stridor

Radiographs*	Swollen epiglottis seen on
	  lateral neck x-ray
		Steeple sign on
		  AP neck x-ray

Differential diagnosis	Bacterial tracheitis, laryngeal foreign body, retropharyngeal abscess, and diptheria	

*Diagnostic procedures and radiography are contraindicated in the presence of respiratory distress. The patient should be emergently brought to the operating room for laryngoscopy and intubation with an experienced anesthesiologist and a surgeon capable of performing cricothyrotomy/tracheostomy.

Peritonsillar Abscess (Quinsy)[47]

1. Peritonsillar abscess tends to occur in older children or young adults. Incision and drainage are required if the response to antibiotic therapy is inadequate.
2. Severe pharyngeal swelling, trismus, distortion of pharyngeal anatomy (shifted uvula), and airway obstruction can occur. Dehydration results from swallowing difficulty and hyperventilation.
3. Aspiration during incision and drainage is best avoided in an older child by keeping the patient awake. A rapid-sequence induction is performed in young children if no airway difficulty is suspected (peritonsillar abscesses rarely obstruct the airway). Alternatively, if significant trismus or a difficult intubation is anticipated, an inhalation induction with spontaneous ventilation can be performed. On rare occasions, an extremely critical airway will require tracheostomy under local anesthesia before general anesthesia.
4. Bleeding can be profuse from the hyperemic, infected area. Inadvertent perforation of an abscess calls for rapid suctioning and immediate placement of the patient in the Trendelenburg position to prevent aspiration.

Ludwig's Angina[48]

Ludwig's angina is a submandibular, sublingual cellulitis. Because the molars are usually the origin of infection, this disease occurs primarily in older children and young adults. Fulminant edema of the mouth, tongue, neck, and deep cervical fascia can occur, making oral or nasal intubation impossible. Tracheostomy under local anesthesia is then indicated to avoid airway obstruction.

Angioneurotic Edema[49,50]

1. Angioneurotic edema is an autosomal dominant disorder of the complement pathway.
2. Clinically, episodic swelling of the extremities, face, and bowel wall is seen. Involvement of the larynx is associated with a mortality of up to 30%.
3. Prophylactic use of purified C1 inhibitor has proven effective in preventing the swelling. Prophylactic fresh frozen plasma (FFP) can supply adequate amounts of C1 inhibitor but may also adversely fuel further pathway activation. Danazol, an androgen, can prevent attacks by stimulating production of the deficient C1 esterase inhibitor.
4. The local trauma of intubation has been known to trigger attacks of edema. Normal levels of C1 inhibitor and C4 should be demonstrated preoperatively before any airway manipulation. Symptomatic airway edema warrants either intubation or tracheostomy.

EARS

Myringotomy with placement of pressure-equalizing tubes helps to control recurrent otitis media in children. The very short time required by this procedure often precludes the need for IV catheter placement. The procedure may be difficult or prolonged in children with dysmorphic syndromes and very small external canals (notably, children with Down syndrome).

The brevity and simplicity of myringotomy are often given as reason for avoiding the use of premedication or analgesia. However, routine doses of preoperative nasal midazolam have not been reported to prolong discharge after myringotomy and tube placement.[51] Likewise, intraoperative ketorolac (IM) or acetaminophen (PR) or postoperative oral ibuprofen or acetaminophen can be used for analgesia without prolonging discharge. The use of preoperative midazolam in flavored ibuprofen or acetaminophen syrup is a technique that provides both preoperative anxiolysis and postoperative analgesia. The addition of codeine to the flavored vehicle may further enhance postoperative analgesia.[52]

Children with complications of chronic otitis may require more complex ear surgery, including mastoidectomy, middle ear exploration, or tympanoplasty. These procedures are generally performed using microsurgical techniques. Muscle relaxation is useful to maintain a quiet operative field. Use of nitrous oxide during reconstruction of the tympanic membrane (TM) may result in expansion of the middle ear space and disruption of the TM repair. Nitrous oxide should be discontinued for approximately 10 minutes before replacement of the TM or graft.

Nausea and vomiting are common after ear procedures. Prophylactic intraoperative treatment is recommended (see p. 101).

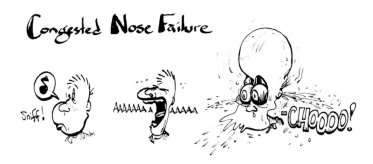

SINUS DISEASE[53]

PATHOPHYSIOLOGY

1. Sinusitis is probably more common in children with defective immunity.
2. Impaired ciliary mobility occurs in children with alterations in the mucus blanket (e.g., asthma, cystic fibrosis). This results in recurrent upper respiratory infections and chronic sinusitis. Treating the sinus disease may lower airway reactivity.[54]
3. Cystic fibrosis patients have abnormal mucus, resulting in sinus polyps, which often require surgical removal. Anesthesia and surgery may be complicated by abnormal pulmonary function and abnormal coagulation (from malabsorption of fat-soluble vitamins) that accompanies cystic fibrosis[55] (see also p. 124).

ANESTHETIC MANAGEMENT

1. Surgery for sinus disease is now largely performed as functional endoscopic sinus surgery (FESS) through the nose, an

outpatient procedure unless contraindicated by coexisting disease.

2. FESS can be performed using local anesthesia and sedation in older, cooperative children or adolescents. This technique may be reasonable in older cystic fibrosis patients, in whom avoidance of general anesthesia may be advisable.

3. Those patients given steroids preoperatively for chronic sinus disease require stress coverage in the perioperative period (hydrocortisone 4 to 8 µg/kg in 3 divided doses).

4. A bloodless field is vital for successful endoscopic sinus procedures. Topical vasoconstrictors used include cocaine, phenylephrine, and epinephrine. Doses should be carefully calculated, particularly in young children, to avoid toxicity. Use of halothane simultaneously with rapidly absorbed vasoconstrictors may precipitate cardiac arrhythmias (doses discussed in Chapter 10; see p. 236).

TRAUMA

Maxillofacial Trauma

Lacerations, bleeding, edema, and fractures of the maxillofacial area make airway management extremely difficult. Blood, vomitus, secretions, and broken teeth or bony fragments can occlude the airway. In general, awake intubation is preferred. Intraoperatively, the use of halothane can trigger dysrhythmias if large amounts of epinephrine have been used to minimize bleeding during surgical repair.[19]

Laryngeal and Tracheal Trauma

Open or closed injuries to the larynx and trachea can occur from direct trauma (usually a steering wheel) but are unusual in children. Closed injury, because it is easily overlooked, can be the more dangerous of the two. Subcutaneous emphysema, dyspnea, hoarseness, cough, hemoptysis, and, in particular, voice changes indicate the possibility of laryngeal damage. Computed tomography is useful in identifying specific injury.

Excessive positive pressure by face mask, coughing, struggling, and nitrous oxide all increase subcutaneous emphysema, which can worsen obstruction. Overzealous attempts at intubation can result in further laryngeal or tracheal damage and create a false passage through a mucosal tear. Cricoid pressure is not used with laryngeal trauma, because it can collapse an incompetent larynx. Blind nasotracheal intubation is also to be avoided because of potential trauma to the larynx. One of the safest approaches to securing the airway is the use of fiberoptic bronchoscopy, especially when the anatomy is grossly distorted. Tracheostomy under local anesthesia below the level of injury may be necessary.

References

1. Tan OT, Sherwood K, Gilchrest BA: Treatment of children with port-wine stains using the flashlamp-pulsed tunable dye laser, *N Engl J Med* 320:416-421, 1989.
2. Rampil IJ: Anesthetic considerations for laser surgery, *Anesth Analg* 74:424-435, 1992.
3. McGoldrick KE, Ho MD: Endoscopy procedures and laser surgery of the airway. In McGoldrick KE, ed: *Anesthesia for ophthalmic and otolaryngologic surgery,* Philadelphia, 1992, WB Saunders, pp 37-63.
4. Sosis MB, Dillon F: Prevention of CO_2 laser–induced endotracheal tube fires with the laser-guard protective coating, *J Clin Anesth* 4:25-27, 1992.
5. Sosis MB: Which is the safest endotracheal tube for use with the CO_2 laser? A comparative study, *J Clin Anesth* 4:217-219, 1992.
6. Pashayan AG, SanGiovanni C, Davis LE: Positive end-expiratory pressure lowers the risk of laser-induced polyvinylchloride tracheal-tube fires, *Anesthesiology* 79:83-87, 1993.
7. Depierraz B, Ravussin P, Brossard E, Monnier P: Percutaneous transtracheal jet ventilation for paediatric endoscopic laser treatment of laryngeal and subglottic lesions, *Can J Anaesth* 41:1200-1207, 1994.
8. Stool SE, Eavey RD: Tracheotomy. In Bluestone CD, Stool SE, Scheetz MD, eds: *Pediatric otolaryngology,* ed 2, Philadelphia, 1990, WB Saunders, pp 1226-1243.
9. McGoldrick KE: Anesthesia for elective ear, nose, and throat surgery. In McGoldrick KE, ed: *Anesthesia for ophthalmic and otolaryngologic surgery,* Philadelphia, 1992, WB Saunders, pp 97-111.
10. Nemechek AJ, Amedee RG: Choanal atresia, *J La State Med Soc* 146:337-340, 1994.
11. Prescott CAJ: Nasal obstruction in infancy, *Arch Dis Child* 72: 287-289, 1995.
12. Glasson MJ, Taylor SF: Cervical, cervicomediastinal and intrathoracic lymphangioma, *Prog Pediatr Surg* 27:62-83, 1991.
13. Baxter MRN: Congenital laryngomalacia, *Can J Anaesth* 41:332-339, 1994.
14. Duncan S, Eid N: Tracheomalacia and bronchopulmonary dysplasia, *Ann Otol Rhinol Laryngol* 100:856-858, 1991.
15. Cotton RT, Reilly JS: Congenital malformation of the larynx. In Bluestone CD, Stool SE, Scheetz MD, eds: *Pediatric otolaryngology,* ed 2, Philadelphia, 1990, WB Saunders, pp 1121-1128.
16. Kaufman FL: Managing the cleft lip and palate patient, *Pediatr Clin North Am* 38:1127-1147, 1991.
17. Nguyen PN, Sullivan PK: Issues and controversies in the management of cleft palate, *Clin Plast Surg* 20:671-682, 1993.
18. Sommerlad BC: Surgical management of cleft palate: a review, *JR Soc Med* 82:677-678, 1989.
19. Karl HW, Swedlow DB, Lee KW, Downes JJ: Epinephrine-halothane interactions in children, *Anesthesiology* 58:142-145, 1983.
20. Ochiai R, Guthrie RD, Motoyama EK: Differential sensitivity to halothane anesthesia of the genioglossus, intercostals, and diaphragm in kittens, *Anesth Analg* 74:338-344, 1992.

21. Bell C, Oh TH, Loeffler JR: Massive macroglossia and airway obstruction after cleft palate repair, *Anesth Analg* 67:1-4, 1988.

22. Fishman SJ, Mulliken JB: Hemangiomas and vascular malformations of infancy and childhood, *Pediatr Surg* 40:1177-1200, 1993.

23. Wahrman JE, Honig PJ: Hemangiomas, *Pediatr Rev* 15:266-271, 1994.

24. Cotton RT: Management and prevention of subglottic stenosis in infants and children. In Bluestone CD, Stool SE, Scheetz MD, eds: *Pediatric otolaryngology,* ed 2, Philadelphia, 1990, WB Saunders, pp 1194-1204.

25. Murthy P, Laing MR: Macroglossia, *Br Med J* 309:1386-1387, 1994.

26. McGoldrick KE: The larynx: normal development and congenital anomalies. In McGoldrick KE, ed: *Anesthesia for ophthalmic and otolaryngologic surgery,* Philadelphia, 1992, WB Saunders, pp 1-14.

27. Iannetti G, Belli E, De Ponte F, Cicconetti A, Delfini R: The surgical approaches to nasopharyngeal angiofibroma, *J Craniomaxillofac Surg* 22:311-316, 1994.

28. Potsic WP, Wetmore RF: Practical aspects of managing the child with apnea, *J Otolaryngol* 21:429-433, 1992.

29. Gaultier CL: Clinical and therapeutic aspects of obstructive sleep apnea syndrome in infants and children, *Sleep* 15:S36-38, 1992.

30. Patel RI, Hannallah RS, Norden J, Casey WF, Verghese ST: Emergence airway complications in children: a comparison of tracheal extubation in awake and deeply anesthetized patients, *Anesth Analg* 73:266-270, 1991.

31. Splinter WM, Rhine EJ, MacNeill HB, et al: The effect of general anaesthesia on post-tonsillectomy vomiting, *Can J Anaesth* 37:S96, 1990.

32. Ferrari LR, Donlon JV: Metoclopramide reduces the incidence of vomiting after tonsillectomy in children, *Anesth Analg* 75:351-354, 1992.

33. Litman RS, Wu CL, Catanzaro FA: Ondansetron decreases emesis after tonsillectomy in children, *Anesth Analg* 78:478-481, 1994.

34. Pandit UA, Malviya S, Lewis IH: Vomiting after outpatient tonsillectomy and adenoidectomy in children: the role of nitrous oxide, *Anesth Analg* 80:230-233, 1995.

35. Jebeles JA, Reilly JS, Gutierrez JF, Bradley EL Jr, Kissin J: Tonsillectomy and adenoidectomy pain reduction by local bupivacaine infiltration in children, *Int J Pediatr Otolorhinolaryngol* 25:149-154, 1993.

36. Rusy LM, Houck CS, Sullivan LJ, Ohlms LA, Jones DT, McGill TJ, Berde CB: A double-blind evaluation of ketorolac tromethamine versus acetaminophen in pediatric tonsillectomy: analgesia and bleeding, *Anesth Analg* 80:226-229, 1995.

37. Richmond KH, Wetmore RF, Baronak CC: Postoperative complications following tonsillectomy and adenoidectomy: who is at risk? *Int J Pediatr Otolaryngol* 13:117-124, 1987.

38. Crysdale WS: Complications of tonsillectomy and adenoidectomy in 9409 children observed overnight, *Can Med Assoc J* 135:1139-1142, 1986.

39. Rosen GM, Muckle RP, Mahowald MW, Goding GS, Ullevig C: Postoperative respiratory compromise in children with obstructive sleep apnea syndrome, *Pediatrics* 93:784-788, 1994.

40. McGoldrick KE: Pediatric airway emergencies: foreign body aspiration, epiglotittis, laryngotracheobronchitis, and bacterial tracheitis. In McGoldrick KE, ed: *Anesthesia for ophthalmic and otolaryngologic surgery,* Philadelphia, 1992, WB Saunders, pp 112-123.

41. Esclamado RM, Richardson MA: Laryngotracheal foreign bodies in children, *Am J Dis Child* 141:259-262, 1987.

42. Holinger LD: Foreign bodies of the larynx, trachea, and bronchi. In Bluestone CD, Stool SE, Scheetz MD, eds: *Pediatric otolaryngology,* ed 2, Philadelphia, 1990, WB Saunders, pp 1205-1214.

43. Cressman WR, Myer III CM: Diagnosis and management of croup and epiglottitis, *Pediatr Clin North Am* 41:265-276, 1994.

44. Walker P, Crysdale WS: Croup, epiglottitis, retropharyngeal abscess, and bacterial tracheitis: evolving patterns of occurrence and care, *Int Anesthesiol Clin* 30:57-70, 1992.

45. Cruz MN, Stewart G, Rosenberg N: Use of dexamethasone in the outpatient management of acute larngotracheitis, *Pediatrics* 96:220-223, 1995.

46. Klassen TP, Feldman ME, Watters LK, Sutcliffe T, Rowe PC: Nebulized budesonide for children with mild-to-moderate croup, *N Engl J Med* 331:285-289, 1994.

47. Weinberg E, Brodsky L, Stanievich J, Volk M: Needle aspiration of peritonsillar abscess in children, *Arch Otolaryngol Head Neck Surg* 119:169-172, 1993.

48. Fritsch DE, Goldenberg-Klein D: Ludwig's angina, *Heart Lung* 21:39-47, 1992.

49. Huston DP, Bressler RB: Urticaria and angioedema, *Med Clin North Am* 76:805-840, 1992.

50. Orfan NA, Kolski GB: Angioedema and C1 inhibitor deficiency, *Ann Allergy* 69:167-174, 1992.

51. Davis PJ, Tome JA, McGowan FX Jr, Cohen IT, Latta K, Felder H: Preanesthetic medication with intranasal midazolam for brief pediatric surgical procedures, *Anesthesiology* 82:2-5, 1995.

52. Tobias JD, Lowe S, Hersey S, Rasmussen GE, Werkhaven J: Analgesia after bilateral myringotomy and placement of pressure equalization tubes in children: acetaminophen vs acetaminophen with codeine, *Anesth Analg* 81:496-500, 1995.

53. Lusk RP, Wolf G: Pathophysiology of chronic sinusitis. In Lusk RP, ed: *Pediatric sinusitis,* New York, 1992, Raven Press, pp 7-13.

54. Slavin RG: Sinusitis and asthma. In Lusk RP, ed: *Pediatric sinusitis,* New York, 1992, Raven Press, pp 59-64.

55. Parson DS: Sinusitis and cystic fibrosis. In Lusk RP, ed: *Pediatric sinusitis,* New York, 1992, Raven Press, pp 65-70.

ANESTHETIC MANAGEMENT OF PEDIATRIC PATIENTS WITH NEUROLOGIC DISEASES

9

Inside Your Head

Tiny one, silent one, face is all red
Tell me what's happening inside your head.

Talk to me, move for me, whisper or bawl
Give me a sign—don't do nothing at all.

Try though we might we can't tell what you're thinking
Your brain could be starving, or watered and sinking

There's nothing more scary to lie there in bed
With scarcely a clue 'bout what's inside your head.

Rivian Bell

INCREASED INTRACRANIAL PRESSURE (ICP) IN CHILDREN[1]

Increased ICP is often the presenting pathophysiology for intracranial lesions of multiple etiologies (traumatic, infectious, vascular, neoplastic). An understanding of the differences and similarities in diagnosis and control of ICP in children as compared to adults helps to determine optimal anesthetic management.

Diagnosis

1. Normal ICP for neonates is 2 to 4 mm Hg and gradually increases with age to adult levels (≤ 15 mm Hg).
2. Increased ICP is often difficult to diagnose in infants and young children because open suture lines increase the compliance of the cranial vault. When pressures are sufficiently high or sustained, there will be bulging of the fontanelle and eyes. Eventually there will be an increase in head circumference and the presence of downward gaze (setting sun sign).
3. Neurologic signs are diffuse and nonspecific. The child may be increasingly irritable or sedated, with slowing of motor responses.

4. The typical Cushing response to raised ICP (hypertension, bradycardia, and irregular breathing) is not usually present in infants because of open sutures. Papilledema is also unusual despite high intracranial pressures.
5. Because of the nonspecific neurologic symptoms and physical signs, increased ICP in infants and children is best diagnosed by computed tomographic (CT) scan. Diffuse edema, small obliterated ventricles, and midline shift are radiologic indications of increased ICP.

Control of ICP

The intracranial vault contains the brain parenchyma and fluid. The three fluid compartments are the interstitial fluid (80%), blood (10%), and cerebrospinal fluid (10%). Increased ICP is treated by manipulation of these three fluid compartments.

Techniques to lower increased ICP[1,2]

Technique	Results/comments
Hyperventilation $Paco_2$ 25-30 mm Hg	Decreases CBF by arteriolar vasoconstriction Vasoconstriction lasts only 24 hr because of readjustment of buffering systems CBF decreases 4% for each 1 mm Hg decrease in $Paco_2$ Cerebral ischemia is associated with a $Paco_2$ < 20 mm Hg
Diuretics Furosemide 0.5-1.0 mg/kg IV	Furosemide decreases: • Production of CSF • Amount of interstitial fluid • Circulating blood volume
Mannitol 0.5-1.0 g/kg IV	Osmotic diuretics such as mannitol initially cause an increase in brain compliance and possibly vasoconstriction; over time they decrease the amount of interstitial fluid and the circulating blood volume
Steroids Hydrocortisone 1.0-1.5 mg/kg/dose IV Dexamethasone 0.5-1.5 mg/kg IV (loading dose) 0.2-0.5 mg/kg/24 hr IV q6h (maintenance)	Restore the integrity of the blood-brain barrier in abnormal/ischemic tissue Decrease production of CSF
CSF drainage HR, BP, and pupils are carefully monitored during removal of CSF	Rapid removal in the presence of elevated ICP can result in tonsillar herniation Careful monitoring is required during removal
Position Elevate head of bed 30 to 45 degrees	Facilitates jugular venous drainage to decrease venous congestion and CBV.

CEREBROSPINAL FLUID (CSF)[1]

Production.   CSF is produced in the choroid plexus and renewed five times a day. An adult will produce as much as 750 ml/day. Production in children varies with age and pathophysiology; infants may produce 100 ml/day.

Production of CSF is not affected by changes in ICP. It can be temporarily decreased by certain drugs such as furosemide, steroids, and acetazolamide.

Reabsorption.   Reabsorption of CSF occurs in the arachnoid villi, which have a limited capacity to increase reabsorption during periods of increased ICP. The rate of CSF absorption may be decreased by intracranial hemorrhage, infection, or congenital malformations.

CEREBRAL BLOOD FLOW (CBF)[1]

Cerebral blood volume (CBV) is determined by cerebral blood flow, which is in turn regulated by cerebral metabolic demand ($CMRO_2$ or cerebral metabolic rate of oxygen consumption). Brain tissue acidosis and hypercapnia will also increase cerebral blood flow. The anesthesiologist's ability to alter cerebral blood flow directly (or indirectly by altering metabolic demand) is a critical tool for controlling intracranial pressure changes in children.

Autoregulation.   The central nervous system is one of the three tissue beds that can auotregulate blood flow in order to maintain perfusion over a wide range of blood pressure (MAP = 50 − 150 mm Hg). Cerebral blood flow is also very reactive to changes in $PaCO_2$. When $PaCO_2$ is between 20 and 80 mm Hg, cerebral blood flow rises proportionally to increases in carbon dioxide tension (see Fig. 9-1).

The immature autonomic nervous system of the premature infant results in impaired myogenic control of arteriolar resistance. Cerebral perfusion in these children depends upon systemic blood pressure. Intracerebral hemorrhages may occur from hypertension or stress.

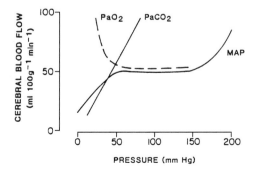

FIG. 9-1.   Cerebral blood flow is influenced by arterial oxygenation (PaO_2), alveolar ventilation ($PaCO_2$), and mean arterial pressure (MAP). (From Stoelting RK: Central nervous system. In *Pharmacology and physiology in anesthetic practice,* Philadelphia, 1987, JB Lippincott, p. 587.)

PREOPERATIVE ASSESSMENT OF THE PATIENT FOR NEUROLOGIC SURGERY

History

1. Associated syndromes (see Chapter 23, p. 520)
   a. Congenital anatomic defects including craniofacial syndromes
   b. Metabolic disorders
2. Previous neurologic deficits
   a. Hypotonia
   b. Localized cranial or peripheral nerve lesions
3. Previous increase in ICP
   a. Changes in mental status
   b. Nausea/vomiting
   c. Increased head circumference
4. Lack of airway protection
   a. Ability to take solids/liquids orally
   b. History of aspiration pneumonia
   c. History of reflux
5. Intellectual and motor development

Physical

1. Ability to understand and cooperate
2. Level of consciousness/mental status
3. Airway protection and anatomy
   a. Gag/swallow/cough
   b. Dysmorphism
   c. Cervical range of motion
4. Neurologic deficits
   a. Hypotonia
   b. Spasticity
   c. Flaccidity
   d. Generalized or localized
5. Signs of increased ICP

Premedication

As with adults, premedication is avoided for pediatric patients at risk for increasing ICP with ventilatory depression. It should also be avoided if continuous neurologic assessment is required and mental status or level of consciousness will be altered by the drug.

Conversely, anxiolysis is particularly useful in patients with vascular anomalies in whom acute anxiety and stress may lead to hypertension and subsequent intracranial hemorrhage. In these situations, intramuscular injections are best avoided.

Oral benzodiazepines (diazepam, midazolam) are useful for

promoting anxiolysis with minimal respiratory depression. Barbiturates potentially lower ICP by decreasing $CMRO_2$ and can be given orally (e.g., pentobarbital) or rectally (e.g., methohexital). (See Chapter 2 for dosing.)

MONITORING

1. Noninvasive monitoring for pediatric neurosurgical procedures includes the following: ECG, blood pressure cuff, pulse oximeter, auscultation of heart and breath sounds, temperature monitoring, and monitoring of expired gas for CO_2.
2. Invasive monitoring with an intraarterial catheter is recommended for close hemodynamic control of blood pressure and frequent sampling of blood for oxygen and carbon dioxide tensions. The transducer level should be adjusted according to the patient's head level; the lateral corner of the eye or the ear can be used as a landmark when the patient's head is elevated during the procedure.
3. A precordial Doppler is recommended for procedures performed in the sitting position to detect venous air embolus.
4. A central venous pressure catheter may be helpful for monitoring circulating blood volume, calculating ICP (MAP − CVP), and removing air should a large venous embolus occur.
5. Cerebral evoked potentials (mapping) are monitored during selected procedures.
6. Urinary output should be measured during major intracranial operations, when diuretics are employed, when a lengthy operation is planned, or when significant blood loss and volume replacement are anticipated.

POSITIONING

Sitting position.   The sitting position is rarely used in young children, because it does little to improve the surgical exposure. Use of the sitting position for older children necessitates monitoring for venous air emboli with a precordial Doppler and placement of a central venous catheter for extraction of air.

Prone position.   The prone position is commonly used for spinal procedures (e.g., repair of meningomyelocele, and release of tethered cord). Attention to endotracheal tube placement and patency is essential in this position. Some advocate the use of a nasotracheal or wire-reinforced tube. Pressure on the posterior pharynx and larynx caused by the natural curve of the endotracheal tube can lead to postoperative airway edema and obstruction.

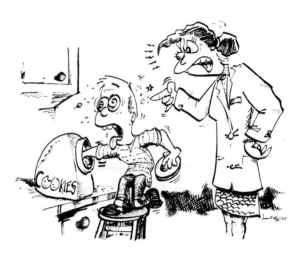

THAT'D BETTER BE A FUGUE STATE BUSTER. WE BEGIN THE WORKUP IMMEDIATELY.

AGENTS FOR INDUCTION AND MAINTENANCE OF ANESTHESIA

1. Laryngoscopy and endotracheal intubation can increase ICP if either coughing or hypertension and tachycardia occur. This response can be attenuated pharmacologically (see table on next page).
2. When increased ICP is suspected, an intravenous induction is ideal to avoid the elevations in $PaCO_2$ seen with an inhalation technique. However, it is not clear if placing an IV catheter in a crying, struggling child is a better technique when ICP is elevated than a calm, controlled inhalation induction.
3. Controlled ventilation with a $PaCO_2$ between 25 and 30 is critically important in the child with elevated ICP, regardless of agents selected.
4. In general, glucose-containing intravenous solutions are avoided if the potential for cerebral ischemia is present. Greater permanent neurologic injury has been noted in animal models when ischemia occurs after the administration of glucose, presumably because of higher postischemic cerebral lactate levels.[3] In infants or during prolonged procedures, blood glucose should be monitored to avoid hypoglycemia when glucose-containing infusions are not used.

Drugs for induction and maintenance of anesthesia in patients with elevated intracranial pressure[4-6]

Drug	Effects
Intravenous	
Barbiturates	Lower ICP by producing dose-dependent depression of CBF and $CMRO_2$ up to a maximum of 40% to 50% of normal, correlating with a quiet EEG
Lidocaine	Can decrease the response to intubation if given intratracheally or intravenously several minutes before intubation
Benzodiazepines	Evidence is controversial regarding the effects on CBF and $CMRO_2$, but both most likely are decreased; probably best used as a premedication
Etomidate	Can produce up to a 50% decrease in CBF and $CMRO_2$, with EEG suppression similar to barbiturates; it is not widely used in pediatrics and can suppress adrenal function
Ketamine	Generally contraindicated because it causes cerebral stimulation; increases ICP, CBF, and $CMRO_2$
Opioids	Increase cerebrovascular resistance and decrease CBF and $CMRO_2$ (fentanyl>morphine>meperidine); very high doses of fentanyl and sufentanil have precipitated seizures in animal models; sufentanil causes minor increases in CBF and ICP, which can be overcome by hypocapnia
Propofol	Reduces $CMRO_2$ and may protect against anoxic injury
Inhalation	
Halothane	Increases ICP by increasing CBV secondary to direct cerebrovasodilation; decreases CSF production, but increases resistance to absorption
Enflurane	Increases ICP by cerebrovasodilation; increases CSF production and decreases CSF absorption; may lower seizure threshold at >2 MAC in the face of hyperventilation
Isoflurane	Produces little change in CBF at 1 MAC; more depression of $CMRO_2$ than halothane; less impairment of autoregulation than halothane
Nitrous oxide	May increase ICP; elevations of ICP can be attenuated with thiopental and hyperventilation; should be discontinued before closure of the dura so that it does not cause expansion of closed, air-filled spaces

CHOICE OF MUSCLE RELAXANTS
Depolarizing

Succinylcholine administration should be avoided unless a rapid-sequence induction is indicated. Succinylcholine is contraindicated in muscular dystrophies, multiple sclerosis, spinal cord injuries, encephalitis, crush injuries, and burn injuries, because of the risk of hyperkalemia.

Increases in ICP have been reported with succinylcholine, although this effect is attenuated by induction doses of thiopental (5 to 10 mg/kg) or pretreatment with nondepolarizing relaxants.[4]

Nondepolarizing

1. Relaxants provide a motionless field for difficult surgical dissections and microscopic or laser procedures.
2. Anesthetic requirements are minimal after skin incision and craniotomy; relaxants ensure absence of movement even when anesthetic doses are reduced.
3. If a preexisting neurologic deficit exists, the neuromuscular blockade monitor should be placed on an unaffected limb.
4. Pancuronium may elevate ICP by increasing heart rate and blood pressure.
5. Curare and atracurium release histamine, causing vasodilation, increased CBV, and decreased cerebral perfusion pressure (CPP).
6. Laudanosine, a metabolite of atracurium, may cause cerebral stimulation. This is probably unimportant clinically.
7. Vecuronium, devoid of hemodynamic effects, may be an ideal relaxant for intracranial procedures.
8. Mivacurium is devoid of many of the undesirable side effects of succinylcholine and may be used for rapid-sequence induction when the use of succinylcholine is contraindicated. Because mivacurium is primarily hydrolyzed by pseudocholinesterase, its duration of action is very brief, necessitating a continuous infusion for muscle relaxation in lengthy procedures.
9. Rocuronium displays a rapid onset with minimal hemodynamic effects in children, but has a longer duration of action than mivacurium (recommended for procedures lasting longer than 30 minutes).
10. The surgical team may request that no muscle relaxants be used, particularly during procedures on the spinal cord, when nerve function needs to be assessed intraoperatively (e.g., meningomyelocele, release of tethered cord). The endotracheal tube can be secured with a short-acting agent (mivacurium or atracurium) and reversed prior to operation and testing of nerve function. Relaxants may be avoided by inducing and intubating with inhalation agents only.

ANESTHETIC MANAGEMENT OF COMMON PEDIATRIC NEUROSURGICAL PROCEDURES

Dysraphism (meningomyelocele, encephalocele)

1. Adequate preoperative hydration is imperative, especially if a CSF leak exists.
2. All antibiotics should be continued.
3. Preexisting neurologic deficits should be documented.
4. Because these infants frequently have lower motor neuron involvement, the use of succinylcholine may precipitate hyperkalemia.
5. To protect the open cord, the trachea may be intubated with the infant in the lateral position (usually awake). If the defect is too large to be safely supported and protected in the lateral position, the infant can be held during intubation.
6. The operation is performed in the prone position, necessitating careful padding of pressure points and a secure airway.
7. The surgeon may request that no muscle relaxant be given, so that nerve function can be tested.
8. These infants will be kept in the prone position postoperatively and may require prolonged mechanical ventilation.

Latex Allergy and Meningomyelocele[7-10]

Up to 50% of children with myelodysplasia, children who require frequent urinary catheterization, and those with history of multiple allergies, atopy, eczema, or repeated latex exposure are at risk for acute anaphylaxis when exposed to latex products in the operating room. Children with cerebral palsy (spastic quadriplegia) have also been identified as being at high risk for latex allergy. A history of facial urticaria after dental visits or when a child is blowing up balloons often means a susceptibility to latex allergy. The allergic reaction appears to be IgE mediated and can cause urticaria, wheezing, and hypotension.

TREATMENT OF THE LATEX-ALLERGY SUSCEPTIBILE PATIENT

1. A detailed history should be obtained regarding previous episodes of urticaria, angioedema, or cardiorespiratory symptoms with latex exposure.
2. Some authors recommend allergy testing in susceptible individuals by skin testing or in vitro radioallergen absorbent testing (RAST). No allergy tests are completely reliable; preoperative testing is not uniformly advocated.
3. Pretreatment 24 hours preoperatively with corticosteroids, antihistamines (diphenhydramine), and H_2 blockers (cimetidine or ranitidine) has also been suggested. Unfortunately, no studies

document that a preoperative regimen alone will prevent anaphylactic reactions or decrease severity. Several cases have been reported of anaphylactic reactions after pretreatment.

4. Complete avoidance of latex-containing products in the operating room is thus far the only technique that uniformly prevents intraoperative latex allergy in susceptible patients.

5. Should anaphylaxis occur, the patient can be treated with 0.1 µg/kg/ IV epinephrine, repeated as needed. An epinephrine or isoproterenol infusion may be required (0.1 µg/kg/min starting dose).

6. An anesthetic technique that avoids drugs that release histamine (e.g., atracurium, morphine) will decrease the likelihood of urticaria being confused with a true allergic reaction.

Potential latex-derived products

The products listed below can be replaced with polyvinylchloride, plastic, or glass alternatives. Cotton placed under blood pressure cuffs or tourniquets prevents contact with skin.

Surgical gloves
Airway devices: masks, oral and nasal airways, endotracheal tubes, breathing circuits, ventilator bellows, anesthesia bag and tubing
Baby bottle nipples, pacifiers
Dental casts, rubber dams, tooth protectors/blocks and mouth gags
Instrument mats, rubber shods, vascular tags
IV administration sets—injection ports/adapters
Syringe barrels
Bulb—irrigation
Multidose drug vials
Blood pressure cuffs
Tourniquets—IV and surgical
Rubber bands
Electrode pads
Stethoscope tubing
Elastic bandages/Elastoplast/adhesive tape/moleskin
Esmarch bandages
Hemodialysis equipment/cardiopulmonary bypass/cell saver
Wound drains
Catheters: CVP/pulmonary artery catheters
Hemodialysis/peritoneal dialysis
VP/VJ shunts
Urinary catheters, including condom collection
Enema tubing
GI/feeding/NG "red rubber" tubes
Bougie dilators
Rubber stoppers on test tubes, culture tubes
Headstraps

IV, intravenous; *CVP,* central venous pressure; *VP,* ventriculoperitoneal; *VJ,* ventriculojugular; *GI,* gastrointestinal; *NG,* nasogastric.

Hydrocephalus

1. Operations for obstructive hydrocephalus or aqueductal stenosis include ventriculoperitoneal (VP) shunt, ventriculoatrial shunt, and third or fourth ventriculostomy.
2. Children with shunts are at risk for developing meningitis/encephalitis; careful aseptic technique should be used during venous cannulation and administration of intravenous drugs.
3. Children may present for emergency shunt placement or revision with acute elevation of intracranial pressure. All precautions for induction and maintenance of anesthesia in the presence of high ICP should apply.
4. Patients are susceptible to hypotension during CSF drainage. Blood pressure should be closely and accurately monitored.
5. Ventriculoatrial shunts pose an increased risk of air emboli. Methods to decrease the size and incidence of air emboli include the following:
   - Avoiding the use of N_2O
   - Maintaining intravenous hydration to ensure that the hydrostatic pressure in the venous circulation is high
   - Controlled positive-pressure ventilation to keep venous pressure high
6. Third ventriculostomy, which drains CSF into the basilar cisterns, may avoid the need for VP shunt placement. Intraoperative complications include cardiac arrhythmias (rarely, asystole) and intraventricular hemorrhage.
7. Most children can be awakened in the operating room after placement of a CSF shunt and do not require prolonged mechanical ventilation.

Tethered Spinal Cord[11]

1. Tethered cord syndrome (or filum terminale syndrome) consists of a low conus medullaris tethered to the dura by fibrous bands or a lipoma.
2. The incidence is higher in females (2:1) than males, as are other forms of dysraphism.
3. Presenting symptoms include gait abnormalities, bowel or bladder dysfunction, sensory or motor deficits, and occasionally visible muscle atrophy.
4. The use of succinylcholine is controversial, especially if muscle wasting is present. The surgeon may request that no muscle relaxant be given, so that nerve function can be tested.
5. These infants will be kept in the prone position postoperatively and may require prolonged mechanical ventilation.

Craniosynostosis

1. Craniosynostosis is often found in children with craniofacial syndromes (e.g., Apert and Crouzon), which are also associated with a difficult airway.

2. Intracranial hypertension can result from untreated craniosynostosis.

3. Craniosynostectomy often results in significant and rapid blood loss. Large-bore intravenous access is essential for volume replacement. An arterial catheter should be considered for blood pressure monitoring and for assessing hematrocrit and blood gases.

4. Patients should be observed in the ICU after surgery because of the high risk of subdural or epidural hematoma formation.

5. Unless other medical problems are present, these children usually do not require prolonged ventilation. However, prolonged ventilation may be required in prolonged procedures when considerable facial and airway swelling is anticipated.

6. Opioids and sedatives should be used judiciously so as not to obscure the postoperative neurologic examination.

Aneurysms and Arteriovenous Malformations (AVM)[12]

1. Premedication of children with intracerebral vascular lesions prior to arrival in the operating room minimizes the risk of bleeding or rupture of the aneurysm as a result of anxiety, crying, and struggling.

2. A variety of induction techniques (steal, inhalation, intravenous, rectal methohexital) can be used to keep the child calm. All are acceptable methods as long as coughing and hypertension, which can lead to vessel rupture, are avoided.

3. The placement of at least two large-bore intravenous catheters will be helpful for volume resuscitation if profuse bleeding occurs.

4. An arterial catheter for blood pressure monitoring and obtaining laboratory data is essential; it is usually placed after induction.

5. The trachea should be intubated after a muscle relaxant has been given to avoid any coughing during endotracheal tube insertion.

6. A hypotensive technique may help reduce bleeding (see p. 264).

7. Tracheal extubation should be accomplished with minimal coughing or straining, to decrease the risk of bleeding. Methods used to achieve a quiet extubation include the following:
   - Deep extubation (not appropriate for an infant)
   - Extubation of the trachea while maintaining tight hemodynamic control with vasodilator agents
   - Administration of intravenous lidocaine before extubation, to depress airway reflexes

8. Opioids and sedatives should be used judiciously so that the child can cooperate fully with a neurologic exam in the postoperative period.

Cerebral Palsy[10,13-15]

1. Cerebral palsy (CP) describes a group of disorders that are associated with motor abnormalities and are commonly ascribed to perinatal asphyxia.
2. Spastic quadriplegia is the most common variety and is directly related to premature birth and low birth weight. Mental retardation may or may not be present. A higher incidence of gastroesophageal reflux and drooling due to inability to clear pharyngeal secretions is characteristic. Asthma often accompanies chronic reflux, and postoperative pulmonary problems are common.
3. The advantages of a rapid-sequence induction in the presence of severe reflux must be weighed against the advantages of a slower induction that avoids bronchospasm (see Chapter 6). Spasticity and limited neck motion may complicate intubation.
4. Children with cerebral palsy may show resistance to nondepolarizing muscle relaxants. They have been found to be only slightly more sensitive to succinylcholine, but not sufficiently to be of clinical importance. Succinylcholine does not cause abnormal potassium release.
5. These children may be susceptible to latex allergy (see p. 213).
6. Hypothermia may occur and necessitates careful temperature monitoring.

Seizure Disorders[16-18]

Commonly used terminology and new classification

Old classification	New classification
Petit mal seizures	Absence seizures
Grand mal seizures	Tonic-clonic seizures
Psychomotor seizures	Complex partial seizures
Temporal lobe seizures	Complex partial seizures
Minor motor seizures	Atonic or akinetic seizures
Focal motor seizures	Simple partial seizures
Jacksonian seizures	Simple partial seizures

Seizures represent an excessive, usually self-limited, neuronal discharge. Epilepsy is a common childhood problem, and approximately 50% of childhood epilepsy is idiopathic, with many clinical forms in existence. Seizures may also occur in patients with disorders of brain metabolism, infections, scarring, edema, tumor, or vascular anomaly.

Febrile seizures.   A febrile seizure is a generalized, tonic-clonic (grand mal) seizure that occurs during a high fever (T>38° C), most commonly in children between 3 months and 6 years of age. Approximately 2% to 5% of all children experience a febrile seizure.

Most febrile seizures are benign, although 33% of patients may have a second episode. The treatment of recurrent febrile seizures is controversial; some children receive prophylactic therapy.

Neonatal seizures. Neonatal seizures are usually seen in the setting of prenatal asphyxia, birth injury, hypocalcemia, or hypoglycemia, or secondary to an intraventricular hemorrhage in a premature infant. The seizure presents as a subtle change in behavior, such as eye fluttering, sucking, drooling, tonic posturing, or apnea. Electroencephalogram (EEG) and CT scan help to confirm the diagnosis.

The prognosis of neonatal seizures largely depends upon the underlying etiology. The outcome cannot be predicted on the basis of borderline abnormal EEGs. Infants whose serial EEGs are normal tend to have only minor sequelae.

Infantile spasms. Infantile spasms are a generalized seizure disorder occurring during the first year of life. A brief flexion contracture of the head, neck, and upper extremity with extension of the extremities (i.e., "jack-knife" spasms) is most common. Invariably, either poor motor function or mental retardation will also be present. Unfortunately, infantile spasms respond poorly to conventional epileptic therapy.

Absence seizures (petit mal). Petit mal seizures usually develop in children before the age of 10 years, but are rare in children less than 3 years old. The child stares off blankly for brief periods and is unaware of these lapses in time. The three-per-second spike pattern is a hallmark EEG finding for this seizure disorder.

Tonic-clonic seizures (grand mal). Grand mal seizures usually present as a loss of consciousness followed by a "cry" during rhythmic tonic contraction of chest wall muscles. Respiratory stridor, cyanosis, and urinary incontinence commonly occur. Similarly, the seizure is followed by a postictal period of confusion or sleep.

Although most grand mal seizures in children are idiopathic, a complete diagnostic evaluation should be undertaken. The onset of seizures in adults (after the age of 20) must be studied for an underlying etiology.

ANTIEPILEPTIC AGENTS

The agents used in the treatment of epilepsy generally include barbiturates, benzodiazepines, succinimides, and hydantoins. The pharmacologic ability to prevent or reduce excessive neuronal discharge is a result of the following neurophysiologic effects: reduction of Na^+ or Ca^{++} fluxes, reduction of evoked responses, and/or potentiation of presynaptic or postsynaptic inhibition.

Antiepileptic drugs: neurophysiologic effects and uses[16]

Drug	Molecular/cellular effect	Use
Phenytoin	Voltage-dependent block of sodium channels Decreases depolarization-dependent calcium uptake	Partial and generalized convulsive seizures
Carbamazepine	Voltage-dependent block of sodium channels	Effective in partial and generalized convulsive seizures
Ethosuximide	Blocks slow calcium curent in thalamic neurons	Absence seizures
Valproic acid	Voltage-dependent sodium channel block Increases calcium--dependent potassium conductance Increases the threshold to produce caudate spindles	Convulsive and nonconvulsive generalized seizures Moderately effective against partial seizures
Barbiturates	Increase chloride conductance Increase GABA binding	Partial and generalized convulsive seizures
Benzodiazepines	Increase chloride conductance Increase GABA binding Increase adenosine effect	Effective in all seizure types

ANESTHETIC IMPLICATIONS OF EPILEPSY

1. The child with epilepsy requires a thorough preoperative history and physical examination with careful scrutiny for many of the common side effects of anticonvulsant therapy (see p. 221). A complete blood count with differential, a platelet count, and liver function tests are often indicated.
2. All anticonvulsant drugs should be continued in the perioperative period to maintain adequate blood levels and seizure control.
3. A discussion with the parents concerning the need to continue anticonvulsant therapy (despite an otherwise NPO status) and the potential for postoperative seizures should take place.
4. Accelerated or altered biotransformation of volatile anesthetic agents as a result of enzyme induction by chronic anticonvulsant therapy may be an important consideration when choosing agents.

5. Practically speaking, all anesthetic agents can be used safely in the child with epilepsy. Controversy surrounds certain agents such as methohexital, meperidine, fentanyl, ketamine, and enflurane (see following table). In general, anesthetic agents cause EEG wave slowing and decrease $CMRO_2$.

Anesthetic agents and seizures[4, 19-22]

Drug	Implications in the seizure patient
Barbiturates	Dose-related effect upon the EEG Isoelectric EEG at high doses Methohexital lowers seizure threshold
Ketamine	Hallucinogenic and convulsant properties can be seen on EEG; however, a predominance of theta activity and loss of alpha rhythm are seen with subsequent doses of ketamine and deeper planes of anesthesia; may actually raise seizure threshold Severe myoclonus in infants with myoclonic encephalopathy Although studies have shown no seizures in patients with known seizure disorders, it may be best to choose an alternative agent that is not as controversial
Benzodiazepines	Primarily used for sedation, anxiolysis, and amnestic properties Significantly raise seizure threshold
Narcotics	Meperidine's metabolite normeperidine is a well-recognized cerebral irritant; its use with MAO inhibitors is contraindicated because of seizures Several case reports of grand mal seizures following fentanyl have been reported; EEG studies have not corroborated these findings, and therefore the use of fentanyl is not contraindicated in a child with seizures
Halogenated agents	Increased and altered biotransformation by liver enzymes may be of concern Enflurane and concomitant hypercarbia can cause audiogenic seizures Isoflurane may produce spikes on EEG without seizures Halothane has no epileptogenic potential Electrical seizure activity (by EEG) without clinical seizures has been reported with sevoflurane
Atracurium	Laudanosine, a product of degradation, may cause cerebral excitation that does not appear to be clinically significant

Complications of anticonvulsant therapy[2,23]

Drug (brand name)	Side effects
Phenytoin (Dilantin)	Nystagmus Gum hyperplasia Hirsutism Encephalopathy Sedation Ataxia Leukopenia, agranulocytosis Decreased cardiac conduction
Phenobarbital (Luminal)	Impaired development of fine motor skills Sedation Nystagmus Hyperkinesis Ataxia
Primidone (Mysoline)	Marked sedation Hyperkinesis Ataxia Nystagmus
Carbamazepine (Tegretol)	Sedation Ataxia Anorexia, nausea and vomiting Diplopia Vertigo Hepatic dysfunction Leukopenia, thrombocytopenia, agranu-locytosis
Ethosuximide (Zarontin)	Abdominal pain, anorexia, nausea and vomiting Headaches, dizziness Leukopenia, agranulocytosis, aplastic anemia Photophobia
Valproic acid (Depakene)	Nausea and vomiting, anorexia Increased appetite and weight gain Thrombocytopenia, anemia, leukopenia Acute hepatic failure, acute pancreatitis Alopecia
Clonazepam (Clonopin)	Sedation Ataxia Behavioral changes Thrombocytopenia, leukopenia

SURGERY FOR SEIZURE CONTROL[24]

The most common surgical procedure for seizure control is temporal lobectomy. These patients are usually 6 to 8 years of age when presenting for surgery. Patients with intractable extratemporal seizures often require surgery as infants or very young children. Non–temporal lobe foci are often difficult to locate in preoperative mapping.

Population

1. Patients with frequent seizures with life impairment
2. Patients who have demonstrated refractoriness to medical therapy
3. Patients for whom therapeutic agents have unacceptable side effects

Anesthetic Management

Initial anesthetic management includes preoperative evaluation of seizure disorder, neurologic deficits, medications, and side effects from medical therapy (including evaluation of hematologic and hepatic function).

CONSCIOUS PATIENT

1. Infiltration of long-acting local anesthesia by surgeon
2. Monitored sedation carefully titrated to maintain patient cooperation (see p. 445)
3. Ability to treat acute seizure activity and manage airway

GENERAL ANESTHESIA

1. Requires use of electrocorticography.
2. Anesthesia may be induced with a short-acting barbiturate and maintained with N_2O/O_2, fentanyl, and muscle relaxants. A narcotic technique allows avoidance of volatile agents that depress electrical activity.
3. Low concentrations of volatile agents may be used; however, the volatile agents should be discontinued during recording of the seizure focus.
4. Anticonvulsant therapy should be resumed immediately after resection of seizure focus, because the incidence of seizure activity is often initially increased.

References

1. Pickard JD, Czosnyka M: Management of raised intracranial pressure, *J Neurol Neurosurg Psychiatry* 56:845-858, 1993.
2. Johnson KB, ed: *The Harriet Lane handbook,* ed. 13, St Louis, 1993, Mosby.
3. Lanier WL, Stangland KJ, Scheithauer BW, Milde JH, Michenfelder JD: The effects of dextrose infusion and head position on neurologic

outcome after complete cerebral ischemia in primates: examination of a model, *Anesthesiology* 66:39-48, 1987.

4. Bendo AA, Kass IS, Hartung J, Cottrell JE: Neurophysiology and neuroanesthesia. In Barash PH, Cullen BF, Stoelting RK, eds: *Clinical anesthesia,* ed 2, Philadelphia, 1992, JB Lippincott.

5. Milde LN, Milde JH, Gallagher WJ: Effects of sufentanil on cerebral circulation and metabolism in dogs, *Anesth Analg* 70:138-146, 1990.

6. Rosenberg RB, Kass IS, Cotrell JC: Propfol improves electrophysiologic recovery after anoxia in rat hippocampal slice, *Anesthesiology* 75:3A, 1991.

7. Holzman RS: Latex allergy: an emerging operating room problem, *Anesth Analg* 76:635-641, 1993.

8. Hancock DL: Latex allergy, *Anesthesiology Rev* 21:153-163, 1994.

9. Hirshman CA: Latex anaphylaxis, *Anesthesiology* 77:223-225, 1992.

10. Dormans JP, Templeton JJ, Edmonds C, Davidson RS, Drummond DS: Intraoperative anaphylaxis due to exposure to latex (natural rubber) in children, *J Bone Joint Surg* 76A:1688-1691, 1994.

11. Harris, M: Neurologic and neuromuscular diseases. In Berry FA, Steward DJ, eds: *Pediatrics for the anesthesiologist,* New York, 1993, Churchill Livingstone.

12. Millar C, Bissonnette B, Humphreys RP: Cerebral arteriovenous malformations in children, *Can J Anaesth* 41:321-331, 1994.

13. Kuban KCK, Leviton A: Cerebral palsy: *N Engl J Med* 330:188-195, 1994.

14. Theroux MC, Brandon B, et al: Dose response of succinylcholine at the adductor pollicis of children with cerebral palsy during propofol and nitrous oxide anesthesia, *Anesth Analg* 79:761-765, 1994.

15. Park TS, Owen JH: Surgical management of spastic diplegia in cerebral palsy, *N Engl J Med* 326:745-749, 1992.

16. Dodson WE, Pellock JM: *Pediatric epilepsy: diagnosis and therapy,* New York, 1993, Demos Publications.

17. Smith MC: Febrile seizures: recognition and management, *Drugs* 47:933-944, 1994.

18. Legido A, Clancy RR, Berman PH: Neurologic outcome after electroencephalographically proven neonatal seizures, *Pediatrics* 88:583-596, 1991.

19. Corssen G, Little SC, Tanakoli M: Ketamine and epilepsy, *Anesth Analg* 53:319-335, 1974.

20. Tommasino C, Maekawa T, Shapiro HM: Fentanyl induced seizures activate sub-cortical brain metabolism, *Anesthesiology* 60:283-290, 1984.

21. Murkin JM, Moldenhauer CC, Hug CD, Epstein CM: Absence of seizures during induction of anesthesia with high dose fentanyl, *Anesth Analg* 63:489-494, 1984.

22. Komatsu H, Taie S, Endo S, Fukuda K, Ueki M, Nogaya J, Ogli K: Electrical seizures during sevoflurane anesthesia in two pediatric patients with epilepsy, *Anesthesiology* 81:1535-1537, 1994.

23. Schweich PJ: Emergency medicine except poisoning. In Oski FA, DeAngelis CD, Feigin DR, McMillan JA, Warshaw JB eds: *Principles and practice of pediatrics,* ed 2, Philadelphia, 1994, JB Lippincott.

24. Holmes GL: Surgery for intractable seizures in infancy and early childhood, *Neurology* 43:S28-S37, 1993.

ANESTHESIA FOR OPHTHALMIC SURGERY

10

Two Times

Sally Ann saw twice as much
As any girl her age
Twice as many suns and moons
And words upon the page.
But everyone thought Sally Ann
Saw nothing much at all,
She couldn't read or write her name
Or catch a basketball.

Twice as sad was Sally Ann
Who figured not a wit
Why what she saw
And how things looked
Were not a perfect fit.

Rivian Bell

PREOPERATIVE PREPARATION

Preoperative preparation of the child for ophthalmologic surgery begins with the establishment of rapport and communication among the anesthesiologist, the surgeon, the patient, and the patient's parents.

1. As always, a thorough history and physical examination with a complete list of medical and appropriate laboratory data are necessary. Any history of allergies to drugs, foods, or adhesive tape should be elicited.

2. A personal or family history of adverse reactions to anesthesia is very important before eye surgery because of the higher incidence of masseter spasm and malignant hyperthermia associated with strabismus.

3. It is important to counsel the child that one or both eyes may be patched postoperatively. Not surprisingly, occluded vision from either patches or ointments may terrify children as they emerge from anesthesia.

Coexisting Problems

The presence of an ocular abnormality always should alert the anesthesiologist to the possibility of other associated anomalies, genetic aberrations, or systemic disease (see box below). Since premature infants or neonates not uncommonly require ophthalmic procedures, special age-related differences in physiology and pharmacology that apply to these groups should be considered.

Ocular anomalies and coexisting disease

Anomalies frequently associated with coexisting problems

Aniridia
Colobomata
Optic nerve hypoplasia
Cataracts
Ectopia lentis
Glaucoma

Partial listing of genetic, metabolic, infectious, and systemic diseases with ocular pathology

Apert syndrome (acrocephalosyndactyly)	Patau syndrome (trisomy 13)
Crouzon syndrome (craniosynostosis)	Edwards syndrome (trisomy 18)
Kartagener's syndrome (immotile cilia)	Down syndrome (trisomy 21)
Lowe syndrome (oculocerebrorenal)	Diabetes mellitus
Marfan's syndrome	Galactosemia
Sturge-Weber syndrome	Gangliosidoses
Riley-Day syndrome (familial dysautonomia)	Lipidoses
	Mucopolysaccharidoses
Wagner-Stickler syndrome (arthroophthalmomyopathy)	Hypercalcemia
	Homocystinuria
Zellweger syndrome (cerebrohepatorenal)	
	Sickle cell disease
	Neurofibromatosis
Cytomegalovirus	Congenital myotonic
Rubella	dystrophies
Herpes	

OPHTHALMIC EFFECTS OF ANESTHETIC AGENTS
Inhalation Agents

Inhalation agents cause dose-related decreases in intraocular pressure (IOP).[1] The precise mechanism(s) remains unclear. However, postulated etiologies are: depression of a central nervous system control center in the diencephalic region; reduced aqueous humor production; enhancement of aqueous humor outflow; or relaxation of extraocular muscle tension. A recent study has demonstrated minimal effect of halothane on IOP when the concentration ranged between 0.5% and 1.0%.[2]

Intravenous Agents

1. Narcotics, barbiturates, propofol, and etomidate all lower IOP, provided that normocapnia is maintained.[3]
2. Ketamine has minimal, if any, effect on IOP, as indicated by recent studies.[4]
3. In general, asphyxia, hypoventilation, or administration of carbon dioxide will raise IOP, while hypothermia, nondepolarizing muscle relaxants, ganglionic blockers, or hypertonic solutions such as dextran, urea, mannitol, or sorbitol will reduce IOP.[3]
4. Atropine premedication administered parenterally in clinically used dosages has no effect on IOP in patients with glaucoma.[5]

Muscle Relaxants

1. Succinylcholine raises IOP as much as 8 mm Hg, and extrusion of vitreous humor following the administration of succinylcholine has been reported.[6] Postulated mechanisms for this phenomenon are: tonic contraction of the extraocular muscles; choroidal vascular dilation; and relaxation of orbital smooth muscle. A recent study speculated that the succinylcholine-induced increase in IOP is multifactorial but is primarily the result of the cycloplegic action of succinylcholine producing a deepening of the anterior chamber and increased outflow resistance.[7] Because they studied eyes with the extraocular muscles detached and still observed an elevation in IOP, these investigators proposed that changes in extraocular muscle tone do not contribute significantly to the increase in IOP observed after succinylcholine administration.
2. The efficacy of pretreatment with nondepolarizing muscle relaxants to prevent increases in IOP caused by succinylcholine is still questionable. Suggested regimens include:
   a. Pretreatment with small amounts of curare or gallamine[8,9]
   b. Premedication with sufentanil (0.05 µg/kg) plus pretreatment with a nondepolarizing relaxant followed by a high-dose thiopental induction (7 mg/kg)[10]
   c. Alfentanil (150 µg/kg) induction following the pretreatment mentioned above[10]
3. Lidocaine is unreliable in preventing the ocular hypertensive response from either succinylcholine or intubation.[11]
4. Nondepolarizing agents will lower IOP, as long as hypercapnia is avoided.[12,13]

Effect of anesthesia on intraocular pressure (IOP)[3]

Raise IOP	Lower IOP	No effect
Asphyxia (hypoxia)	Hypocapnia	Ketamine
Hypercapnia	Hypothermia	Lidocaine†
Succinylcholine	Inhalation agents	Atropine
	Barbiturates	
	Neuroleptics	
	Opioids	
	Hypnotics	
	Etomidate*	
	Propofol	
	Ganglionic blockers	
	Hypertonic solutions:	
	Dextran	
	Urea	
	Mannitol	
	Sorbitol	
	Nondepolarizing neuromuscular	
	blockers	

*Myoclonus may be hazardous in presence of open globe.
†May protect from increase in IOP if 1.5 mg/kg given IV 1 min prior to thiopental/succinylcholine for rapid-sequence induction.[14]

INDUCTION TECHNIQUES

A broad spectrum of induction techniques exists. In the appropriate settings, methohexital per rectum, thiopental (or another barbiturate) intravenously, propofol intravenously, and inhalation induction (usually with halothane because it is less irritating to airways) are all acceptable methods. Flexibility is essential because the induction plan may have to be modified depending upon ophthalmic pathology, patient age and physiology, and NPO status.

A recent report indicates that the laryngeal mask airway (LMA) may be useful for certain ophthalmic surgeries.[15] Less time was required for insertion than with tracheal intubation, and insertion of the LMA did not increase IOP, heart rate, or arterial blood pressure.

ANESTHETIC CONSIDERATIONS FOR SPECIFIC OPHTHALMIC SURGERIES
Strabismus

1. Strabismus surgery is the most common pediatric ocular operation. Approximately 3% of the population has malalignment of the visual axes.
2. Strabismus is associated with an increased incidence of malignant hyperthermia (MH), and some studies show a three-times-higher incidence of masseter spasm in children undergoing strabismus repair than in the general population.[16]
3. The forced duction test (FDT), which is used to determine

whether the muscle is paretic as opposed to restricted in motion, will not be possible if succinylcholine has been used within 20 minutes of the test.

4. Intubation of the trachea can be achieved under deep inhalational anesthesia or with the use of a nondepolarizing agent. Such problems as succinylcholine-induced masseter spasm and FDT invalidation can be circumvented with these techniques.

5. Oculocardiac reflex prophylaxis is advised before intubation of the trachea and surgical manipulation. Intravenous atropine 0.02 mg/kg or glycopyrrolate 0.01 mg/kg can be used (see p. 234).

6. Postoperative nausea and vomiting are common. Prophylactic administration of droperidol, [17] metoclopramide, [18] or ondansetron [19] is useful. A total intravenous technique with propofol has also been associated with a low incidence of emesis following pediatric strabismus surgery. [20] The antiemetic effects of prophylactic lidocaine are questionable. [21]

Antiemetics useful for strabismus surgery	
Droperidol	0.075 mg/kg IV
Metoclopramide	0.25 mg/kg IV
Ondansetron	0.05 to 0.15 mg/kg IV (maximum dose 4 mg)
Lidocaine	1 to 2 mg/kg IV

Congenital Cataracts

1. Fifty percent of the cases of congenital cataracts are idiopathic. The remainder are associated with chromosomal disorders, inborn errors of metabolism such as galactosemia, intrauterine infections, trauma, and drugs such as corticosteroids.

2. Surgical removal is indicated as early as possible because the clouded lens will impede retinal stimulation and proper visual development. Visual outcome is compromised severely if surgery is delayed beyond 6 months of age.

3. Optimal surgical conditions include an immobile eye and a maximally dilated pupil that permits adequate observation of the red reflex to ensure complete removal of the affected lens. Additionally, once the eye is open a uniform intraocular pressure should be maintained. Any coughing or "bucking" on the endotracheal tube could produce loss of the intraocular contents.

4. Mydriasis can be achieved with preoperative topical 2.5% phenylephrine and 1% cyclopentolate. Additional intraoperative mydriasis is induced by continuous infusion of epinephrine 1:200,000 in a balanced salt solution in the anterior chamber. The drug is simultaneously removed from the chamber by aspi-

ration. The intense vasoconstriction of the iris and ciliary body is felt to limit any uptake of epinephrine. Certainly systemic uptake of epinephrine is always of concern. Nonetheless, under halothane anesthesia, in both children and adults, no increased incidence of dysrhythmias has been reported following direct instillation of epinephrine into the anterior chamber.

5. Paralysis with a nondepolarizing muscle relaxant is advocated strongly to maintain a motionless eye with stable IOP. A sufficiently deep level of anesthesia is indicated for similar reasons until the wound has been closed completely. If the patient should move unexpectedly when the eye is open, intravenous thiopental should be given immediately. Succinylcholine is contraindicated when the eye is surgically open.

6. Any inhalation agent, a balanced technique, or total intravenous anesthesia with propofol may be appropriate. Hypercapnia-associated elevations in IOP should be avoided by means of adequate ventilation. Many patients are neonates; an unnecessarily high FIO_2 should be avoided because of the potential for retinopathy of prematurity (ROP).

7. The goal is safe extubation of the trachea without coughing. Intravenous lidocaine and extubation in the lateral position while the patient is still deeply anesthetized are current recommendations. Alternatively, a laryngeal mask airway is generally associated with minimal coughing upon removal.

8. Intravenous antiemetic therapy with droperidol, metoclopramide, or ondansetron is used to prevent increases in IOP caused by vomiting. (This should be administered at the start of the case, before ocular manipulation.)

Corneal Transplant

The anesthetic considerations for a penetrating keratoplasty are similar to those for cataract surgery. Both are exquisitely delicate intraocular procedures that demand meticulous attention to appropriate anesthetic depth.

Retinoblastoma

1. Retinoblastoma is the most common pediatric ocular malignancy. It usually is diagnosed during the first 3 years of life. Despite their relative rarity, these aggressive tumors account for 1% of all cancer-related pediatric deaths.

2. Common presenting symptoms include white pupillary reflex, strabismus, ocular inflammation, and glaucoma.

3. Treatment varies depending upon the grade and involvement of the tumor. Cryotherapy, photocoagulation, enucleation, chemotherapy, and radiation are current therapies. If enucleation is required, it is advisable to administer intravenous at-

ropine prophylactically because of the relatively high incidence of oculocardiac reflex (see p. 234).

4. Daily irradiation for a period of weeks is common therapy for these children (see Chapter 19 for details of anesthetic techniques during radiation therapy).

Open-Eye and Full-Stomach Situations

1. This clinical situation has become a frequent conundrum for the anesthesiologist. Methods and agents useful in protecting against aspiration of gastric contents must be balanced against their potential to increase IOP.

2. Trauma is the typical cause of the open globe. Simultaneous injuries, such as intracranial trauma producing subdural or epidural hematoma, skull or orbital fractures, and thoracic or abdominal trauma, need to be excluded before operation.

3. Any unnecessary stimulation should be avoided because coughing or vomiting can raise IOP as much as 40 mm Hg or more. The stomach should not be emptied by a nasogastric

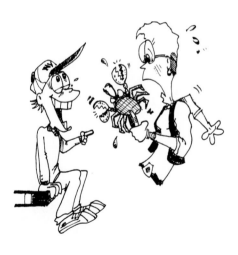

I told you there was something in my eye...

tube. Additionally, any external pressure on the globe by aggressive placement of an anesthetic mask or increase in venous pressure (as may result from narcotic-induced vomiting, coughing, or struggling) must be avoided. The use of a slightly larger mask with the inferior aspect placed under the chin will help to avoid pressure on the eyes (see Fig. 10-1).

4. Aspiration prophylaxis with an H_2-receptor antagonist is advised. Metoclopramide (0.15 mg/kg IV) is also useful to help stimulate peristalsis.

5. After pretreatment with a nondepolarizing agent, rapid-sequence induction is generally the method of choice for an open-globe injury in a patient with a full stomach (see table on next page).[22] It is recommended that the patient be extubated in the lateral position when the patient is fully awake. Suction of gastric contents while the child is still deeply anesthetized is advised before reversal of muscle relaxation.

6. Rocuronium, with its purportedly rapid onset, may prove to be a useful drug in this setting. Recent evidence suggests that a generous dose of 1.2 mg/kg IV may be necessary to ensure adequately smooth and rapid intubating conditions.

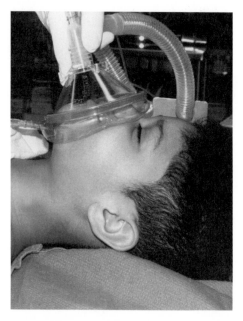

FIG. 10-1. For ophthalmic procedures, placing the inferior aspect of the face mask under the chin helps to avoid direct pressure on the eyes during induction or emergence.

Induction techniques for open globe/full stomach

Technique	Advantages	Disadvantages
Technique I		
1. Pretreatment with nondepolarizing relaxant 2. Barbiturate (thiopental) 7 mg/kg 3. Succinylcholine 1-2 mg/kg	Rapid onset Excellent intubating conditions Short duration No report of extruded intraocular contents with this technique	Slight elevations in IOP may occur Bradycardia associated with succinylcholine necessitates pretreatment with atropine
Technique II		
1. Barbiturate (thiopental) 7 mg/kg 2. Pancuronium 0.15 mg/kg	Pancuronium lowers IOP	Possible aspiration and death during 75-150 sec of unprotected airway Dramatic increase in IOP if intubation attempts produce coughing or straining Prolonged muscle relaxation beyond length of procedure Duration problematic with a difficult airway
Technique III		
1. Barbiturate 2. High-dose vecuronium (0.4 mg/kg)	Minimal cardiac effects	Variability in onset Duration problematic with a difficult airway
Technique IV		
1. Priming dose ($\frac{1}{10}$ of intubating dose of nondepolarizer) 2. Barbiturate 3. Intubating dose of nondepolarizer 4 min after priming dose	May be able to intubate within 90 sec	Wide variability in onset of relaxation Aspiration and respiratory dysfunction can occur with priming dose Duration problematic with a difficult airway
Technique V		
1. Barbiturate (thiopental) 7 mg/kg 2. Rocuronium (0.6-1.2 mg/kg)	1. Rapid onset 2. Minimal hemodynamic perturbation	Intermediate duration problematic with a difficult airway Quality of airway intubating conditions

OCULOCARDIAC REFLEX
Underlying pathology
1. The oculocardiac reflex has trigeminal (V) afferent and vagal (X) efferent pathways.
2. It is triggered by pressure on the globe or traction of the extraocular muscles, the conjunctiva, or orbital structures. It can be elicited by performance of a retrobulbar block, by ocular trauma, or by direct pressure on remaining tissue in the orbital apex following an enucleation.
3. The most common manifestation is sinus bradycardia. However, a vast array of dysrhythmias may occur, including junctional rhythm, ectopic atrial rhythm, atrioventricular block, ventricular bigeminy, multifocal premature ventricular contractions, wandering pacemaker, idioventricular rhythm, asystole, and ventricular tachycardia.
4. Hypercapnia, hypoxemia, or inappropriate depth of anesthesia can augment the severity of the problem.

Incidence
The incidence ranges from 16% to 82%.[23,24] Strabismus patients can have an incidence as high as 90%, if not pretreated with atropine.

Prophylaxis
1. For strabismus surgery, most anesthesiologists favor routine prophylaxis with atropine 0.02 mg/kg IV before commencement of surgery. Alternatively, glycopyrrolate 0.01 mg/kg IV can be administered.
2. Because nearly complete vagolytic blockade requires 0.03 to 0.05 mg/kg of atropine, and because the peak action of intramuscular atropine occurs approximately 30 minutes following administration, it is not surprising that the much smaller doses of atropine historically given more than 1 hour before surgery by the intramuscular route have afforded inconsistent protection.
3. Recently, investigators in Germany reported that the topical administration of 1 ml of 2% lidocaine onto the medial aspect of the eye following induction of anesthesia significantly attenuated the oculocardiac reflex and prevented severe bradydysrhythmias.[25] However, this intervention has not been widely studied.

Treatment
1. Treatment of the oculocardiac reflex depends upon its nature and severity. Small decrements in cardiac rate are acceptable if unaccompanied by hypotension. Severe bradycardia or hypotension is treated by asking the surgeon to stop ocular ma-

nipulation. If the heart rate does not return to normal, atropine (0.01 mg/kg IV) should be given.
2. Ventricular dysrhythmias triggered by the reflex may require the administration of 1 to 2 mg/kg of IV lidocaine.

ANESTHETIC IMPLICATIONS OF TOPICAL OCULAR DRUGS
Absorption of Topical Drugs

1. Systemic absorption occurs from either the conjunctiva or nasal mucosa (following drainage through the nasolacrimal duct). Absorption is more rapid and extensive from nasal mucosal surfaces and can be reduced by application of digital pressure to the inner canthus of the eye for 3 to 5 minutes.
2. The lacrimal apparatus is dependent upon an active blink reflex and muscle action. Systemic absorption, therefore, is decreased significantly under general anesthesia. Nasolacrimal duct occlusion is still advisable, even in the anesthetized state, since small children are more vulnerable to the toxic side effects of certain ocular drugs.
3. Topical ocular drugs with systemic toxicity to which the anesthesiologist should be alert are found among commonly used mydriatics (atropine, scopolamine, cyclopentolate), antiglaucoma agents (echothiophate iodide, epinephrine, timolol, betaxolol), and vasoconstrictors (cocaine and phenylephrine).

Topical ocular medication

Drug	Concentration (%)	Amount per drop (mg)	Pediatric dose	Indication(s)
Atropine	1	0.5	1 drop	Mydriasis Cycloplegia
Cocaine	4	2	<1.5 mg/kg	Vasoconstriction during dacryocystorhinostomy
Cyclopentolate	0.5-1	0.25-0.5	1 drop	Mydriasis Cycloplegia
Echothiophate iodide	0.03-0.125	0.015-0.0625	1 drop bid	Antiglaucoma
Epinephrine	0.25-1	0.125-0.5	1 drop bid	Antiglaucoma
Phenylephrine	2.5	1.25	1 drop	Mydriasis Vasoconstriction Decongestion
Scopolamine	0.5	0.25	1 drop	Mydriasis Cycloplegia
Timolol	0.25, 0.5	0.125, 0.25	1 drop bid	Antiglaucoma
Betaxolol	0.5	0.25	1 drop bid	Antiglaucoma

Mydriatics

Mydriatics are primarily anticholinergic agents, and, as such, anesthesiologists can predict systemic effects. CNS effects can be anticipated in those drugs which cross the blood-brain barrier (scopolamine and cyclopentolate). See table, p. 237.

Antiglaucoma Agents

Commonly used antiglaucoma agents achieve their effects through different mechanisms (see descriptions in table on next page). Potential complications from β-agonist/antagonists should be considered before administration to children with congenital heart disease. Likewise, consideration should be given to the potential respiratory effects of β-blockade in children with reactive airway disease. See table, p. 237.

Vasoconstrictors

Both cocaine and phenylephrine are known for the severity of systemic reactions (particularly cardiac) that can occur. Consequently, careful attention to dosing should be given by the anesthesiologist and ophthalmologist prior to administration. Cocaine has limited topical ocular use because of its corneal toxicity, but it is used in nasal packing during dacryocystorhinostomy for vasoconstriction and shrinkage of nasal mucosa. One drop of 4% cocaine solution contains 2 mg of cocaine. The maximum safe dosage is 3 mg/kg, but 1.5 mg/kg is recommended if a volatile anesthetic is being used. Furthermore, it must be appreciated that systemic reactions may transpire with as little as 20 mg of cocaine; there is, unfortunately, a narrow range from safety to toxicity to death with cocaine usage. Cocaine should not be administered in combination with epinephrine because of the facilitation of dysrhythmias, especially during halothane anesthesia. Cocaine is contraindicated in patients with hypertension or those receiving adrenergic modifying drugs. To avoid cocaine toxicity the physician should search out possible contraindications and then administer meticulously calculated doses of dilute solutions. See table, p. 238.

Mydriatics

Drug	Description	Toxicity
Atropine	Anticholinergic: long-acting mydriatic, cycloplegic	Systemic reactions include flushing, thirst, tachycardia, dry skin, temperature elevation, and agitation.
Scopolamine	Anticholinergic: produces potent mydriasis, cycloplegia	CNS toxicity: excitation and disorientation (may be seen with 1 drop of 0.5% solution [0.25 mg])
Cyclopentolate	Synthetic antimuscarinic: short-acting mydriatric	CNS toxicity manifests as dysarthria, disorientation, seizures, and frank psychosis. Concentrations of 1% or less are advised for pediatric use.

Antiglaucoma agents

Drug	Description	Toxicity
Echothiophate iodide	Long-acting anticholinesterase	Cholinergic side effects: vomiting, hypotension, and abdominal pain Preoperative IV atropine prevents severe bradydysrhythmias Drugs metabolized by plasma pseudocholinesterase (succinylcholine, procaine, cocaine, and chloroprocaine) should be reduced in dosage or avoided if the patient has received echothiophate iodide within the last 5 weeks
Epinephrine	β-agonist used to treat open-angle glaucoma	Side effects: hypertension, tachycardia, dysrhythmias (associated with higher concentrations)
Timolol maleate (Timoptic)	Nonselective β-blocker	Exacerbation of myasthenia gravis Postoperative apnea in neonates Extreme caution advised in patients with known contraindications to β-blockade (i.e., asthma, congestive heart failure, heart block)
Betaxolol hydrochloride	$β_1$-blocker	Side effects are rare Contraindicated in patients in whom cardiac β-blockade is potentially dangerous

Vascoconstrictors

Drug	Description	Toxicity
Cocaine	Ester-linked local anesthetic Sympathomimetic properties secondary to its ability to block the reuptake of catecholamines	Severe sympathomimetic reactions include: tachycardia, hypertension, dysrhythmias, and seizures Treatment: IV barbiturates (CNS complication), IV labetalol (cardiac complications)
Phenylephrine (Neo-Synephrine)	α-agonist: produces pupillary dilation and capillary decongestion	Children are especially vulnerable to overdose and manifest severe bradycardia, hypertension, ST-segment depression, and asystole. Only the 2.5% solution is recommended for pediatric use, with one drop (1.25 mg)/eye/hr.

POSTOPERATIVE PROBLEMS
Nausea and Vomiting

The high incidence of nausea and vomiting associated with pediatric strabismus has been reduced dramatically by the prophylactic use of droperidol (0.075 mg/kg IV), metoclopramide (0.25 mg/kg IV), or ondansetron (0.05 to 0.15 mg/kg IV).[19,26] Further postoperative nausea and vomiting can be treated with low dosages of droperidol (0.010 mg/kg IV), or with dimenhydrinate (Dramamine) in doses of 1 mg/kg IM or 2 mg/kg per rectum. If the patient appears excessively drowsy, metoclopramide 0.15 mg/kg or ondansetron 0.05-0.1 mg/kg may be administered instead. Small doses of benzodiazepines (midazolam 0.01 mg/kg IV) may also be useful.

Pain

Strabismus surgery, cryotherapy, and retinal detachment surgery frequently are associated with considerable postoperative pain. Analgesics such as codeine or morphine are helpful, if rectal Tylenol does not provide adequate analgesia (see p. 459 for analgesic doses). A recent study indicated that administration of the nonopioid analgesic ketorolac, in a dose of 0.75 mg/kg IV, provided analgesia comparable to morphine 0.1 mg/kg IV but with a much lower incidence of nausea and vomiting in the first 24 hours.[26, 27]

References

1. Al-Abrak MH, Samuel JF: Effects of general anesthesia on intraocular pressure in man: comparison of tubocurarine and pancuronium in nitrous oxide and oxygen, *Br J Ophthalmol* 58:806, 1974.
2. Watcha MF, Chu FC, Stevens JL, et al: Effects of halothane on intraocular pressure in anesthetized children, *Anesth Analg* 71:181, 1990.
3. McGoldrick KE: Anesthesia and the eye. In Barash PG, Cullen BJ, Stoelting RK, eds: *Clinical anesthesia,* ed 3, JB Lippincott (in press).
4. Ausinisch B et al: Ketamine and intraocular pressure in children, *Anesth Analg* 55:773-775, 1976.
5. Duncalf D, Foldes FF: Effect of anesthetic drugs and muscle relaxants on intraocular pressure. In Smith RB, ed *Anesthesia in ophthalmology,* Boston, 1973, Little, Brown & Co, p 21.
6. Lincoff HA et al: Effect of succinylcholine on intraocular pressure, *Am J Ophthalmol* 40:501, 1955.
7. Kelly RE, Dinner M, Turner LS, Haik B, Abramson DH, Daines P: Succinylcholine increases intraocular pressure in the human eye with the extraocular muscles detached, *Anesthesiology* 79:948-952, 1993.
8. Miller RD, Way WL, Hickey RF: Inhibition of succinylcholine-induced increased intraocular pressure by nondepolarizing muscle relaxants, *Anesthesiology* 29:123-126, 1968.
9. Meyers EF et al: Failure of nondepolarizing neuromuscular blockers to inhibit succinylcholine-induced increased intraocular pressure: a controlled study, *Anesthesiology* 48:149-151, 1978.
10. Badrinath SK, Braverman B, Ivankovich AD: Alfentanil and sufentanil prevent the increase in IOP from succinylcholine, *Anesth Analg* 67:S5, 1988.
11. Smith RB, Babinski M, Leano N: Effect of lidocaine on succinylcholine-induced rise in IOP, *Can Anaesth Soc J* 26:482, 1979.
12. Duncalf D, Weitzner SW: Ventilation and hypercapnia on intraocular pressure in children, *Anesth Analg* 43:232, 1963.
13. Litwiller RW, Difazio CA, Rushia EL: Pancuronium and intraocular pressure, *Anesthesiology* 42:750, 1975.
14. Grover VK, Lata K, Sharma S, et al: Efficacy of lidocaine in the suppression of the intraocular pressure response to suxamethonium and tracheal intubation, *Anaesthesia* 44:22, 1989.
15. Watcha MF, White PF, Tychsen L, Stevens JL: Comparative effects of laryngeal mask airway and endotracheal tube insertion on intraocular pressure in children, *Anesth Analg* 75:355-360, 1992.
16. Carroll JB: Increased incidence of masseter spasm in children anesthetized with halothane and succinylcholine, *Anesthesiology* 67:559-661, 1987.
17. Lerman J. Eustis S, Smith DR. Effect of droperidol pretreatment on postanesthetic vomiting in children undergoing strabismus surgery, *Anesthesiology* 65:322-325, 1986.
18. Lin DM, Furst SR, Rodarte A: A double-blinded comparison of metoclopramide and droperidol for prevention of emesis following strabismus surgery, *Anesthesiology* 76:357-361, 1992.
19. Rose JB, Martin TM, Corddry DH, Zabnoev M, Kettrick RG: Ondansetron reduces the incidence and severity of poststrabismus repair vomiting in children, *Anesth Analg* 79:486-489, 1994.

20. Watcha MF, Simeon RM, White PF, Stevens JL: Effect of propofol on the incidence of postoperative vomiting after strabismus surgery in pediatric outpatients, *Anesthesiology* 75:204-209, 1991.
21. Christensen S, Farrow-Gillespie A, Lerman J: Incidence of emesis and postanesthetic recovery after strabismus surgery in children: a comparison of droperidol and lidocaine, *Anesthesiology* 70:251-254, 1989.
22. Linbonati MM, Leahy JJ, Ellison N: Use of succinylcholine in open eye surgery, *Anesthesiology* 62:637, 1985.
23. Berler DK: Oculocardiac reflex, *Am J Ophthalmol* 12:56, 954, 1963.
24. Taylor C et al: Prevention of the oculocardiac reflex in children: comparison of retrobulbar block and intravenous atropine, *Anesthesiology* 24:646, 1963.
25. Möllhoff T, Ruta U, Markodimitrakis H, et al: Attenuation of the oculocardiac reflex after topical administration of lidocaine in children undergoing surgery for strabismus, *Anesthesiology* 77:A1188, 1992.
26. Watcha MF, Bras PJ, Cieslak GD, Pennant JH: The dose-response relationship of ondansetron in preventing postoperative emesis in pediatric patients undergoing ambulatory surgery, *Anesthesiology* 82:47-52, 1995.
27. Munro HM, Rieger LQ, Reynolds PI, Wilton NCT, Lewis IH: Comparison of the analgesic and emetic properties of ketorolac and morphine for paediatric outpatient strabismus surgery, *Br J Anaesth* 72:624-628, 1994.

Suggested Readings

Abramowitz MD, Oh TH, Epstein BS: Antiemetic effect of droperidol following outpatient strabismus surgery in children, *Anesthesiology* 59:579-583, 1983.

France NK: Ophthalmological disease. In Katz J, Steward DJ, eds: *Anesthesia and uncommon pediatric diseases,* Philadelphia, 1987, WB Saunders.

McGoldrick KE: Anesthetic implications of congenital and metabolic diseases. In Bruce RA, McGoldrick KE, Oppenheimer P, eds. *Anesthesia for ophthalmology,* Birmingham, 1982, Aesculapius.

McGoldrick KE: Ocular pathology and systemic diseases: anesthetic implications. In McGoldrick KE: *Anesthesia for ophthalmic and otolaryngologic surgery,* Philadelphia, 1992, WB Saunders, pp. 210-226.

ANESTHESIA FOR GASTROINTESTINAL DISORDERS

11

When you're in a boring meeting
When your best team takes a beating
Even though your funds are fleeting
Just try eating.

Try some fowl that's finger lickin'
With a spread or sauce for dipping
There are scores of sweets and fixings
Just for eating.

Have a roast or chop so tasty
Choose a flaky pie or pastry
Even pudding known as Hasty
Just for eating.

But if you are allergic
Or your stomach walls aren't too thick
You can make yourself feel more sick
Just by eating.

It's no fun to moan and mumble
When your guts begin to grumble
Your whole life can take a tumble—
Forget eating!

Rivian Bell

GUT EMBRYOLOGY AND CONGENITAL DEFECTS[1]

During the third gestational week the primitive gut tube is formed extending from mouth to cloaca. Three separate branches from the aorta provide blood to the foregut (celiac artery), midgut (omphalomesenteric or superior mesenteric artery), and hindgut (inferior mesenteric artery).

The foregut is the precursor for pharynx, esophagus, stomach, and the first part of the duodenum. Liver, gallbladder, and pancreas also develop from foregut.

Developing canaliculi and *bile ducts* are susceptible to injury by maternal drugs, toxins, and viruses during this period. *Duodenal atresia,* frequently seen with trisomy 21 (Down syndrome) may also occur. See Fig. 11-1.

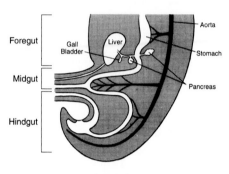

5 WEEKS

FIG. 11-1.   Fifth week of gestation.

During the fifth to tenth week of gestation, the midgut (second portion of duodenum to proximal large bowel) grows rapidly and the part connected to the yolk sac returns to the body. Interruption of the blood supply as the gut rotates around the omphalomesenteric artery can lead to *bowel atresia.* Abdominal wall defects may result in *umbilical hernia, omphalocele,* and *gastroschisis.* Incomplete rupture of the cloacal membrane (9 weeks) is associated with *anorectal anomalies* and *bladder exstrophy.* See Fig. 11-2.

Rotation of the bowel and mesenteric attachment (cecum and appendix to right lower quadrant) occur by 11 weeks. Anomalous rotation causes *bowel obstruction* and *strangulation.*

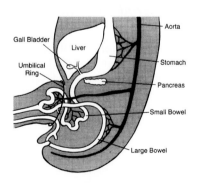

10 WEEKS

FIG. 11-2.   Tenth week of gestation.

NORMAL PATTERNS OF GASTROINTESTINAL (GI) FUNCTION IN THE NEWBORN

Swallowing

The fetus is able to swallow in utero; esophageal peristalsis also begins at this time. It is not until the seventh month of age that the infant can coordinate the movement of solid food from the front of the tongue to the pharynx.[2] When chronic illness prevents the introduction of solid foods beyond 15 months of age, many infants will have difficulty accepting solids in their diet.

Gastric Emptying

The gastric emptying time for a healthy full-term infant is highly variable. Gastric emptying is slow in the first 12 hours of life, and "full stomach" precautions prevail for any anesthesia conducted in a neonate during this period of time. Because of the high closing capacity relative to functional residual capacity (FRC) in the neonate and high oxygen consumption, a rapid-sequence induction usually results in marked desaturation before the succinylcholine is effective. Therefore, awake intubation is usually advocated for newborns.

Intestinal Motility

Intestinal motility is disorganized in the preterm infant until about 34 weeks of gestation, when a more cyclical pattern of smooth muscle activity develops with corresponding neurologic development. It is not until the end of the first year of life that a normal adult pattern of gastrointestinal motility is present.

Gastroesophageal Reflux (GER)

Passive gastrointestinal reflux is a common condition in a newborn infant. As many as 40% of infants will regurgitate or "spit up" gastric contents.[3] This results from an immature gastroesophageal sphincter, absent or disorganized peristaltic waves, and a lower pressure in the esophagus than in the stomach. Normal passive GER will either improve or resolve in most children during the first year of life.[4]

COMMON GASTROINTESTINAL DISORDERS

Gastroesophageal Reflux[3,5]

Clinically significant GER will often present as failure to thrive, recurrent pulmonary infections, asthma, irritability, or GI bleeding. Secondary GER may be caused by severe neurologic impairment, esophageal atresia repair, or large hiatal hernia. Localized complications include esophageal stricture, ulceration, bleeding, and Barrett's esophagus.

Complications of gastroesophageal reflux in children

Nutritional

Failure to thrive
Rumination
Vomiting

Respiratory/Cardiac

Aspiration
Recurrent upper
  respiratory infections
Asthma
Apnea/bradycardia
Cyanosis and respiratory
  distress
"Near dying" spells
Chronic cough
Laryngospasm
Stridor

Esophageal

Esophagitis
Hiatal hernia with reflux
Dysphagia
Esophageal stricture
Odynophagia or unresponsive heart-
  burn
Bleeding or anemia
Barrett's esophagus and premalignant
  changes

Other

Torticollis (Sandifer"s syndrome)

ANESTHETIC CONSIDERATIONS FOR GER

1. Preoperative medical management should aim to resolve any respiratory infections, maintain adequate fluid and electrolyte balance, and treat acidic reflux with H_2 antagonists and metoclopramide.
2. A child with severe reflux is usually considered to require "full-stomach" precautions, and either a rapid-sequence induction or awake intubation should be considered.
3. An inhalation induction may be appropriate in the child whose symptoms are well controlled or when airway management supersedes GI concerns.
4. A Nissen fundoplication is the most common operative procedure for correction of GER. The surgeon may approach the operative site through either a high midline abdominal or a thoracic incision. A gastrostomy tube may be placed. The patient may require prolonged postoperative ventilation, depending on age, weight, site of incision, preoperative pulmonary status, and anticipated postoperative analgesic needs.
5. Attention to adequate postoperative pain management, by either regional or parenteral techniques, is an important adjunct to minimize postoperative pulmonary complications (see Chapter 20).

6. Reactive airway disease (bronchospasm) and chronic cough are common problems in children with reflux and are not necessarily due to aspiration.[3] The decision to avoid intubation to minimize bronchospasm (or utilize a deep extubation technique) vs. securing the airway to minimize aspiration risks must be individualized for each patient.

Drug therapy for reflux[6]

Medication	Dose	Comments
Cimetidine	7.5 mg/kg PO/IV	Reduced gastric acid secretion by antagonism of H_2 receptors Given 1-3 hr before induction Inhibits cytochrome P_{450} oxidase system
Ranitidine	0.5 mg/kg PO/IV	Reduced gastric acid secretion by antagonism of H_2 receptors Given 1-3 hr before induction Binds minimally to P_{450} system May increase serum levels of theophylline and warfarin
Metoclopramide	0.1-0.2 mg/kg IV	Improves gastric emptying Given 30 min before induction Effects may be offset by simultaneous use of atropine Should not be given to patients receiving MAO inhibitors or tricyclic antidepressants

Nausea and Vomiting

The causes of nausea and vomiting are numerous. Because young infants have high caloric and fluid requirements, they can rapidly develop dehydration, starvation ketosis, and hypochloremic/hypokalemic metabolic alkalosis from persistent vomiting. An assessment of the degree of dehydration and adequate fluid and electrolyte therapy are necessary.

Diarrhea

Diarrhea is a major cause of infant mortality. Common etiologies include infection, inborn errors of metabolism, food allergy, carbohydrate intolerance, and inflammatory bowel disease. Children have a large intestinal surface/body weight ratio and large extracellular fluid compartment, making them particularly susceptible to dehydration and increased morbidity and mortality from diarrhea. Evaluation of a child with diarrhea includes assessment of fluid and electrolyte imbalances and proper replacement therapy.

Metabolic disturbances associated with diarrhea
(see also Dehydration in Chapter 4, p. 73)

Metabolic disturbance	Etiology	Treatment
Metabolic acidosis	Bicarbonate loss in stool	If pH <7.29, HCO_3^- 1 mEq/kg
Ketosis	Malabsorption; poor oral intake	Glucose-containing IV
Hypokalemia	Potassium loss in stool or emesis	K^+ 0.5 mEq/kg/hr IV over 30 min after the patient has voided twice
Hypoglycemia	Prolonged diarrhea	Glucose 0.5-1.0 g/kg
Hypocalcemia	Ca^{++} loss in stool	Calcium gluconate 100 mg/kg IV slowly
Hypernatremia	Severe fluid losses	IV therapy with D_5W

Inguinal hernias

1. The incidence of inguinal hernias is 1 to 2 per 100 live births; the condition is more commonly seen in males. Sixty percent of hernias appear on the right side, 30% on the left side, and 10% bilaterally.
2. Associated conditions include prematurity, undescended testes, positive family history, presence of ventricular peritoneal shunt (due to excessive fluid in peritoneal cavity), hypospadias, hydrocele, connective tissue disorders, and cystic fibrosis.
3. Most hernias are repaired electively soon after diagnosis to avoid potential incarceration. The incidence of incarceration is 32% in infants under 3 months of age and 66% in infants under 1 year of age.[7]
4. If strangulation or incarceration occurs, then the patient is treated as for a bowel obstruction. Age and overall condition will determine whether a rapid-sequence induction or awake intubation is indicated.
5. The preterm infant with inguinal hernia is at increased risk for postoperative apnea and pulmonary complications (see p. 5). Use of regional techniques (spinal or caudal anesthesia) without additional sedation reportedly decreases the incidence of postoperative respiratory complications (see p. 466 for technique of spinal anesthesia).
6. Postoperative inpatient monitoring for former preterm infants has been advocated in a variety of studies (detailed in Chapter 1, p. 6).
7. The use of sedation is controversial during spinal anesthesia, because of increased risk of apnea, and should be avoided when possible.[8]

8. Postoperative pain can be managed by an ilioinguinal and iliohypogastric nerve block, local infiltration of the wound, caudal blockade, or local anesthetics dripped into the wound before closure. Opioids are usually avoided in infants at risk for apnea.

SEVERE GASTROINTESTINAL DISORDERS

Necrotizing Enterocolitis (NEC)

Necrotizing enterocolitis is a disease process of premature infants characterized by varying degrees of bowel necrosis. It is the most common acquired gastrointestinal emergency in the intensive care nursery. The infant at greatest risk is less than 32 weeks of gestational age and weighs less than 1500 g, although the disease may occur in full-term infants. The exact cause remains an enigma and is probably multifactorial.

Features of necrotizing enterocolitis (NEC)

Etiologies

Asphyxia, polycythemia, hyperosmolar feedings, umbilical artery catheterization, respiratory distress syndrome, exchange transfusions, congenital cardiac disease; an ischemic insult to the intestine is the final common pathway

Clinical features

Irritability and/or lethargy, abdominal distention, bloody mucus in stool, vomiting, high gastric residuals

Associated problems

Acidosis, hypothermia, apnea and bradycardia, thrombocytopenia, disseminated intravascular coagulation (DIC), septic/hypovolemic shock

Radiographic findings

Pneumatosis intestinalis (presence of air within the bowel wall); pneumoperitoneum

Medical management

Antibiotics, nasogastric suction, discontinuation of enteral feedings, IV fluids; medical therapy is successful in avoiding surgery in 85% of all cases

Surgical intervention

Indications for surgery include: intestinal perforation, mechanical obstruction, peritonitis, progressive acidosis, and failed medical therapy

---

ANESTHETIC MANAGEMENT OF NEC

Preoperative management. Only those infants failing medical therapy proceed to surgical intervention, so these infants by definition are critically ill and often moribund. Most infants are hypovolemic with a metabolic acidosis requiring colloid and crystalloid resuscitation. Coagulopathy and hypocalcemia also must be corrected. An arterial catheter allows direct blood pressure monitoring and frequent measurement of arterial blood gases, pH, hematocrit, coagulation parameters, and electrolytes to guide resuscitation efforts. The necessary blood and blood products should be ordered, especially if thrombocytopenia or coagulopathy is present.

Airway management. If the infant has not yet been intubated in the intensive care unit, the airway must be established by either a rapid-sequence induction or awake intubation. Although awake intubations carry the risk of intracranial hemorrhage from increased intracranial pressure, most anesthesiologists believe this is the safest technique in the premature infant with an acute abdomen and marginal respiratory reserve.

Anesthetic agents. Appropriate anesthetic agents include opioids and ketamine. Inhalation agents should be used judiciously in these critically ill infants, who may not tolerate the cardiovascular depressant effects of these anesthetics. Nitrous oxide should be avoided because of bowel distention and the frequent presence of pneumatosis intestinalis. An air/oxygen mixture is used to maintain arterial oxygen tension between 50 and 70 mm Hg or SpO$_2$ around 90%.

Intraoperative management. During the operation, attention must be paid to adequate fluid replacement, electrolyte deficiencies, acid-base balance, serum glucose, coagulation abnormalities, and hematocrit level. Inotropic support (usually dopamine) may be needed, particularly in severe sepsis.

Temperature maintenance. Hypothermia is a common problem in septic infants and worsens with bowel exposure during surgery. Normothermia is maintained with increased room temperature, radiant heat lamps, warming blankets, warmed and humidified gases, wrapping the extremities in plastic wrap, covering the head, and warmed-air delivery systems.

Postoperative management. The infant requires ventilatory assistance in the postoperative period and should be transported back to the intensive care unit in a warm isolette with full monitoring, resuscitative drugs, and oxygen. A prolonged ileus is expected and will likely necessitate placement of a central venous catheter for parenteral hyperalimentation.

Pyloric Stenosis

1. Pyloric stenosis is the most frequent cause of gastrointestinal obstruction seen in infants.[1] Congenital hypertrophy of the pyloric sphincter causes a gradual obstruction of the gastric outlet,

commonly in male infants. Symptoms of nonbilious, persistent or projectile vomiting usually present in the fourth to sixth week of life. An olive-sized mass is classically palpable in the pyloric region. Diagnosis can be confirmed by ultrasonography.

2. Dehydration and hypochloremic, hypokalemic metabolic alkalosis may develop if vomiting has been severe or prolonged.[9] It must be emphasized that pyloric stenosis is first a medical emergency, requiring correction of fluid and electrolyte abnormalities, and then a surgically treatable condition.

3. Preoperative management includes continuous nasogastric suction and intravenous replacement of fluids and electrolytes (see page 74).

4. Before induction of general anesthesia, the stomach must be emptied with a 10 or 12 French suction catheter. Despite continuous low-pressure nasogastric suction, these infants will commonly have a large amount of fluid in their stomachs. The presence of large volumes of residual barium if a diagnostic upper GI series has been performed makes these infants particularly susceptible to aspiration.

5. The airway is secured either by an awake intubation or rapid-sequence induction. The age, size, and overall medical condition of the child, as well as the experience and expertise of the anesthesiologist, will determine which method is more suitable.

6. Because pyloromyotomy is a relatively short procedure, short-acting muscle relaxants are useful in this setting.

7. Extubation of the trachea should follow when the child is wide awake and the stomach has been emptied.

8. Postoperative apnea has been reported in healthy, full-term infants after pyloromyotomy.[10] The actual etiology is unknown but may be due to changes in cerebrospinal fluid pH secondary to hyperventilation or alkalosis. For this reason, opioids are avoided or minimized and short-term apnea monitoring may be indicated in the postoperative period.

Bowel Obstruction

1. Etiologies of bowel obstruction in children include congenital bands, malrotation, intestinal atresia, volvulus, appendicitis, meconium inspissation, intussusception, Hirschsprung's disease, imperforate anus, meconium ileus and meconium peritonitis, and mucosal cysts and polyps (see tables on pp. 252 and 253).

2. Preoperative management consists of nasogastric suction and intravenous replacement of fluids and electrolytes.

3. A rapid-sequence induction or awake intubation is indicated.

4. Appropriate anesthetic agents include inhalation or intravenous agents. Nitrous oxide can be used judiciously once the abdomen is open. However, it may cause increased bowel disten-

tion and make the surgical closure of the abdomen more difficult in a small infant. An air/oxygen mixture is a better choice
in the small infant and child.

5. Stomach contents should continue to be aspirated via an orogastric or nasogastric suction catheter after the airway is secured. This is an important maneuver before any surgical
manipulation of the gut, since regurgitation and leakage of
stomach contents beyond an uncuffed endotracheal tube consti-
tute an ever-present hazard.

6. The trachea should be extubated when the child is fully awake.
The lateral position is advised for transport to the recovery
room.

Bowel obstruction in older children

Disorder	Signs and symptoms	Surgical management
Intussusception	Inversion of loop of bowel into the next one; usually at ileocecal valve Currant jelly stools caused by blood and mucus secreted into bowel lumen Usually male, 5 to 9 months of age	Often can be reduced with barium enema Surgical intervention necessary for about 25% of patients
Appendicitis	Low-grade fever, mild leukocytosis Guarding and rebound on examination	Immediate operative intervention (morbidity and mortality greatly increase if appendix ruptures) Rarely, a profoundly dehydrated child requires normalization of fluids and electrolytes preoperatively
Colonic polyps Juvenile	Never malignant Rarely prolapse through rectum	Removal of polyps during sigmoidoscopy
Multiple polypoid adenomatosis	Genetically determined All result in malignant conversion	Total proctocolectomy
Peutz-Jeghers syndrome	Hamartomatous bowel or stomach polyps; will occasionally bleed, causing anemia Pigment spots on skin and mucosa Not associated with malignancy	Treatment indicated if persistent bleeding

Bowel obstruction in neonates

Disorder	Signs and symptoms	Surgical management
Intestinal atresia Duodenal atresia	Absence of abdominal distension because of proximal obstruction X-ray findings: double-bubble (air/fluid levels in stomach and proximal duodenum)	Duodenoduo-denostomy
Ileal and jejunal atresia	High incidence of associated anomalies Abdominal distention Multiple loops of small bowel on x-ray; no air in colon	Duodenojejunos-tomy or ileal resection
Malrotation and volvulus	Duodenal obstruction because of anomalous peritoneal bands Volvulus of entire small bowel with early signs of necrosis as superior mesenteric vessels twist with unfixed mesentery May present with distention and bloody stools	Exploration, Ladd procedure to lyse band and fix mesentery (see table on p. 258)
Meconium ileus	Obstruction caused by unusually thick meconium Most often associated with cystic fibrosis	May resolve with hyperosmolar enemas of meglumine diatrizoate (Gastrograffin) Often requires bowel resection or colostomy
Meconium peritonitis	Caused by intrauterine intestinal rupture X-ray: spotty calcification in an area that does not contain loops of bowel	Exploration; correct cause of rupture
Hirschsprung's disease	Clinical symptoms range from constipation to severe colonic obstruction X-ray: narrowed distal segment of colon with proximal dilation Aganglionic section of bowel is usually segmental	Colostomy and biopsy Later, pull-through procedure (see table on p. 258)
Imperforate anus	May be accompanied by fistula into bladder or vagina High incidence of associated renal or GI problems	May require colostomy Later, surgical reconstruction
Mucosal cysts	Obstruction by torsion or by compression from the cystic mass Hemorrhage occurs in cysts lined with gastric mucosa	Resection of cyst or associated bowel

Gastrointestinal Bleeding

1. Gastrointestinal pathology that can lead to bleeding includes intussusception, Meckel's diverticulum, polyps, hereditary telangiectasias, inflammatory lesions (ulcerative colitis, peptic ulcer disease), and trauma.

2. Melena is characteristic of upper GI bleeding, while bright red blood or bloody diarrhea is seen with lower GI bleeding. Currant jelly stools (bloody mucus) are present with intussusception.

3. Preoperative treatment consists of the establishment of a reliable intravenous line (not smaller than 22 gauge) that will be adequate for fluid resuscitation and the administration of blood products. Gastric decompression by continuous nasogastric suction or the passage of an orogastric catheter before the induction of anesthesia is indicated. Appropriate blood products should be ordered and available before the child is brought to the operating room.

4. "Full stomach" considerations apply; the airway is secured either by an awake intubation or rapid-sequence induction with cricoid pressure. Awake intubation can be performed in the lateral position to decrease the likelihood of aspiration.

5. The trachea is extubated when the child is fully awake and in the lateral position.

Inflammatory Bowel Disease

1. Inflammatory bowel disease (IBD) refers to colitis or ileitis of unknown etiology. The most common types in developed countries are ulcerative colitis (UC) and Crohn's disease. The diagnosis is made on the basis of clinical, radiologic, colonoscopic, and pathologic findings.

2. Ulcerative colitis involves only the mucosa of the colon. It most commonly presents as bloody diarrhea.

3. Crohn's disease differs from UC in that there is transmural involvement of the bowel wall and involvement of the entire intestine.

4. Patients with IBD are prone to develop the following problems: anemia, leukocytosis, hypoalbuminemia, hypokalemia, and hypomagnesemia.

5. Preoperative laboratory tests that will help assess the severity of either disease include leukocyte count and determination of hematocrit, albumin, and electrolyte levels.

6. Steroids and antibiotics are used to treat IBD. Stress dose coverage may be required in the perioperative period. Hydrocortisone 4 to 8 mg/kg/day in three divided doses will cover surgical stress in the child. Similarly, any antibiotics should be continued through the operative period.

7. Patients with IBD frequently present to the operating room on

an emergency basis for bowel obstruction or bleeding. The same principles concerning airway management in the child with a full stomach apply.

8. It is not uncommon for the patient with IBD to receive total parenteral nutrition (TPN), to promote bowel rest and a favorable nutrition status. (see Chapter 4).

Complications of inflammatory bowel disease

	Crohn's disease	Ulcerative colitis
Intestinal	Fistula formation Obstruction secondary to fibrous adhesions	Toxic megacolon Carcinoma
Extraintestinal	Arthritis Uveitis Nephrolithiasis Liver dysfunction Cholelithiasis Skin lesions	Arthritis Uveitis Nephrolithiasis Liver dysfunction Growth retardation

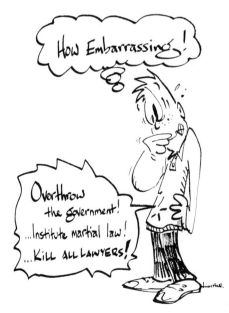

Inflammatory Bowel Disease

Jaundice[11,12]

Physiologic jaundice (neonatal hyperbilirubinemia) is a commonly seen and self-limiting process that usually appears on day 2 or 3 of life and usually resolves in 7 to 10 days. In preterm infants resolution may take 2 to 3 weeks. Pathologic jaundice is noted within 36 hours of birth with a total bilirubin >12 mg/dl (direct >1.5 mg/dl), persisting past the 7- to 10-day interval. The use of halothane in children with chronic liver dysfunction is controversial, although there is evidence to indicate that preexisting liver disease in children does not predispose to worsening hepatic injury after halothane anesthesia.[13]

Pathologic jaundice
Increased unconjugated (indirect) bilirubin

Cause	Characteristics
Rh/ABO incompatibility	First 36 hours Hemolysis secondary to maternal antibodies Anemia
Extravasation of blood	Caused by neonatal hematoma or ecchymosis Accelerated destruction of RBCs
Polycythemia	Elevated hematocrit (>65%) Normal rate of RBC destruction
Breast milk jaundice	Competitive inhibition of glycuronyl transferase Decreased conjugation
Hemoglobinopathies, spherocytosis, enzyme deficits	Hemolysis, anemia Crisis rarely occurs in neonatal period
Crigler-Najjar syndrome (familial non-hemolytic icterus)	Absence of bilirubin UDP-glucuronyl transferase
Gilbert's syndrome	Decreased activity of bilirubin UDP-glucuronyl transferase Not usually seen in neonatal period
Hypothyroidism	Decrease in bile flow

Pathologic jaundice
Increased conjugated (direct) bilirubin

Cause	Characteristics
Alagille syndrome	Hypoplastic intrahepatic bile ducts Cholestatic jaundice Developmental delay Associated anomalies
Hypopituitarism	Cholestasis Hypoglycemia Seizures Nystagmus
TPN-associated jaundice	Usually preterm
Infectious disease	Bacterial Viral (neonatal) Congenital cytomegalovirus, herpes
Biliary atresia	Absence of extrahepatic biliary tree
Bile plugs	Usually seen in patients at risk for increased viscosity (e.g., cystic fibrosis, hemolytic disorders)
Inborn errors of metabolism	Fructosemia Galactosemia α_1 antitrypsin deficiency Tyrosinemia
Dubin-Johnson syndrome	>2 yr of age Defect in canalicular secretion
Rotor syndrome	>2 yr of age Defect in hepatic storage
Bile duct perforation/ choledochal cyst	Probable biliary tract congenital anomalies Necessitate surgical exploration

Biliary Atresia

1. Biliary atresia is the obliteration of the extrahepatic bile ducts by a progressive inflammatory process of unknown etiology. It may be due to viral or ischemic causes or the congenital failure of the biliary tree to canalize.[11,14] The incidence is 1 in 15,000 live births, and 15% of these infants will have other congenital anomalies: absent inferior vena cava, malrotation of the bowel, polysplenia, or a preduodenal portal vein.[15]

2. Management and prognosis are determined by the type of atresia:

    Type I: atresia limited to common bile duct
    Type II: atresia limited to the hepatic duct
    Type III: atresia extends to the porta hepatis

In Types I and II, bile duct to bowel anastomosis may be possible. Type III may be corrected by the Kasai procedure (see table below), which creates a conduit from a segment of jejunum to residual patent bile duct tissue at the porta hepatis.

3. These infants are quite ill and generally debilitated. Associated problems include hyperbilirubinemia (conjugated type), increased liver enzymes (AST, ALT, alkaline phosphatase), abnormal coagulation studies (prothrombin time, partial thromboplastin time, dysfunctional platelets, prolonged bleeding time), severe malnutrition (hypoalbuminemia), and anemia.

4. Preoperative management of the infant with biliary atresia includes correction of any associated physiologic abnormalities before starting surgical repair. Antibiotics and red blood cell transfusions are often required, along with vitamin K or platelet/FFP transfusions to treat coagulopathies. Administration of TPN promotes a positive nitrogen balance and therefore healing.

5. Besides standard monitoring, placement of arterial and central venous catheters in the child undergoing the Kasai procedure is useful for close hemodynamic monitoring, frequent blood sampling, and infusion of inotropic or resuscitative drugs.

6. The Kasai procedure is 90% successful if performed before 2 months of age. 40% of these patients will have an excellent prognosis, while 60% of patients will continue to have progressive liver failure despite successful drainage.[11,14]

7. Postoperative complications include ascending cholangitis, portal hypertension, esophageal varices, and malabsorption.

8. Two thirds of all patients with biliary atresia require an eventual liver transplant because of progressive hepatic fibrosis.[16] Controversy exists as to whether the first treatment should consist of liver transplantation rather than the Kasai procedure.[17]

Eponyms for surgical procedures for GI disorders

Diagnosis/eponym	Procedure	Comments
Hirschsprung's disease Swenson's procedure	1. Resection of aganglionic intestine 2. Eversion of rectal stump through anus 3. Anastomosis of stump and normal colon 4. Posterior sphincterotomy	Lengthy procedure Difficult pelvic dissection

Eponyms for surgical procedures for GI disorders—cont'd

Diagnosis/eponym	Procedure	Comments
Duhamel's procedure	1. Aganglionic intestine resected to peritoneal reflection 2. Rectum sutured closed 3. Wide anastomosis of end of normal colon to posterior rectal wall	Eliminates much pelvic dissection Decreased blood and fluid losses Shorter procedure Preserves aganglionic rectum Sphincter mechanism is undisturbed
Soave, State, Soper, Ikeda, Martin	Modifications of Duhamel	
Biliary atresia Kasai (portoenterostomy)	1. Removal of extrahepatic bile ducts 2. Bile drainage established by anastomosis of intestinal conduit to transected duct (usually, Roux-en-Y jejunostomy) 3. Temporary exteriorization of conduit (decreases pressure and stasis, and allows monitoring of adequate function)	Cholangitis is a frequent complication (caused by stasis and contamination by enteric bacteria)
Malrotation; division of Ladd's bands (peritoneal bands) Ladd's procedure	1. Reduction of volvulus (coils of intestine wrapped around root of unanchored mesentery) 2. Resection of peritoneal bands 3. Fixation of mesentery 4. Appendectomy (cecum ends up in left lower quadrant; appendicitis in future may be misdiagnosed)	May need to be done emergently if obstructed Fluid, blood, and electrolyte losses may be severe, particularly if significant ischemia, or necrotic bowel
Gastroesophageal reflux Nissen fundoplication	1. Wrapping gastric fundus around gastroesophageal junction 2. May include gastrostomy	Assume "full stomach" precautions Patients often have a history of respiratory dysfunction from recurrent aspiration pneumonia Complications include inability to vomit and gas bloat syndrome
Thal-Ashcraft procedure	270-degree wrap of gastric fundus around gastroesophageal junction	Avoids complications of Nissen

References

1. Holl JW: Anesthesia for abdominal surgery. In Gregory GA, ed: *Pediatric anesthesia,* ed 3, New York, 1994, Churchill Livingstone, pp 549-570.
2. Gilger MA: Normal gastrointestinal function. In Oski FA ed: *Principles and practice of pediatrics,* ed 2, Philadelphia, 1994, JB Lippincott, pp 1838-1843.
3. Orenstein SR: Gastroesophageal reflux disease, *Sem Gastrointest Dis* 5:2-14, 1994.
4. Yemen TA: Gastrointestinal diseases. In Berry FA, Steward DJ, eds: *Pediatrics for the anesthesiologist,* New York, 1993, Churchill Livingstone, pp 101-127.
5. Bernard F, Dupont C, Viala P: Gastroesophageal reflux and upper airway diseases, *Clin Rev Allergy* 8:403-425, 1990.
6. Johnson KB, ed: *The Harriet Lane handbook,* ed 13, St Louis, 1993, Mosby.
7. Harvey MH, Johnstone MJS, Fossard DP: Inguinal herniotomy in children: a five year survey, *Br J Surg* 72:485-487, 1985.
8. Welborn LG, Rice LJ, Hannallah RS, Broadman LM, Ruttiman UE, Fink R: Postoperative apnea in former preterm infants: prospective comparison of spinal and general anesthesia, *Anesthesiology* 72:838-842, 1990.
9. Bissonnette B, Sullivan PJ: Pyloric stenosis, *Can J Anaesth* 38:668-676, 1991.
10. Andropoulous DB, Heard MB, Johnson KL, Clarke JT, Rowe RW: Postanesthetic apnea in full-term infants after pyloromyotomy, *Anesthesiology* 80:216-219, 1994.
11. Hicks BA, Altman RP: *The jaundiced newborn,* Pediatr Surg 40:1161-1175, 1993.
12. Molteni RA: The newborn infant. In Ziai M, ed: *Pediatrics,* ed 3, Boston, 1984, Little, Brown & Co, pp 151-200.
13. Wark H, Earl J, Cooper M, Overton J: Halothane in children with chronic liver disease, *Anaesth Intensive Care* 19:9-16, 1991.
14. Altman RP, Stylianos S: Pediatric surgery, *Pediatr Clin North Am* 40:1161-1175, 1993.
15. Spear RM, Deshpande JK, Davis PJ: Anesthesia for general, urologic and plastic surgery. In Motoyama EK, Davis PJ: *Smith's anesthesia for infants and children,* ed 5, St Louis, 1990, Mosby, pp 591-610.
16. Wood RP, Langnas AN, Stratta RJ, et al: Optimal therapy for patients with biliary atresia: portoenterostomy ("Kasai" procedures) versus primary transplantation, *J Pediatr Surg* 25:153-162, 1990.
17. Ryckman F, Fisher R, Pedersen S, et al: Improved survival in biliary atresia patients in the present era of liver transplantation, *J Pediatr Surg* 28:382-386, 1993.

ANESTHESIA FOR CHILDREN WITH MUSCULOSKELETAL DISORDERS

12

Zach's back was out of whack
It swerved and curved like a railroad track
Where most backs lie in a line so straight
Zach's formed an S or a figure eight.
Zach discovered when he lay face down
That his back was used by the kids in town
Who played Parcheesi and other games
Or tattooed maps on his vertebrae.

There was nothing else
With quite the knack
As that
Singularly
Interesting
Back of Zach's.

Rivian Bell

DISEASES OF BONES AND JOINTS

Scoliosis

Scoliosis is defined as lateral deviation of the spine. Severity of the curve is determined by the degree of angulation measured on the x-ray by the Cobb method (see Fig. 12-1). Curves of less than 20 degrees usually cause few physiologic effects and therefore rarely require operative intervention.

Classification of scoliosis

Type	Age	Sex	Associated problems
Congenital	Birth	M=F	Results from vertebral abnormalities (e.g., hemivertebra)
Idiopathic: Infantile	Birth to 2 yr	M>F	Mental retardation, congenital anomalies, inguinal hernias. Eighty to ninety percent of cases of infantile scoliosis resolve spontaneously.
Juvenile	3-6 yr 7-10 yr	M>F F>M	Rarely self-resolving
Adolescent	Postpuberty	F>M	Curve may progress if >60 degrees at spinal maturation.

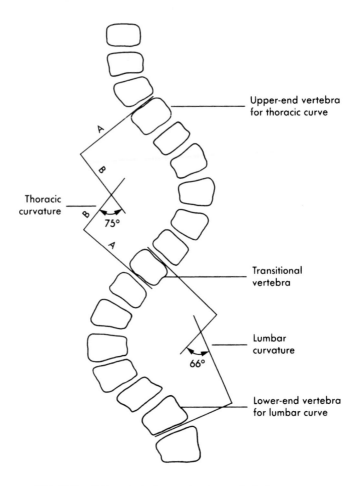

FIG. 12-1. Cobb method of measuring degree of spinal angulation in scoliosis. Lines are drawn parallel to the upper border of the highest vertebral body and lower border of the lowest vertebral body of the curve (*A*). Lines drawn perpendicularly to *A* will intersect *B*, forming an angle equal to the degree of curvature. (Adapted from Bernstein RL: Anaesthetic management of patients with scoliosis, ASA Refresher Courses, vol 16, Chapter 2, Philadelphia, 1988, JB Lippincott.)

Physiologic Effects[1-3]

Spinal deformity must be moderately severe before it interferes with respiratory function, causing a restrictive process. As the degree of spinal curvature increases, lung compliance and lung volumes (especially VC and FRC) decrease, predisposing to airway closure, ventilation/perfusion mismatch, increased alveolar-arterial gradient, and scattered atelectasis. When the curvature approaches 65 degrees with a long-term history of scoliosis, pulmonary hypertension may develop.

Cardiorespiratory effects of scoliosis

- Ventilation/perfusion abnormality
   $\uparrow$Alveolar-arterial oxygen gradient (A-aDO_2)
   $\uparrow$Dead space (V_D/V_T)
- Total lung volume (TLV)
   $\downarrow$Vital capacity (VC)
   $\downarrow$Functional residual capacity (FRC)
- $\downarrow Pao_2$ normal $Paco_2$ (may increase with advanced disease)
- $\downarrow$Ventilatory response to CO_2
- Pulmonary hypertension, cor pulmonale (secondary to chronic hypoxia and low lung volumes)
   Right ventricular enlargement
   Right atrial enlargement
   Pulmonic insufficiency
- Tracheal shortening or distortion, pulmonary artery kinking

---

Operative Treatment[4,5]

Anterior approach (Luque instrumentation). This approach is used mainly when posterior fusion is not possible (e.g., spinal cord defects). The technique requires a thoracotomy with division of the diaphragm to gain access to the vertebrae. Bleeding, postoperative pain control, and respiratory dysfunction are significant problems. One-lung ventilation should be considered to improve surgical exposure.

Posterior approach (Harrington rod placement and spinal fusion). This technique involves placement of a hook into the facet joints of the upper and lower vertebrae to hold a distraction rod along the concave aspect of the curve. A compression rod may be placed on the convex side. Vertebrae are decorticated, and spinous processes, intraspinal ligaments, and facet joints are obliterated. Bone graft, usually from the iliac crest, is used to fuse the spine. The procedure may be lengthy, requiring multiple transfusions, and the recovery is prolonged. Fixed, rigid curves may first require an anterior approach for discectomy before attempting distraction by the posterior approach. Both procedures may be done during the same operation or in two separate staged operations.

ANESTHETIC MANAGEMENT[6]

Positioning.   The Relton-Hall operation frame provides four padded supports—paired and V-shaped.[7] The upper support should be at the anterior/lateral part of the thorax, while the lower supports the anterior/lateral aspects of the pelvis. This minimizes abdominal pressure and inferior vena cava (IVC) compression so that functional residual capacity remains near normal. IVC compression can lead to blood diversion into the vertebral venous system, resulting in increased bleeding. Maintenance of FRC minimizes atelectasis. Care should be taken to pad the legs and avoid knee contact with the table.

Blood loss.   Blood loss usually is dependent on venous engorgement of the vertebrae and the extent and difficulty of the operative procedure, not the severity of the curve.[4-6] Blood loss can be minimized by the following:

1. Correct positioning with minimal pressure on the IVC.
2. Infiltration of the operative site with large volumes of dilute epinephrine solution (1:500,000). On the rare occasion when larger epinephrine doses are used (greater than 1.5 μg/kg or 0.15 ml/kg of 1:100,000 solution), then prophylactic β-blockade may be indicated.
3. Hyperventilation to $PaCO_2$ of 25 to 30 mm Hg can cause peripheral vasoconstriction that reduces blood loss. However, a low $PaCO_2$ decreases spinal cord blood flow, thus making ischemia possible.
4. Autologous storage for intraoperative transfusions.
5. Hemodilution results in a lower viscosity of blood, which improves microcirculation and reduces afterload of the left ventricle. Stroke volume and cardiac output increase to compensate for the decreased oxygen content in blood.[8] Routine clinical use of normovolemic hemodilution should only be recommended to hematocrit levels of about 20%.[9]
6. Use of cell saver-retrieved blood.
7. Controlled hypotension[6,10]
   a. Controlled hypotension is a technique that may reduce blood loss and decrease operative time. When this technique is used, arterial monitoring is essential for beat-to-beat observation of blood pressure because cardiopulmonary resuscitation would be nearly impossible in the prone position. After determination of the patient's baseline mean arterial pressure, a decrease of 25% to 30% generally is well tolerated if gradual in onset (over 10 to 15 minutes). This technique allows time for cerebral, renal, and coronary vascular beds to dilate and maintain adequate perfusion.
   b. Hyperventilation with hypotension may lead to spinal cord ischemia. The FIO_2 should be increased to compen-

sate for physiologic shunting and a near-normal $PaCO_2$ maintained. Assessment of arterial blood gases reveals adequacy of oxygenation/ventilation and possible metabolic acidosis caused by low perfusion or nitroprusside toxicity.

   c. Agents used to induce controlled hypotension include the following:

Agents used to induce controlled hypotension	
Sodium nitroprusside (SNP)	**Nitroglycerin**
Requires placement of intraarterial catheter Has a rapid onset of action—within 30 seconds after starting infusion Infusion rate is titrated easily to the desired level of hypotension Combination with a β-blocking agent (propranolol or esmolol) prevents reflex tachycardia (which increases oxygen consumption) and decreases the amount of drug required to produce hypotension Recommended maximal dose limit is 8 to 10 µg/kg/min Tachycardia, tachyphylaxis, and acidosis may indicate early toxicity May increase intracranial pressure by vasodilation	Decreases preload and cardiac output Reflex tachycardia can be limited by β-blockade Usual dosage range is 1 to 10 µg/kg/min
Trimethaphan Infusion maximum is 100 µg/kg/min Avoids reflex tachycardia because of ganglionic blocking activity Slower onset than sodium nitroprusside Slight reverse-Trendelenburg is needed to enhance hypotensive effect Causes pupillary dilation	**Inhalation agents (enflurane, isoflurane)** For desired level of hypotension, cardiac depression may be significant Onset is slower than with nitroprusside

MONITORING SPINAL CORD FUNCTION

Intraoperative "wake-up" test.[6,11]   The "wake-up" test requires the patient to move his extremities on command after placement of the distraction rod, testing gross spinal motor function. Preoperative discussion with the patient is essential to ensure full cooperation. The test is relatively contraindicated in the mentally retarded, young children, paraplegics, the hearing impaired, or children with emotional or behavioral disorders. Continuous somatosensory evoked potential monitoring is a prudent alternative to the "wake-up test" and eliminates the risk of accidental extubation intraoperatively with the patient in the prone position.

Nitrous-narcotic (balanced) technique.   To awaken the patient, approximately half the calculated neuromuscular reversal dose is given and titrated over 5 minutes until spontaneous respiration returns. If spontaneous respirations do not occur in the presence of adequate twitch response, small amounts of naloxone (20-µg aliquots) should be titrated slowly. At this point, nitrous oxide is discontinued and the airway should be monitored closely. Extubation may occur or the rod may dislodge if there is excessive movement. The patient is asked to move his or her hands and feet sequentially. Absence of movement or weakness of one or both feet indicates that rod adjustment is necessary. After the test is completed, thiopental should be given to induce rapid loss of consciousness and amnesia.

Inhalation technique.   If an inhalation agent is being used, the agent should be discontinued at least 10 minutes before planned awakening. The patient should be reanesthetized using a rapid-acting intravenous induction agent with amnestic properties (i.e., thiopental) after the test is completed.

Somatosensory corticol evoked potential (SSEP).   This technique involves electrical stimulation of at least two peripheral nerves from surface electrodes, one above the lesion and one below the lesion.[12-14] The nerves used most frequently are the posterior tibial and median. Surface electrodes are placed over the contralateral cortex of the respective somatosensory areas preoperatively. Many drugs and conditions affect SSEPs, including inhalation agents, nitrous oxide, etomidate, large doses of thiopental, incomplete muscle relaxation, hypotension, hypothermia, and hypoxia. Although this test may help predict postoperative outcome, SSEPs monitor only dorsal column function (not motor function), so that postoperative neurologic defects may result without significant intraoperative SSEP changes.

POSTOPERATIVE CARE

The operative correction of scoliosis may be a lengthy surgical procedure accompanied by significant blood loss and large intraoperative fluid and transfusion requirements. Preoperative criteria that indicate a need for prolonged postoperative mechanical ventilation include:

1. VC < 50% predicted value (functional VC < 2.0 L)
2. Elevated baseline $PaCO_2$ (>45 mm Hg)
3. Decreased baseline PaO_2
4. Pulmonary hypertension

Dysplastic Disease of Bone and Cartilage; Dwarfism (Osteochondrodystrophies)[15,16]

Dwarfism should not be considered a single disease entity. There are over 100 different types of dwarfism, and the associated abnormalities of the respiratory, circulatory, and physiologic systems pose specific challenges to the anesthesiologist. The most common disorder is achondroplasia and occurs in approximately 1.5 per 10,000 births. Camptomelic dwarfism is a lethal form of the disease. Other disorders known to cause dwarfism include the diseases of mucopolysaccharide metabolism.

CLASSIFICATION

Persons of short stature are usually divided into two categories:
1. Persons with proportionate growth and a normal ratio of trunk-to-limb length
2. Persons with disproportionate development, characterized by either short limbs or short trunks

PHYSIOLOGIC MANIFESTATIONS

Physiologic manifestations of dwarfism

Airway	• Upper airway obstruction • Cervical abnormalities impede direct laryngoscopy • Laryngomalacia, laryngotracheal stenosis, micrognathia
Respiratory	• Restrictive lung disease from thoracic cage dystrophy, kyphosis, scoliosis • Obstructive central and mixed sleep apnea (more common with achondroplasia and MPS*)
Cardiovascular	• Atrial or ventricular septal defects • Valvular stenosis • Cardiomyopathy (MPS) • Pulmonary hypertension
Neurologic	• Association with hydrocephalus • Spinal stenosis contributes to spinal cord and nerve root compression

*MPS, Mucopolysaccharidoses.

ANESTHETIC MANAGEMENT

Airway
1. Suspicion of an anatomically abnormal airway should be confirmed with computed tomography, magnetic resonance imaging, or neck radiographs.
2. Preoperative sedation should not be given, in order to avoid upper airway obstruction.
3. Antisialagogues are particularly useful in children with copious secretions.

4. Both awake intubation and mask inhalation induction with spontaneous ventilation have been used successfully.
5. A short-handled laryngoscope may be useful in patients with pectus carinatum.
6. Muscle relaxants are avoided until the airway is secured. Tracheostomy may be extremely difficult because of chest deformities and tracheal stenosis.

Respiratory

1. Preoperative pulmonary function tests, blood gases, and flow-volume loops will help to quantitate respiratory insufficiency and obstruction.
2. Restrictive lung disease may prolong inhalation induction.
3. Arterial cannulation for blood gas analysis is recommended for all but the shortest and simplest surgical procedures.
4. Patients may require postoperative ventilation.

Cardiovascular

1. Preoperative echocardiography can diagnose valvular lesions and ventricular dysfunction. Prophylactic antibiotics may be required (see Appendix F, p. 666, for cardiac prophylaxis).
2. Invasive monitoring is mandatory in patients with valvular disease, pulmonary hypertension, or impaired myocardial function.
3. Agents and techniques that aggravate pulmonary vasoconstriction should be avoided.

Neurologic

1. Neck radiographs help to determine cervical stability and range of motion.
2. Neck manipulation should be avoided to prevent neurologic damage.
3. Positioning is of utmost importance in avoiding extremes of flexion or extension.
4. Succinylcholine is avoided if muscle wasting because of spinal cord compression has occurred.

Dysplastic disease of bone and cartilage[15-19]

Type/clinical manifestations	Anesthetic considerations
Achondroplasia Proximal limb shortening, long trunk Frontal bossing, large head Prominent mandible Short neck Reduced lung volumes and pulmonary hypertension CNS: dilated ventricles, small foramen magnum, hydrocephalus, spinal cord compression Bone: narrow spinal canal, lumbar lordosis, kyphoscoliosis	• Difficult intubation • Neck instability • May have increased risk of neurologic deficit after regional techniques • Spine and bone deformities cause technical difficulties for regional techniques • Predisposition to sleep apnea

Dysplastic disease of bone and cartilage[15-19]—cont'd

Type/clinical manifestations	Anesthetic considerations
Asphyxiating thoracic dystrophy (Jeune syndrome) Stiff, small thorax with short ribs Short, broad hands and feet Postaxial polydactyly Respiratory dysfunction (may improve with age) Pulmonary hypertension Cardiac defects Renal disease	• Small larynx • May need invasive monitors for cardiopulmonary disease • May require cardiac prophylaxis • Baseline pulmonary and renal function tests needed • May have decreased renal clearance of anesthetic drugs
Ellis–van Creveld syndrome Polydactyly Mesomelic dwarfism Long, narrow thorax Nail/teeth abnormalities Absence of tracheal cartilage causes airway collapse and tension lobar emphysema Cardiac defects (usually septal)	• Abnormalities of dentition and upper/lower airway may result in difficult airway • High airway pressures may cause barotrauma • Nitrous oxide should be avoided with emphysema • May need invasive monitors for cardiopulmonary involvement
Chondrodysplasia punctata (stippled epiphyses) Frontal bossing Hypertelorism High palate/saddle nose Short neck and stature Tracheal stenosis Atlantoaxial instability Cardiac defects Hydrocephalus or other CNS abnormalities Associated renal anomalies	• Difficult intubation (facial and neck abnormalities) • Renal, cardiac function need to be assessed • Possible elevated intracranial pressure
Osteogenesis imperfecta Brittle bones with multiple fractures Blue sclera Scoliosis Deafness Intracranial hemorrhages Impaired platelet function	• Difficult intubation (short neck, teeth easily broken) • Extra padding and careful positioning required • Respiratory dysfunction caused by scoliosis • Succinylcholine fasciculations may cause fractures • Propensity for temperature increase during anesthesia (responds to cooling, unlike malignant hyperthermia)
Osteopetrosis (Albers-Shönberg disease) Failure to thrive Ecchymoses Megalocephaly Hepatosplenomegaly Pancytopenia Low serum calcium Brittle bones	• Careful positioning required • May have coagulopathy and thrombocytopenia • Serum calcium deficit may cause arrhythmias, seizures, or prolonged neuromuscular blockade

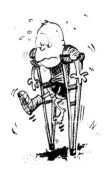 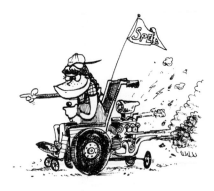

Juvenile Rheumatoid Arthritis[20,21]

Juvenile rheumatoid arthritis (JRA), or Still's disease, is an autoimmune disease associated with chronic nonsuppurative inflammation of synovioum and connective tissue. JRA is defined as continuously active arthritis involving one or more joints for a minimum of 6 weeks in a child younger than 16 years of age who has no other etiology for the symptoms.

INCIDENCE

1. Females affected more commonly than males
2. Rarely occurs in children younger than 6 months
3. Usually occurs between 1 and 3 years of age

PHYSIOLOGIC MANIFESTATIONS

Airway

1. Temporomandibular joint involvement limits aperture.
2. Extreme mandibular hypoplasia occurs because of growth impairment.
3. Narrowing of the glottis, anterior fixation of the cords, and rotation of the larynx are common.
4. Cervical spine inflammation results in limitation of neck movement. Subluxation of atlantoaxial joint occurs more commonly after 5 years of age and may result in cord compression, quadriplegia, and possibly death.

Respiratory

Common findings include the following:

1. Pleural effusions
2. Pneumonia
3. Pleuritis
4. Classic adult rheumatoid pulmonary nodules are rare in children.

Cardiovascular
1. Pericarditis is found by echocardiography in almost half the children with JRA.
2. The conduction system of the heart may be involved.
3. Cardiac valves may reflect inflammatory changes.

Renal
1. Impaired creatinine clearance is common.
2. Renal failure is rare.

Hematologic
1. Anemia is typically microcytic, hypochromic, and refractory to iron therapy.
2. Bleeding resulting from platelet dysfunction is caused by chronic use of antiinflammatory agents.
3. Neutrophilia may be associated with a high fever.
4. Splenomegaly may be associated with thrombocytopenia.

ANESTHETIC MANAGEMENT

Preoperative evaluation
1. Indirect laryngoscopy may help to evaluate glottic position. Cervical spine x-rays should include flexion and extension films for evaluation of atlantoaxial joint stability.
2. Cardiac examination should include careful auscultation for murmurs, a chest x-ray if clinically indicated, and an electro-cardiogram for conduction delays. An echocardiogram can pro-vide information on the extent of pericardial effusions and cardiac valve involvement.
3. Recommended laboratory tests include blood count with platelet count and differential, coagulation parameters, elec-trolytes, creatinine, urea nitrogen, and urinalysis.
4. Perioperative stress steroid coverage is indicated if the patient is on chronic steroid therapy or if a recent history of steroid use is present (hydrocortisone 4 to 8 mg/kg/day in three divided doses). Premedication should be conservative because the air-way may be difficult to secure.
5. Preoperative transfusion may be required, depending on the de-gree of anemia and cardiorespiratory function.

Intraoperative management
Airway. Inhalation induction with face mask followed by nasal or oral intubation, awake fiberoptic intubation, or any combination of the above is advisable when a difficult airway is anticipated. Muscle relaxants should be used only after securing the airway.
Vascular access. Chronic illness and chronic steroid use can lead to difficult access. Alternative plans (cutdown or indwelling central venous catheter) should be considered preoperatively.
Positioning. All pressure points should be padded carefully. The degree of cervical spine involvement determines head positioning.

Anesthetic agent. A marginal airway necessitates an awake, alert patient before tracheal extubation. Cardiac and respiratory involvement may limit anesthetic dosages. Infusion of short-acting agents may provide the most titratability without prolonged effects. Opioid analgesics are recommended in small, divided doses.

Slipped Capital Femoral Epiphysis[22]

This condition occurs when the proximal femoral plate weakens, permitting the femoral head to slip off, usually posteriorly and medially.

Patient Characteristics

1. Adolescents
2. More common in males than in females
3. Bilateral involvement occurs in 25% to 30% of patients
4. Most patients fall into one of two body types:
   a. Short, obese, prepubescent
   b. Tall and thin

Anesthetic Considerations

The primary anesthetic considerations are those that apply to obese children. The airway should be assessed; inhalation induction is often disastrous in the obese child with redundant soft tissue. An obstructed airway results in rapid desaturation because of marginal pulmonary reserve. It is unwise to rely on the ability to place an intravenous catheter in the obese child rapidly during a difficult induction. Furthermore, details surrounding gastric emptying in obese children are limited, but it is anticipated that the risks of acid aspiration are increased. For these reasons, a rapid-sequence induction with preoperative placement of the intravenous catheter is recommended. The IV also permits premedication with an H_2 antagonist and metoclopramide. The judicious use of narcotics is recommended, especially if any history of obstructive sleep apnea or snoring is present. The trachea should not be extubated until the child is fully awake and alert.

NEUROMUSCULAR DISORDERS
Von Recklinghausen Disease (Neurofibromatosis)[23]

Von Recklinghausen disease (VRD) is an autosomal dominant trait with new mutations being common. The hallmark of the disease is café-au-lait spots (more than six that are greater than 1.5 cm in diameter) and neurofibromas.

ASSOCIATED CONDITIONS

1. Laryngeal and tracheal compression secondary to tumor
2. High incidence of kyphosis and progressive scoliosis
3. Increased incidence of neural tumors such as glioma, meningioma, acoustic neuroma, and pheochromocytoma (which may present as sustained hypertension)
4. Compression of spinal roots, cerebello-pontine angle, medulla oblongata, and other nonneural structures
5. Impaired mental function (usually mild)
6. Megalocephaly
7. Malformations of the greater wing of the sphenoid bone with pulsating exophthalmos
8. Congenital pseudoarthrosis (commonly tibia and radius)
9. Increased incidence of cancer

ANESTHETIC CONSIDERATIONS

1. Airway abnormalities may lead to difficulties with intubation and ventilation.
2. Patients may have a prolonged response to nondepolarizing muscle relaxants.
3. Hypertension, tachycardia, or arrhythmias may indicate pheochromocytoma.
4. Increased intracranial pressure may require appropriate treatment.

Tuberous Sclerosis[24]

Tuberous sclerosis is an autosomal dominant disease, best known for its cutaneous and neurological manifestations and described classically as a triad of mental retardation, epileptic seizures, and facial angiofibromas. It is often associated with spinal deformities, especially scoliosis.

ANESTHETIC CONSIDERATIONS

1. Respiratory compromise should be anticipated in the presence of scoliosis.
2. Antiepileptic medications should not be discontinued prior to surgery.
3. Anesthetic considerations for patients with seizure disorders should be followed (see p. 217).

Myotonic Dystrophy[25]

Myotonic dystrophy is an autosomal dominant trait affecting primarily the limb muscles but also with extraocular and facial involvement. Clinical features can include poor sucking/swallowing, muscle atrophy, facial weakness, ptosis, cataracts, frontal baldness, gonadal atrophy, endocrine failure, and mental retardation.

ANESTHETIC CONSIDERATIONS

1. Poor sucking/swallowing predisposes these patients to aspiration. "Full-stomach" premedication (antacids, H_2 antagonists, gastric motility stimulants) and induction techniques apply.
2. Patients may have a poor cough and gag reflex, resulting in an increased incidence of atelectasis, pneumonia, and aspiration.
3. Bradycardia and intraventricular conduction delays are common. Death has been described due to arrythmias. The extent of cardiac involvement does not correlate with the extent of muscle involvement.
4. A depressed respiratory response to CO_2 with pulmonary hypertension and weakened respiratory muscles can cause serious hypoxemia and hypercapnia. Respiratory dysfunction dictates the judicious use of preoperative medications, narcotics, benzodiazepines, barbiturates, and inhalation agents.
5. Myotonia worsens with hypothermia. Maintenance of normothermia is essential.
6. Muscle spasms may complicate airway management.
7. Succinylcholine may precipitate a myotonic crisis. General and spinal anesthesia cannot break a myotonic contracture. Nondepolarizing neuromuscular agents do not elicit contractures and can be used safely.
8. Reversal with neostigmine and an antimuscarinic can precipitate myotonic contracture. The use of newer short-acting nondepolarizing agents and close monitoring of twitch response are recommended.
9. Patients frequently require postoperative mechanical ventilation. The trachea should not be extubated until the patient has completely recovered.

Less common myotonias

Type	Features	Anesthetic considerations
Myotonic chondrodystrophy (Schwartz-Jampel syndrome)	Progressive Autosomal recessive Dwarfism Muscle stiffness Skeletal abnormalities	Same as myotonic dystrophy Predisposed to malignant hyperthermia
Myotonia congenita (Thomsen disease)	Not progressive Autosomal dominant Myotonia and hypertrophy of voluntary muscle (decrease with exercise) No cardiac involvement No dystrophic changes	Same as myotonic dystrophy
Paramyotonia	Similar to myotonia congenita	Myotonia develops with exposure to cold

Muscular Dystrophy
DUCHENNE (PSEUDOHYPERTROPHIC)[26,27]

Duchenne muscular dystrophy is an X-linked recessive trait that usually presents with a waddling gait, appearing in a child between the ages of 3 and 5 years. The hallmark of the disease is muscle degeneration, a process of atrophy that confines the patient to a wheelchair by the early teens. Death is usually secondary to congestive heart failure, cardiomyopathy, or pneumonia, and usually occurs by 20 years of age.

Anesthetic considerations

1. Succinylcholine may cause hyperkalemia, myoglobinemia, cardiac arrest, and rhabdomyolysis and should therefore be avoided. These effects can be seen in the absence of clinical disease and in relatives of affected patients.
2. Sensitivity to nondepolarizing neuromuscular blockers is common.
3. As the disease progresses, patients are unable to protect their airways from secretions, resulting in frequent pneumonia.
4. Worsening kyphoscoliosis with advancing disease impairs pulmonary function. Spinal fusion can reduce the rate of advancement of pulmonary disease. Surgical risk is related to vital capacity (VC). For VC greater than 45% of that predicted, postoperative ventilation normally is not necessary. For VC less

than 30% serious postoperative complications are more common, even with supportive postoperative ventilation.

5. Cardiac muscle degeneration can lead to decreased contractility, right ventricular outflow obstruction, and mitral regurgitation. Anesthetics with the potential for myocardial depression should be used judiciously.

6. A nasogastric tube may prevent the acute gastric dilatation that has been associated with cardiovascular compromise.

7. Muscular dystrophy may be associated with malignant hyperthermia, so triggering agents should be avoided. Dantrolene may cause significant muscle weakness in these patients.

8. Use of atropine and scopolamine should be avoided if possible.

9. Hypomotility and delayed gastric emptying increase the risk of aspiration. Administration of H_2 antagonists, neutralization of gastric acidity, agents to increase gastric emptying, possible rapid-sequence induction with a nondepolarizing agent, and/or awake intubation should be considered.

Less common muscular dystrophies

These muscular disorders are characterized by specific clinical features, although they share the same anesthetic considerations as Duchenne

Type	Features
Limb-girdle (Erb's, Leyden-Möbius)	Autosomal recessive Involves hips and shoulders Presents in second decade with severe involvement by third decade Rare cardiac involvement
Late onset X-linked	Onset occurs after age 10 Slower onset and lesser severity than Duchenne
Facioscapulohumeral	Autosomal dominant Onset after age 10 Normal life expectancy Affects arms, shoulders, face; later may involve back and hips Atria may lack electrical activity and not respond to pacing; severe bradycardia may require ventricular pacing Weak accessory muscles may increase pulmonary complications
Distal	Autosomal dominant Seen only in people of Swedish descent
Ocular	Begins with ptosis and extraocular muscle weakness, necessitating special care to eyes and facial pressure points Onset before age 30 Slow progression with limited muscular involvement Extreme sensitivity to curare (paralysis can occur with 10% of usual dose)

Myasthenia Gravis [28-31]

CHARACTERISTICS

Myasthenia gravis is an autoimmune disorder that results in a decrease in the number of acetylcholine receptors at the neuromuscular junction. Antibodies to the receptors may be present.

Symptoms include weakness and fatiguability of voluntary muscles. Such symptoms worsen with exercise. Ptosis, diplopia, and dysphagia are common, and a significant decrease in respiratory function may occur. Three forms of the disease occur in children:

1. Neonatal transient myasthenia, seen in infants born to mothers with the disease. Symptoms are usually transient.
2. Congenital myasthenia has symptoms first noticeable in infancy that persist throughout life and are usually mild.
3. Juvenile myasthenia occurs after age 10 and closely resembles the adult form of the disease. It has a female predominance.

TREATMENT

Drug therapy.   Oral neostigmine and pyridostigmine are used to elevate levels of acetylcholine by inhibiting cholinesterase. Side effects include increased secretions, sensitivity to narcotics, and prolongation of succinylcholine and ester local anesthesia.

Operative.   In up to 25% of patients, thymectomy eliminates the need for further drug therapy.

ANESTHETIC MANAGEMENT

Preoperative

1. Anticholinesterase therapy should be continued if generalized symptoms are present.
2. Discontinuation of therapy with 24 hours of bed rest may be appropriate for patients with only ocular symptoms.
3. Premedication should be avoided.

Intraoperative

1. Inhalation anesthesia with spontaneous ventilation using a face mask or laryngeal mask airway obviates the need for muscle relaxation for intubation. The use of halothane will have less effect on muscle relaxation than will other inhalation agents.
2. If absolutely necessary, nondepolarizing relaxants should be used in $^1/_{20}$ of the usual dose and titrated to effect. Reversal of neuromuscular blockade may be ineffective.
3. Hypothermia and hypokalemia can further decrease respiratory function and reserve.
4. Narcotics should be titrated carefully in the postoperative period.
5. Patients should meet the following criteria prior to tracheal extubation:

a. Awake and alert
b. Adequate head lift
c. Vital capacity >15 ml/kg
d. Negative inspiratory force > -30 cm H_2O
e. Ability to swallow and handle secretions

Myasthenic Syndrome (Eaton-Lambert)[32]

Myasthenic syndrome differs from myasthenia in that it primarily involves proximal limb muscles, not ocular or bulbar muscles. It is caused by a decrease of acetylcholine at the end plate, probably due to impaired acetylcholine esterase activity. Associated diseases include leukemia, neuroblastoma, systemic lupus erythematosus, rheumatoid arthritis, hypothyroidism, and hyperthyroidism. Anesthetic management should parallel that for myasthenia gravis.

References

1. Bentley G, Donell ST: Scoliosis in childhood and its management, *Br J Rheum* 33:486-494, 1994.
2. Lonstein JE: Adolescent idiopathic scoliosis, *Lancet* 344:1407-1412, 1994.
3. Day GA, Upadhyay SS, Ho EK, Leong JC, Ip M: Pulmonary functions in congenital scoliosis, *Spine* 19:1027-1031, 1994.
4. King HA: Analysis and treatment of Type II idiopathic scoliosis, *Orthop Clin North Am* 25:225-237, 1994.
5. Puno RM, Mehta S, Byrd JA III: Surgical treatment of idiopathic thoracolumbar and lumbar scoliosis in adolescent patients, *Orthop Clin North Am* 25:275-286, 1994.
6. Salem MR, Klowden AJ: Anesthesia for orthopedic surgery. In Gregory GA, ed: *Pediatric Anesthesia,* ed 3, New York, 1994, Churchill Livingstone, pp 607-656.
7. Relton JE, Hall JE: An operation frame for spinal fusion: a new apparatus designed to reduce haemorrhage during operation, *J Bone Joint Surg* 49B:327-332, 1967.
8. Fontana JL, Welborn L, Mongan PD, Sturm P, Martin G, Bünger R: Oxygen consumption and cardiovascular function in children during profound intraoperative normovolemic hemodilution, *Anesth Analg* 80:219-225, 1995.
9. Lindahl SG: Thinner than blood, *Anesth Analg* 80:217-218, 1995.
10. Wildsmith JA, Sinclair CJ, Thorn J, MacRae WR, Fagan D, Scott DB: Haemodynamic effects of induced hypotension with a nitroprusside-trimethaphan mixture, *Br J Anaesth* 55:381-389, 1983.
11. Hall JE, Levine CR, Sudhir KG: Intraoperative awakening to monitor spinal cord function during Harrington instrumentation and spine fusion, *J Bone Joint Surg* 60:533-536, 1978.
12. Helmers SL, Hall JE: Intraoperative somatosensory evoked potential monitoring in pediatrics, *J Pediatr Ortho* 14:592-598, 1994.
13. Black S, Mehla ME, Cucchiara RF: Neurologic monitoring. In Miller RD, ed: *Anesthesia,* ed 4, New York, 1994, Churchill Livingstone, pp 1319-1344.

14. Grundy BL: Intraoperative monitoring of sensory-evoked potentials, *Anesthesiology* 58:72-87, 1983.
15. Berkowitz ID, Raja SN, Bender KS, Kopits SE: Dwarfs: pathophysiology and anesthetic implications, *Anesthesiology* 73:739-759, 1990.
16. Clark RN: Congenital dysplasias and dwarfism, *Pediatr Rev* 12:149-159, 1990.
17. Brueton LA, Dillon MJ, Winter RM: Ellis–van Creveld syndrome, Jeune syndrome, and renal-hepatic-pancreatic dysplasia: separate entities or disease spectrum? *J Med Genet* 27:252-255, 1990.
18. Singer FR, Chang SS: Osteoporosis, *Sem Nephrol* 12:191-199, 1992.
19. Byers PH, Steiner RD: Osteogenesis imperfecta, *Ann Rev Med* 43:269-282, 1992.
20. Leak AM: The management of arthritis in adolescence, *Br J Rheumatol* 33:882-888, 1994.
21. Miller ML: Juvenile rheumatoid arthritis, *Curr Probl Pediatr* 24:190-198, 1994.
22. Crawford AH: Slipped capital femoral epiphysis, *J Bone Joint Surg* 70:1422-1427, 1988.
23. Listernick R, Charrow J: Neurofibromatosis type 1 in childhood, *J Pediatr* 116:845-853, 1990.
24. Lee JJ, Imrie M, Taylor V: Anaesthesia and tuberous sclerosis, *Br J Anaesth* 73:421-425, 1994.
25. Russell SH, Hirsch NP: Anaesthesia and myotonia, *Br J Anaesth* 72:210-216, 1994.
26. Iannaccone ST: Current status of Duchenne muscular dystrophy, *Pediatr Clin North Am* 39:879-894, 1992.
27. Sethna NF, Rockoff MA, Worthen HM, Rosnow JM: Anesthesia-related complications in children with Duchenne muscular dystrophy, *Anesthesiology* 68:462-465, 1988.
28. Richman DP, Agius MA: Myasthenia gravis: pathogenesis and treatment, *Sem Neurol* 14:106-110, 1994.
29. Nilsson E, Muller K: Neuromuscular effects of isoflurane in patients with myasthenia gravis, *Acta Anaesthesiol Scand* 34:126-131, 1990.
30. Nilsson E, Meretoja OA: Vecuronium dose-response and maintenance requirements in patients with myasthenia gravis, *Anesthesiology* 73:28-32, 1990.
31. Saito Y, Sakura S, Takatori T, Kosaka Y: Epidural anesthesia in a patient with myasthenia gravis, *Acta Anaesthesiol Scand* 37:513-515, 1993.
32. Sanders DB: Lambert-Eaton myasthenic syndrome: pathogenesis and treatment, *Semin Neurol* 14:111-117, 1994.

ANESTHETIC MANAGEMENT OF CHILDREN WITH HEMATOLOGIC AND ONCOLOGIC DISORDERS

13

daniel was a real lightweight
cranky and fussy
hardly ever ate
depleted iron was the worm
iron sulfate made it turn

Adrienne Coleman

ANEMIA[1]

As more restrictions are placed on the current blood supply, the contemporary anesthesiologist caring for children needs to increase his or her understanding of anemia in order to narrowly define the indications for transfusion.

Anemia can be classified into three major physiologic categories: decreased production, increased destruction, or blood loss. Knowledge of the cause of a child's low hemoglobin (Hb) level is considerably more important than merely knowing the absolute Hb level. For example, the anesthetic implications for a child with sickle cell anemia should focus on end-organ damage and the potential for intraoperative sickling rather than on the absolute Hb level, which might be only 6 to 7 g/dl. In general, a thorough investigation is warranted in the child who is discovered to have a hemoglobin level below 9 g/dl in the preoperative assessment.

Normal hemoglobin levels

Age	Hemoglobin values (g/dl)
Neonate	17
3 months	10-11
2 years	12.5
3-5 years	12.5-13.0
5-10 years	13.0-13.5
>10 years	14.5

Decreased Production
PHYSIOLOGIC ANEMIA

Fetal hematopoietic physiology undergoes a dramatic change in the extrauterine oxygen-rich environment. In the normal newborn, erythropoietin levels drop and β-chain production shifts from Hb F to Hb A. Over the first few weeks of life, Hb levels fall to an average nadir of 11 g/dl. The lowest levels are usually seen between 8 and 12 weeks of age. It is rare for infants to develop any clinically significant symptoms from physiologic anemia of the newborn.

Premature infants experience a more rapid and precipitous drop in postnatal Hb levels, not uncommonly to 6 to 8 g/dl by 4 to 6 weeks of age. These low Hb levels may be a factor in apnea and bradycardia of the premature infant.[2] In addition, anemia in the premature infant may cause poor feeding and growth, decreased activity, and, rarely, congestive heart failure. Treatment of symptomatic premature infants with fresh packed red blood cells in the nursery is indicated.

Iron-deficiency anemia is not typically seen in either term or preterm neonates, as adequate iron stores are present at birth unless there are significant blood losses.

PATHOLOGIC ANEMIA

Aplasias.   Bone marrow aplasia can affect all of the hematopoietic progenitors or only a single cell line. Congenital inherited aplastic disorders as well as acquired idiopathic or drug- or infection-associated aplastic anemias are rare. Aplasia in the perioperative setting is usually a result of chemotherapy or radiation therapy. Furthermore, with the increasing prevalence of infection with the human immunodeficiency virus (HIV), aplasia due to antiviral therapy, direct bone marrow suppression, or bone marrow infiltration by opportunistic infection has become more common. Patients with bone marrow aplasia are often seen for placement of central venous catheters, for infectious complications, or because of internal bleeding. Anesthetic considerations include:

- Transfusional support with packed red cells or platelets as dictated by the nature of the operative procedure and the institutional guidelines for blood product use
- Avoidance of intramuscular injections
- Stress dose coverage for patients receiving corticosteroids
- Judicious use of nitrous oxide, which can suppress bone marrow activity

Aplastic anemias

	Disease	Clinical manifestation
Single cell line	Blackfan-Diamond anemia	Pure red cell asplasia
	Congenital neutropenia (Kostmann's) Cyclic neutropenia	Chronic or intermittent reduction in the number of neutrophils
	TAR syndrome: congenital thrombocytopenia with absent radii	Thrombocytopenia
	Parvovirus	May cause red cell aplasia in some cases of sickle cell anemia
	Transient erythroblastopenia of childhood	Self-limited red cell anemia resembling newborn physiologic anemia, with Hb levels of 4-6 g/dl
Multiple cell lines	Fanconi's anemia	Autosomal recessive disorder with multiple organ system dysfunction
	Dyskeratosis congenita	Mostly neutropenia
	Schwachmann's syndrome	Pancreatic insufficiency and bone marrow hypoplasia
	Viral disease	Multi–cell line aplasia
	Drugs • Chemotherapeutic agents • Chloramphenicol • Trimethoprim-sulfamethoxazole • Anticonvulsants • Antiviral compounds	Multi–cell line aplasia

Iron deficiency. Iron-deficiency anemia is the most common hematologic disease of childhood. It is most often seen in children between the ages of 1 and 3 years, but can occur at any age. The otherwise healthy neonate is born with sufficient iron stores to last about 9 months. Any newborn with increased blood losses, such as with fetal-maternal transfusion or prematurity necessitating blood sampling, will be at increased risk of developing iron-deficiency anemia because of depletion of red cell iron stores. Exhaustion of iron stores may also be seen with inadequate dietary intake or various chronic disease states.

Symptoms include pallor, irritability, pica, tachycardia, systolic murmurs, and, less commonly, congestive heart failure. Anemia is hypochromic and microcytic, with a low reticulocyte count. Oral ferrous sulfate is the usual therapy of choice. A prompt reticulocytosis is seen by 3 to 5 days, and the Hb levels begin to rise 1 to 2 days thereafter.

Elective surgery should be postponed if the Hb level is sufficiently low to cause concern about oxygen-carrying capacity. Maximizing oxygen delivery by increasing cardiac output and delivered FIO_2 can compensate for mild anemia when emergent surgery is indicated. The need for transfusion must be individualized. Children with chronic anemia have an expanded intravascular volume and cardiac output, and rapid transfusion may induce congestive heart failure.

Chronic renal failure. Anemia due to the lack of production of erythropoietin is virtually universal in children with chronic renal failure. The anemia is most often normochromic and normocytic, with Hb levels between 5 and 8 g/dl. In addition, these patients may have circulating erythropoiesis inhibitors and decreased red cell survival due to uremia and microangiopathy. These intrinsic problems are often compounded by blood loss anemia (from dialysis, bleeding, or sampling) or nutritional anemias. Current therapy incorporates recombinant erythropoietin, which has lessened the need for traditional transfusion support.

Children with chronic anemia are usually well compensated hemodynamically. A shift of the oxyhemoglobin curve to the right improves oxygen delivery to tissues. Assuming normal cardiopulmonary function, transfusion is not usually required for surgery if significant blood loss is not anticipated.

Megaloblastic. Megaloblastic anemias are rare in children and are usually seen with dietary folic acid deficiency (goat's milk or phenylketonuric diets) or occasionally as a result of trimethoprim-sulfamethoxazole administration. The anemia is treated by replacement of vitamin B_{12}. As the hematologic response to therapy takes about a week, transfusion support may be required for emergent procedures. Patients who have recently started therapy for one of these nutritional anemias may become hypokalemic, so that potassium levels should be assessed preoperatively.

Nitrous oxide.[3] Administration of nitrous oxide may be associated with inhibition of methionine synthetase activity, which can impair DNA synthesis, inactivate viatmin B_{12}, and result in megaloblastic anemia. These biochemical changes appear to be related to the duration of N_2O administration. Folinic acid can prevent bone marrow toxicity; however, avoidance of N_2O may be preferable in patients who already have compromised erythropoiesis.

Increased Destruction

Intravascular red cell destruction is accompanied by hemoglobinemia, hemoglobinuria, and hemosiderinuria. Extravascular hemolysis is usually accompanied by jaundice (unconjugated bilirubin), splenomegaly, and cholelithiasis. In both intravascular and extravascular destruction, reticulocytosis is common and circulating haptoglobin, which combines with free hemoglobin, will fall to quite low levels.

INTRINSIC TO RED CELL

Membranes

Hereditary spherocytosis.   This autosomal dominant disorder is caused by a deficiency of spectrin in the membrane of the erythrocyte. The cells assume a more rigid spherical shape, which leads to fragmentation and loss of membrane in the spleen. The spherical cells are susceptible to lysis by hypotonic solutions, forming the basis of the osmotic fragility test. Infants may present with marked jaundice in the newborn period.

Patients may present with reticulocytosis and a characteristic elevation in the mean corpuscular hemoglobin concentration (MCHC) because of the relative loss of red cell membrane. Because of the high rate of red cell turnover, excessive amounts of bilirubin are produced and the majority of these patients will develop bilirubin cholelithiasis. Since red blood cell survival returns to normal in the absence of the spleen, elective splenectomy has become the treatment of choice, usually between the ages of 5 and 12 years. The anesthesiologist should maximize O_2 delivery if significant anemia is present.

Enzyme deficiency

Pyruvate kinase deficiency.   This autosomal recessive disorder is caused by a deficiency in glycolytic enzymes of the Embden-Meyerhof pathway, causing hemolysis in infancy or early childhood. Most patients require only supplementation with folic acid and rarely red cell transfusions. If the disease is severe, splenectomy may be indicated.

Glucose-6-phosphate dehydrogenase (G6PD) deficiency.   This disorder is X-linked and prevalent in the African-American (15%), Mediterranean, and Chinese populations. Drugs that form peroxides are usually implicated as triggering agents, which can induce hemolysis. Fava beans may also cause acute hemolytic reactions, depending on the penetrance. See box on next page.

Drugs associated with hemolysis in patients with G6PD deficiency

Drug class[4]	Drugs
Antimalarials (aminoquilones)	Pentaquine Primaquine Quinine
Antibiotics/antiparasitics	Doxorubicin Nalidixic acid Niridazole
Nitrofurans	Furazolidone Nitrofurantoin
Sulfonamides	Sulfacetamide Sulfamethoxazole Sulfanilamide Sulfapyridine
Sulfones	Dapsone Thiazolsulfone
Miscellaneous	Fava beans Toluidine blue

Hemoglobin[5]

Sickle syndromes[6,7]

Pathophysiology: The single-gene amino acid substitution of valine for glutamic acid at position 6 in the β-hemoglobin chain results in the production of Hb S. Other hemoglobin variants, such as Hb C, D, E, or β-thalassemia, may be seen in patients who also have a gene expressing Hb S. About 10% of the African-American population has the Hb S gene, with increased prevalence also noted in those of Middle Eastern, Indian, or Mediterranean descent.

Common sickle syndromes

Phenotype (β-locus)	Description	Hb present
Hb A/Hb A	Normal	Hb A, A_2, F
Hb A/Hb S	Sickle cell trait	Hb A, S, A_2, F
Hb S/Hb S	Sickle cell anemia	Hb S, A_2 F
Hb A/Hb C	Hemoglobin C trait	Hb A, C, A_2, F
Hb S/Hb C	Sickle C disease	Hb S, C, A_2, F
Hb C/Hb C	Homozygous hemoglobin C disease	Hb C, A_2, F
Hb S/β-thalassemia	Sickle β-thalassemia	Hb S,($\pm$A), A_2, F

Hb S, when deoxygenated, can polymerize with itself, leading to damage to the red cell that causes it to assume the sickled shape. These cells can hemolyze or they can become entrapped in the small capillaries and arterioles to form microaggregate emboli. Vasoocclusive symptoms predominate after the first year of life. As early as 12 to 18 months of age, many children have completely autoinfarcted their spleens. Splenic entrapment and sequestration of blood in infants can cause profound hypovolemic shock.

Sickle cell disease: organ system dysfunction

Hematologic	Hemolysis, anemia, leukocytosis, jaundice
Renal	Loss of concentrating ability
Immunologic	Splenic autoinfarction, immunoincompetence
Pulmonary	Diminished function due to recurrent infarcts
Cardiac	Cor pulmonale
Neurologic	Stroke, seizures
Dermatologic	Chronic leg ulcers
Endocrine	Growth retardation, delay in sexual maturity
Skeletal	Osteomyelitis (femoral head)
Genital	Priapism
Gastrointestinal	Cholelithiasis, bowel infarcts

Diagnosis: Many states routinely screen newborns for sickling diseases. Tests will reliably detect the presence of Hb S, but they cannot distinguish diseased patients from those with trait. Hemoglobin electrophoresis remains the benchmark standard test to identify affected children.

Treatment[7,8]:

- Supportive care includes hydration, analgesics, transfusion.
- Bone marrow transplantation.
- Oral hydroxyurea to stimulate endogenous production of hemoglobin F has decreased the prevalence of painful crisis in many patients.[9]

Anesthetic Management: Cholecystectomy for pigment stones, splenectomy for recurrent sequestration, plastic surgery for leg ulcers, and urologic surgery for priapism are common procedures in the sickle cell population. Vasoocclusive episodes with severe abdominal pain can sometimes be confused with the acute abdomen that requires operation. In general, anesthetic techniques should be designed to minimize the possibility of hypoxia, vascular stasis, hypothermia, and catecholamine production, which can trigger vasoocclusive episodes.

1. Ideally, it is recommended that the percentage of Hb S be decreased below 50%, and if possible to about 30% before operation. In addition to decreasing abnormal hemoglobin, preoperative transfusion improves the anemia typically

found among sickle cell patients. Recent data suggest that preoperative transfusion that increases the Hb level to 10 g/dl is just as effective in preventing perioperative complications as transfusions designed to establish an Hb level of 10 g/dl *and* an Hb S level below 30%.[10] Controversy arises concerning the relative risks of transfusion for simple, brief operative procedures in patients who are minimally symptomatic and considered at low risk for intraoperative vasoocclusive crisis. Unfortunately, there are no data that identify which patients will have intraoperative crises or anesthetic techniques that will absolutely avoid this complication. Furthermore, pulse oximetry is not accurate for Hb S during crisis, as the aggregation of cells seems to interfere with LED reception. It therefore becomes difficult intraoperatively to identify crisis and hypoxia in patients with mostly Hb S. If patients, parents, or referring physicians request that preoperative transfusion be avoided, they must be willing to share the risks as explained by the anesthesiologist.[10,11]

2. Aggressive hydration with crystalloid or colloid is recommended except in the presence of congestive heart failure.

3. Intraoperative normothermia is maintained with fluid warmers, breathing circuit humidification, warming blankets, forced-air warmers, and a heated operating room.

4. Preoxygenation and an increased delivered FIO_2 minimize the opportunity for hypoxia.

5. Traditionally, spinal anesthesia has been avoided because of the potential complications of hypotension and sickling. Since hypotension is unusual in children under 5 years of age, spinal anesthesia may be considered. In addition, epidural techniques for anesthesia and analgesia may be used.

6. Tourniquet use is avoided, especially with limb exsanguination.

7. Postoperative pain should be managed aggressively to avoid catecholamine-mediated vasoconstriction and hypoventilation (with resultant hypoxia and respiratory acidosis).

Sickle Cell Trait: Although these individuals would be expected to have equal concentrations of Hb S and A, the ratio is usually about 60% A and 40% S. Life expectancy is normal, and the only common clinical manifestation is a mild impairment of the concentrating abilities of the renal medulla. It is rare for sickling of red cells to occur with Hb AS, as markedly decreased oxygen tensions would be required for such an event. This may, however, occasionally occur in the perioperative setting with cardiopulmonary bypass or prolonged application of a tourniquet.[6,12]

Thalassemias.[13-15]   These are a diverse group of congenital disorders of globin chain synthesis leading to microcytic, hypochromic

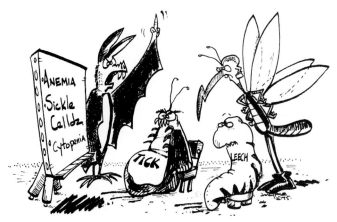

"FRIENDS, this has got to stop ... Our livelihoods are at stake here.....!"

red cells. The affected genes may control synthesis of α- or β-chains. The phenotypic expression of the disorder will depend upon the number and severity of affected genes. Alpha-chain production is regulated by 4 gene alleles, all or some of which may be affected. Beta-chain production is regulated by 2 alleles, but clinically gene expression is either silent (β°) or partially impaired (β^+).

α-*Thalassemia:* This defect is found primarily in people of Mediterranean, African, or Asian descent. Its clinical manifestations relate to the number of inactive α-alleles.

1. Carriers have a single defective gene and are asymptomatic, with a very mild, iron-resistant hypochromic, microcytic anemia.

2. If two alleles are inactive, patients demonstrate a modest anemia, resembling iron deficiency although resistant to iron therapy.

3. When three alleles are missing or defective, β-chain production so greatly exceeds α-chain production that Hb H disease results. This Hb consists of tetramers of β-chains. These patients have a hemolytic anemia with Hb levels between 5 and 10 g/dl. There is usually jaundice, splenomegaly, and signs of marrow hyperplasia.

4. If all four alleles are absent, there is usually fetal demise.

β-*Thalassemia:* This disorder occurs most frequently in individuals of Mediterranean extraction; however, it is also present in Africans, Asians, and Pacific Islanders. Since there are only two β-chain alleles, the disorder follows simple mendelian inheritance. Patients are often classified as having thalassemia minor, if they have one abnormal gene, or thalassemia major (Cooley's anemia)

if they have two abnormal genes. Patients described as having thalassemia intermedia can belong to a number of categories, including those with:

1. Two abnormal β genes, which produce some β chains
2. An unusually high level of Hb F with otherwise abnormal β
   alleles
3. δβ-thalassemia
4. β-thalassemia associated with α-thalassemia, which leads to
   a better balance of α- and β- chain production
5. Sickle β-thalassemia, which clinically resembles sickle cell
   disease

Pathophysiology: Patients with thalassemia major have a severe
hemolytic anemia usually apparent by 3 to 4 months of age and necessitating frequent transfusions. Splenomegaly and bone marrow
hyperplasia are present. Iron overload with the development of he-
mosiderosis was previously the most common complication of
therapy and the usual cause of death in adolescence. Desferox-
amine chelation therapy has dramatically altered the progressive
accumulation of iron in these patients. In addition, some centers
are now treating with allogeneic bone marrow transplantation
pending availability of more directed genetic therapy.

Anesthetic Management:

1. Hemoglobin levels must be maintained at a level acceptable for
   the specific surgical procedure. In addition, blood product support with fresh frozen plasma and platelets may be dictated by
   coagulopathies present in these patients.
2. Careful clinical assessment for signs and symptoms of iron
   toxicity must be sought.
3. Maxillary overgrowth due to marrow hyperplasia may hamper
   direct laryngoscopy.
4. Patients with sickle β-thalassemia should be managed like
   those with sickle cell anemia.

EXTRINSIC TO RED CELL

1. Mechanical red cell trauma (e.g., from artificial heart valves)
   causes microangiopathic hemolytic anemia, which can usually
   be treated with iron replacement.
2. Immune hemolytic anemia is usually caused by autoantibodies.
   - Treatment consists of steroids, splenectomy, gammaglobu-
     lins, or antimetabolites to suppress antibody production.
   - It may be difficult to maintain adequate hemoglobin levels
     perioperatively, as transfused blood is quickly consumed by
     the hemolytic process.
   - Stress coverage steroids are usually required.
   - End-organ damage (most commonly renal) from circulating
     free hemoglobin should be evaluated.

POLYCYTHEMIA[16]

Definition. Polycythemia is described as an Hb concentration in excess of 17 g/dl in the child or 22 g/dl in the neonate.

Etiology. Although polycythemia vera does not occur in childhood, secondary polycythemia from prolonged arterial oxygen desaturation is common in children with cyanotic congenital heart disease or chronic pulmonary disease (e.g., cystic fibrosis) or in children living at high altitudes. Hb levels rise about 4% per 1000-meter increase in altitude. Neonatal polycythemia, which predisposes to intracerebral and renal vein thrombosis, can be caused by fetal hypoxia, maternal-fetal transfusion, or twin-twin transfusion.

Pathophysiology. The elevated hematocrit may lead to increased blood viscosity with increased cardiac work and red blood cell sludging and thrombosis. In the chronically cyanotic child, tissue oxygen delivery is dependent upon the increased Hb mass. Therefore, acute hemodilution can result in severe hypoxia. When the hematocrit is above 60% to 70%, thrombotic sequelae can occur. Partial exchange transfusion with fresh frozen plasma or 5% albumin is indicated.

$$Vol_E = \frac{BV \times (Hct_o - Hct_d)}{Hct_o}$$

where

Vol_E = Volume of exchange

BV = Blood volume

Hct_o = Observed hematocrit

Hct_d = Desired hematocrit

COAGULATION
Defects in the Plasma Coagulation Cascade

Disorders of coagulation result from an imbalance in the coagulation cascade or from deficiencies of any of the components of these interactive pathways.

Normal values for coagulation tests[17]

	Child/adolescent	Newborn
Platelet count	150,000-400,000/mm^3	100,000-400,000/mm^3
Bleeding time	4-9 min	Not applicable
Prothrombin time	10-12 sec	10-13 sec
Activated partial thromboplastin time	25-35 sec	31-54 sec
Fibrinogen level	200-400 mg/dl	150-400 mg/dl
Fibrin split products	<40 mg/ml	<40 mg/ml

HEMOPHILIA[18]

The hemophilias are the most common of the inherited coagulation disorders. They are inherited as X-linked disorders and do occur without any family history in about one third of affected patients. Patients with hemophilia A have a deficiency in factor VIII, while those with hemophilia B (Christmas disease) are deficient in factor IX. Although these diseases are clinicallly indistinguishable, they are easily separated by laboratory testing and require different therapy.

Diagnosis of hemophilia

Symptoms

Usually normal hemostasis with minor cuts
Bleeding with circumcision as a neonate
Joint and muscle bleeding by age 1 year
Spontaneous hemorrhage into deep tissues (e.g., psoas muscle, bladder, retroperitoneum)

Diagnostic tests

Normal prothrombin time (PT)
Prolonged partial thromboplastin time (PTT)
Normal platelet count
Normal bleeding time
Reduced amounts of factor VIII (A) or IX (B)
Normal amount of von Willebrand factor

Anesthetic management

1. Intramuscular injections should be avoided.
2. Replacement with factor VIII or IX 15 to 20 minutes before invasive procedures or intravascular catheter placement is recommended.

Replacement guidelines (approximate level of plasma factor activity desired)

Minor bleeds (hemarthrosis)	30%
Moderate bleeds (deep muscle, minor superficial surgery)	50%
Severe bleeds (head trauma, major closed-space surgery)	100%
Postoperative	Maintain between 25% and 100% for 7-10 days

3. Factors VIII and IX can be administered as boluses or by continuous infusion; specific therapy should be established in consultation with the referring hematologist.
4. Patients should be screened for the presence of anti-factor VIII or anti-factor IX antibodies (7 to 10% of patients).
5. All patients who have been treated with products derived from plasma are at risk for having and transmitting HIV, and hepatitis B and C.

Factor VIII replacement: 1 Unit factor VIII activity/kg = 2% increase in plasma factor VIII level

Sources of factor VIII	Factor VIII activity level
Fresh frozen plasma	1 unit/ml
Cryoprecipitate	75-100 units/bag (20-30 ml)
Factor VIII concentrate (heat treated)	25 units/ml (reconstituted in bottles of 400-1000 U)
Factor VIII concentrate (immunoaffinity purified)	25 units/ml (reconstituted in bottles of 400-1000 U)
Factor VIII concentrate (recombinant)	25 units/ml (reconstituted in bottles of 400-1000 U)
Desmopressin (DDAVP)	Increases factor VIII levels 100%-600% from baseline

Factor IX replacement: 1 unit factor IX activity/kg = 1% increase in plasma factor IX level

Sources of factor IX	Factor IX activity level
Fresh frozen plasma	1 unit/ml
Factor IX concentrate (heat treated)	25 units/ml (reconstituted in bottles of 400-1000 U)

VON WILLEBRAND'S DISEASE[19]

Von Willebrand's disease (vWD) is an autosomal dominant coagulation defect caused by deficiency of von Willebrand factor (vWF); found in platelets, plasma, and endothelial cells, it serves to mediate platelet adhesion. There is variable penetrance of the defective gene and thus considerable variability in clinical manifestations, classified into types I, II, and III. The majority of patients (about 90%) have type I disease in which there is a quantitative decrease in vWF with a prolonged bleeding time and partial thromboplastin time.

Clinical manifestations. Patients typically have a history of abnormal bleeding that dates back to early childhood. Epistaxis, mucosal and gum bleeding, bruising, and menorrhagia are common. Excessive bleeding can be expected with surgery, especially if mucosal surfaces are involved.

Anesthetic management[20,21]

1. The perioperative management of patients with vWD requires consultation with the hematologist. Many patients can achieve adequate plasma levels of vWF after administration of DDAVP alone. Other patients will require replacement with specially prepared factor concentrates that are relatively rich in vWF. Patients with type IIb vWD should not receive DDAVP.

2. DDAVP is given as 0.3 μg/kg intravenously over 20 minutes in 50 ml of normal saline. If necessary, coagulation tests can be repeated after 1 hour.

3. If more than three doses of DDAVP are required in 48 hours, the risk of hyponatremia and fluid retention is increased.

4. Cryoprecipitate or fresh frozen plasma can provide a source of vWF if DDAVP is contraindicated or ineffective.

PLATELET DEFECTS

Pathophysiology. Thrombocytopenia can be caused by decreased production of platelets (aplastic anemia, megaloblastic anemia, bone marrow infiltration, post-chemotherapy), increased peripheral destruction (hypersplenism, consumption coagulopathies, immune thrombocytopenic purpura, prosthetic heart valve, cardiopulmonary bypass), or dilution (massive blood transfusions). Clinical manifestations of thrombocytopenia are usually absent until the platelet count falls significantly below 100,000/μl, with bleeding rarely occurring until platelet levels fall below 20,000/μl. Therapy is directed at correcting the underlying pathology, with judicious use of platelet replacement therapy for bleeding.

Immune thrombocytopenic purpura (ITP).[22] This disorder usually presents in early childhood with frank and severe thrombocytopenia after a minor viral illness. It is self-limited in approximately 80% to 85% of patients. Diagnosis is established by the presence of thrombocytopenia with an otherwise normal bone marrow and increased numbers of megakaryocytes. The presence of antiplatelet antibodies may also be documented. Treatment consists of corticosteroids, intravenous gammaglobulin, and occasionally splenectomy.

Anesthetic management

1. Intramuscular injections should be avoided if the platelet count is decreased.

2. Except for emergency procedures, attempts should be made preoperatively to increase the platelet count. High doses of intravenous methylprednisolone and intravenous gammaglobulin have proven useful in acutely elevating the platelet count.[23,24]

3. Patients with a history of chronic corticosteroid use should receive stress doses.
4. Platelet transfusions (0.2 U/kg) should be available to correct serious bleeding.
5. Thrombocytopenia often improves dramatically after the splenic artery is clamped.

ONCOLOGY

Children with malignant diseases often come to the operating room for tumor surgery, central venous catheter placement, and diagnostic procedures such as bone marrow aspiration/biopsy or lumbar puncture. In some situations, such as the presence of an anterior mediastinal mass, the disease process itself presents an anesthetic challenge. More frequently, side effects of antineoplastic therapy must be considered in determining the anesthetic plan.

Leukemias[25]

Leukemia accounts for about 50% of pediatric malignancies; about 80% of the leukemias are acute and 20% are chronic. Of the acute leukemias, 80% are lymphoid (acute lymphocytic leukemia or ALL) in origin and about 20% myeloid (acute myelocytic leukemia or AML). Almost all of the chronic leukemias in childhood are myeloid (CML).

It is not unusual for life-threatening systemic illness to be present at the onset of the disease when children are seen in the operating room for diagnostic procedures or central venous catheter placement.

1. Varying degrees of pancytopenia are common, requiring component replacement blood products.
2. Disseminated intravascular coagulation is universally seen in children with AML and may be seen with other leukemias as well.
3. Massive hepatosplenomegaly or cervical adenopathy may exert mass effects in their individual anatomic locations.
4. Signs and symptoms of an anterior mediastinal mass can be present in as many as 20% of newly diagnosed patients with ALL (see p. 297).
5. Electrolyte abnormalities including hyponatremia, hyperkalemia or hypokalemia, hypercalcemia, and hyperphosphatemia may be present.
6. Renal function may be significantly compromised because of direct tumor infiltration or because of the presence of tumor lysis syndrome. In these patients, high serum levels of uric acid are present from tumor degradation products that precipitate in the kidneys, leading to a tubular obstructive uropathy. Allopurinol is given to treat or prevent this problem.

7. As many as 5% of newly diagnosed leukemias have an active life-threatening infection at diagnosis, particularly pneumonia or septicemia.

8. Central nervous system involvement (meninges) is present in as many as 10% of children at diagnosis and during the course of therapy.

Treatment of leukemias

Systemic chemotherapy

Corticosteroids
Vincristine
Cyclophosphamide
Daunorubicin
L-Aspariginase
Methotrexate
6-Mercaptopurine

Prophylactic antibiotics

Trimethoprim-sulfamethoxazole *(Pneumocystis carinii)*

Craniospinal irradiation

Bone marrow transplant

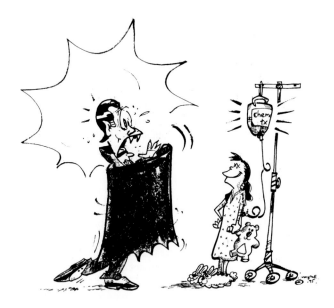

Solid Tumors
LYMPHOMAS[26]

Tumors in this group are classified as either Hodgkin's or non-Hodgkin's lymphomas. The non-Hodgkin's lymphomas usually occur as widely disseminated diseases with many of the life-threatening problems common to the leukemias. Hodgkin's lymphomas are often more indolent, arising in childhood in the mediastinum and cervical lymph glands.

Mediastinal masses.[27,28] Masses occur in all of the anatomic compartments of the mediastinum, but those of the anterior mediastinum are the most challenging to the anesthesiologist.

Mediastinal location	Types of masses
Anterior	Hodgkin's and non-Hodgkin's lymphoma Teratoma Thymoma Ectopic thyroid Cystic hygroma Pericardial cysts
Middle	Lymphomas Infectious lesions (tuberculosis, histoplasmosis) Bronchogenic cysts Esophageal duplications
Posterior	Neurogenic tumors (neuroblastoma) Esophageal duplications Diaphragmatic hernias

1. Cardiopulmonary arrest and death during induction of anesthesia have been reported in patients with anterior mediastinal masses. [29,30]
   - Compression of the trachea and larger bronchi by tumor mass has contributed to anesthetic difficulty or poor outcome.
   - Compression of the distal airways can occur precipitously, often at the time of conversion of spontaneous ventilation to positive pressure. Because small airway collapse is distal to the trachea and main bronchi, it is unrelieved by the passage or prior placement of an endotracheal tube or rigid bronchoscope.
   - Vascular collapse due to loss of cardiac output from acute compression of the great vessels or superior vena cava has also been observed.
2. In patients with severe airway/respiratory compromise, pre-anesthesia radiation therapy has been advocated. This option should be reserved for extreme circumstances, as the radiation may obliterate the opportunity for an accurate tissue diagnosis of the tumor.[31]

3. It has been advocated that induction of general anesthesia is probably safe in asymptomatic patients. Unfortunately, intraoperative death has been reported even in children without symptoms.[32]

4. Along with clinical evaluation for signs and symptoms of airway or major vessel compromise, preoperative assessment should include computed tomographic (CT) or magnetic resonance imaging (MRI) of the chest. Since many of these tumors are lymphomas and rapid doubling times are not uncommon, the diagnostic imaging should take place as close to the anticipated procedure time as possible.

5. *Anesthetic Management* [31,33]

   Preoperative evaluation must include assessment for clinical signs of airway or cardiac obstruction and CT or MRI of the chest. Arterial blood gases and flow volume loops to differentiate intrathoracic and extrathoracic obstruction are recommended.

   - The initial operative procedure should be reserved for tissue biopsy. More elective procedures (e.g., placement of indwelling central venous catheters) can be delayed until treatment has decreased the mass effect.

   - Semi-Fowler's position is recommended, especially for patients with dyspnea and orthopnea.

   - A slow, gentle inhalation induction, with oxygen and halothane maintaining spontaneous ventilation, is preferred. It has been suggested that positive-pressure ventilation may convert adequate laminar flow in the smaller compressed airways to turbulent flow without effective air exchange. Muscle relaxants should be avoided even after endotracheal intubation if small airway compression is present. Judicious doses of intravenous propofol may help to maintain anesthetic depth and spontaneous ventilation if airway obstruction impedes gas delivery.

   - Fiberoptic bronchoscopy is recommended if tracheal deviation is seen on diagnostic imaging. Rigid bronchoscopy may be necessary if tracheal compression and collapse hinders passage of the endotracheal tube. Both bronchoscopes and a wide variety of emergency airway equipment should be available for induction.

   - In some reports, the ability to rapidly connect the patient to cardiopulmonary bypass when ventilation or cardiac output is severely impaired has been life-saving. Preparation of the patient for femoral-femoral bypass before beginning induction facilitates the ability to rapidly bypass the patient's circulation should disaster occur.

ABDOMINAL TUMORS[34]

Wilms' tumor (nephroblastoma). Wilms' tumor is the most commonly occurring childhood abdominal malignancy, with an incidence of 1:15,000 live births. It usually affects preschool-age children, with bilateral involvement in about 10% of patients. The tumor may be associated with aniridia, hemihypertrophy, neurofibromatosis, Beckwith-Wiedemann syndrome, and anomalies of the genitourinary tract.

Clinical findings. Wilms' tumor is usually diagnosed when a large intrabdominal mass is discovered. There may be associated hematuria, weight loss, and abdominal pain. Hypertension from renal artery compression or direct tumor invasion into the hilar vascular structures can occur.

Treatment. Prognosis is related to staging, with greater than 96% survival reported for Stage I disease. Complete surgical resection remains the mainstay of treatment, usually followed by chemotherapy and radiation.

Neuroblastoma.[35] Neuroblastoma is the most common tumor of infancy, usually diagnosed in children less than 2 years of age. The tumor is derived from neural crest cells (sympathoblasts). Although most commonly found in the abdomen (70%) and more specifically the adrenal medulla, neuroblastoma is not uncommonly found in the mediastinum (usually posterior). Intracranial tumors also occur and may cause increases in intracranial pressure.

Clinical findings

1. Children frequently have a painful abdominal mass, neurologic findings (gait disturbances, bowel or bladder dysfunction), and nonspecific symptoms such as fever, weight loss, and lymphadenopathy.
2. Anemia, thrombocytopenia, and pancytopenia are not uncommon.
3. Neuroblastomas synthesize and secrete dopamine, epinephrine, and norepinephrine, with increased urinary catecholamines (vanilmandelic acid [VMA] and homovanillic acid [HVA]) present in over 90% of patients.
4. Preoperative hypertension and intravascular volume reduction may be seen as a result of increased catecholamine secretion.
5. Wheezing and stridor from tracheobronchial compression in children with thoracic lesions have been reported.

Treatment. Staging is the major determinant of survival. Conventional treatment remains surgical excision followed by chemotherapy and radiation. In patients with advanced metastatic disease, chemotherapy is often initiated prior to surgical resection of the mass. A type of advanced disease that has been known to undergo spontaneous regression may be seen in children less than 1 year of age.

Hepatic tumors. Primary tumors of the liver are uncommon in children, so that most hepatic tumors represent metastatic disease. Hepatoblastoma is seen usually in males less than 5 years of age. It is associated with Wilms' tumor, fetal alcohol syndrome, polyposis coli, and Beckwith-Wiedemann syndrome. Physical findings include a palpable abdominal mass, with weight loss, pain, and vomiting seen with more advanced disease. These tumors may secrete β human chorionic gonadotropin (HCG), causing precocious puberty. Resection when possible is considered optimal treatment.

Anesthetic management of abdominal tumors

Preoperative considerations

1. The mass effect of the tumor, abdominal distension, and vomiting place most patients at risk for aspiration on induction. Aspiration prophylaxis with H_2 blockers, metoclopramide, and nonparticulate antacids should be considered. A rapid-sequence induction with cricoid pressure may also be indicated.

2. Patients who received preoperative chemotherapy should be evaluated for organ system dysfunction (see table p. 303). Most notably, patients who have received adriamycin are at risk for dose-dependent cardiomyopathy, necessitating cardiac consultation and echocardiographic evaluation.

3. Mediastinal and intracranial involvement should be considered in patients with neuroblastoma and verified by computed tomography or magnetic resonance imaging. The anesthetic plan may require modification if lower airway compromise or increased intracranial pressure is present.

4. Systemic hypertension in patients with catecholamine-secreting tumors must be treated. Preoperative hydration and volume expansion may also be indicated.

5. Blood should be available for transfusion.

Anesthetic technique

1. For patients at risk for aspiration, a rapid-sequence induction is preferred. However, large abdominal masses often cause loss of functional residual capacity and lower ventilatory volume. Thus, rapid desaturation may occur during even brief periods of apnea.

2. Large fluid shifts should be anticipated because of preoperative fluid losses (bowel preparation, vomiting, etc.), the large abdominal incision usually required, and bleeding during resection. Multiple large-bore intravenous catheters are recommended, preferably above the diaphragm in case clamping of the inferior vena cava is necessary. As indwelling central venous catheters are usually needed after surgery for chemotherapy, placement at the beginning of the procedure provides central access for volume replacement and central venous pressure monitoring.

3. Intraarterial catheters are needed for continuous assessment of blood pressure, as significant bleeding from major retroperitoneal vessels is not uncommon. Futhermore, intraoperative hypertension can occur from secretion of vasoactive substances during tumor manipulation or by kinking of the renal artery.

4. Heat loss from surgical exposure and fluid infusions will make it difficult to maintain normothermia. Heating blankets, forced-air warmers, or fluid/blood warmers should be used at the outset of the procedure to prevent hypothermia.

5. Nitrous oxide should be avoided to prevent bowel distension. There may be an association between hepatic toxicity and repeated halothane exposure in children receiving high-dose chemotherapy.[36,37] There are no reports, however, of increased arrhythmogenicity in patients with neuroblastoma and halothane despite increased catecholamine secretion.

6. Postoperatively, mechanical ventilation should be considered for patients with compromised pulmonary function prior to surgery. Placement of indwelling neuroaxis catheters for pain management will also allow for improved pulmonary toilet in children with large abdominal incisions.

INTRACRANIAL TUMORS

Brain tumors of childhood are catalogued into those primarily of neural origin (e.g., astrocytoma, glioma, medulloblastoma) versus those arising from nonneural tissue (e.g., meningioma, lymphoma, germ cell tumor, craniopharyngioma, metatastic).

Anesthetic management

1. The preoperative assessment should include documentation of any neurologic deficits and signs and symptoms of elevated intracranial pressure (ICP).

2. The induction technique selected should consider the presence of increased ICP from the mass (see p. 205). In the absence of mass effect, an induction suitable for the child's age and associated medical conditions is selected.

3. Invasive monitoring is recommended. An intraarterial catheter helps to maintain tight hemodynamic control and allows for easy access to the circulation for monitoring arterial blood gases and other laboratory data.

4. Central venous pressure monitoring is useful for fluid management, particularly when diuretics are used to decrease ICP. A central venous catheter also supplies access to the circulation for volume or pharmacologic resuscitation. The CVP catheter will be easier to access if placed in the femoral vein. Jugular catheters may kink or become dislodged during craniotomy, or they may worsen jugular venous drainage.

5. Placement of a Foley catheter is also necessary for fluid management.

6. As microsurgical techniques are often used, muscle relaxants are critical to maintain a motionless field during resection.
7. Many children can be awakened at the end of the surgical procedure, and the anesthetic administered should be geared toward this option. Having an alert child in the postoperative period permits close monitoring of the neurologic status.
8. Prolonged intubation and mechanical ventilation are common after resection of posterior fossa tumors; airway edema from neck flexion in the prone position may be present postoperatively and preclude early tracheal extubation.

Chemotherapy

Cytotoxic therapy for children with malignancies has evolved into the delivery of complex combinations of chemotherapeutic agents and supportive drugs. Many of these drugs will have major systemic or target organ–specific toxicity that will affect the anesthetic plan. The anesthesiologist must pay particular attention to patients who have received anthracyclines (doxorubicin, daunorubicin), bleomycin, and cyclophosphamide (see table, p. 303). The following are general guidelines for children receiving chemotherapy.

- Administration of most chemotherapeutic agents will result in a dose-dependent suppression of the bone marrow, leading to pancytopenia.
- Many agents also produce anorexia, nausea, and vomiting, causing dehydration and potential electrolyte imbalances.
- Painful stomatitis and alopecia are common among these patients.
- All patients are immunocompromised from either their underlying disease or their therapy, necessitating strict asepsis.
- In addition to chemotherapy, patients may also receive prophylactic antibiotics or antiviral agents. Immunosuppressive agents are routine after bone marrow transplantation. Most children with malignancies who receive chemotherapy are treated with prophylactic trimethoprim-sulfamethoxazole to prevent *Pneumocystis carinii* pneumonia.
- Treatment with high-dose corticosteroids is common in children with leukemias or brain tumors and necessitates perioperative stress-dose coverage.

The following table highlights side effects of the more common chemotherapeutic agents that may have implications for anesthesia care.

Implications of cancer chemotherapy

Class	Drug	Specific toxicity
Alkylating agents	Cyclophosphamide (Cytoxan)	Hemorrhagic cystitis Pulmonary fibrosis/infiltrates Inhibition of plasma cholinesterase Cardiomyopathy at high doses
	Chlorambucil	Hepatitis Pulmonary fibrosis/infiltrates
	Melphalan	Pulmonary fibrosis/infiltrates
	Busulfan	Pulmonary fibrosis/infiltrates Inhibition of plasma cholinesterase
	Ifosfamide	Hemorrhagic cystitis Renal tubular/glomerular damage
Nitrosoureas	Carmustine (BCNU) Lomustine (CCNU)	Pulmonary fibrosis Delayed marrow suppression
Antimetabolites	Methrotrexate	Hepatitis Nephrotoxicity Pulmonary fibrosis/infiltrates
	Cytosine arabinoside (Ara-C)	Hepatitis Neuropathy with high-dose or intrathecal use
	5-Flourouracil (5-FU)	Cerebellar ataxia
	6-Mercaptopurine (6-MP)	Hepatitis/cholestasis Pancreatitis
	6-Thioguanine	Hepatitis
	5-Azacytidine	Hepatitis Central nervous system depression
Antibiotics	Doxorubicin (Adriamycin) Daunorubicin (Daunomycin)	Cardiomyopathy; acute or chronic (cumulative dose dependent: >350-400 mg/m^2); ECG and assessment of cardiac ejection fraction are helpful
	Actinomycin D (Dactinomycin)	Radiation dermatitis
	Bleomycin (Blenoxane)	Anaphylactic reactions Pulmonary fibrosis

Continued.

Implications of cancer chemotherapy—cont'd

Class	Drug	Specific toxicity
Vinca alkaloids	Vincristine (Oncovin)	Peripheral neuropathies; include ileus, cranial nerve palsies, foot drop, paresthesias Syndrome of inappropriate antidiuretic hormone secretion Seizures
	Vinblastine (Velban)	Peripheral neuropathies Syndrome of inappropriate antidiuretic hormone secretion
Epidophyllotoxins	Etoposide (VP-16)	Hypotension Hepatitis
	Teniposide (VM-26)	Hypersensitivity reaction Peripheral neuropathy
Enzyme	L-aspariginase (Elspar)	Hemorrhagic pancreatitis Anaphylactic reactions Coagulopathy: hypofibrinogenemia and decreased antithrombin III Hyperglycemia (hypoinsulinemia) Hepatitis
Synthetics	Cisplatin (Cis-DDP)	Renal tubular damage with hyponatremia, hypocalcemia, and hypomagnesemia Ototoxicity Peripheral neuropathy
	Carboplatin	Ototoxicity Rare peripheral neuropathy
	Hydroxyurea (Hydrea)	Hepatitis
	Procarbazine (Matulane)	Lethargy Peripheral neuropathy Myopathy/myalgia
	Dacarbazine (DTIC)	Hepatitis

Chronic Cancer Pain/Terminal Care

Anesthesia consultation may be sought for the management of pain in children with cancer. Pain present at the time of diagnosis can often be improved by initiation of specific antitumor therapy. Much of the initial pain experienced by children with cancer will be from diagnostic procedures (bone marrow aspirations, lumbar punctures, intravenous cannulations, etc.). Occasionally tumors may impinge on major neurovascular structures, resulting in neuropathic pain syndromes.

Therapy with a nonsteroidal anti-inflammatory agent is the usual first step, particularly for patients with bone pain. Because of the antiplatelet effects of the drugs in this class, acetaminophen may be selected. In most circumstances, oral therapy is the preferred route; the less potent opioids such as codeine or oxycodone may be added to nonopiod regimens. Potent narcotics (morphine, hydromorphone, and methadone) can also be given orally.

Intravenous administration of the opioids is advised for children with severe vomiting, ileus, or stomatitis. Drugs can be given intermittently, by continous infusion, or by patient-controlled analgesia pumps. The intramuscular route, which causes bleeding in patients with thrombocytopenia and pain universally, is not recommended. In children without intravenous access, small-gauge butterfly needles or catheters over a needle can be placed for subcutaneous infusions of opioids. Occasionally, children with intractable pain requiring extremely high doses of opioids, or intolerance to systemic opioids, will require therapy with neuraxial opioids and/or local anesthetics.

Adjuvant therapy with corticosteroids may prove quite helpful for bone pain and nerve root entrapment pain. Local radiation therapy can often be used to alleviate discrete symptoms caused by a radiosensitive tumor in specific locations.

Anticipated side effects of the opioids (e.g., constipation) can be treated prophylactically. Side effects of analgesic therapy should be treated aggressively so that the quality of life of the child is not compromised by the pain relief. Many children in the terminal phases of their illness will be managed at home. It is common to continue opioid infusions at home under the supervision of the oncology care team or a pediatric hospice program.

HUMAN IMMUNODEFICIENCY VIRUS (HIV)

Incidence.[38,39] Infection with HIV has become the leading cause of immunodeficiency in children. Over 1000 cases of acquired immunodeficiency syndrome (AIDS) in children under the age of 13 years were reported to the Centers for Disease Control in 1994.

Etiology. Greater than 90% of cases of HIV infection in children are caused by perinatal transmission. Infection in teenagers is becoming more prevalent, occurring most frequently as a result of sexual transmission.

Pathophysiology. Primary HIV infection usually causes an acute illness resembling mononucleosis. During this period there is widespread dissemination of virus and the onset of a serologic immune response. The acute phase is followed by the clinical latency period, which can last for several years. Ultimately, CD4 T lymphocytes are depleted with the progressive onslaught of opportunistic infections or malignancies.[40]

Clinical manifestations

1. Craniofacial abnormalities may be present in cases of early antenatal infection, with microcephaly, frontal bossing, ocular hypertelorism, nasal and ocular anomalies, and patulous lips.
2. Congenitally infected infants may develop symptoms by 4 to 6 months of age. Lymphadenopathy, hepatomegaly, and opportunistic infections are common. Signs of growth failure and progressive dementia seen in early infancy may be reversible with antiviral therapy.
3. HIV-infected children frequently develop a progressive encephalopathy, which causes developmental delay, behavioral abnormalities (including extreme irritability), paresis, palsy, and ataxia.
4. Children are more likely than adults to develop serious bacterial infection, especially with *Streptococcus, Haemophilus, Staphylococcus, Salmonella,* and *Pseudomonas.*
5. Lymphoid interstitial pneumonia (LIP) can cause severe hypoxemia. Treatment with corticosteroids is usually beneficial. *Pneumocystis carinii* pneumonia (PCP) may also be life threatening, causing high fever, dyspnea, cough, and severe hypoxemia. Treatment consists of trimethoprim-sulfamethoxazole or pentamidine.
6. Minor childhood viral illnesses (varicella, herpes zoster, rubeola) can cause severe morbidity in these children.
7. Multiple organ systems are usually affected; hepatic dysfunction as well as azotemia are common. Severe progressive cardiomyopathy has also been reported.[41]
8. The bone marrow can be either suppressed or infiltrated with opportunistic infections causing pancytopenia or single-line anemias.

Anesthetic management[41,42]

1. Strict adherence to universal precautions is required.
2. A careful preoperative assessment of organ system function will direct anesthetic techniques and specific agents.
3. A slow inhalation induction is usually helpful, as many HIV-infected children have extreme airway irritability.
4. Regional techniques may be used if contraindications (such as coagulopathy and local infection) are absent.
5. Concern for postoperative analgesia and adequate sedation for painful procedures can greatly contribute to the quality of life for these children.

Drug treatment for children with AIDS [43-45]

Treatment	Comments
Antiviral therapy	
AZT (zidovudine, ZDV)	Reduces HIV transmission in families Anemia and leukopenia are common Myopathy may develop Resistance to the drug may develop over time
DDI (didanosine)	May be used alone or in combinations with AZT Peripheral neuropathy is a common side effect Pancreatitis is present in 5% to 10% of patients Diarrhea and headache are also seen
Prophylactic antibiotics	
Trimethoprim-sulfamethoxazole	Also used to treat PCP Leukopenia, rash, and hepatic dysfunction are common
Pentamidine	May be used in the intravenous or nebulized form May cause leukopenia, thrombocytopenia, hypoglycemia, and hepatic dysfunction
Intravenous immunoglobulin	Appears to decrease the risk of bacterial infections in children with advanced HIV

References

1. Oski FA: Differential diagnosis of anemia. In Nathan DG, Oski FA, eds: *Hematology of infancy and childhood,* Philadelphia, 1993, W.B. Saunders.
2. Welborn LG, Hannallah RS, Luban NL, Fink R, Ruttiman UE: Anemia and postoperative apnea in former preterm infants, *Anesthesiology* 74:1003-1006, 1991.
3. Frasca V, Riazzi BR, Matthews RG: *In vitro* inactivation of methionine synthase by nitrous oxide, *J Biol Chem* 261:15823-15826, 1986.
4. Beutler E: The genetics of glucose-6-phosphate dehydrogenase deficiency, *Semin Hematol* 27:137-164, 1990.
5. Bunn HF: Human hemoglobins: normal and abnormal methemoglobinemia. In Nathan DG, Oski FA, eds: *Hematology of infancy and childhood,* Philadelphis, 1993, WB Saunders.
6. Gill FM, Sleeper LA, Weiner SJ, Brown AK, Bellevue R, Grover R, Pegelow CH, Vichinsky E: Clinical events in the first decade in a cohort of infants with sickle cell disease: Cooperative Study of Sickle Cell Disease, *Blood* 86:776-783, 1995.
7. Steingart R: Management of patients with sickle cell disease, *Med Clin North Am* 76:669-682, 1992.
8. Buchanan GR: Sickle cell disease: recent advances, *Curr Probl Pediatr* 23:219-229, 1993.
9. Charache S: Hydroxyurea as treatment for sickle cell anemia, *Hematol Oncol Clin North Am* 5:571-583, 1991.

10. Vichinsky EP, Haberkern CM, Neumayr L, et al: A comparison of conservative and aggressive transfusion regimens in the perioperative management of sickle cell disease, *N Engl J Med* 333: 206-213, 1995.

11. Esseltine DW, Baxter MRN, Bevan JC: Sickle cell states and the anaesthetist, *Can J Anaesth* 35: 385-403, 1988.

12. Banerjee AK, Layton DM, Rennie JA, Bellingham AJ: Safe surgery in sickle cell disease, *Br J Surg* 78:516-517, 1991.

13. Giardina PJ, Hilgartner MW: Update on thalassemia, *Pediatr Rev* 13: 55-62, 1992.

14. Piomelli S, Loew T: Management of thalassemia major (Cooley's anemia), *Hematol Oncol Clin North Am* 5:557-569, 1991.

15. Higgs DR: The thalassaemia syndromes, *Q J Med* 86:559-664, 1993.

16. Black VD: Neonatal hyperviscosity syndromes, *Curr Probl Pediatr* 17: 73-130, 1987.

17. Andrew M, Paes B, Milner R, et al: The development of the human coagulation system in the full term infant, *Blood* 70:165-172, 1987.

18. Hoyer LW: Hemophilia A, *N Engl J Med* 330:38-47, 1994.

19. Cameron CB, Kobrinsky N: Perioperative management of patients with von Willebrand's disease, *Can J Anaesth* 37:341-347, 1990.

20. Bloom DA: The American experience with desmopressin, *Clin Pediatr,* Spec No, pp. 28-31, 1993.

21. Lethagen S: Desmopressin (DDAVP) and hemostasis, *Ann Hematol* 69: 173-180, 1994.

22. Kurtzberg J, Stockman JA III: Idiopathic autoimmune thrombocytopenic purpura, *Adv Pediatr* 41:111-134, 1994.

23. Bussel JB: Autoimmune thrombocytopenic purpura, *Hematol Oncol Clin North Am* 4:179-191, 1990.

24. Van Hoff J, Ritchey AK: Pulse methylprednisolone therapy for acute childhood idiopathic thrombocytopenic purpura, *J Pediatr* 113: 563-566, 1988.

25. Pui CH: Childhood leukemias, *N Engl J Med* 332: 1618-30, 1995.

26. Kwak LW, DeVita VT Jr, Longo DL: Lymphomas, *Cancer Chemother Biol Response Modif* 14:383-426, 1993.

27. Shamberger RC, Holzman RS, Griscom NT, Tarbell NJ, et al: Prospective evaluation by computed tomography and pulmonary function tests of children with mediastinal masses, *Surgery* 118:468-471, 1995.

28. Shamberger RC, Holzman RS, Griscom NT, Tarbell NJ, Weinstein HJ: CT quantitation of tracheal cross-sectional area as a guide to the surgical and anesthetic mangement of children with anterior mediastinal masses, *J Pediatr Surg* 26: 138-142, 1991.

29. Wolfe TM, Rao CC: Anesthesia for selected procedures, *Semin Pediatr Surg* 1:74-80, 1992.

30. Robie DK, Gursoy MH, Pokorny WJ: Mediastinal tumors: airway obstruction and management, *Semin Pediatr Surg* 3:259-266, 1994.

31. Sibert KS, Biondi JW, Hirsch NP: Spontaneous respiration during thoractomy in a patient with a mediastinal mass, *Anesth Analg* 66:904-907, 1987.

32. Viswanathan S, Campbell CE, Cork RC: Asymptomatic undetected mediastinal mass: a death during ambulatory anesthesia, *J Clin Anesth* 7:151-155, 1995.

33. Ferrari LR, Bedford RF: General anesthesia prior to treatment of anterior mediastinal masses in pediatric cancer patients, *Anesthesiology* 72:991-995, 1990.

34. Caty MG, Shamberger RC: Abdominal tumors in infancy and childhood, *Pediatr Clin North Am* 40:1253-1271, 1993.

35. Kain ZN, Shamberger RS, Holzman RS: Anesthetic management of children with neuroblastoma, *J Clin Anesth* 5:486-491, 1993.

36. Gentet JC, Bernard JL, Aimard L, Alfonsi SM, Raybaud C: Venoocclusive disease in children after intensive chemo- and radiotherapy and repeated halothane anesthesias, *Acta Oncol* 27:579-581, 1988.

37. Spiegel RJ, Pizzo PA, Fantone JC, Zimmerman HJ: Fatal hepatic necrosis after high dose chemotherapy following haloalkane anesthesia, *Cancer Treat Rep* 64:1023-1029, 1980.

38. Centers for Disease Control: Update: acquired immunodeficiency syndrome—United States, 1994, *MMWR* 44:664-671, 1995.

39. Ammann AJ: Human immunodeficiency virus infections/AIDS in children: the next decade, *Pediatrics* 93:930-935, 1994.

40. Pantaleo G, Graziosi C, Fauci AS: The immunopathogenesis of human immunodeficiency virus infection, *N Engl J Med* 328:327-335, 1993.

41. Luginbuhl LM, Orav J, McIntosh K, Lipschultz SE: Cardiac morbidity and related mortality in children with HIV infection, *JAMA* 269:2869-2875, 1993.

42. Shapiro HM, Grant I, Weinger MB: AIDS and the central nervous sytem, *Anesthesiology* 80:187-200, 1994.

43. Husson RN, Mueller BU, Farley M, et al: Zidovudine and didanosine combination therapy in children with human immunodeficiency virus infection, *Pediatrics* 93: 316-322, 1994.

44. Hirsch MS, D'Aquila RT: Therapy for human immunodeficiency virus infection, *N Engl J Med* 328:1686-1695, 1993.

45. Spector SA, Gelber RD, McGrath N, et al: A controlled trial of intravenous immune globulin for the prevention of serious bacterial infections in children receiving zidovudine for advanced human immunodeficiency virus infection, *N Engl J Med* 331:1181-1187, 1994.

ANESTHETIC MANAGEMENT OF CHILDREN WITH RENAL AND ENDOCRINE DYSFUNCTION

14

seasaw susie
swallowed sweet
swinging high and low
soaring solo
endocrine
swimming to and fro

Adrienne Coleman

RENAL DEVELOPMENT AND THE INFANT KIDNEY [1,2]

Renal function is depressed in the newborn infant, particularly in the premature population. The glomerular filtration rate (GFR) in an infant is approximately one third that of adult levels (30 to 35 ml/min/1.73 m^2), approaching adult levels by the first year of life. The GFR of the premature infant may be as low as one tenth of adult levels. Although this rate of filtration is sufficient to meet demands of homeostasis and growth, it allows for minimal reserve for circumstances that may compromise renal function (e.g., perinatal asphyxia, hypotension, respiratory distress syndrome, renal vein thrombosis, and surgical procedures with general anesthesia).

The neonate has a decreased resorptive capacity, seen as a decreased ability to concentrate urine and to excrete a solute load, and a lower renal threshold for bicarbonate, which leads to increased filtration. Plasma bicarbonate levels are thus lower than those of adults (18 to 22 mEq/L).

By nine months of age, the normal infant has renal function approaching 80% to 90% of adult levels, with adult renal function achieved by 1 year of age. Fluid replacement for infants less than 1 year of age should approximate fluid loss, with careful monitoring of electrolyte levels in serum and urine.

Assessment of renal function in infants and children[3]

Parameter (normal values)	Etiology of abnormal value

Urine output
(0.5-1.5 ml/kg/hr)
	Causes of decreased output include:
	  Hypoperfusion
	  Persistent fetal circulation
	  Renal vein thrombosis
	  Hemolytic transfusion reaction
	  Obstructed catheter
	  Malignant hyperthermia

Urine specific gravity (SG)
Urine osmolarity (Osm)
(Newborn:
SG=1.004-1.020;
Osm=100-600 mOsm/L)
	SG may be increased by:
	  Glucose
	  Protein
	  Mannitol
	  Radiographic contrast
	SG may be decreased by nonosmotic
	  diuretics.

Proteinuria
(Infants: 240 mg/m²/day)
(Children: 100 mg/day;
  10-20 mg by dipstick)
	Albumin is not completely resorbed in
	  newborns.
	Nonrenal causes of proteinuria include
	  exercise, dehydration, fever, and
	  orthostatic proteinuria.
	Renal causes of proteinuria include
	  nephrotic syndrome, glomeru-
	  lonephritis, interstitial nephritis, uri-
	  nary tract infection, renal vein
	  thrombosis, hypertension, diabetes,
	  and collagen vascular disease.

Serum creatinine
(Newborn: approximates
  maternal values)
(One week of age:
  0.25-0.4 mg/dl)
(1-10 years: 0.4-0.9 mg/dl)
	Creatinine reflects glomerular filtration
	  rate (GFR).

Blood urea nitrogen (BUN) (Newborn: 25-31 mg/dl) (Preterm: 16-22 mg/dl) (1-16 years: 8-12 mg/dl)	BUN is a function of dietary protein intake and renal clearance.

Creatinine clearance
(Newborn: 1.07±0.12 ml/min/kg)
(5-8 months: 87.7±11.9
  ml/min/m²)
(1-5 year to adolescent:
  124±25 ml/min/m²)
	Levels affected by patient age, muscle
	  mass, and GFR

ACUTE RENAL FAILURE (ARF)[1,2,4,5]

Marked oliguria is the predominant sign of acute renal failure. Prerenal, renal, or postobstructive conditions may cause acute renal failure, and treatment is dependent on elucidating the primary etiology.

Prerenal Causes of ARF

ETIOLOGY

The most common cause of prerenal ARF is renal hypoperfusion, which may result from hemorrhage, dehydration, sepsis, hypotension, or intravascular volume depletion. ARF may also be caused by renal vein thrombosis (associated most often with birth asphyxia), cyanotic heart disease, maternal diabetes, and polycythemia, particularly in premature infants.

DIAGNOSIS

A clinical history is necessary, as is physical evidence of heart failure, cardiac tamponade, shock, sepsis, bleeding, dehydration, or third-space losses that may be present. Blood pressure and central venous pressure may be decreased. Heart rate may be increased. A urine output less than 0.5 ml/kg/hr by bladder catheterization, with elevated urine specific gravity and osmolarity, is also present. Initially, electrolytes and creatinine may be normal, but BUN may be elevated. Metabolic acidosis is present if systemic perfusion is compromised (see box on p. 315 for complications of acute renal failure). Invasive monitors are rarely necessary for diagnostic purposes.

TREATMENT

1. Intravascular volume should be immediately restored with normal saline or lactated Ringer's, followed by replacement of estimated deficits. Appropriate rehydration should be accompanied by improved perfusion and hemodynamics and restoration of urine flow.
2. If no improvement in urine output is seen after appropriate restoration of the intravascular volume, a diuretic trial of mannitol (0.5 g/kg IV) or furosemide (1 to 2 mg/kg IV) is recommended.
3. If there is no improvement in the oliguria/anuria, cessation of further diuretic or aggressive fluid management should be considered, and the patient evaluated for renal and postrenal causes of the oliguria.

Renal Causes of ARF

ETIOLOGY

The most common renal cause of ARF in children is kidney ischemia caused by hypoperfusion with resultant parenchymal damage. Children with right-to-left shunting and cyanosis from congenital heart disease may be at high risk. Other renal causes of ARF include nephrotoxins, acute tubular necrosis, hemolytic-uremic syndrome, immunologic diseases, hemoglobinuria, myoglobinuria, heart failure, and fresh water near-drowning.

DIAGNOSIS

The diagnosis of ARF secondary to parenchymal disease must exclude prerenal or postrenal causes. These patients have markedly diminished creatinine clearance and elevated serum creatinine. Hyponatremia, hyperkalemia, hypervolemia, metabolic acidosis, and uremia are often present.

A renal ultrasound helps to exclude obstruction. Radionuclide renal scanning will evaluate renal perfusion. The clinical history may provide clues about the cause (e.g., severe trauma and shock, drug ingestion, crush injury with rhabdomyolysis, vasculitis, tumor lysis secondary to chemotherapy).

TREATMENT

1. Initial treatment should be as for prerenal azotemia, ensuring adequate intravascular volume and renal perfusion.
2. Urinary and serum electrolytes should be closely monitored and potassium omitted from replacement regimens. Any predisposing causes should be vigorously treated.
3. Attempting to alkalinize the urine and promote diuresis may be useful if myoglobin, hemoglobin, or tumor lysis is a causative factor.
4. Dopamine infused at 3 to 5 µg/kg/min will augment renal perfusion.
5. Urgent hemodialysis or peritoneal dialysis is indicated for the following:
   a. Volume overload leading to congestive heart failure or malignant hypertension
   b. Severe hyperkalemia (see box, p. 81 for treatment of hyperkalemia)

Postrenal Causes of ARF
ETIOLOGY

The most common cause of postrenal failure is obstruction as a result of congenital anomalies, with posterior urethral valves the most frequently occurring anomaly in male infants. Other causes include tumor, trauma, retroperitoneal fibrosis, uric acid crystals, and kidney stones.

DIAGNOSIS

Examination may reveal abdominal, flank, or bladder masses. An abdominal ultrasound is often diagnostic.

TREATMENT

1. Therapy for postrenal obstruction consists primarily of repair or bypass of the obstructed area.
2. In cases of bilateral obstruction, the phenomenon of postobstructive diuresis may occur. This entity is characterized by a transient (12 to 48 hour) diuresis, the consequence of excretion of salt, water, urea, and other products that accumulated during the obstruction. Natriuretic factor and damage to the tubules and collecting duct may also play a role.
3. Treatment initially involves replacement of electrolyte and water losses, according to plasma and urine electrolyte values. Gradually restricting water and electrolyte replacement will progressively encourage the kidney to resume tubular and concentrating duties.

Complications of ARF

Hypovolemia

Present as a result of fluid restriction in renal or postrenal ARF, or after hemodialysis

Hypervolemia

More common in renal or postrenal ARF
May be treated with diuretics or dialysis

Hypertension

Seen with volume overload and activation of renin-angiotensin system
Treated with fluid and salt restriction and antihypertensive agents
Dialysis may be necessary

Hyperkalemia

$K^+ > 5.5$ mEq/L necessitates monitoring
$K^+ > 6.5$ mEq/L requires urgent treatment with close ECG monitoring

Metabolic acidosis

Worsens as a result of hypothermia, dehydration, bleeding, poor perfusion or inadequate ventilation
Intraoperative use of hyperventilation will increase pH
Administration of HCO_3^-, citrate, or lactate will also increase pH (lactate and citrate require liver metabolism for conversion to HCO_3^-,)

CHRONIC RENAL FAILURE (CRF)[1,2,4]

CRF in children is most commonly due to congenital anomalies, including polycystic kidney disease, renal dysplasia, and obstructive uropathy. Other causes include glomerulonephritis, hemolytic-uremic syndrome (HUS), and nephritis from systemic diseases. The chronicity and typical irreversibility of the disease process often result in multisystem disease.

Clinical manifestations of chronic renal failure

Neurologic	Fatigue and lethargy
	Somnolence
	Muscle weakness
	Uremic or hypertensive encephalopathy
	Peripheral neuropathy
	Autonomic nervous system dysfunction
Pulmonary	Pulmonary edema
	Pleural effusions
Cardiac	Hypertension
	Congestive failure
	Peripheral edema
	Uremic pericarditis
	Pericardial effusion and tamponade
Metabolic	Acidosis
	Hyperkalemia
	Hypocalcemia
	Hyperphosphatemia
	Hyperuricemia
	Secondary hyperparathryoidism
Hematologic	Anemia (often with Hct in low 20s)
	Platelet dysfunction (less than 100,000/mm^3)
	Coagulopathy
	Decreased immune function
Bone	Rickets
	Osteomalacia
	Osteitis fibrosa
Growth	Somatic growth retardation

PATHOPHYSIOLOGY

Knowledge of the type of defect can help guide fluid and drug therapy. Inappropriate administration of fluid/electrolyte solutions may easily worsen these patients' marginal homeostatic reserve.

1. Glomerulonephritis is a glomerulotubular imbalance leading to sodium and water retention, hypertension, edema, and occasionally congestive heart failure.
2. Renal dysplastic and obstructive lesions cause defective concentrating mechanisms, resulting in obligate free water loss.
3. Medullary cystic disease, sickle cell nephropathy, and hydronephrosis exhibit defective distal sodium resorption, resulting in obligate sodium and free water requirements.
4. End-stage renal disease (ESRD) exhibits severely limited GFR, which disables the filtering of sodium, water, potas-

sium, acid, and other products of metabolism. Calcium and vitamin D metabolism are also impaired.

SYSTEMIC EFFECTS OF CHRONIC RENAL FAILURE

Cardiopulmonary sequelae. Increased work of breathing and decreased reserve during induction result from an increased respiratory rate present to compensate for metabolic acidosis. Acidosis and volume overload may cause congestive heart failure. Decreased myocardial contractility due to uremia, pericardial effusion and tamponade, pleural effusions, and pulmonary edema may also occur.

Anemia. Normochromic, normocytic anemia with a hematocrit in the low 20s is common. To compensate for the anemia, there is an increase in cardiac output and a rightward shift of the oxyhemoglobin dissociation curve secondary to metabolic acidosis and increased 2,3-DPG levels (see Fig. 6-2, p. 118). Prophylactic transfusion is not usually recommended, but, when necessary, frozen washed RBCs, which have the lowest volume and potassium level, are selected.

Dialysis. Patients with chronic renal failure often require long-term peritoneal dialysis or hemodialysis. The systemic complications of dialysis may well affect the anesthetic care of the patient who requires a surgical procedure.

Platelet dysfunction (both qualitative and quantitative) can be improved after dialysis. Desmopressin (DDAVP), 0.2 to 0.4 µg/kg IV over 30 minutes (peak effect in 60 to 90 minutes and a 4-hour duration), is used to correct platelet dysfunction preoperatively. Coagulation factors may be altered.

Relative intravascular volume depletion or overload is dependent on dialysis. Appropriate timing of dialysis is needed relative to the surgical procedure. The patient may experience electrolyte imbalances or recurrent septicemia. There is an increased risk of hepatitis or HIV because of multiple exposures to blood and blood products.

HYPERTENSION (HTN)[6-8]

Unlike essential hypertension in adults, hypertension in childhood is generally caused by renovascular or renal disease. Etiologies include: renal artery stenosis; polycystic kidney disease; glomerulonephritis; renal vein thrombosis; malignancies such as Wilms' tumor and neuroblastoma; Williams syndrome; aortic coarctation; congenital adrenal hyperplasia; and immunosuppressant therapy with cyclosporine or steroids.

DIAGNOSIS

HTN is defined as a blood pressure greater than 2 standard deviations above the mean for age or above the 95th percentile for age. Hypertensive crisis is defined by values *significantly* greater than 2 standard deviations above the mean, in which diastolic blood pressure is greater than 95 mm Hg in an infant or >110 mm Hg in an older child. Cardiac symptoms (heart failure, angina) or neurologic symptoms (visual disturbances, headaches) may be present with hypertensive crisis.

Treatment of hypertension is guided by knowledge of age-appropriate blood pressures (see p. 13). Proper-size blood pressure cuffs are needed in the pediatric population to prevent erroneous diagnosis of HTN. Additionally, Doppler techniques provide reliable noninvasive means of measuring systolic blood pressure (i.e., DINAMAP) (see p. 54). If HTN is severe and requires immediate intervention with pharmacologic agents, then invasive blood pressure monitoring is prudent.

Treatment of hypertensive crises in children[3,4,8,9]

Drug	Dose (IV)	Comments
Vasodilators		
Sodium nitroprusside	0.5-8.0 µg/kg/min	Rapid onset Tachyphylaxis may develop if use is prolonged Potential for cyanide toxicity
Diazoxide	2-6 mg/kg bolus	Should be given rapidly with furosemide (1-2 mg/kg) IV to limit fluid retention; hyperglycemia may occur
Calcium channel blockers		
Nifedipine	0.25-0.5 mg/kg sublingual (up to 10 mg in older children)	May have rapid onset and marked lowering of blood pressure
α-Blocker		
Phentolamine	Initial bolus 1.0 mg, then 0.1-0.2 mg/kg (max 10 mg)	Used for pheochromocytomas (see p. 332)
β-Blocker		
Esmolol	0.5 mg/kg bolus; 50-200 µg/kg/min infusion	Rapid onset and short half-life (9 min) Decreased myocardial O_2 consumption
α, β–Blocker		
Labetolol	0.1 mg/kg bolus; 1-3 mg/kg/hr infusion	Peak onset: 10 min Duration: 4-5 hr

TREATMENT

1. In the presence of acute or chronic renal failure, fluid and salt restrictions are advised.
2. If hypertension is severe, dialysis may be useful.
3. Long-term antihypertensive therapy includes diuretics, β-blockers, ACE inhibitors, and calcium channel blockers.

Antihypertensive agents used in children[3,8,9]

Initial dosages are listed; some children may require gradual increasing dosages.

Drug	Dose (mg/kg)	Comments/side effects
β-blockers		
Propranolol	0.5-1.0 mg/kg/day divided q6-12h PO	Contraindicated in asthma and congestive heart failure Use heart rate as guide to degree of β-blockade Blood pressure rebounds if stopped acutely
Metoprolol and atenolol	1.0-2.0 mg/kg/day divided q12h PO	More β_1-specific; otherwise as above
Vasodilators		
Hydralazine	0.75-3.0 mg/kg/day divided q6-12h PO	May cause lupus-like syndrome, tachycardia, volume retention
Diuretics		
Hydrochlorothiazide	2.0-3.0 mg/kg/day divided q12h PO	May cause hyperuricemia, photosensitivity, hypokalemia
Chlorothiazide	20-30 mg/kg/day divided q12h PO	May cause hypokalemia
Furosemide	0.5-2.0 mg/kg/dose given q6-12h PO	May cause hypokalemia
Spironolactone	1.0-2.0 mg/kg/day divided q6-12h PO	K^+ sparing; avoid in hyperkalemia
Angiotension-converting enzyme (ACE) inhibitors		
Captopril	<6 months: 0.05-0.5 mg/kg/day divided q6-12h PO >6 months: 0.5-2.0 mg/kg/day divided q8h PO	May precipitate renal failure with renal artery stenosis; monitor BUN and Cr levels May cause neutropenia
Centrally acting agents		
Clonidine	5-7μg/kg/day divided q6h PO	Rebound hypertension when stopped Can be given as a transdermal patch

ANESTHETIC CONSIDERATIONS FOR RENAL FAILURE PATIENTS (see also p. 354)[10-13]

Renal failure presents a twofold problem to the anesthesiologist: (1) the effects of anesthetic agents on the dysfunctional kidney; and (2) the effect of marginal renal function on drug metabolism and excretion. Often, the anesthesiologist must also consider other organ system involvement as part of the anesthetic plan.

Anesthetic Pharmacology for Renal Failure Patients (see table, pp. 357-358, in Chapter 15)

In the presence of renal failure, many drugs have altered metabolism that includes decreased renal excretion of drugs and drug metabolites. The blood-brain barrier is more permeable, increasing patient sensitivity to the drug administered. Optimal drugs are those that do not rely on renal metabolism for excretion.

Inhalational anesthetic agents. Pulmonary uptake and distribution are relatively unaffected in renal disease. All inhalational agents decrease GFR by decreasing cardiac output. Fluoride ion accumulation may occur with prolonged use of enflurane and halothane when GFR <16 ml/min.

Opioids. The effects of opioids may be potentiated by changes in mental status and the blood-brain barrier present in the severely uremic patient. Hemodynamic stability is achieved with judicious use of fentanyl. It is best to avoid the use of meperidine, as its metabolite, normeperidine, may accumulate and can lead to seizure activity.

Sedative-hypnotics. Propofol shows a slight prolongation of effect. Thiopental should be used in a reduced induction dose because of decreased protein binding. Etomidate has a stable cardiovascular profile but a slight prolongation of effect.

Muscle relaxants. Succinylcholine may cause hyperkalemia in children with renal failure. The optimal relaxant may be atracurium (which requires virtually no renal excretion) or the new isomer cisatracurium (which has minimal cardiovascular effects). Increased sensitivity to nondepolarizers may be due to acidosis and electrolyte disturbances, such as hypokalemia, hypermagnesemia, and hypokalemia. Redosing of all muscle relaxants should not occur without monitoring of neuromuscular function.

ANESTHETIC MANAGEMENT OF SPECIFIC PEDIATRIC RENAL SYNDROMES

Hemolytic-Uremic Syndrome (HUS)[14,15]

HUS occurs most often in infants and young children. It is usually preceded by a prodromal illness, such as diarrhea, vomiting, or upper respiratory infection. Infectious causes such as viruses, *Shigella,* and *Salmonella* have also been implicated.

Acute renal failure, thrombocytopenia, and hemolytic anemia are due to microangiopathic disruption. Renal involvement can range from mild, transient depression of function to development of renal necrosis and chronic renal failure in approximately 20% to 30% of the cases. Severe hypertension, hypovolemia, electrolyte imbalance, anemia, congestive heart failure, seizures, lethargy, and coma may accompany renal failure.

TREATMENT

Causes of infection must be identified and treated. Early aggressive, supportive therapy with red cell and platelet transfusions is necessary, as consumptive coagulopathy may decrease the life span of transfused blood products. Dialysis is required for the treatment of hyperkalemia, volume overload, acidosis, congestive heart failure, and hypertension.

ANESTHETIC MANAGEMENT

1. Large-bore venous catheters and arterial and central venous access may help to maintain intraoperative fluid and electrolyte balance.
2. Treatment of children with renal failure complicated by coagulopathy and anemia includes preoperative dialysis, blood pressure control, and blood component therapy as indicated.

Nephrotic Syndrome[16,17]

Nephrotic syndrome is defined as proteinuria, hypoalbuminemia, hyperlipidemia, and edema caused by increased glomerular permeability to plasma proteins. Its most common causes in children are idiopathic or primary glomerular lesions, as well as lupus, the glomerulonephritides, diabetes mellitus, sickle cell disease, and amyloidosis.

Intravascular volume depletion is often associated with ascites and gastrointestinal mucosal edema, resulting in nausea and vomiting. Decreased drug protein binding is present. Respiration may be compromised by ascites and pleural effusions. There is a decrease in total serum calcium, although ionized calcium is usually normal because of decreased albuimin. Coagulopathy is usually present.

ANESTHETIC MANAGEMENT

1. Intravascular volume is usually contracted and must be re-expanded to preserve GFR. Placement of a central venous catheter is indicated for central pressure monitoring if a major surgical procedure is planned.
2. Sodium-poor albumin (10 to 20 ml/kg infused slowly) helps to mobilize ascites and edema fluid and restore intravascular volume. Furosemide (1 to 2 mg/kg PO or IV) may be used in sequence with albumin to promote diuresis.
3. Immunosuppressants and steroid therapy should be continued perioperatively. Stress dose steroids may also be required.
4. A reduction in thiopental dosage is warranted because of decreased protein binding and tenuous volume status.

Proximal Renal Tubular Acidosis (RTA)[18]

Proximal RTA is frequently seen in Fanconi syndrome, cystinosis, Wilson's disease, heavy metal poisoning, and medullary cystic disease. The renal resorptive threshold for bicarbonate is lowered (16 to 18 mEq/L) so that there is bicarbonate wasting in urine. Distal hydrogen ion and acidification of urine are not affected. The major clinical manifestations are metabolic and include: hyperchloremic acidosis; hypocalcemia; probable alkalotic urine pH; Na^+ and H_2O wasting. Rickets and osteomalacia are late findings with disease progression.

Bicarbonate replacement and potassium supplementation are usually necessary. Hydrochlorothiazide has been used to increase the bicarbonate threshold. Volume expansion with normal saline may paradoxically worsen acidosis by increasing bicarbonate wasting. However, fluid expansion may be necessary in the perioperative period.

Distal Renal Tubular Acidosis[18]

Distal RTA results from the distal tubules' inability to secrete hydrogen ions. Failure to acidify the urine renders the urine alkaline (pH usually greater than 6), potentiating the occurrence of nephrocalcinosis, osteomalacia, growth retardation, and progressive renal insufficiency. Acidosis, hypocalcemia, and polyuria may also be found.

Treatment consists of bicarbonate replacement. Response to treatment is generally greater in distal RTA patients than in those with proximal RTA.

Sickle Cell Nephropathy[19]

Sickle cell nephropathy occurs primarily in homozygous (HbSS) patients, but has also been reported in those with sickle cell trait (HbAS). A progressive decrease in urine concentrating ability occurs, producing a dilute urine. Therefore, urine osmolarity and specific gravity are not good indicators of volume status. Treatment should follow the basic tenets for children with sickle disease (see p. 286) and those with chronic renal failure (p. 315).

Diabetic Nephropathy[20]

Diabetic nephropathy rarely occurs in children, usually requiring a minimum of 10 to 15 years of disease progression to develop. The pathognomonic lesion is nodular intercapillary glomerulosclerosis (Kimmelstiel-Wilson lesions).

The initial indication of diabetic nephropathy is proteinuria, followed by a declining GFR and a rising serum creatinine. Patients may also develop nephrotic syndrome (see p. 321). Hypertension is a frequently associated finding. In diabetics with renal failure, myocardial infarction is a major cause of morbidity and mortality.

Anesthetic management includes routine care of the diabetic patient as well as considerations for those with chronic renal failure.

ANESTHESIA FOR MISCELLANEOUS UROLOGIC PROCEDURES

Cystoscopy and Urodynamic Studies

As cystoscopy and urodynamic studies are usually brief procedures, general anesthesia administered by face mask may be sufficient for infants and children. Alternatively, a laryngeal mask airway (LMA) or propofol infusion may be used.

Thiopental, deep inhalation anesthesia, opioids, and atropine may inhibit bladder and sphincter tone and interfere with urodynamic studies.

Hypospadias, Chordee, and Undescended Testicles

Procedures for hypospadias, chordee, and undescended testicles are usually performed using general anesthesia. The major anesthetic concerns relate to the status of any coexisting disease. Caudal/epidural anesthesia is now a common adjunct to urologic surgery to minimize depth of general anesthesia and provide postoperative pain relief. An undescended, unlocated testicle may require an intraabdominal approach, necessitating muscle relaxation and intubation.

Manipulation of the testicles and the peritoneum that occurs during undescended testicle repair can produce profound vagal stimulation. Atropine or glycopyrrolate is effective in preventing this response when given prior to surgical manipulation, but has little effect if given after bradycardia occurs. Regional anesthetic techniques (caudal anesthesia) are also effective in preventing vagal symptoms.

If bradycardia occurs, a rapid intravenous fluid bolus (10 to 20 ml) can reverse the vagal tone and increase heart rate by stimulating right atrial baroreceptors. Rarely, a small bolus of epinephrine (10 to 20 μg IV) may be required if bradycardia is severe and unresponsive.

ENDOCRINE DISEASES
Diabetes Mellitus[21-23]

Diabetes mellitus is the most common childhood endocrine disorder. A chronic metabolic disease, it is frequently genetic in origin and results in deranged metabolism of carbohydrates, protein, and fat. Insulin-dependent diabetes mellitus (IDDM), sometimes referred to as juvenile-onset or type I diabetes, is most often diagnosed in children and shows no sexual predilection. These patients have pancreatic β-cell destruction that ablates the ability to synthesize and release insulin. Non–insulin-dependent diabetes mellitus (NIDDM), formerly referred to as maturity-onset or type II diabetes, is more commonly diagnosed in the adult. These patients have normal or high insulin levels and do not usually develop ketoacidosis.

CLINICAL MANIFESTATIONS

Children with new-onset IDDM commonly have a history of lethargy, polyuria, polydipsia, weakness, weight loss, and polyphagia. Renal insufficiency or failure may also be present. Diabetic ketoacidosis (DKA), a catabolic state often precipitated by trauma, infection, vomiting, or psychological stress, is the initial presentation in 10% to 30% of children with diabetes mellitus.

Symptoms of diabetes mellitus
Hyperglycemia (serum glucose greater than 300 mg/dl)
Dehydration
Ketonemia
Metabolic acidosis
Hypokalemia
Hyperlipidemia
Abdominal pain
Leukocytosis

Insulin replacement in children is approximately 0.5 to 1.0 units/kg/day initially and often declines after initial therapy to 0.3 units/kg/day or less. Hypoglycemia is a frequent complication of insulin therapy, manifested by trembling, diaphoresis, tachycardia,

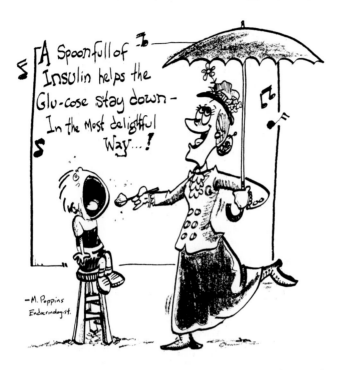

and nervousness. Symptoms may progress to a change in mental status, seizures, or coma. Treatment of hypoglycemia is oral or intravenous dextrose and glucagon (0.1 mg/kg/dose).

ANESTHETIC MANAGEMENT[23,24]

Preoperative assessment

1. The preoperative assessment of a diabetic requires the following information:
   - Age of onset of diabetes
   - Type and dosage of insulin
   - Dietary habits
   - Frequency of DKA and/or hypoglycemic episodes
2. Unstable diabetic patients should be admitted to the hospital before surgery so that their insulin therapy can be optimized and their serum glucose controlled. Children with stable diabetes undergoing surgical procedures of less than 1 hour's duration may be admitted on the day of surgery. Surgery should be scheduled as early as possible on the day of admittance.
3. Preoperative laboratory measurements include:
   - Serum glucose, electrolytes, creatinine, and blood urea nitrogen (BUN)
   - Urinary glucose and ketones
   - Glycosylated hemoglobin (Hgb A1c) may be helpful in evaluating blood sugar control for the preceding 3-month period.

4. The preoperative visit provides an opportunity to allay concerns and develop rapport with the patient. Anxiety associated with surgery may heighten sympathetic or neuroendocrine activity, which will result in an elevated serum glucose level.

5. Preoperative sedatives should be prescribed in their usual dosages. Delayed gastric emptying due to gastroparesis is often present; maintenance of usual NPO times and use of H_2 antagonists and metoclopramide preoperatively are recommended.

Intraoperative management.   Anesthesia and sedation may mask the occurrence of hypoglycemia. Regional anesthesia offers the advantage of assessment of the child's mental status if hypoglycemia should occur. One of the following three protocols may be used for the management of insulin therapy in the perioperative period. All treatment options demand frequent measurement of blood glucose and treatment of hypoglycemia or hyperglycemia as indicated.

1. The most common method uses a D_5.25 NS intravenous infusion begun early in the morning on the day of surgery at a maintenance rate. One-half the usual NPH insulin dosage is given after the dextrose infusion is begun. Blood glucose levels are measured before induction and frequently during the operative procedure. Plasma glucose should be maintained between 100 and 250 mg/dl. Regular insulin doses of 0.1 units/kg are given when plasma glucose exceeds 250 mg/dl.

2. An alternative method is to begin simultaneous insulin and glucose infusion on the morning of surgery. The insulin infusion rate allows for 0.2 to 0.4 units of regular insulin per gram of glucose. This infusion results in 1 to 2 units of insulin per 100 ml of D_5W. Once again, blood glucose levels are maintained between 100 and 250 mg/dl by adjusting the insulin infusion rate.

3. The third method of preoperative diabetes management is to withhold both insulin and glucose infusions. This technique may be used for short procedures that occur early in the morning and permit oral intake in the recovery room. After oral intake is resumed, 40% to 50% of the usual insulin dose is given. Serum glucose should be monitored intraoperatively and postoperatively.

Postoperative management.   Blood glucose should be measured every 4 to 6 hours beginning in the recovery room and continuing postoperatively. A sliding scale for insulin administration is frequently used until the usual oral intake is resumed.

Hyperthyroidism[25]

Hyperthyroidism in children is most commonly congenital or a result of Graves' disease. Congenital hyperthyroidism is caused by the transfer of maternal thyroid-stimulating immunoglobulins in utero. These infants may be premature, and tachycardia, respiratory distress, and congestive heart failure may be present along with the physical appearance of goiter. Conversely, Graves' disease occurs more frequently among adolescents than children and 4 to 5 times more frequently among females.

CLINICAL MANIFESTATIONS

1. Signs and symptoms of hyperthyroidism in children include goiter, exophthalmos, hypertension, tachycardia, widened pulse pressure, and tremor.
2. Levels of serum thyroxine (T_4) and triiodothyronine (T_3) are elevated. Age-adjusted normal values are needed because thyroid hormone levels are higher in children.
3. Treatment of hyperthyroidism in children includes propylthiouracil and radiolabeled iodide (^{131}I). Although symptoms will resolve in 1 to 2 weeks, laboratory values may not normalize for 4 to 6 weeks. Propranolol is useful for controlling symptoms of nervousness, tremor, and tachycardia.

ANESTHETIC MANAGEMENT[24, 26]

The child should have received ablation treatment to ensure a euthyroid state confirmed by preoperative thyroid function tests. One week before surgery, administration of Lugol's iodine solution should be initiated to decrease vascularity and hyperplasia of the overreactive gland. A larger goiter requires a computed axial tomography (CAT) scan to determine if tracheal compression or deviation exists. Propranolol may be used preoperatively to control tachycardia.

Anticholinergics are best avoided because they can worsen tachycardia and interfere with heat dissipation by blocking the ability to perspire. Likewise, ketamine and pancuronium may increase heart rate and sympathetic tone. Conversely, vecuronium, rocuronium, atracurium, and mivacurium offer minimal cardiovascular effects.

Increased cardiac output prolongs induction time with inhalation agents. Isoflurane dose not sensitize the myocardium to catecholamines and has minimal metabolism, making it a recommended choice for maintenance of anesthesia. Intravenous techniques (particularly high-dose fentanyl) also offer hemodynamic stability.

Thyroid storm (an acute release of thyroid hormone) can mimic malignant hyperthermia, with hyperpyrexia, tachycardia, congestive heart failure, increased $ETCO_2$ and creatine phosphokinase (CPK), dehydration, and shock.[27] Treatment is initially supportive, with reduction of heart rate by β-blockade. Sodium iodide, cortisol, and propylthiouracil (PTU) are also used to control acute hyperthyroidism.

Perioperative complications of thyroidectomy

Corneal dessication and abrasions from inadequate eye care in the
 presence of exophthalmos
Unilateral or bilateral recurrent laryngeal nerve injury
Hypoparathyroidism, hypocalcemia
Airway obstruction from edema, hematoma, or tracheomalacia

Hypothyroidism[24-26, 28]

Females are affected by hypothyroidism twice as often as
males. Congenital hypothryoidism usually occurs as a result of
thyroid dysgenesis, and is not as common as acquired hypothyroidism. Acquired hypothyroidism results from chronic lymphocytic thyroiditis (Hashimoto's), radioactive iodine therapy,
infiltrative diseases, hypopituitarism, surgical excision, or sick euthyroid syndrome.

Clinical manifestations of hypothyroidism

Puffy face
Wide fontanelle and sutures
Flat nasal bridge
Large tongue
Hoarse cry
Cold, mottled, or jaundiced skin
Reduced growth
Protuberant abdomen with umbilical hernia
Poor muscle tone
Sluggish reflexes
Lethargy
Hypothermia
Goiter
Myxedema
Precocious sexual development
Bradycardia
Low pulse pressure
Elevated thyroid-stimulating hormone (TSH)
Low or normal T_3 resin uptake (T_3RU)
Low serum thyroxine (T_4)

ANESTHETIC MANAGEMENT

Preoperative management.   At least 2 weeks of thyroxine therapy is necessary to establish a euthyroid state. When cardiac involvement is present, treatment should begin gradually because of
the risk of sudden death. Thyroid medications should be continued
preoperatively.

Reductions in heart rate and stroke volume may result in a significant reduction in cardiac output, making hypothyroid children
more sensitive to the depressant effects of medications on the res-

piratory and cardiovascular systems. Preoperative sedation is best avoided or should be carefully titrated.

Hydrocortisone may be given (2 mg/kg every 6 hours) because of the increased incidence of adrenocortical insufficency and impaired response to adrenocorticotropic hormone (ACTH).

Intraoperative management.   Before induction, atropine or glycopyrrolate may be used. Other anesthetic doses should be reduced intraoperatively because of heightened sensitivity, attributed to decreased cardiac output, reduced intravascular volume, and altered baroreceptor function. There may also be a reduction in hepatic metabolism and renal excretion.

Decreased intravascular volume may result in hypotension when vasodilating agents are used. Preemptive volume loading (10 to 20 ml/kg) may prevent a fall in blood pressure at induction. Use of arterial and central venous pressure catheters is recommended for hemodynamic monitoring in major surgical procedures. To prevent hyponatremia and hypoglycemia, intravenous solutions of sodium and dextrose along with frequent monitoring of sodium and glucose levels are necessary.

Since the risk of hypothermia is high, operating room temperatures should be maintained at a minimum of 25°C. All fluids should be warmed, and heating mattresses and forced-air warmers can be used when appropriate.

Postoperative management.   Emergence from anesthesia may be prolonged. Compromised pulmonary and cardiac function should be anticipated. The child's ventilatory response to hypercapnia and hypoxia may be impaired, necessitating ventilatory assistance. Body temperature and serum glucose should be monitored into the postoperative period. The administration of corticosteroids and thyroid medications should be resumed as soon as the patient begins accepting oral fluids. Intravenous forms of these drugs should be given to fasted patients.

Hypoparathyroidism[26]

Primary hypoparathyroidism is caused by a decrease in parathyroid hormone (PTH) production and commonly results from surgical excision of the glands during thyroid surgery. Pseudohypoparathyroidism is an inherited disorder resulting from decreased end-organ responsiveness to PTH despite elevated hormone levels. Physical characteristics include short stature, thick neck, short metacarpals and metatarsals, and often mental retardation.

The clinical manifestations of hypoparathyroidism include a low serum Ca^{++} (positive Chvostek or Trousseau sign), seizures, muscle spasms, prolonged QT interval on ECG, chronic diarrhea, skin changes, and cataracts in older children.

ANESTHETIC MANAGEMENT

Surgery should be delayed until the serum calcium level approximates normal. If emergent surgery is required, calcium gluconate (30 mg/kg) or calcium chloride (10 mg/kg) should be given with ECG monitoring, and pH should be measured frequently to avoid alkalosis.

1. Serum ionized calcium should be monitored intraoperatively and treated when necessary.
2. Intraoperative hypotension may occur as a result of myocardial depression from anesthetic agents coupled with low serum ionized calcium.
3. Responses to nondepolarizing muscle relaxants may be potentiated in the presence of decreased serum ionized calcium levels.
4. Laryngospasm may result from an acute decrease in ionized calcium, especially after thyroid surgery.

Hyperparathyroidism[24,26,29]

Hyperparathyroidism is classified as primary or secondary, or as pseudohyperparathyroidism. Primary hyperparathyroidism is usually due to a parathyroid adenoma during childhood. The infant has poor muscle tone, dehydration, and poor feeding habits with resultant weight loss. Poor rib development causes respiratory dysfunction. An elevated ionized serum calcium level with an increased parathyroid hormone level is diagnostic, and metabolic acidosis with hyperchloremia and hyperphosphatemia are often seen. Secondary hyperparathyroidism results from renal or gastrointestinal disease. Pseudohyperparathyroidism is due to an ectopic release of parathyroid hormones or a parathyroid-like substance usually secreted from tumors.

ANESTHETIC MANAGEMENT

The preoperative electrocardiogram of the patient with hyperparathyroidism reveals a prolongation of the PR interval and a shortening of the QT interval inversely proportional to the serum calcium. T wave changes may appear with acute elevations in serum calcium. Blood pressure and electrolytes should be evaluated. Preoperative hydration is often necessary. Serum calcium may be lowered by normal saline infusions, furosemide, mithramycin, and calcitonin.

Intravenous or inhalation agents can be used for induction. Hypercalcemic crisis can occur intraoperatively and requires blood pressure support, hyperventilation, hydration, and monitoring of urine output.

After parathyroid resection, airway obstruction secondary to hematoma, edema, or recurrent laryngeal nerve injury may occur.

Hypocalcemia may be present, with cramps, paresthesias, and a widened QT interval. Treatment with calcium gluconate (30 mg/kg) or calcium chloride (10 mg/kg) is recommended.

Pituitary Disease[24,26]

Children with pituitary pathology may have elevated intracranial pressures (ICP) with headache, vomiting, tense fontanelle, and behavioral changes (see p. 205).

Hypopituitarism in children is often secondary to compression by craniopharyngioma, a malignancy that accounts for 10% of all brain tumors in children less than 14 years of age. The tumor results in failure to grow, elevated intracranial pressure, and visual losses. There is a higher incidence in males than in females, with a peak incidence at 7 years of age.

Physical characteristics of hypopituitarism include short stature, lack of sexual development, and obesity. Hypothyroidism, adrenal insufficiency, and diabetes insipidus may also be present.

Hyperpituitarism may involve excesses of growth hormone, resulting in gigantism associated with glucose intolerance and hyperinsulinemia. Excessive secretion of ACTH results in Cushing's disease, which is characterized by obesity, reduced growth, and osteoporosis. The posterior pituitary may produce excessive antidiuretic hormone secretion (SIADH), with hyponatremia, reduced serum osmolality, elevated urine osmolality, and decreased urine output.

ANESTHETIC MANAGEMENT

Preoperative sedation is best avoided in patients with elevated ICP. Corticosteroids and thyroid hormones should be given when indicated.

Surgical removal of pituitary tumors includes three approaches: stereotactic, transsphenoidal, and frontal craniotomy. An induction technique designed to lower ICP with hyperventilation and thiopental is recommended, with intravenous lidocaine or fentanyl to blunt the cardiovascular response to laryngoscopy. Mannitol may be used to reduce cerebral edema (see p. 206).

Invasive arterial monitoring permits continuous blood pressure monitoring and frequent blood sampling. Nasogastric tubes are contraindicated in patients with pituitary tumors. If necessary, the stomach may be decompressed with an orogastric tube.

Involvement of the cavernous sinus implies a significant risk of air embolism and bleeding. Venous air embolism is a potential complication, particularly if the sitting position is used for the craniotomy. Precordial Doppler monitoring will help to diagnose the presence of intracardiac air.

Postoperative complications include thyroid and ACTH deficiency, hyperthermia, and seizures. Serum sodium, osmolality and glucose, and urine output, must be measured frequently for possible diabetes insipidus (DI), which may be present in about 20% of patients.

Diabetes insipidus as a complication of pituitary disease

Clinical signs and symptoms

Polyuria and polydipsia
Urine output greater than 3 ml/kg/hr
Elevated serum sodium
Decreased urine osmolality
Increased plasma osmolality
Ratio of serum to urine osmolality greater than 1:1

Treatment

Desmopressin acetate
   >3 months: 5-30 µg per 24h qd-bid intranasally
Hypotonic fluids
Potassium

Pheochromocytoma[24,26,30,31]

Pheochromocytoma is a catecholamine-secreting tumor that originates in the adrenal medulla (90%), but may also be found wherever chromaffin tissue is present (as in the sympathetic chain extending from the base of the skull to the pelvis). Approximately 10% of tumors are bilateral. In nearly 20% of patients, functional tumors occur at multiple sites. Malignant pheochromocytomas rarely occur in children (<10%), with a greater incidence in puberty than in childhood. The tumor may be one of the diseases in multiple endocrine neoplasia (MEN) type IIa or IIb.

Clinical manifestations of pheochromocytoma: symptomatology of elevated plasma norepinephrine and epinephrine

Headaches
Nausea
Vomiting
Diaphoresis
Visual complaints
Tremors
Weight loss
Pallor
Cool extremities
Anxious appearance
Intermittent or persistent hypertension
Reduced intravascular fluid volume resulting in orthostatic
   hypotension

ANESTHETIC MANAGEMENT

Preoperative management.   Serum electrolytes and creatinine, fasting blood sugar, and possibly a glucose tolerance test should be obtained preoperatively. Hyperglycemia results from adrenergic inhibition of insulin release and glycogenolysis. Chronically elevated plasma catecholamines may result in a cardiomyopathy, necessitating an ECG and echocardiogram. α-adrenergic blockade should be instituted several days before surgery. Phenoxybenzamine, an α_1 and α_2 receptor antagonist, or prazosin, an α_1 receptor antagonist, prevents vasoconstriction in response to catecholamines and facilitates insulin release. Initial doses are administered cautiously, as marked hypotension can occur. Since the child's blood volume is contracted, a reduction in hematocrit indicates a return to normal blood volume. Although cardiac arrhythmias and tachycardia are rare in the pediatric population, the administration of β-adrenergic blockade may be necessary. β-adrenergic blocking drugs should not be used in the absence of α-adrenergic blockade. Unopposed α-adrenergic vasoconstriction increases systemic vascular resistance (afterload) and prevents the β-blocked heart from maintaining adequate cardiac output.

Preoperative sedation serves to reduce anxiety and the associated catecholamine release.

Intraoperative management[32,33]

1. Medications that stimulate the sympathetic nervous system should be avoided, and medications to blunt stimulation of laryngoscopy may be used.
2. β-adrenergic blockade should be continued until the day of surgery.
3. An arterial catheter may be placed prior to induction.
4. Anesthesia may be induced with a balanced technique using lidocaine, benzodiazepines, sedative-hypnotics (thiopental or propofol), or inhalation agents. Halothane is best avoided because of the likelihood of arrhythmias in the presence of excess circulating cathecholamines.
5. Theoretically, succinylcholine-induced fasciculations could increase catecholamine release by the tumor, but this effect is not clinically apparent.
6. Vecuronium and atracurium are the recommended muscle relaxants because they produce minimal cardiovascular side effects.
7. Lidocaine or fentanyl given intravenously 1 minute before laryngoscopy may diminish an increase in blood pressure and prevent cardiac arrhythmias.
8. Anesthesia can be maintained with nitrous oxide, oxygen, enflurane, or isoflurane.
9. Hypertension is controlled by the use of sodium nitroprusside (1 to 4 μg/kg/min) or phentolamine (0.1 to 0.2 mg/kg).

10. As the veins draining the pheochromocytoma are ligated, a decline in blood pressure may result from the decrease in plasma catecholamines.
11. An infusion of norepinephrine may be necessary if hypotension persists.
12. Intravascular volume is evaluated by means of a central venous pressure catheter.
13. Serial arterial blood gases should be obtained and frequent measurements of electrolytes taken.
14. Hyperglycemia is common before surgery. Hypoglycemia is evident after the tumor has been removed.

Postoperative management. Invasive monitoring should be maintained until the child's cardiovascular and pulmonary statuses stabilize. Between 24 and 48 hours postoperatively, blood pressure returns to normal values if the entire tumor has been excised. Plasma catecholamine concentrations should normalize in 7 to 10 days.

References

1. Berry FA: Anesthesia for the genitourinary system. In Gregory GA, ed: *Pediatric anesthesia,* ed 3, New York, 1994, Churchill Livingstone.
2. Berry FA: Renal diseases. In Berry FA, Steward DJ, eds: *Pediatrics for the anesthesiologist,* New York, 1993, Churchill Livingstone.
3. Johnson KB, ed: *The Harriet Lane handbook: a manual for pediatric house officers,* ed 13, St Louis, 1993, Mosby.
4. Cramolini, GM: Diseases of the renal system. In Katz J, Steward DJ, eds: *Anesthesia and uncommon pediatric diseases,* ed 2, Philadelphia, 1993, WB Saunders.
5. Kellen M, Aronson S, Roizen MF, Barnard J, Thisted RA: Predictive and diagnostic tests of renal failure: a review, *Anesth Analg* 78:134-142, 1994.
6. Morgenstern BZ: Hypertension in pediatric patients: current issues, *Mayo Clin Proc* 69:1089-1097, 1994.
7. Daniels SR: Primary hypertension in childhood and adolescence, *Pediatr Ann* 21: 224, 226-229, 231-234, 1992.
8. Task Force on Blood Pressure Control in Children, National Heart, Lung, and Blood Institute, Bethesda, Maryland: Report of the Second Task Force on Blood Pressure Control in Children—1987, *Pediatrics* 79:1-25, 1987.
9. *Drug facts and comparisons,* ed 49, St. Louis, 1995, Facts and Comparisons.
10. Weir PH, Chung FF: Anaesthesia for patients with chronic renal disease, *Can Anaesth Soc J* 31:468-480, 1984.
11. Prielipp RC, Coursin DB, Scuderi PE, et al: Comparison of the infusion requirements and recovery profiles of vecuronium and cisatracurium 51W89 in intensive care unit patients, *Anesth Analg* 81:3-12, 1995.
12. Loehning RW, Mazze RI: Possible nephrotoxicity from enflurane in patients with severe renal disease, *Anesthesiology* 40:203-205, 1974.

13. Don HF, Dieppa RA, Taylor P: Narcotic analgesics in anuric patients, *Anesthesiology* 42:745-747, 1975.

14. Grimm PC, Ogborn MR: Hemolytic uremic syndrome: the most common cause of acute renal failure in childhood, *Pediatr Ann* 23: 505-511, 1994.

15. Stewart CL, Tina LU: Hemolytic uremic syndrome, *Pediatr Rev* 14:218-225, 1993.

16. Salcedo JR, Thabet MA, Latta K, Chan JC: Nephrosis in childhood, *Nephron* 71:373-385, 1995.

17. Warshaw BL: Nephrotic syndrome in children, *Pediatr Ann* 23: 495-497, 500-504, 1994.

18. Zelikovic I: Renal tubular acidosis, *Pediatr Ann* 24: 48-54, 1995.

19. Falk RJ, Scheinman J, Phillips G, et al: Prevalence and pathologic features of sickle cell nephropathy and response to inhibition of angiotensin-converting enzyme, *N Engl J Med* 326:910-915, 1992.

20. Sowers JR, Epstein M: Diabetes mellitus and associated hypertension, vascular disease, and nephropathy: an update, *Hypertension* 26:869-879, 1995.

21. Bland GL, Wood VD: Diabetes in infancy: diagnosis and current management, *J Natl Med Assoc* 83: 361-365, 1991.

22. Ginsberg-Fellner F: Insulin-dependent diabetes mellitus, *Pediatr Rev* 11: 239-247, 1990.

23. Walts LF, Miller J, Davidson MB, Brown J: Perioperative management of diabetes mellitus, *Anesthesiology* 55:104-109, 1981.

24. Keon TP, Templeton JJ: Diseases of the endocrine system. In Katz J, Steward DJ, eds: *Anesthesia and uncommon pediatric diseases,* ed 2, Philadelphia, 1993, WB Saunders.

25. Lee WN: Thyroiditis, hyperthyroidism, and tumors, *Pediatr Clin North Am* 26:53-64, 1979.

26. Scott GM, Steward DJ: Diseases of the endocrine system. In Berry FA, Steward DJ, eds: *Pediatrics for the anesthesiologist,* New York, 1993, Churchill Livingstone.

27. Peters KR, Nance P, Wingard DW: Malignant hyperthyroidism or malignant hyperthermia? *Anesth Analg* 60: 613-615, 1981.

28. Murkin JM: Anesthesia and hypothyroidism: a review of thyroxine physiology, pharmacology, and anesthetic implications, *Anesth Analg* 61:371-383, 1982.

29. Bronsky D, Dubin A, Waldstein SS, Kushner DS: The electrocardiographic manifestations of hyperparathyroidism and of marker hypercalcemia from various other etiologies, *Am J Cardiol* 7:833-839, 1961.

30. Ram CV, Fierro-Carrion GA: Pheochromocytoma, *Semin Nephrol* 15: 126-137, 1995.

31. Werbel SS, Ober KP: Pheochromocytoma: update on diagnosis, localization, and management, *Med Clin North Am* 79:131-153, 1995.

32. Strebel S, Scheidegger D: Propofol-fentanyl anesthesia for pheochromocytoma resection, *Acta Anaesthesiol Scand* 35:275-277, 1991.

33. Jovenich JJ: Anesthesia in adrenal surgery, *Urol Clin North Am* 16:583-587, 1989.

ANESTHETIC MANAGEMENT OF TRANSPLANT PATIENTS

15

tired, weak
so hook me up
organ, wait
with some luck
running, jumping
spirits high
kidney transplant
now I fly...

Adrienne Coleman

Over the last decade, organ transplantation has become a standard therapy for treating incurable diseases in several organ systems. Pediatric patients in particular have benefited from the progress in organ transplantation.[1] As increasing numbers of organ transplants occur in children, anesthesiologists must care for them not only during organ transplantation but also during subsequent surgical procedures.

Principles of perioperative anesthetic management for solid organ transplantation

Limited time is available for preoperative preparation (fasting, correction of laboratory abnormalities).

Successful fluid management necessitates adequate vascular access, placement of invasive monitors, and availability of blood products.

An understanding of physiologic changes associated with the underlying disease and those imposed by the surgery is required.

Strict aseptic technique must be applied in managing these immunosuppressed patients during vascular catheter insertion and endotracheal intubation.

Acute intraoperative physiologic changes should be anticipated by heightened vigilance, appropriate selection of vasoactive drugs for circulatory support, and invasive monitors.

Because laboratory results must be obtained with rapid turnaround time throughout the intraoperative period, the anesthesiologist must actively organize ancillary services in caring for these patients.

DONOR MANAGEMENT

The potential heart or liver donor must meet the criteria of brain death, which is defined as the absence of cortical and cerebral function without preservation of brainstem function.[2] Brain death may result in profound hemodynamic and metabolic disturbances, which in turn can lead to somatic death with loss of valuable organs.[3] Therefore, the most important objective of the perioperative management of the donor is to maintain hemodynamic stability and whole-body homeostasis during retrieval of donor organs.

Anesthetic Goals for Organ Retrieval

With improvements in core cooling and en bloc harvesting, surgeons are able to shorten the warm ischemia time (ischemia time at normal body temperature), decrease excessive manipulation of the organs, and improve the quality of the donated organs. The anesthesiologist contributes significantly to donor organ viability by meeting the following goals during the harvesting procedure:

1. Maintenance of hemodynamic stability
2. Maintenance of normal pH, $PaCO_2$, PO_2, and body temperature
3. Maintenance of hematocrit at 28% to 30% by red cell transfusion
4. Heparinization to prevent microvascular thrombosis, promoting even flushing and eventual organ reperfusion
5. Administration of additional drugs to the donor, which may include antibiotics, allopurinol (free radical scavenger), chlorpromazine (vasodilation), PGE_1 (vasodilation), dextran 40 (hemodilution, to improve microcirculation), lidocaine (vasodilation), and T_3 (to improve hemodynamic stability)[4]
6. Maintenance of strict aseptic techniques to avoid infection
7. Communication with members of the surgical team, to keep them informed as problems develop so the surgical approach may be altered in urgent situations in order to salvage the organ

Problems of anesthetic management during organ retrieval

Problem	Cause	Management
Hypotension	Neurogenic shock Hypovolemia Myocardial injury Loss of sympathetic tone Endocrine disturbances	Maintenance of in- travascular volume Inotropic support, in order of preference (μg/kg/min): Dopamine ≤ 10 Dobutamine ≤ 15 Epinephrine ≤ 0.1
Arrhythmia- bradycardia	Central nervous system injury Hypothermia Electrolyte imbalance Myocardial ischemia Brain herniation	Bradycardia may be atropine resistant Direct chronotropic drugs (isoproterenol) or temporary venous pacing Electrolytes corrected to normal values
Hypoxemia	Aspiration pneumonia Bacterial pneumonia Pulmonary contusions Neurogenic pulmonary edema Atelectasis	Pulmonary status opti- mized with these goals: PaO_2: 100-150 mm Hg $PaCO_2$: 35-45 mm Hg
Diabetes insipidus	Pituitary or hypothalamic dysfunction	Volume replacement Vasopressin (0.1 U/min infusion) DDAVP (0.3 μg/kg/IV) to maintain urine output of 1.5-3.0 ml/kg/hr Correction of electrolytes Inotropic support
Hypothermia	Loss of hypothalamic temperature regulation	Early aggressive warm- ing to maintain the temperature above 34°C
Anemia	Hemorrhage Hemodilution	Transfusion to keep the hematocrit at 28%- 30%
Unopposed spinal reflexes	Loss of cerebral and brainstem reflexes	Neuromuscular activity can be controlled with nondepolarizing relaxants
Coagulopathy	Release of thromboplas- tic, fibrinolytic sub- stances or plasminogen	Transfusion of blood products

Adapted from Robertson KM: Logistics of donor procurement, management of the donor organ, and organ preservation. In Cook DR, Davis PJ,
eds: *Anesthetic principles for organ transplantation*, New York, 1994,
Raven Press.

HEART TRANSPLANTATION
IN CHILDREN AND NEONATES

At present, infants and children receive approximately 15% of all heart transplants performed annually.[5] The most common indications for heart transplantation in the pediatric age group are congenital heart diseases such as hypoplastic left heart syndrome (HLHS) and complex single-ventricle lesions.[6] Regardless of the etiology, these patients have little or no cardiac reserve, may have secondary organ system dysfunction, and are extremely sensitive to any stimulus, including anesthetic agents or operative manipulation.[7] Often respiratory and inotropic support is needed before transplantation.

Preoperative Management

1. A thorough evaluation of cardiac function, and other organ function (liver, kidney, and pulmonary), is indicated.[2]

2. Preoperative workup should include electrocardiogram, echocardiogram, cardiac catheterization, history of medical treatments, and routine hematologic and chemistry analysis. Immunosuppressive therapy (cyclosporine, 15 mg/kg PO) should be administered preoperatively.

3. Most children, regardless of whether they have fasted, should probably be considered to have a full stomach because of their poor perfusion and preoperative administration of a cyclosporine "milkshake." The administration of nonparticulate antacids or H_2 antagonists and metoclopramide is therefore advisable.

4. Children with HLHS require patency of the ductus arteriosus for the continued ejection of blood from the right ventricle into the aorta and systemic and pulmonary circulation. Ductal patency is maintained with continuous PGE_1 infusion (0.05 to 0.1 µg/kg/min). Metabolic acidosis due to systemic hypoperfusion may be severe and should be corrected with bicarbonate and volume expansion.[8]

5. When HLHS is present, maintaining a careful balance between systemic and pulmonary perfusion becomes the most important preoperative goal. Maintenance of a Q_p/Q_s ratio at or close to 1 is vital for survival. Although increased FIO_2 does not improve oxygenation with a fixed shunt, high concentrations of inspired oxygen will dilate the pulmonary vasculature, increasing pulmonary blood flow at the expense of systemic blood flow. An FIO_2 sufficient to maintain an O_2 saturation of 75% to 80% is satisfactory to ensure adequate tissue oxygenation. Ventricular dysfunction can be treated with either digoxin or inotropic agents such as dobutamine. Extra attention should be paid to the effects of the inotropic agent on the equilibrium between pulmonary vascular resistance (PVR) and systemic vascular re-

sistance (SVR). Agents such as peripheral vasoconstrictors (phenylephrine, norepinephrine) should be avoided because they increase SVR, leading to the imbalance of Q_p/Q_s (see also p. 141).

Intraoperative Management
VASCULAR ACCESS

1. A central venous catheter should be inserted in the left internal jugular vein for infusion of fluids and vasopressor or inotropic agents. The right internal jugular vein is left for access for the frequent postoperative myocardial biopsies.
2. A radial arterial catheter should be placed to continuously monitor blood pressure and to obtain samples of blood for gas and laboratory analysis.

MONITORS AND EQUIPMENT

Along with standard noninvasive monitoring and those mentioned above, a pulmonary artery catheter may be inserted in teenagers and older children. Multiple infusion pumps should be available, and transesophageal echocardiography can be helpful. A heating/cooling blanket is also required.

ANESTHETIC AGENTS

1. Opioids (fentanyl, 50 to 100 µg/kg, or sufentanil, 10 µg/kg) are the preferred anesthetic agents for cardiac surgery in infants, since they cause minimal changes in resistance, inotropy, and heart rate.[9]
2. Inhalation agents are usually avoided, as they depress the myocardium and decrease SVR. A slow, judicious inhalational induction with a low concentration of halothane may be used to induce anesthesia in patients without intravenous access, appreciating that the failing ventricle may be exquisitely sensitive to halothane's negative inotropy and ability to slow conduction.
3. Pancuronium (0.1 to 0.2 mg/kg) or vecuronium (0.1 to 0.2 mg/kg) is used to provide muscle relaxation.
4. Ketamine (1 to 2 mg/kg) or etomidate (0.3 mg/kg) can be combined with succinylcholine or high-dose vecuronium or rocuronium if a rapid-sequence induction is required.
5. Scopolamine may be used to supplement amnesia when an opiate technique is used.
6. Benzodiazepines can cause significant reductions in myocardial contractility and SVR when given in combination with potent opioids. Acute hemodynamic decompensation with induction of anesthesia may be caused by changes in PVR, SVR, heart rate, or myocardial depression. Inotropic agents such as dopamine, isoproterenol, and epinephrine may help maintain ventricular function.

Weaning from Cardiopulmonary Bypass (CPB)[7]

The requirements prior to weaning from CPB include: adequate anesthesia with muscle relaxation, good oxygenation with mild to moderate hyperventilation (PaCO$_2$ of 25 to 30 mm Hg), no metabolic acidosis, and normothermia. In most cases, allograft performance is quite good after reeperfusion, although chronotropic support with a pacemaker is often needed transiently. If inotropic support is needed, an infusion of dobutamine or dopamine is initiated. Increases in postbypass PVR will compromise right ventricular function, since the allograft may have difficulties adjusting acutely to a high right ventricular afterload. Ventilatory manipulations are the initial approach to reducing PVR (thereby optimizing right ventricular performance). If right ventricular failure occurs, additional pharmacologic interventions such as PGE$_1$ and prostacyclin,[10] or inhaled nitric oxide,[11] may be indicated.

Post-CPB Period

After successful weaning from CPB, attention should focus on adequate hemostasis. Protamine sulfate is used to reverse heparinization (1 mg per mg heparin); clotting factors and platelets may be needed to correct coagulation defects. Problems associated with closure of the chest include: (1) discrepancy in size between donor and recipient and (2) direct compression of the heart or pulmonary outflow, which may interfere with systemic pressure and/or right heart function.[1]

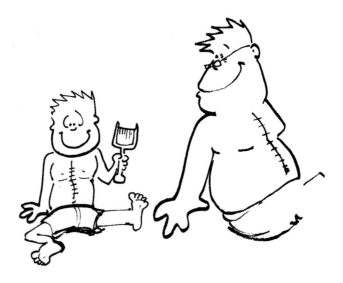

PEDIATRIC LUNG TRANSPLANTATION

Improved outcome with lung transplantation has encouraged wider applications of this procedure for children with end-stage lung disease. To date, cystic fibrosis is by far the most common indication, followed by primary pulmonary hypertension (PPH). Because of shortages in appropriately sized donor organs and because the above diseases are slow in progression, fewer than 4% of all lung transplant procedures are performed in patients under 12 years of age.[12] The majority of children undergo double-lung transplantation (DLT). In the past, DLT was performed as an en bloc procedure requiring cardiopulmonary bypass (CPB); however, the development of bilateral sequential lung transplantation (BSLT) has allowed for this procedure without CPB.

Anesthetic Considerations[6]

1. Time available for preoperative preparation is brief because of the short preservative life of the donor lung.
2. Premedication is seldom administered, but an antacid with cyclosporine is usually given prior to induction of anesthesia.
3. Patients with cystic fibrosis tend to have a permanent intravenous catheter in situ prior to operation, as frequent pulmonary infections require intravenous antibiotic treatment.
4. Respiratory compromise usually precludes an anesthetic induction with the patient lying supine; anesthesia must often be initiated with the patient in the sitting position.[13]
5. A ventilator capable of administering high respiratory rates and inflation pressures, as well as high levels of PEEP, should be available.
6. Fiberoptic bronchoscopes are also essential to facilitate double-lumen or single-lumen tube mainstem bronchial placement, or to perform therapeutic bronchoscopy and clear secretions and assess anastomotic patency and integrity.

Monitoring and Vascular Access

1. Standard, noninvasive monitors should be placed prior to induction.
2. As with other forms of transplantation, significant blood losses can be anticipated, and at least two large-bore peripheral intravenous catheters are needed, as well as a continuous central venous pressure monitor. A pulmonary artery catheter may also be beneficial; however, the catheter must be inserted after reperfusion or else be withdrawn to the central venous pressure position during the pneumonectomies.
3. In the hemodynamically stable patient, the indwelling arterial catheter is inserted after induction. If the surgeon plans to clamp the right subclavian artery, the right radial artery should

be avoided as a potential monitoring site, and the left radial or femoral artery selected instead.

Anesthetic Induction

1. Because all pulmonary transplants are urgent procedures, fasting guidelines cannot be followed and anesthesia is induced with intravenous agents using a rapid-sequence technique. Etomidate may provide the best overall combination of hemodynamic stability and airway control. Opioids and lidocaine can blunt the pulmonary hypertension caused by intubation. Ketamine should be avoided because it can aggravate preexisting pulmonary hypertension and because of direct negative inotropic effects that may be pronounced in patients with chronic ventricular failure.

2. Intubation should be performed with meticulous sterile technique, demanding sterile gloves, laryngoscope, and endotracheal tube (ETT). The largest possible ETT that the trachea accommodates is used, to facilitate postintubation bronchoscopy, lavage, and suction. A fiberoptic bronchoscope verifies ETT position initially and again after the tracheal anastomosis is completed. A standard ETT placed in the upper third of the trachea is used for en bloc DLT. A left-sided double-lumen endotracheal tube may be selected for older children having a single-lung transplant. At the conclusion of surgery, the double-lumen tube is changed to a standard single-lumen ETT for postoperative care.[10]

3. A thoracic, lumbar, or caudal epidural catheter may be inserted for intraoperative anesthesia and for postoperative pain management. The risk of epidural hematoma must be considered if heparinization and bypass are planned and if coagulation abnormalities are present in patients with cystic fibrosis.

Intraoperative Management

1. Positive-pressure ventilation sufficient to achieve normal blood gases may cause air-trapping or severe hypotension from the decrease in cardiac output caused by the high intrapulmonary pressures. Intentional hypoventilation may therefore improve overall cardiorespiratory stability.[14] Sudden hemodynamic decompensation after positive-pressure ventilation may indicate a pneumothorax in these high-risk patients. If a BSLT is being performed, it is necessary to attempt a short trial of one-lung ventilation to determine tolerance during insertion of the donor lung.

2. If CPB is needed, an extensive dissection of adhesions and di-

vision of bronchial collateral vessels can cause significant blood loss necessitating transfusion.

3. Cross clamping of the pulmonary artery is usually done in a stepwise fashion. Pulmonary artery pressure, right ventricular function, and systemic cardiac output (blood pressure and perfusion) are carefully monitored during clamping. Vasodilators such as PGE_1 may be needed to decrease pulmonary artery pressure and right ventricular afterload.

4. If a BSLT is performed, the anastomoses are completed in the following order: left atrial cuff, bronchus, and finally branch pulmonary artery. The endotracheal tube is then withdrawn into the trachea, and ventilation can begin.

5. Hypotension caused by retraction of the heart and lung is treated with vasopressors (phenylephrine). Aggressive hydration can cause posttransplantation pulmonary edema. When fluid resuscitation is absolutely necessary, blood products are preferred to crystalloid.

6. All newly reperfused lungs must be reexpanded with several sustained, high-pressure (40 cm H_2O) breaths, and then ventilated while maintaining at least 7 to 10 cm H_2O of PEEP. This high level of PEEP is used to minimize atelectasis and the accumulation of edema fluid. Deteriorating lung compliance, increasing peak airway and pulmonary artery pressures, and frank pulmonary edema are all indicative of either reperfusion injury or stenosis of the pulmonary venous anastomoses. Aggressive treatment with increased levels of PEEP, diuretics, and, if necessary, pulmonary vasodilators (PGE_1) is often necessary.

Postoperative Management

1. Hemorrhage, bacterial infection, and difficulties with mechanical ventilation are the most common complications after lung transplant.

2. The FIO_2 is gradually decreased to reduce the risk of oxygen toxicity while maintaining the PaO_2 at 90 to 120 mm Hg. Peak airway pressures $\leq$ 40 cm H_2O and positive end-expiratory pressure of about 5 cm H_2O are recommended. Tracheal extubation is usually accomplished in the first 48 hours after operation.

3. These patients are prone to posttransplantation intersitial pulmonary edema so that fluid administration is often restricted. It is important to achieve a negative fluid balance as soon as the patient is hemodynamically stable.

4. The postoperative course is usually complicated within the first month with at least one episode of rejection and/or infection.

PEDIATRIC LIVER TRANSPLANTATION

Increasingly, liver transplantation has become an accepted modality for the treatment of end-stage liver disease in children. Between 1980 and 1995 over 2000 pediatric patients have successfully received liver, multivisceral, and small bowel transplants in the United States,[15] and the long-term survival rate for children approaches 70% at 5 years.[15,16] The majority of liver transplants are received by patients less than 5 years old.[16]

Indications for liver transplantation in children

Congenital biliary atresia (50% to 60%)

Biliary hypoplasia
Alagille syndrome

Inborn errors of metabolism (20% to 40%)

Hemophilia A
Tyrosinemia
Glycogen storage diseases types I or IV
Antithrombin III (Budd-Chiari syndrome)
Hydroxyoxaluria type I

Metabolic disorders (10% to 15%)

Reye's syndrome
α_1-Antitrypsin deficiency
Wilson's syndrome
Hemachromatosis
Cystic fibrosis

Cryptogenic cirrhosis

Chronic hepatitis

Tumors

Adapted from Scott V, Firestone S, Robertson KM, Borland LM: Pediatric organ transplantation. In Motoyama EK, Davis PJ, eds: *Smith's anesthesia for infants and children,* ed 6, St. Louis, 1996, Mosby.

Pathophysiology of End-Stage Liver Disease

Regardless of the underlying disease process, patients with end-stage liver disease (ESLD) share several common pathophysiologic characteristics. (See table on next page.)

Pathophysiology of end-stage liver disease

Clinical conditions	Pathologic manifestations
Hematologic problems	Anemia (decreased production, bone marrow suppression) Thrombocytopenia (70% of patients) Increased protime (PT) and partial thromboplastin time (PTT) Disseminated intravascular coagulation (DIC) Diminished hepatic synthesis of factors I, II, V, VII, IX, X Dysfibrinogenemia; fibrinolysis; increased levels of fibrinogen and factor VII
Cardiovascular changes	Hyperdynamic circulation (supranormal left ventricular ejection fraction) Decreased systemic vascular resistance (shunts, vasodilation) Right-to-left shunts with increased risk of air emboli
Respiratory problems	Restrictive defect from ascites Increased alveolar-arterial O_2 difference from pulmonary shunting; clubbing and cyanosis Decreased pulmonary diffusing capacity
Renal failure	Prerenal azotemia Hepatorenal syndrome Acute tubular necrosis (ATN)
Encephalopathy	Increased blood ammonia and other endotoxins False neurotransmitters GABA hyperactivity
Glucose	Decreased stores of glycogen; insulin resistance; hypoglycemia
Electrolyte disorders	Hyponatremia Hypokalemia Hyperphosphatemia Hypocalcemia Hypomagnesemia Alkalosis or acidosis
Changes in pharmacokinetics	Decreased protein binding Increased volume of distribution Decreased hepatic blood flow and hepatic enzyme activity, resulting in decreased clearance and increased half-life of drugs dependent on liver metabolism

The Surgical Technique

The intraoperative anesthetic management is dependent on the three distinct phases of the surgical procedure. Stage 1, the *preanhepatic stage,* occurs from the induction of anesthesia to the devascularization of the liver. Stage 2, the *anhepatic stage,* occurs during the removal of the native liver and attachment of the donor liver prior to reperfusion of the graft. Stage 3, the *neohepatic stage,* begins immediately after the new graft is reperfused, lasting until the end of the surgical procedure.

Stages of liver transplantation

Stage	Surgical procedure	Anticipated sequelae
I. Preanhepatic	1. Bilateral subcostal incision 2. Liver freed to its vascular pedicle 3. Veno-venous bypass (patients > 20 kg) by cannulating and draining portal/femoral veins into axillary vein 4. Preparation of donor homograft	Hypotension due to surgical bleeding or drainage of ascites Potential hypothermia from massive fluid exchanges, use of veno-venous bypass, evaporative loss
II. Anhepatic	1. Diseased organ's vessels are clamped and bile duct transected 2. Vascular anastomoses: a. Suprahepatic IVC b. Infrahepatic IVC 3. Liver perfused by unclamping of infrahepatic IVC and portal vein 4. Hepatic artery anastomosed (may require aortic cross-clamp in small children)	Reduced renal perfusion from cross-clamping Cardiovascular changes: • A decrease in cardiac output, central venous pressure, pulmonary artery pressure, and mean arterial pressure • Arrhythmias (bradycardia, tachycardia, heart block, arrest) • Cardiac decompensation Pulmonary edema Hypoxemia from diaphragmatic retraction, emboli, pulmonary edema Hyperkalemia after reperfusion Hypothermia Hypoglycemia

Stages of liver transplantation—cont'd

Stage	Surgical procedure	Anticipated sequelae
III. Neohepatic	1. Reperfusion and hemostasis control 2. Hepatic artery anastomosis is completed 3. Biliary reconstruction: Roux-en-Y-choledochojejunostomy 4. Incision closure	Postreperfusion syndrome: • Hypotension • Bradycardia • Occasional cardiac arrest (< 1%) Persistent myocardial depression from lowered calcium levels, hypotension, and acidosis Worsened coagulopathy from massive transfusion Respiratory insufficiency caused by large donor liver after incision closure

Anesthetic Management[17]
PREOPERATIVE EVALUATION AND PREPARATION

1. Most recipients arrive at the transplant center on very short notice, leaving limited time for preparation. Even with improvements in preservative solutions, the donor liver can be safely preserved for only 24 hours after retrieval. This brief period may not allow time for complete correction of the abnormalities in the patient's coagulation or electrolyte status.

2. Liver transplantation is a lengthy procedure. Additional anesthesiologists should be available to assist with the procedure to prevent fatigue and manage the extensive complications that can arise during the operation.

3. A preoperative visit should include a detailed history and physical examination.

4. Laboratory data (complete blood count, liver function tests, coagulation, electrolytes), chest radiograph, electrocardiogram, and arterial blood gases should be obtained and reviewed.

5. Depending on the emotional and physical status of the child, premedication can be administered.

6. There should be continuous communication with the retrieval team to predict a starting time. The anesthetic team may need 1 to 2 hours for induction and completion of catheter insertions before incision is made.

Vascular Access and Monitors

Two or more large-bore intravenous catheters for fluid infusion and a central venous catheter for central monitoring and pressor infusion are needed. Also, two arterial catheters, one for blood pressure monitoring and the other for blood gas and laboratory blood sampling, should be available. If vascular access in the arms is difficult, the lower extremities may be used, with the knowledge that during the anhepatic stage venous return to the heart depends on veno-venous bypass or collateral flow. A rapid-infusion device may be useful for larger children or when rapid blood loss is expected. In addition, multiple infusion pumps and a cell saver device should be available. The use of a thromboelastogram (TEG) is highly recommended because it distinguishes the particular clotting defect (e.g., thrombocytopenia versus fibrinolysis).

Induction and Maintenance
of Anesthesia

1. Intravenous inductions are common in children because IV access is usually in place to administer preoperative immunosuppressive medication and antibiotics. In nonfasted children, a rapid-sequence induction with a sedative hypnotic agent, i.e., thiopental (3 to 5 mg/kg), etomidate (0.2 to 0.3 mg/kg), or ketamine (1 to 2 mg/kg), and a depolarizing or nondepolarizing muscle relaxant is administered.

2. If succinylcholine is used, two potential problems should be considered:
   a. ESLD may be associated with decreased plasma levels of pseudocholinesterase.[18] Prolonged effect of succinylcholine, however, is of little clinical consequence because of the prolonged duration of perioperative ventilation required and the dilutional effect of the massive intraoperative blood replacement.
   b. Preoperative hyperkalemia may be seen in patients with severe liver disease, and administration of succinylcholine may increase the serum potassium concentration by 0.5 to 0.7 mmol/L, predisposing these patients to cardiac arrhythmias.

3. Since most of the muscle relaxants are metabolized and/or eliminated by the liver or kidney, the duration of nondepolarizing muscle relaxants can be prolonged. For example, pancuronium has an increased volume of distribution, prolonged elimination half-life, and decreased plasma clearance in patients with cirrhosis. These patients may need more pancuronium initially to achieve muscle relaxation, and still have a prolonged recovery of blockade between doses.[19] Longer duration of action, however, rarely poses a problem, as postoperative ventilation is usually required for at least 24 hours.

4. Although inhalation induction is rarely needed, brief use of halothane has been reported without complications. Sevoflurane may offer the same advantages as halothane in terms of decreasing airway irritability without the metabolic implications. Nitrous oxide can be used to speed induction, but should then be discontinued to avoid bowel distension and expansion of air emboli.

5. Isoflurane with supplementary opioid/amnestic agents and a nondepolarizing muscle relaxant is the current choice for maintenance of anesthesia.

6. Hypothermia commonly occurs because of the large abdominal incision, prolonged procedure time, and massive intravenous infusions. Aggressive efforts to maintain normothermia are required, and include the use of blood/fluid warmers and forced-air warmers.

PROBLEMS ENCOUNTERED DURING THE INTRAOPERATIVE PERIOD

Blood loss.   The greatest blood loss occurs during the preanhepatic stage and the beginning of the anhepatic stage. Several factors influence surgical blood loss, with portal vein hypoplasia, presence of severe hepatic failure requiring inpatient support, and use of a reduced-size liver graft carrying the greatest predictability.[20] Replacement of as much as 0.5 to 25 blood volumes may be required.

Replacement of blood products and fluids requires constant assessment of numerous patient variables, including coagulation status, hematocrit, blood pressure, filling pressures, cardiac output, and urine output. Before skin incision, fresh frozen plasma (FFP), packed red blood cells (RBC), and platelets should be available. Filtered and warmed packed red blood cells and fresh frozen plasma (FFP) are administered in a 1:1 ratio by either rapid transfusion device or large-bore IV catheters to maintain a hematocrit of 28% to 30%. Separate IV catheters should be used to administer platelets and cryoprecipitate.

Coagulopathy.   Coagulation defects are caused by dilutional coagulopathy, progressive thrombocytopenia, primary fibrinolysis, disseminated intravascular coagulation (DIC), and secondary fibronlysis. Activity from heparin given during donor organ harvesting may also inhibit clotting.

Because of the high incidence of hepatic artery thrombosis (5% to 10%) in children receiving liver transplants, treatment of coagulopathy dictates that less FFP and platelets are given.[21] Thus, in some institutions, aggressive correction of coagulation is pursued only when there is diffuse bleeding after graft reperfusion or if monitoring reveals fibrinolysis that is not reversible by the new liver. Ongoing bleeding or coagulopathy necessitates repeat thromboelastograms, fibrin split products, and factor VII levels to direct pharmacologic and transfusion therapy.

Metabolic abnormalities

Hypocalcemia and hypomagnesemia.   Massive blood transfusion in patients with ESLD may result in citrate toxicity with low ionized calcium and magnesium levels. A prolonged QT interval, A-V dissociation, myocardial depression, hypotension, or even asystole may be initial manifestations of hypocalcemia. Treatment, based on measured ionized calcium levels, consists of calcium chloride IV bolus (10 to 20 mg/kg) or infusion (approximately 10 mg/kg/hr). Calcium chloride should be given through a central catheter. Calcium gluconate is not used, as it is metabolized by the liver.

Hyperkalemia and hypokalemia.   Hypokalemia is present in most patients with ESLD but rarely requires treatment. Acute hyperkalemia (7 to 11 mEq/L) is always anticipated after reperfusion even though the liver is flushed to remove the potassium-rich solution. Treatment of hyperkalemia consists of glucose, insulin, and bicarbonate (see p. 81).

Altered glucose metabolism.   Glucose levels remain normal or high during transplantation as a result of decreased utilization and the continuous infusion of blood products (one unit of red cells contains 0.5 g of glucose). Levels should be monitored often, although insulin infusions are rarely required. The high glucose levels decrease spontaneously after revascularization, as the new liver begins effective metabolism.

Acid-base balance.   Metabolic acidosis resulting from hypoperfusion and continuous transfusion peaks during graft reperfusion. A base deficit of greater than 5 mmol/L should be treated using either bicarbonate or THAM (tris[hydroxymethyl]–aminomethane). With reperfusion, however, metabolic alkalosis may occur from the metabolism of citrate to bicarbonate and furosemide-induced chloride loss. The alkalosis usually persists postoperatively and occasionally requires treatment.

Intraoperative laboratory data obtained during liver transplantation*

Blood gases, pH[†]
Electrolytes: sodium, potassium, ionized calcium[†]
Glucose[†]
Hematocrit[†]
Hemoglobin
Colloid osmolarity
Platelet count
Protime
Partial thromboplastin time
Fibrinogen

---

*Results should be available within 10 minutes after samples are obtained.
[†]Data should be procured at least hourly.

Hypothermia.   Methods to prevent hypothermia, including radiant and forced-air warmers, should be instituted early. Although esophageal temperatures below 35.5° C are common, hypothermia below 34° C is not well tolerated.

Cardiovascular changes.   After the native liver is removed, the cardiac output (CO), central venous pressure (CVP), and mean arterial pressure (MAP) decrease, with a compensatory increase of the systemic vascular resistance (SVR). Also, CO_2 production ($\dot{V}CO_2$) and $\dot{V}O_2$ are decreased. There is a decreased $\dot{V}O_2$ during the anhepatic stage as well.[15]

During the neohepatic stage, mismatch of the size of the donor liver's vascular bed compared with the recipient's total blood volume often results in significant hemodynamic instability. With graft reperfusion, cold, acidotic hyperkalemic solution (cardioplegia) is released directly into the right heart, resulting in a phenomenon called the postperfusion syndrome (hypotension, bradycardia, and occasionally cardiac arrest (<1%). The postperfusion syndrome is observed in up to 30% of patients, and aggressive treatment with epinephrine (5 to 10 μg/kg bolus) may be required to prevent cardiovascular collapse.[22] Although the manifestations of postperfusion syndrome are usually temporary and short lived (lasting less than 5 min), continued inotropic support with dopamine, dobutamine, or epinephrine may be required in the neohepatic stage for up to 2 to 3 hours postoperatively.

Pulmonary changes

1. Hypoxemia due to parenchymal disease, pulmonary arteriovenous shunting, and pleural effusions may exist preoperatively.
2. If possible, the delivered oxygen concentration should be maintained below 50% to prevent further pulmonary damage from oxygen toxicity and atelectasis.
3. Pulmonary edema may occur with reperfusion of the donor liver and should be treated with PEEP, diuretics, and decreasing volume replacement.
4. The proximity of the surgical field makes pneumothorax a potential problem.
5. Abdominal closure may be impossible because of gut distention and a large donor liver, resulting in increased airway pressure and inadequate ventilation. In this situation, a temporary closure can be utilized.

Renal function[23].   Low urine output at the start of the procedure is usually caused by hepatorenal syndrome or acute tubular necrosis (ATN). Most patients are anuric or oliguric during the anhepatic phase because of increased venous pressure in renal beds. Urine output usually improves after revascularization. After ensuring adequate hydration and perfusion pressures, dopamine (3 μg/kg/min) and furosemide (0.5 to 1.0 mg/kg) are utilized if urine output does not improve.

POSTOPERATIVE COURSE

1. The most common complication seen after liver transplantation is persistent hypertension, frequently associated with underlying renal dysfunction, increased circulating catecholamines, steroids, and cyclosporine therapy. Aggressive treatment is required to prevent irreversible organ system injury.
2. Persistent bleeding is common, especially with split liver transplant, and may necessitate reexploration.
3. Other complications include vascular thrombosis of the transplanted liver, renal insufficiency, and hepatic dysfunction. Bacterial sepsis is often seen in the immediate postoperative period. Viral infections may occur later in the chronically immunosuppressed patient.

PEDIATRIC RENAL TRANSPLANTATION

Children with chronic renal failure suffer stunted growth, multiorgan disturbances, and social maladjustment despite recent improvements in dialysis techniques.[24, 25] Kidney transplants account for two thirds of all solid organ transplants in the United States,[26] and about 500 to 700 kidney transplants are performed annually in children. As a result of the introduction of cyclosporine, survival after kidney transplant has improved dramatically, and graft survival is now reported at 88% to 100% at 1 year and 80% to 90% at 5 years.[27]

Indications for Renal Transplant

In the neonate and small infant, congenital and anatomic abnormalities of the kidney are the most common causes of renal failure. In older children renal failure is mainly due to immunologic and metabolic disease processes, which can cause a recurrence of renal failure after transplantation.

Etiology of chronic renal failure in children leading to transplantation

Disease	Percent of transplants resulting from disease
Pyelonephritis	20-30
Glomerulopathies	20-30
Hereditary nephropathies, cystic kidney, hypoplasia	30-50
Vascular nephropathies	5
Other	5-10

Adapted from Caldwell JE, Cook RD: Kidney transplantation. In Cook DR, Davis PJ, eds: *Anesthetic principles for organ transplantation,* New York, 1994, Raven Press.

Manifestations of End-Stage Renal Disease (ESRD)

Perioperative management of the transplant recipient requires a thorough understanding of the multiple organ derangements characteristic of end-stage renal disease.

Pathology associated with end-stage renal disease[6]

System	Pathologic feature
Neurologic	Peripheral neuropathy (median and common peroneal nerves are most commonly involved) Uremic encephalopathy; seizures; psychosis Developmental delay Autonomic dysfunction
Hematologic	Anemia Platelet dysfunction Hemolysis
Cardiovascular	Increased cardiac output Hypertension Congestive heart failure Arrhythmia
Gastrointestinal	Delayed gastric emptying Anorexia Nausea; vomiting
Hepatic	Decreased serum protein Reduced plasma cholinesterase level Possible hepatitis caused by frequent blood transfusion
Fluid and electrolytes	Volume overload Hyperkalemia Hypocalcemia Hyperphosphatemia Hyponatremia Hypermagnesemia Hypoglycemia or hyperglycemia
Other	Metabolic acidosis Lethargy; fatigue Failure to thrive Dry skin

Surgical Considerations

1. The size of the recipient determines the operative approach and the positioning of the donor kidney. In children and infants weighing less than 20 kg, adult kidneys are placed in the retroperitoneal space or intraabdominally through a transperitoneal midline incision. In recipients weighing more than 20 kg the abdominal extraperitoneal operative approach is used, with placement of the organ in the iliac fossa.

2. For infants or small children, the procedure is complicated by the technical difficulties of vascular anastomosis associated with small body size and the relatively large donor kidney.[28] The donor renal vein is anastomosed to the side of the distal aspect of the recipient's inferior vena cava, common iliac vein, or

external iliac vein, and the donor renal artery is anastomosed to the common iliac artery, hypogastric artery, or side of the aorta. Urinary drainage is completed by an end-to-end anastomosis of the donor and recipient ureters, by ureteral implantation into the bladder with an antireflux procedure, or rarely by urinary diversion.

Preoperative Management

1. Regardless of the source of the donor (cadaveric or living re-lated), improvements in kidney preservation have resulted in the ability to delay transplant time for 48 hours after harvest-ing. This provides ample time to correct metabolic abnormali-ties such as fluid overload or electrolyte disturbances in the recipient.[1]

2. A detailed history and physical examination including all major organ systems is obtained with particular attention to the patient's current state of hydration. The dialysis records should be reviewed, including electrolyte levels, blood pressure before and after dialysis, dry weight of the patient, complications as-sociated with dialysis, the date of last dialysis, and postdialysis hematocrit. Electrocardiogram and chest radiograph are rou-tinely obtained. Antihypertensive medications are continued until surgery, to avoid rebound hypertension. Patients on steroid therapy receive perioperative stress doses.

3. Previous blood transfusions and complications (hepatitis, viral infections, febrile reactions) are noted.

4. Preoperative sedatives may be indicated to decrease anxiety. The clearance of midazolam is relatively unchanged in patients with ESRD.[29] Morphine, however, can produce severe respira-tory depression because of decreased protein binding and changes in the blood-brain barrier.

5. Renal transplantation is a semi-urgent procedure, allowing ade-quate time for preoperative fasting in children who do not have significant gastroparesis or gastroesophageal reflux. However, since delayed gastric emptying can occur in patients with ESRD, H_2 blockers and metoclopramide to increase gastric motility are usually given with preoperative sedation.[1]

Monitoring and Vascular Access

In addition to the standard noninvasive monitors, an intraarter-ial catheter may be needed for continuous pressure monitoring and serial sampling of serum electrolytes, hematocrit, pH, and blood gases. The location of the dialysis catheter or shunt should be pro-tected and frequently inspected during the operation. A large-bore peripheral intravenous catheter for volume administration is placed away from the site of permanent vascular shunts. Jugular veins are preferred for central venous access for pressure monitoring and inotropic support. Femoral veins are avoided, as the inferior vena cava may be clamped during surgery. Special care should be taken in the use of forearm vessels, as they may be needed for future shunts or fistulas.

Induction and Maintenance of Anesthesia

1. No specific drug regimen demonstrates superiority for induction or maintenance of anesthesia in patients with ESRD. Induction may be accomplished by inhalation of a volatile agent or by preoxygenation followed by a rapid-sequence induction (if indicated). Usual induction doses of thiopental or etomidate are used. Although the unbound portion of thiopental is increased in ESRD, the volumes of distribution and clearance are also increased, and the half-life remains unchanged. Also, the pharmacokinetics of propofol are unaltered by renal failure.[26]

2. Succinylcholine is acceptable with ECG monitoring if the potassium is less than 5.5 mEq/L. Because of minimal requirements for renal excretion, vecuronium, rocuronium, or atracurium is recommended for muscle relaxation. Pancuronium in a single dose to last the duration of the procedure can be used; use of a neuromuscular blockade monitor is required for repeat dosing or for assessing the effectiveness of reversal. Both depolarizing and nondepolarizing neuromuscular blockade may be potentiated by acidosis, hypocalcemia, hypermagnesemia, and hypovolemia, so that intraoperative monitoring of acid-base status and serum electrolyte levels is critical.

3. Isoflurane with supplementary opioids/amnestic agents and an intermediate-duration nondepolarizing muscle relaxant are recommended for maintenance of anesthesia.

Implications of ESRD for anesthetic pharmacology

Drugs	Effects of ESRD
Neuromuscular blockers	Blockade may be potentiated by: • Acidosis • Increased serum magnesium • Hypocalcemia • Hyponatremia • Mycin antibiotics Usual doses of atropine and neostigmine, edrophonium, or pyridostigmine can be used for reversal.
Succinylcholine	Use is contraindicated if potassium is greater than 5.5 mEq/L.
Pancuronium, d-tubocurarine	$T_{1/2}$ increased up to 500%. The same initial loading dose (pancuronium 0.1 mg/kg, d-tubocurarine 0.5 mg/kg) is needed to produce intubating conditions. Interval dosing requires adjustment to avoid prolonged relaxation.

Implications of ESRD for anesthetic pharmacology—cont'd

Drugs	Effects of ESRD
Neuromuscular blockers—cont'd	
Vecuronium	Normally 10% to 25% excreted in urine, the remainder in bile. Accumulation can occur as $T_{1/2}$ is increased about 30% in patients with ESRD. Interval dosing should be titrated to twitch response.
Atracurium	Essentially unaffected by hepatorenal function. No cumulative effect with dosing.
Rocuronium	Alternative to succinylcholine for rapid-sequence induction (0.6-1.2 mg/kg). Interval dosing should be titrated to twitch response.
Intravenous hypnotic/ analgesics	
Thiopental	Induction dose is unchanged. Twice as much thiopental exists in the unbound state in patients with ESRD. An increased volume of distribution and increased clearance cause no change in $T_{1/2}$.
Midazolam	Primarily metabolized by the liver. No change in clearance or $T_{1/2}$ of a single dose.
Etomidate, fentanyl, alfentanil	Short acting, with minimal change in duration caused by ESRD.
Inhalation anesthetics	
Enflurane	Metabolized to fluoride, which is nephrotoxic and relies on glomerular filtration for elimination.
Halothane	Metabolized to fluoride but to a much lesser extent than enflurane. May cause myocardial depression and subsequent hypotension, which decreases glomerular filtration rate.
Isoflurane	No known renal side effects and therefore useful for anesthetic maintenance.
Sevoflurane	Metabolized to fluoride and hexafluoroisopropanol. The peak plasma concentration of fluoride is proportional to the duration of exposure. However, no instance of nephrotoxicity occurred after more than 2 million anesthetics with sevoflurane in Japan to date.[30]
Desflurane	No known renal side effects.

Intraoperative Considerations

1. Fluid administration should be based on central venous pressure, with awareness that false elevations can occur during abdominal retraction. Blood pressure, CVP, venous PO_2, and urine output help to monitor volume status. Lactated Ringer's should be avoided because of the potassium content. Large amounts of normal saline solution may cause hypernatremia. When blood products are indicated, washed red blood cells provide the greatest number of red cells and the least amount of potassium per unit. Blood should be irradiated to minimize graft-versus-host (GVH) reaction.

2. Prior to releasing of the vascular clamps, the CVP should be raised with crystalloid to 12 to 16 cm H_2O to prevent hypotension with ischemic injury to the kidney and/or vascular thrombosis. A higher CVP may be needed if false elevations exist because of abdominal retractors or packs.

3. Intraoperative doses of immunosuppressive agents and antibiotics are administered as per institutional protocol. These can be prepared preoperatively.

4. Electrolytes, glucose, pH, and oxygen tension are monitored frequently. The perfusate solution is flushed from the donor kidney and replaced with cold lactated Ringer's before transplantation, in order to avoid high potassium concentrations released in the vascular space.

5. Furosemide, 1 mg/kg, may be given prior to clamp release to improve urine output. Ischemic injury may be attenuated by furosemide's inhibition of cell transport activity.

6. Mannitol, 125 to 200 mg/kg, given before clamp release increases plasma volume, filling pressures, and cardiac output and decreases systemic vascular resistance. It is a renal vasodilator, has osmotic action in the tubules, and will increase plasma potassium slightly.

7. Vascular clamps are released slowly. After unclamping, a fall in CVP with resultant hypotension is due to the following factors:
   a. A significant portion of the child's blood volume (up to 300 ml) may be diverted to the new adult kidney.
   b. Hyperkalemia caused by various endogenous and exogenous vasodilating agents released during washout of the graft preservative.
   c. Lactic acidosis from an ischemic lower body.

8. Treatment includes volume expansion and judicious use of dopamine (3 to 5 µg/kg/min).

9. The living-related adult donor kidney begins to function immediately after unclamping of the renal artery and continues to produce adult volumes of urine. One should replace urine output ml-for-ml with crystalloid to prevent a decrease in central venous pressure.

10. After surgery, neuromuscular blockade is reversed with standard doses of reversal agents. Prolonged mechanical ventilation is not usually needed except in situations of residual muscle relaxation or inadequate oxygenation/ventilation. Rarely, a large kidney placed in a small child compromises pulmonary function in the immediate postoperative period and necessitates gradual weaning from mechanical ventilation.

11. Lumbar and caudal epidural techniques may be used in children as an adjunct to general anesthesia for intraoperative and postoperative pain management.[31] However, residual heparinization and other ESRD coagulation abnormalities should be assessed carefully before using regional techniques.

12. Continued postoperative monitoring of the heart rate, arterial blood pressure, and central venous pressure is necessary for meticulous fluid management. Potassium, calcium, phosphorus, and magnesium levels should be determined at 2- to 4-hour intervals.

BONE MARROW TRANSPLANTATION[32, 33]

Bone marrow transplantation (BMT) is becoming an increasingly important therapeutic intervention in the treatment of various hematologic malignancies. In 1990, more than 5000 cases were reported to the International Bone Marrow Transplant Registry.[34]

Indications

1. Bone marrow transplantation is the treatment of choice for severe combined immunodeficiency syndrome (SCIDS), aplastic anemia, Wiskott-Aldrich syndrome, and other lethal hematopoietic disorders when a histocompatible donor is available.

2. For hematologic malignancies, bone marrow transplantation is used after failure of traditional chemotherapy or for "poor-risk" leukemias in first remission.

Anesthesia for Donors

Donors are generally healthy HLA-matched siblings from 5 to 6 months of age and older. The volume of marrow required for transplantation is 10 ml/kg body weight of the recipient. To minimize dilution of the marrow aspirate by peripheral blood, individual aspirates are limited to 2 to 3 ml per puncture, necessitating 100 to 400 separate aspirates per harvest, depending on the size of the recipient. Major complications occur rarely in the donor (0.3% incidence).

ANESTHETIC CONSIDERATIONS

1. General anesthesia is usually selected for young children donating bone marrow, as multiple needle aspirations are required (may be > 100), potentially over several hours. A regional technique (caudal or epidural) for postoperative pain management is recommended.

2. Nitrous oxide use has been controversial because of the potential for stem cell suppression. Recent evidence negates this belief.[35]

3. It is often necessary to harvest bone marrow from both anterior and posterior iliac crests, making it necessary to adjust the patient's position during the operation from supine to prone or vice versa.

4. About 25% to 35% of the patient's blood volume may be removed by a single bone marrow harvest. Volume of marrow taken should be replaced as if it were blood lost directly from the intravascular space.

Anesthesia for Recipients

Marrow is given to the recipient intravenously after suitable marrow ablation with high-dose chemotherapy and/or total body irradiation. Should the recipient require surgery following transplantation, certain BMT complications are of concern.

1. Profound immunosuppression is present until effective hematopoiesis begins around 3 to 5 weeks after BMT.

2. Acute graft-versus-host disease (GVHD) can appear 10 days to 6 weeks after BMT, causing skin, liver, and gastrointestinal (GI) complications.

   a. Chronic GVHD also involves the skin, liver, and gastrointestinal tract and is associated with more profound immunosuppression after BMT.

   b. GVHD has a very low incidence among young children, but the incidence increases with age.

3. There is a 50% incidence of interstitial pneumonitis after a bone marrow transplant, which may result in severe hypoxemia. Opportunistic infections are most serious in the first weeks immediately following transplant, prior to effective granulopoiesis.

4. Chemotherapeutic toxicity may be particularly severe, in part because of the marrow-ablative doses required. The most commonly used agent is cyclophosphamide, associated with pulmonary, GI, hepatic, and renal toxicity. Total-body irradiation may lead to hypothyroidism in approximately 50% of transplant recipients.

ANESTHETIC CONSIDERATIONS FOR THE PREVIOUSLY TRANSPLANTED PATIENT[36, 37]

With the improvement of immunosuppressive agents and technical expertise, there is an increasing number of transplant survivors who experience nontransplant surgery.

Preoperative Management

Of primary concern for the anesthesiologist is the function of the graft and related organ systems and the effects of immunosuppression (see p. 363).

(see p. 363)

1. Prior to surgery, information regarding the transplanted organ function, patient's post-transplant course, graft function, and recent diagnostic results from the transplant center should be obtained.
2. If there is any sign of infection or rejection, one should postpone the elective surgery and contact the physician in charge until further workup and results are completed.
3. All medications, including immunosuppressive agents, should be continued throughout the perioperative period.

Intraoperative Anesthetic Management

1. Aseptic technique should be used during all instrumentation (including insertion of intravenous cannulas).
2. If tracheal intubation is indicated, the oral route is preferable to nasal to decrease contamination caused by nasal flora.
3. Antibiotic administration should be dictated by the surgical procedure.
4. Anesthetic technique should be selected based on the transplanted organ function.
5. The transplanted heart has no sympathetic, parasympathetic, or sensory innervation. Therefore, carotid massage and the Valsalva maneuver have no effect on heart rate.[38]
   a. Drugs that have direct chronotropic effect (isoproterenol or epinephrine) can change the heart rate of the transplanted heart, while drugs with indirect action (pancuronium, gal-

lamine, atropine, glycopyrrolate, scopolamine, and anti-cholinesterases) have no effect on the heart rate. Transvenous pacing may also be utilized to control heart rate. External thoracic pacing is useful in children over 10 kg.

b. The transplanted heart has a high resting heart rate (90 to 100 beats per minute) and two P waves on ECG, and shows no response to laryngoscopy and intubation.

c. Anesthetic agents that maintain heart rate are ideal (e.g., ketamine). Inhalation agents that may cause myocardial depression or slow conduction should be used with caution.

6. The transplanted lung is denervated distal to the bronchial anastomosis, so that these patients have no cough reflex and are prone to retained secretions and aspirations. Patients whose chest radiographs show hilar opacity or infiltration need bronchoscopy and lavage prior to surgery. Postoperatively, aggressive chest physical therapy, postural drainage, and incentive spirometry are indicated to reduce pulmonary complications.

IMMUNOSUPPRESSANT DRUGS[39]

Cyclosporine. Cyclosporine interferes with release of interleukin-2, which normally stimulates antigen-activated helper and cytotoxic T cells to begin DNA synthesis. Cyclosporine also inhibits activation of B and T lymphocytes and certain macrophage functions.

Cyclosporine is extensively metabolized in the liver to inactive metabolites by the cytochrome P_{450} microsomal enzyme system. 99% undergoes biliary elimination and 1% renal elimination. 90% is normally bound to serum proteins. When given simultaneously, the following drugs increase the nephrotoxic potential of cyclosporine: trimethoprim, amphotericin B, aminoglycosides, melphalan, cotrimoxazole, indomethacin. The following drugs will increase cyclosporine levels by enzyme inhibition: ketoconazole, allopurinol, phenylbutazone, chloramphenicol, ethanol, cimetidine, erythromycin. The following drugs will decrease cyclosporine levels by enzyme induction: phenytoin, barbiturates, carbamazepine, rifampin, griseofulvin, primidone, glutethimide.

Cyclosporine is insoluble in water. Oral preparations are mixed with olive oil and ethanol and intravenous preparations with ethanol. Because of the ethanol vehicle, nausea and vomiting may result when cyclosporine is administered with metronidazole, cefamandole, moxalactam, or chlorpropamide. Intravenous preparations should be given slowly over 2 to 4 hours, as hypotension can occur. Desired whole blood levels are 200 to 600 ng/ml.

Side effects of cyclosporine

Nephrotoxicity
Hypertension
Hepatotoxicity
Increased susceptibility to infection
Bone marrow toxicity
Tremors, hyperesthesia
Encephalopathy and seizures have been reported in patients with low
   serum cholesterol after liver transplantation
Gingival hyperplasia
Hirsutism
Gastrointestinal upset: nausea, vomiting, diarrhea (usually mild)
Hyperuricemia
Lymphadenopathy and adenotonsillar hypertrophy
Myocardial fibrosis
Increased incidence of lymphoid tumors

Glucocorticoids.   Glucocorticoids may act synergistically with other immunosuppressants, possibly by inhibiting interleukin production. They will not prevent rejection when used alone. Their use decreases the number of antigen-activated lymphocytes by removing helper inducer lymphocytes from circulation. A high dose is given daily during the first post-transplant week; doses are rapidly tapered. Eventually, transition to an alternate-day regimen to promote growth is ideal. Intravenous high-dose boluses are used during episodes of rejection.

Side effects of glucocorticoids

Suppression of pituitary adrenal function, requiring perioperative
   steroid coverage
Fluid and electrolyte disturbances
Hyperglycemia and glycosuria
Infection
Peptic ulcer disease
Osteoporosis
Myopathy
Behavioral changes
Cataracts
Cushingoid habitus
Inhibition of growth in children
Skin fragility

Azathioprine.   Azathioprine is a derivative of 6-mercaptopurine. It interferes with DNA synthesis of rapidly dividing cells, and is used primarily to decrease the dose of cyclosporine. It is administered in a dose of 1.5 to 5 mg/kg/day IV or PO. Clearance is reduced in the presence of renal insufficiency.

Side effects of azathioprine include myelosuppression (dose related and reversible); cholestatic jaundice (dose related and reversible); and hepatitis. Stomatitis, dermatitis, fever, alopecia, and gastrointestinal disturbances are infrequent side effects.

Antilymphocyte globulin (ALG).   ALG is primarily used for treatment of acute rejection unresponsive to steroids and cyclosporine. Derived from animals inoculated with human lymphocytes, it varies widely in potency and effectiveness. Polyclonal composition allows for repeated use without developing resistance. Pretreatment with steroids, antihistamines, and acetaminophen will attenuate side effects, which include fever, chills, rash, dyspnea, anaphylaxis, and thrombocytopenia. ALG shares the side effects of transfusion of heterologous serum.

Monoclonal antibodies (OKT-3).   OKT-3 is a murine-derived antibody that recognizes the gamma portion of the T cell. Complete disappearance of circulating T cells occurs within 15 minutes of administration. Development of antimurine antibodies limits its repeated use. The antibody does not fix complement. Side effects of monoclonal antibodies include pulmonary edema and a flu-like syndrome often present at initial dosage that will decrease with time. Histamine release can be blocked by pretreatment with H_1 and H_2 antagonists.

Methotrexate.   Methotrexate has been used alone or with cyclosporine for prophylaxis against graft-versus-host disease in patients after bone marrow transplantation. Methotrexate's selective action on DNA synthesis inhibits the replication and function of T and B cells, resulting in immunosuppression. There is some evidence suggesting that recurrence of leukemia in patients after receiving bone marrow transplants may be reduced if methotrexate, rather than cyclosporine, is used.[40]

Methotrexate is also used for severe rheumatoid arthritis and refractory psoriasis. Patients treated with methotrexate for autoimmune diseases requiring long-term low-dosage administration appear to be more susceptible to hepatic fibrosis and nonseptic pneumonitis.[41, 42]

FK506.   FK506 is a relatively new immunosuppressant similar to cyclosporine, yet with greater potency and diminished side effects.[43] Nephrotoxicity, diabetes, and hyperkalemia may be seen as with cyclosporine.[44, 45] However, extreme hypertension is rarely a problem.[45] Drugs that induce or inhibit the cytochrome P_{450} system probably have the same effect on serum levels of FK506 as on cyclosporine.

References

1. Kelley SD, Cauldwell CB: Anesthesia for transplantation. In Gregory GA, ed: *Pediatric anesthesia,* ed. 3, New York, 1994, Churchill Livingstone.
2. Zales VR, Stapleton PL: Neonatal and infant heart transplantation. *Pediatr Clin North Am* 40:1023-1046, 1993.
3. Ali MG. Essentials of organ donor problems and their management, *Anesth Clin North Am* 12:655-671, 1994.
4. Robertson KM: Logistics of donor procurement, management of the donor organ, and organ preservation. In Cook DR, Davis PJ, eds: *Anesthetic principles for organ transplantation,* New York, 1994, Raven Press.
5. Hosenpud JD, Novick RJ, Breen TJ, et al: The registry of the International Society for Heart and Lung Transplantation: eleventh official report—1994, *J Heart Lung Transplant* 13: 561-570, 1994.
6. Frankville DD: Special considerations for pediatric transplantation, *Anesth Clin North Am* 12:767-787, 1994.
7. Zickmann B, Boldt J, Hempelmann G: Anesthesia in pediatric heart transplantation, *J Heart Lung Transplant* 11:S272-S276, 1992.
8. Zahka KG, Spector M, Hanisch D: Hypoplastic left-heart syndrome: Norwood operation, transplantation, or compassionate care, *Clin Perinatol* 20: 145-154, 1993.
9. Hickey PR, Hansen DD: Fentanyl- and sufentanil-oxygen-pancuronium anesthesia for cardiac surgery in infants, *Anesth Analg* 63:117-124, 1984
10. McGowan FX, Baily PL: Heart, lung, heart-lung transplantation. In Cook DR, Davis PJ, eds: *Anesthetic principles for organ transplantation.* New York, 1994, Raven Press, pp 85-157.
11. Mandell MS, Duke J: Nitric oxide reduces pulmonary hypertension during hepatic transplantation, *Anesthsiology* 81:1538-1542, 1994.
12. Starnes VA, Lewiston N, Theodore J, et al: Cystic fibrosis: target population for lung transplantation in North America in the 1990s, *J Thorac Cardiovasc Surg* 103:1008-1014, 1992.
13. Gayes JM, Giron L, Nissen M, Plut D: Anesthetic considerations for patients undergoing double-lung transplantation, *J Cardiothorac Anesth* 4: 486-498, 1990.
14. Quinlan JJ, Buffington CW: Deliberate hypoventilation in a patient with air trapping during transplantation, *Anesthesiology* 78:1177-1180, 1993.
15. Scott V, Firestone S, Robertson KM, Borland LM: Pediatric organ transplantation. In Motoyama EK, Davis PJ, eds: *Smith's anesthesia for infants and children,* ed 6, St. Louis, 1996, Mosby.
16. Whitington PF, Balistreri WF: Liver transplantation in pediatrics: indications, contraindications, and pretransplant management, *J Pediatr* 118:169-176, 1991.
17. Carton EG, Plevak DJ, Kranner PW et al: Perioperative care of the liver transplant patient, part II, *Anesth Analg* 78:382-399, 1994.
18. Khoury GG, Brill J, Walts L, Busuttil RW: Atypical serum cholinesterase eliminated by orthotopic liver transplantation, *Anesthesiology* 67:273-274, 1987.

19. Duvaldestin P, Agoston S, Henzel E, et al: Pancuronium pharmacokinetics in patients with liver cirrhosis, *Br J Anaesth* 50:1131-1136, 1978.

20. Ozier YM, Le Cam B, Chatellier G, et al: Intraoperative blood loss in pediatric liver transplantation: analysis of preoperative risk factors, *Anesth Analg* 81:1142-1147, 1995.

21. Langnas AN, Marujo W, Stratta RJ, et al: Hepatic allograft rescue following arterial thrombosis, *Transplantation* 51:86-90, 1991.

22. Aggarwal S, Kang Y, Freeman JA, Fortunato FL, Pinsky MR: Postreperfusion syndrome: cardiovascular collapse following hepatic reperfusion during liver transplantation, *Transplant Proc* 19: 54-55, 1987.

23. Swygert TH, Roberts LC, Valek TR, et al: Effect of intraoperative low dose dopamine on renal function in liver transplant recipients, *Anesthesiology* 75: 571-576, 1991.

24. Warady BA, Kriley M, Lovell H, et al: Growth and development of infants with end-stage renal disease receiving long-term peritoneal dialysis, *J Pediatr* 112: 714-719, 1988.

25. McGraw ME, Haka-Ikse K: Neurologic-developmental sequelae of chronic renal failure in infancy, *J Pediatr* 106: 579-582, 1985.

26. Caldwell JE, Cook RD: Kidney transplantation In Cook DR, Davis PJ, eds: *Anesthetic principles for organ transplantation,* New York, 1994, Raven Press.

27. Najarian JS, Matas AJ: The present and future of kidney transplantation, *Transplant Proc* 23: 2075-2082, 1991.

28. Bebbe DS, Belani KG, Mergens P, et al: Anesthetic management of infants receiving an adult kidney transplant, *Anesth Analg* 73: 725-730, 1991.

29. Vinik HR, Reves JG, Greenblatt DJ, et al: The pharmacokinetics of midazolam in chronic renal failure patients, *Anesthesiology* 59:390-394, 1983.

30. Cook DR, Davis DJ, Lerman J: Pharmacology of pediatric anesthesia. In Motoyama EK, Davis PJ, eds: *Smith's anesthesia for infants and children,* ed 6, St. Louis, 1996, Mosby.

31. Murakami M, Nomiyama S, Ozawa A, et al: Anesthetic management of pediatric renal transplantation for renal failure, *Jpn J Anesth* 42: 263-270, 1993.

32. Strauss SG, Lynn AM: Autologus bone marrow harvesting. In Stehling L, ed: *Common problems in pediatric anesthesia,* St Louis, 1992, Mosby.

33. Rappaport JM: Bone marrow transplantation. In Oski FH, Nathan DJ, eds: *Hematology of infancy and childhood,* Philadelphia, 1983, WB Saunders.

34. Gronert BJ, Neudorf S: Bone marrow transplantation. In Cook DR, Davis PJ, eds: *Anesthetic principles for organ transplantation,* New York, 1994, Raven Press.

35. Lederhaas G, Brock-Utne GJ, Negrin RS, et al: Is nitrous oxide safe for bone marrow harvest? *Anesth Analg* 80:770-772, 1995.

36. Sharpe MD, Gelb AW: Anesthetic considerations for the previously transplanted patients, *Anesth Clin North Am* 12:827-843, 1994.

37. Reicheld PA, Bell C: Posttransplant patients. In McGoldrick KE, ed: *Ambulatory anesthesiology: a problem-oriented approach,* Baltimore, 1995, Williams & Wilkins.

38. Cheng DCH, Ong DD: Anesthesia for noncardiac surgery in heart transplanted patients, *Can J Anaesth* 40:981-986, 1993.

39. Handschumacher RE: Drugs used for immunosuppression. In Goodman Gilman A, Rall TW, Nies AS, Taylor P, eds: *Goodman and Gilman's The pharmacological basis of therapeutics,* New York, 1990, Pergamon Press.

40. International Bone Marrow Transplant Registry: Effect of methotrexate on relapse after bone-marrow transplantation for acute lymphoblastic leukaemia, *Lancet* 1:535-537, 1989.

41. Roenigk Jr HH, Auerbach R, Maibach HI, Weinstein GD: Methotrexate in psoriasis: revised guidelines, *J Am Acad Dermatol* 19: 145-156, 1988.

42. Shergy WJ, Polisson RP, Caldwell DS, Rice JR, Pietesky DS, Allen NB: Methotrexate-associated hepatotoxicity: retrospective analysis of 210 patients with rheumatoid arthiritis, *Am J Med* 85: 771-774, 1988.

43. Starzl TE, Todo S, Fung J, et al: FK506 for liver, kidney, and pancreas transplantation, *Lancet* 2: 1000-1004, 1989.

44. Miiles, L, Todo S, Fung JJ, et al: Oral glucose tolerance test in liver recipients treated with FK506, *Transplant Proc* 22: 41-43, 1990.

45. McCauley J, Fung J, Jain A, et al: The effects of FK506 on renal function after liver transplantation, *Transplant Proc* 22:17-20, 1990.

THE URGENT OPERATIVE PATIENT

16

> strange faces
> scary places
> lights and white
> helpless fright
> VOICES . . . .
>
> Andrienne Coleman

In many childhood emergencies, the anesthesiologist is consulted to assist with securing the airway, ventilation, placement of intravenous catheters, and invasive monitoring as part of the resuscitation before the patient actually comes to the operating room. For the critical patient, the continuity of care from the emergency department or neonatal unit to diagnostic facilities to the operating room and ultimately the intensive care setting falls under the direction of the anesthesiologist.

THE RESPIRATORY SYSTEM AND THORAX

Airway Emergencies

Refer to Chapter 8.

Congenital Pulmonary Defects[1]

BRONCHOGENIC AND PULMONARY CYSTS[2]

1. Congenital bronchogenic cysts are formed by primordial respiratory tissue isolated from the developing lung. The location and size of the cyst are critical determinants of respiratory compromise. Carinal cysts can cause dramatic respiratory decompensation, as the cyst enlarges to obstruct the mainstem bronchi and cause air trapping. This situation may occur in the neonate, necessitating emergency decompression of the cyst to allow adequate ventilation. Bronchogenic cysts of the hilum or parenchyma often cause chronic infections with abscess formation. The cyst is resected in late infancy or early childhood to prevent recurrent pulmonary infections.
2. Pulmonary cysts may have no significant systemic effect until expanded by N_2O, or until gas trapping with adjacent atelectasis is caused by positive-pressure ventilation. If these occur, mediastinal shifting and cardiac compromise are possible.

LOBAR EMPHYSEMA

Congenital lobar emphysema occurs in the neonatal period as progressive respiratory distress. Chest radiographs reveal unilateral thoracic hyperexpansion with mediastinal shift and contralateral atelectasis. High intrathoracic pressures generated by the emphysematous lobe may decrease cardiac output. Because most commonly only the left upper lobe is affected, the condition can usually be treated successfully by lobectomy. Congenital heart disease coexists in about 15% of patients.

ANESTHETIC MANAGEMENT: CONGENITAL PULMONARY DEFECTS

1. Anesthesia is usually induced with halothane and oxygen by mask inhalation with spontaneous ventilation. If assisted ventilation is necessary, low peak inspiratory pressures should be used, with adequate time allowed for exhalation. Positive-pressure ventilation may increase intrathoracic pressure and worsen air trapping.
2. N_2O should be avoided because it can cause expansion of the emphysematous lobe or cyst. Oxygen and air mixtures should be used to maintain an adequate FIO_2 and saturation.
3. The trachea can be intubated without muscle relaxants, and spontaneous ventilation is maintained until the chest is opened. Alternatively, titrated doses of propofol or ketamine may be used to maintain spontaneous ventilation, combined with local anesthetic infiltration at the incision site.
4. One-lung ventilation may be useful to isolate an infected cyst or to improve visualization of the surgical field. In the neonate, it may be necessary to advance the endotracheal tube into the selected bronchus under direct vision of the surgeon. Alternatively, a Fogarty catheter may be placed in the bronchus through the surgical field. Usually, flow to the ipsilateral pulmonary artery also must be restricted during the procedure to decrease shunting.

Congenital Diaphragmatic Hernia (CDH)
INTRODUCTION[3-5]

1. The incidence of herniation of bowel contents into the chest in utero with concurrent lung hypoplasia is approximately 1:2000 to 1:5000 live births. It occurs more often in males than females (2:1). The most common form is the posterolateral or Bochdalek hernia, which is seen in 85% to 90% of patients. Approximately 80% of hernias occur on the left side.
2. Associated anomalies are observed in 25% to 30% of babies with diaphragmatic herniation and may increase morbidity and mortality significantly. These include: anencephaly, meningomyelo-

cele, hydrocephalus, encephalocele, ventricular septal defects, vascular rings, coarctation, trisomy 13, trisomy 18.
3. Polyhydramnios on prenatal sonogram is an early indicator of herniation. Respiratory distress is usually apparent within the first 24 hours of life. Rarely, a small hernia may be asymptomatic, but classically, CDH presents with dyspnea, cyanosis, and apparent dextrocardia as the heart is displaced rightward by the presence of bowel in the left chest. On examination, the infant shows scaphoid abdomen and barrel chest. Radiographs reveal bowel in the chest with mediastinal shift and absence of intraabdominal air.

Pathophysiology[3,4,6]

1. In the hypoplastic lung, vessels are histologically smaller in diameter and possess a thicker region of smooth muscle. The thickened smooth muscle also extends farther distally into the bronchioles. As a result, the pulmonary vasculature becomes hyperactive, displaying an exaggerated vasoconstrictive response to hypoxia, hypercapnia, acidosis, pain, or positive-pressure ventilation. This hyperactive pulmonary vasculature may also be present in the normal lung.
2. Usually, a brief "honeymoon" period of stability exists immediately after birth, during which the infant has adequate respiration before the development of pulmonary hypertension. With the onset of hypertension, an increase in pulmonary vascular resistance elevates pulmonary artery pressure. Venous blood is then preferentially shunted across the patent ductus arteriosus or patent foramen ovale into the systemic circulation (right-to-left shunt). This constellation is referred to as persistent fetal circulation (PFC) or primary pulmonary hypertension of the newborn (PPHN). The major determinants of outcome are the degree and reversibility of the pulmonary hypertension.

Preoperative Management[3,4,7-10]

1. Historically, CDH has been considered a surgical emergency. However, the hernia repair does not actually increase pulmonary surface area for gas exchange in the hypoplastic lung. Further, more recent evidence indicates that the mechanics of surgery may actually be deleterious to pulmonary compliance. Since pulmonary hypertension and shunting are responsible for outcome, a period of medical stabilization before operation may be important to allow for normal neonatal lung remodelling, which decreases muscle thickness in pulmonary vessels. The decision to operate immediately or postpone remains controversial.
2. If immediate respiratory support is required, the baby's trachea is intubated awake. Mask ventilation is avoided to prevent fur-

ther dilation of the stomach, and an orogastric or nasogastric catheter should be used to evacuate the stomach immediately after intubation.

3. The neonate's lungs are immature and as such are susceptible to barotrauma and oxygen toxicity. Peak inspiratory pressures are kept low (<30 cm H_2O) to avoid contralateral pneumothorax, as higher pressures are preferentially deferred to the larger-diameter airways. High-frequency oscillating ventilation (HFOV) may decrease the possibility of barotrauma.

4. Extracorporeal membrane oxygenation (ECMO) was first used in 1975 to treat acute respiratory failure in neonates. It is a form of cardiopulmonary bypass whereby a portion of the cardiac output is diverted to a membrane oxygenator to meet oxygen demands and allow the lungs to "rest." Infants at highest risk for mortality are frequently treated with ECMO prior to hernia repair. The anesthesia team may be asked to participate in catheter placement before beginning ECMO or to assist at any time while the patient is connected to the oxygenator. Frequently, the actual surgical repair is performed in the neonatal intensive care unit while the infant remains on partial bypass. These infants have been anesthetized using high-dose fentanyl or sufentanil to block the stress response and concomitant catecholamine release. Larger than usual doses are required to counteract the increased volume of distribution of the oxygenator and binding of the opiates to the membrane.

5. Treatment modalities for PPHN are listed in the box at right.

ANESTHETIC MANAGEMENT[6,12,13]

1. Intraoperative goals of diaphragmatic hernia repair consist of maximizing arterial oxygenation while minimizing pulmonary vasoconstriction from hypoxia, hypercapnia, acidosis, pain, and physiologic stress.

2. If the infant trachea has not already been intubated, the technique outlined above under Preoperative Management is recommended.

3. Hyperventilation at rapid rates and low inspiratory pressures will help maintain oxygenation, while avoiding hypercapnia and barotrauma.

4. Standard monitors and a preductal (right radial) arterial catheter for monitoring blood pressure and blood gas analysis are required. Central venous catheters are helpful for volume replacement and monitoring. A precordial stethoscope in the contralateral axilla will help to monitor for pneumothorax in the "good" lung.

5. Anesthesia can be maintained with high-dose opiates (e.g., fentanyl, 50 µg/kg) to block the stress response and muscle relaxants. Inhalation agents are usually avoided because of their

Congenital diaphragmatic hernia: treatment modalities for primary pulmonary hypertension of the newborn (PPHN)[11,12]

Modalities	Drug or techniques	Comments
Pharmacologic	Vasodilators: tolazoline, nitroglycerin, nitroprusside, prostaglandin, isoproterenol (see Appendix E, p.664, for infusion doses)	Dilate systemic vasculature while dilating pulmonary vasculature
	Nitric oxide	Selective pulmonary vasodilation with minimal systemic effects May cause methemoglobinemia
	Bicarbonate infusion	Alkalosis decreases pulmonary vascular resistance
	Vasopressors: dopamine, epinephrine	Although these may worsen PPHN, they are sometimes needed to support circulation with vasodilator therapy
Ventilatory	Low peak inspiratory pressures (<30 cm H_2O) High-frequency oscillating ventilation (HFOV)	These techniques help to avoid barotrauma in the "good" lung
Operative	ECMO	Increases survival in high-risk infants Infants require continuous sedation over days
	Closure of patent ductus	Decreases pulmonary blood flow

hypotensive and cardiac depressant effects. Nitrous oxide is rarely used, because it can expand bowel and because most of these patients require high concentrations of inspired oxygen.

6. Intraoperative treatment of pulmonary hypertension with vasodilators and bicarbonate (as discussed above) may be necessary. Inotropic agents should be available for circulatory support.

7. After hernia reduction, the temptation to "expand" the hypoplastic lung must be avoided, as this maneuver may cause contralateral pneumothorax. Since the "good" lung is responsible for nearly all gas exchange, pneumothorax can cause immediate and profound decompensation.

8. Mechanical ventilation, treatment of pulmonary hypertension, and circulatory support will be required in the postoperative period. If surgery is performed immediately, the postoperative course is heralded by a "honeymoon" period of 1 to 24 hours where improvement is seen, followed by rapid deterioration with potentially irreversible hypoxemia and acidosis as pulmonary hypertension develops.

Esophageal Atresia[13-15]

1. The incidence of esophageal atresia (EA) with tracheo-esophageal fistula (TEF) is approximately 1:3000 to 1:4000 live births.

2. There are five major presentations of EA and TEF (see Fig. 16-1). The most common type is IIIB, which consists of a proximal esophageal blind pouch with the distal esophagus connected to the trachea by a fistula close to the carina (80%). As a result gastric secretions may reflux into the trachea and lungs, producing severe chemical pneumonitis.

3. Almost 50% of infants with EA have associated congenital anomalies significant enough to affect survival.

Congenital defects associated with esophageal atresia

Cardiac—ventricular septal defect, patent ductus arteriosus, tetralogy of Fallot
Gastrointestinal—imperforate anus, duodenal atresia, malrotation
Genitourinary—ureteral reflux, horseshoe kidney, renal agenesis
Musculoskeletal—vertebral, rib, or extremity defects
Chromosomal abnormalities
VATER syndrome:
  Vertebral defects
  Anal atresia
  Tracheoesophageal fistula
  Esophageal atresia
  Renal defects/Radial abnormalities

---

4. Although polyhydramnios may be present during gestation, the diagnosis of TEF usually is made at birth upon failure to pass a catheter into the stomach. Excessive oral secretions are noted, and coughing, cyanosis, and choking occur with first feeding. Chest radiograph shows the catheter coiled in the blind esophageal pouch. Radiographic contrast through the nasogastric tube should be avoided, as it may lead to aspiration.

5. When TEF is suspected, the infant's head is elevated to prevent aspiration, oral feeding is stopped, and an intravenous catheter is placed. Evaluation for coexistent anomalies should include echocardiography.

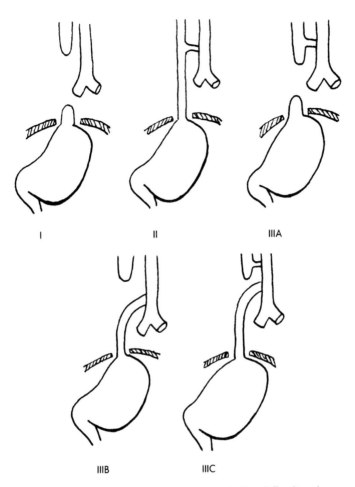

FIG. 16-1. Classification of tracheoesophageal fistula. Type I: Esophageal atresia with no esophageal communication with the trachea. Type II: Esophagus has no disruption of its continuity but has tracheoesophageal fistula. Type IIIA: Esophageal atresia with proximal esophageal fistula to trachea. Type IIIB: Proximal esophageal blind pouch with distal esophageal tracheal fistula. Type IIIC: Esophageal atresia with tracheal fistula from proximal and distal esophageal segments. (Adapted from Dierdord SF, Krishna G: Anesthetic management of neonatal surgical emergencies, *Anes Analg* 60:208, 1981.)

6. Positive-pressure ventilation may be required for the infant in respiratory distress. If so, an emergent gastrostomy may become necessary to decompress the stomach. If the treatment plan includes delay of primary repair, gastrostomy can be placed under local anesthesia, regional anesthesia, or general anesthesia. Aggressive pulmonary toilet, broad-spectrum an-

tibiotics, and total parenteral nutrition are indicated if the definitive repair is delayed.

ANESTHETIC MANAGEMENT

1. Awake tracheal intubation after suction of the esophageal pouch minimizes the possibility of gastric distension during mask ventilation.
2. The endotracheal tube (ETT) is positioned distal to the fistula and above the carina and secured well. Correct tube position can be ensured by several techniques:
   a. Placing the ETT into the right mainstem bronchus and slowly withdrawing until bilateral breath sounds are confirmed. Leaving the ETT in the right bronchus intraoperatively may result in severe hypoxia, as the right lung is compressed during thoracotomy.
   b. A left mainstem intubation throughout the repair is theoretically possible, although usually neonates have insufficient pulmonary reserve to tolerate one-lung ventilation.
   c. If the gastrostomy tube is present, the end of the tube can be placed in a beaker of sterile water. The presence of bubbles during ventilation indicates the ETT is above the fistula. The bubbles disappear as the ETT is advanced.
   d. The gastrostomy tube may be connected to the capnograph. ETT placement above the fistula will be indicated by a CO_2 curve, which disappears as the tube is advanced below the fistula.
3. If not already present, the gastrostomy tube is placed as soon as possible after intubation to avoid gastric distension, which may decrease ventilation and venous return to the heart.
4. The patient is placed in the left lateral decubitus position for right thoracotomy (fistula ligation and primary esophageal anastamosis). Standard monitors should include continuous capnography and placement of a precordial stethoscope in the left axilla. High-risk patients may also require placement of a radial or umbilical artery catheter to continuously monitor blood pressure and to facilitate monitoring arterial blood gases.
5. Intravenous or inhalation agents with muscle relaxation may be used. High-dose opioid techniques may be more effective at blocking the physiologic stress response in high-risk infants, particularly those with coexistent cardiac disease.
6. During the repair, the trachea may obstruct from bleeding or technical problems. Frequent endotracheal suction is usually necessary.

POSTOPERATIVE CONSIDERATIONS

1. Tracheal extubation is encouraged as soon as possible to avoid prolonged pressure on suture lines. Tracheomalacia is a com-

mon finding, and the infant must be observed carefully after extubation for signs of tracheal collapse. Some advocate leaving the ETT in place for 24 to 48 hours postoperatively to avoid trauma to the anastomosis if reintubation due to tracheomalacia is required.

2. Endotracheal suction is performed only with catheters no longer than the distance to the anastomotic line.

3. The esophagus is carefully observed for an anastomotic leak. Total parenteral nutrition is required during the NPO interval.

4. The most frequent complication is pneumonitis or atelectasis. Broad-spectrum antibiotics are usually recommended in the postoperative period.

OUTCOME

Survival of infants with EA is reported as high as 85% to 90%, with associated congenital anomalies being the main cause of death. Esophageal dysmotility and reflux are common. Chronic stricture formation at the esophageal anastomosis is also common, necessitating frequent trips to the operating room for dilatation throughout infancy and childhood. Persistent tracheomalacia is seen in less than 20% of patients.

GASTROINTESTINAL EMERGENCIES
Omphalocele and Gastroschesis[14-17]

Omphalocele and gastroschesis (see box on p. 378 for characteristics) are defects of the anterior abdominal wall with herniation or evisceration of bowel contents through the defect.

PREOPERATIVE CONSIDERATIONS

The prevention of infection and minimization of heat and fluid loss are major concerns. The following measures should be instituted at birth, and continued until the defect is closed:

1. In patients with gastroschesis and ruptured omphalocele, considerable protein loss and fluid translocation can occur because of the absence of a protective membranous sac. Colloid should be given to maintain normal oncotic pressure. Hemoconcentration and metabolic acidosis may be evident, and aggressive fluid therapy should be based on urine output, measurement of serial hematocrit, and arterial blood gases.

2. The herniated viscus should be covered with warm sterile saline-soaked gauze and plastic wrap to minimize fluid and heat loss, as well as infection and bowel injury.

3. A neutral thermal environment should be maintained.

4. A nasogastric tube should be placed to prevent regurgitation and aspiration.

5. Systemic antibiotics should be started early.

Characteristics of abdominal wall defects

	Omphalocele	Gastroschesis
Defect	Herniation of the viscera into the base of the umbilical cord through a central defect; membranous sac covers and protects gut; however, the sac may rupture	Evisceration of gut through 2-5 cm defect in abdominal wall lateral to the umbilicus; no sac covers viscera; viscera directly exposed to chemical burn from amniotic fluid and environment
Embryologic process	Failure of the gut to migrate back into abdominal cavity and thus failure of abdominal wall to develop	Intrauterine occlusion of the omphalomesenteric artery, resulting in a defect of the abdominal wall lateral to the umbilicus
Incidence	1/5000-1/10,000	1/15,000-1/30,000
Incidence of prematurity	30%	60%
Associated congenital anomalies	80% incidence, including: Chromosomal—trisomy 13, 15, 21 Cardiac Genitourinary—bladder exstrophy Craniofacial—cleft palate, jaw and tongue tumors, hemangiomas Diaphragm anomalies Pentalogy of Cantrell— ectopia cordis, sternal cleft, diaphragmatic defect, cardiac disease, omphalocele Beckwith-Wiedemann syndrome—macroglossia, gigantism, hypoglycemia, umbilical anomalies	Rare

ANESTHETIC MANAGEMENT

1. After decompression of the stomach and preoxygenation the awake infant's trachea is intubated.
2. Because prolonged postoperative ventilation usually is required, an opiate technique is reasonable for maintenance of anesthesia. Inhalation agents may be used judiciously in the well-hydrated infant. Muscle relaxants are used to facilitate closure of the defect. N_2O should be avoided because of bowel distention.

3. Primary closure depends on the size of the defect and the development of the anterior abdominal wall. Small defects can be closed primarily. Larger defects require a staged reduction over several days or weeks.

4. Changes in pulmonary compliance will help guide the surgical repair. When the abdomen is closed tightly, peak inspiratory pressures rise, impairing diaphragmatic excursion. A tight repair can impede venous return and thereby reduce cardiac output by caval compression. Bowel ischemia and eventual wound dehiscence may result. Airway pressures, oxygen saturation, and arterial blood gases should be observed carefully during closure of the defect. An intraabdominal or bladder pressure less than 20 mm Hg (or a CVP <4 mm Hg) has been advocated as an indicator of successful primary closure.[18,19] If pressures exceed these limits, staged repair may improve outcome. Heart rate, blood pressure, and systemic vascular resistance have not been shown to be reliable indicators of successful closure.[18]

5. In a staged procedure a dacron-reinforced Silastic silo is placed over the defect and reduced gradually. These procedures can be performed on the intubated infant quite expeditiously with small doses of ketamine or opioid. Muscle relaxation may be required.

6. In addition to standard monitoring, all infants should have airway pressures followed carefully. The use of invasive monitoring depends upon the size of the defect. A large defect requires arterial cannulation for blood gas analysis to guide fluid resuscitation and respiratory support.

7. Successful use of spinal anesthesia for primary repair of small defects has been reported. This technique avoids intubation while allowing for maximal abdominal wall relaxation.[20]

POSTOPERATIVE MANAGEMENT

1. Most infants require postoperative mechanical ventilation. Airway pressures, oxygenation, and respiratory efforts should be observed carefully, and sedation and muscle relaxation provided as needed. Respiratory insufficiency in infants with abdominal wall defects may be due to impaired antenatal lung growth, as these infants are found to have a significantly lower functional residual capacity than normal infants.[21]

2. Prolonged postoperative ileus is not unusual and may necessitate parenteral alimentation.

TRAUMA

Trauma continues to be responsible for 50% of deaths in United States children between the ages of 1 and 14 years.[22] Victims of major trauma usually sustain injuries to more than one organ system, making rapid assessment and evaluation of the entire patient essential. Life-threatening injuries must be identified and treated rapidly; young trauma patients often stabilize vital signs with initial resuscitation and then rapidly decompensate if the injury is not repaired.

Pediatric trauma: children are not just small adults

Anatomic feature of infants and children	Susceptibility to trauma
Relatively large occiput	Prominence of head injuries with motor vehicle accidents and falls is due to: • Greater head-body ratio • Position of head in slight flexion because of large size
Cervical spine • More flexible ligaments • Flatter facets with horizontal orientation • Incomplete ossification	C-spine injuries less common in children than adults In children < 8 yr, injuries are more common at C1-C3 level because of horizontal facets Incomplete ossification and pseudosubluxation (C2-C3) mimic fractures
Airway (infants) • Obligate nasal breathing • Relatively large tongue	Airway obstruction more likely due to nasal passage obstruction or tongue resting against palate.
Greater body surface area–mass ratio	More susceptible to dehydration More susceptible to hypothermia
Mediastinum more mobile	Greater displacement of heart and great vessels by tension pneumothorax
Skeletal elasticity	Kinetic energy absorbed by soft tissue structures rather than bones

Assessment: Trauma Scores[23,24]

Trauma scores were originally designed to provide rapid assessment, simplify triage, and help predict outcome. They are useful for overall management, but are less sensitive for specific organ injury. Initial trauma scores will help guide the anesthesiologist regarding severity of injury, but will not give sufficient information to dictate induction techniques (e.g., presence of increased intracranial pressure versus hypovolemia).

The Pediatric Trauma Score[25] considers the child's size, airway stature, neurologic status, systolic blood pressure, and presence of skeletal injuries and open wounds.

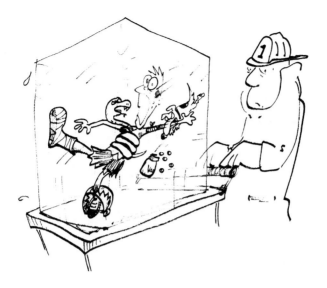

Pediatric trauma score*

Variable	+2	+1	−1
Weight (kg)	>20	10-20	<10
Airway patency	Normal	Maintained	Unmaintained
Systolic blood pressure (mm Hg)	>90	50-90	<50
Neurologic status	Awake	Obtunded	Comatose
Open wound	None	Minor	Major
Skeletal trauma	None	Closed	Open or multiple

*A score of +2, +1, or −1 is given for each variable listed. The scores are then added (range, −6 to +12). A score ≤8 indicates potentially significant trauma.

Preoperative Management

The anesthetic management of the acutely injured child begins with the anesthesiologist's first consultation for assessment and control of the ABCs: airway, breathing, circulation. Vital signs, ventilatory function, level of consciousness, potential for closed head injury, and presence of thoracic or abdominal injuries should be quickly evaluated on initial inspection.

AIRWAY[22,24,26-28]

Airway obstruction by blood, vomitus, foreign body, edema, or the tongue is the most common cause of respiratory failure in pediatric trauma patients. Immediate treatment should proceed in the following order:

1. Clearing the airway of secretions
2. Jaw thrust; open mouth
3. Administration of supplemental oxygen
4. Endotracheal intubation
5. Cricothyrotomy

Oral or nasal airways may produce gagging or vomiting and should be used with caution. The indications for emergent endotracheal intubation for pediatric trauma patients should be carefully delineated by discussion with the trauma team at each institution. It has been retrospectively shown that as many as 25% of infants and children emergently intubated for trauma have serious complications of airway management.[27,28]

Indications for emergent intubation of pediatric trauma patients

Inability to maintain an adequate airway
Hypoxia
Abnormal respiratory pattern
Shock
Coma
Increased risk of aspiration
Inability to clear secretions
Need to contol ventilation (decrease Pa_{CO_2})

The technique of emergent intubation should be selected based on patient injuries and condition. Awake intubation is usually reserved for infants with severe airway obstruction or infants and children with sufficiently depressed consciousness that no resistance is offered that may cause airway trauma during intubation.[27] Atropine is often advocated to avoid reflex bradycardia, particularly in infants and younger children.

Most commonly, orotracheal intubation with a rapid-sequence induction is selected, consisting of atropine pretreatment and preoxygenation, a rapid-onset induction agent (thiopental, ketamine, propofol), and succinylcholine. Succinylcholine should be used with extreme caution in burn patients or those with massive crush injury, who may be hyperkalemic, or in patients with intracranial injuries or open globe (see pp. 212 and 231). Rapid-onset nondepolarizing muscle relaxants (rocuronium, 0.6 to 1.2 mg/kg) may be used alternatively. Cricoid pressure is advocated unless laryngeal trauma is present. In patients at risk for cervical spine injuries, the neck should be immobilized in a neutral position with manual stabilization by a trained assistant during intubation.

Emergent nasotracheal intubation is not recommended, as it may cause nasal bleeding or plugging of the endotracheal tube from adenoidal tissue. It is also more difficult in young children because of the more cephalad larynx.[27]

Recommended techniques for emergent intubation of the trauma patient (see also The Difficult Airway, p. 182)

	Advantages	Disadvantages
Rapid sequence	Rapidly secures airway under direct vision and controlled circumstances	Spontaneous respiration halted prior to checking ability to ventilate Increased risk of aspiration
"Awake"	Usually saved for the extremely obtunded or apneic patient Whatever reflexes or spontaneous respiration are present are preserved	Increased risk of laryngospasm and vomiting if reflexes still present May be traumatic
Laryngeal mask airway (LMA)	Easy to place blindly when glottis is poorly visualized An endotracheal tube over a fiberoptic bronchoscope may be directed through the LMA lumen	Does not guard against aspiration in patients at risk May not be effective for positive-pressure ventilation
Lighted stylet	Can be used for blind placement when glottis poorly visualized Can be placed without manipulating cervical spine	Requires knowledge of technique and experience Does not decrease risk of aspiration Can dislodge foreign body
Fiberoptic bronchoscopy	Allows for visualization of the glottis without neck manipulation Can be performed in the awake patient with topical anesthetics	Visualization difficult with blood and debris in airway Requires knowledgeable practitioner and expensive equipment Time consuming Difficult in the uncooperative child
Needle cricothyrotomy	Can be performed rapidly even by a minimally trained practitioner	May be difficult in very small children Easier to perform with the neck extended Must have an avenue for egress of air, especially if used with jet ventilation, to avoid barotrauma

BREATHING[22,26,27]

After airway obstruction, pneumothorax and hemothorax are the next most common causes of ventilatory failure in pediatric trauma patients. Absence of equally bilateral breath sounds and chest expansion, hypoxemia, cyanosis, neck vein distension, and tracheal deviation may all indicate lung collapse due to air or blood. Pulse oximetry is not always useful in patients with decreased peripheral perfusion; clinical signs may dictate placement of a chest tube.

CIRCULATION

Shock.   For trauma patients, the most common form of shock is hypovolemic or hemorrhagic. Hypotension may also occur with pneumothorax, pericardial tamponade, acidosis, and intracranial hypertension.

Assessing the child for acute hypovolemia[26,29]

1. Actual intravascular volume loss is usually greater than anticipated.
2. Blood pressure is a poor indicator of hypovolemia, as children will maintain a near normal central blood pressure even with an acute 25% loss of intravascular volume, because of a compensatory baroreceptor-mediated response.
3. Marked tachycardia, particularly with an increased systemic vascular resistance (cool extremities, mottling, delayed capillary refill), is a better prognostic indicator of hypovolemia.
4. Differential pulse assessment (central compared to peripheral) is also an indicator of acute volume loss.
5. Tachypnea and dyspnea are seen with hypovolemic shock as the patient tries to increase oxygen delivery.
6. Agitation, lethargy, and/or hypotonia are neurologic signs of severe hypovolemia (see also Massive Hemorrhage, p. 386, for treatment protocols).

Head Trauma

1. The most common cause of morbidity and mortality in salvageable head injuries is acute hypoxia caused by the tongue obstructing the airway in the unconscious patient.
2. Immediate intubation ensures a patent airway, limits the risks of aspiration, and allows for hyperventilation to decrease intracranial pressure.
3. Cervical spine injuries often accompany head trauma. Although cervical spine radiographs are helpful for determining possible fractures, airway management should never be neglected while films are being obtained. A trained assistant can hold the head in a neutral position, with immobilization during intubation of necessary. Blind nasal intubations may cause bleeding or further intracranial trauma through undiagnosed facial fractures. Fiberoptic or awake intubations are difficult in an uncooperative child.
   a. If cervical spine injury is clinically apparent, It is important to document the level of spinal cord injury and the extent of deficit before performing intubation or operative procedures.

Children less than 8 years of age tend to have higher-level injuries (C1 to C3), which probably explains the high rate of fatalities (60%).[30]

    b. Intraoperatively, neuromuscular blockade may interfere with the surgeon's assessment of cord injury. Somatosensory-evoked potentials may be useful to monitor nerve and spinal cord integrity in the presence of neuromuscular blockade.

4. The presence of elevated intracranial pressure (ICP) should be determined quickly (hypertension, bradycardia, irregular respiration, pupil dilatation, posturing).

    a. The most common initial finding on computed tomography (CT) is diffuse cerebral swelling, which mandates early and aggressive treatment. As with adults, these measures include hyperventilation and diuresis.

    b. Systemic hypertension must be avoided, and the head should be carefully elevated and positioned, without any obstruction to venous outflow.

    c. Patients with high ICP should be tracheally intubated with atropine 0.02 mg/kg, thiopental 5 to 10 mg/kg, and succinylcholine 2 mg/kg with cricoid pressure. Thiopental should not be used in the presence of significant hypovolemia, hypotension, or shock. Succinylcholine should be avoided in crush injuries because of the potential for hyperkalemia.

5. It is rare to have hypotension with head injury except as a terminal event. Other sources of bleeding should be suspected.

6. Neurologic function after injury can be described and documented by the *Glasgow Coma Scale* (see box). Although this

Glasgow coma scale[31]	
Eye opening	
Spontaneous	4
To speech	3
To pain	2
None	1
Verbal response	
Oriented	5
Confused conversation	4
Inappropriate words	3
Incomprehensible sounds	2
Nil	1
Best motor response	
Obeys	6
Localizes	5
Withdraws	4
Abnormal flexion—decorticate	3
Extensor response—decerebrate	2
Nil	1
Total	3-15

scale allows uniformity in evaluating level of consciousness, it does not necessarily correlate with the CT scan findings or predict outcome. It is best used for following the progression of neurologic symptoms.

Massive Hemorrhage (see also Assessing the Child for Acute Hypovolemia, p. 384)

Patients with massive hemorrhage usually will stabilize briefly with crystalloid infusion. If necessary, type-specific blood is given. Time is of the essence. It usually is not possible to continuously replace volume losses from an unrepaired major vascular injury. The anesthesiologist must be prepared for rapid volume replacement and transport to the operating room.

TREATMENT OF HYPOVOLEMIC SHOCK: FLUID RESUSCITATION[32]

Obtaining intravenous access is often the most challenging part of acute fluid resuscitation in pediatric trauma patients.

1. Since speed of fluid flow is inversely related to catheter length, resuscitation may proceed more rapidly with two large-bore peripheral catheters than with a single-lumen central catheter.
2. Fluid delivery to the central circulation is essentially the same whether it is delivered above or below the diaphragm, even if the inferior vena cava is occluded.[33,34]
3. A suggested order for accessing the venous circulation is listed below. Techniques for insertion of catheters at these sites may be found in Appendix C, p. 655.

Order of sites for access to venous circulation for trauma patients

---

Percutaneous sites in the distal forearm and hand
Percutaneous saphenous vein
Distal saphenous vein cutdown
Percutaneous femoral vein[35]
Jugular and subclavian catheter placement is difficult with CPR in progress and carries significant risks of complications, notably pneumothorax
Intraosseous

Intraosseous infusion.[36-38]   Intraosseous infusion enables temporary access to the venous circulation for resuscitation. It is generally recommended for life-threatening situations in patients less than 6 years of age, when three attempts to achieve venous access have failed or more than 90 seconds has elapsed. The needle is inserted into the bone marrow of the proximal tibia (see Appendix C,

p. 661); therefore the procedure is contraindicated in the presence of fracture or vascular disruption to the extremity. Reported complications include compartment syndrome, fat embolism, tibial fracture, growth plate injuries, cellulitis, and osteomyelitis.

Fluid selection and administration

1. Intravenous fluids are administered to maintain plasma oncotic pressure, which can successfully be accomplished using crystalloid or colloid. Since no advantage of one over the other has been proven, crystalloid is usually administered because it is significantly more cost effective. Approximately 2 to 3 times the volume of crystalloid is needed as compared to colloid.[29]

2. Isotonic fluids (lactated Ringer's or normal saline) are generally recommended for pediatric resuscitation, using boluses of 20 ml/kg by rapid infusion. If there is no improvement after 3 boluses of crystalloid, red blood cells (10 to 20 ml/kg) are given.[22,26]

3. The use of hypertonic saline (7.5%) may improve survival in patients with head injuries and raised intracranial pressure.[39,40]

4. Glucose-containing infusions are avoided, as glucose can act as an osmotic diuretic and be detrimental to initial resuscitative efforts. Further, glucose infusions have been associated with poorer outcome when administered prior to global cerebral ischemia.[41]

5. Dextran and hetastarch, synthetic colloids, are effective at acutely increasing oncotic pressure. They are, however, associated with decreased platelet function and not generally advocated for the acute trauma patient.[29]

INTRAOPERATIVE ANESTHETIC MANAGEMENT[42-44]

Monitoring

1. As an important member of the trauma team, the anesthesiologist is responsible for continuously monitoring the patient while performing resuscitation, during transport to the operating room, intraoperatively, and postoperatively for transport to the ICU or PACU.

2. In addition to standard monitors (ECG, oximetry, blood pressure, and capnometry), invasive monitors (arterial and central venous catheters) are usually needed to rapidly assess blood pressure and intravascular volume. In children, CVP monitoring is as reliable in the inferior vena cava (by femoral vein catheter) as in the superior vena cava.[45]

3. When speed is essential, some monitors can perform more than one function. An oximeter with plethysmograph can give heart rate, oxygen saturation, and a rough estimate of peripheral perfusion. Capnography supplies both end-tidal CO_2 measurements and an estimate of cardiac output. Rapidly applying

these two monitors may allow the surgical team to proceed in a life-theatening situation while the anesthetists continue to resuscitate and apply remaining monitors.

4. Temperature monitoring often is overlooked in a crisis situation. However, hypothermia from exposure and massive infusion of cold fluids is a common problem in trauma victims. Besides increasing acidosis, hypothermia may result in cardiac fibrillation or arrest.

Induction.   Severely injured children have usually undergone tracheal intubation as part of the resuscitative process (see Airway, p. 381). A more controlled induction of anesthesia in the operating room may be appropriate for more stable patients. Nevertheless, all trauma patients are presumed to have a "full stomach" and are at risk for aspiration, dictating a rapid-sequence induction. The choice of induction agent depends upon the child's neurologic and volume status.

Common induction agents: pediatric trauma

	Advantages	Disadvantages
Sodium thiopental	Rapid acting No pain on injection Lowers intracranial and intraocular pressure	Depresses myocardial function May cause marked hypotension if inadequate volume resuscitation
Ketamine	Usually raises heart rate and blood pressure Analgesic properties	May cause hypotension if catecholamines depleted Usually causes dysphoria Probably raises intracranial and intraocular pressure
Propofol	Lowers intracranial and intraocular pressure Rapid emergence	May be more painful when injected into small vessels May cause hypotension, especially if hypovolemia is present

Maintenance.   If hemodynamically unstable, trauma patients may tolerate very little anesthesia. Volatile agents may worsen hypotension. Ketamine or fentanyl may be used judiciously. At the very least, amnestic agents (scopolamine, benzodiazapines) should be administered, as recall during trauma surgery is not uncommon.

Inotropic agents (dopamine or dobutamine at 3 to 12 μg/kg/min) may be used to support blood pressure. Sodium bicarbonate will correct severe metabolic acidosis. Transfusion techniques and requirements are discussed in Chapter 4.

Emergence and extubation.   Children with minor trauma may tolerate tracheal extubation after fully emerging to the awake state with intact reflexes. These patients should exhibit cardiovascular stability, normothermia, and spontaneous ventilation with adequate oxygenation.

Continued mechanical ventilation is recommended for patients with the following:

- Cardiovascular instability
- Respiratory insufficiency
- Increased intracranial pressure
- Extensive trauma
- Pain associated with respiration
- Metabolic derangement
- Sepsis
- Hypothermia
- Coagulopathy
- Continuing fluid shifts

BURNS[46-49]

Burn injuries in the United States claim the lives of 3000 children and disable 9000 others under the age of 15 each year. Because of the prolonged treatment process, intense pain and suffering, and potential for disfigurement, both children who suffer burns and their parents require special support and attention. The anesthesiologist has the expertise in fluid resuscitation, transfusion therapy, and pain management to assist in the ongoing management of these patients, as well as caring for them in their frequent trips to the operating room.

History

1. The history must include details of the burn injury, especially the amount of time elapsed since the burn and the type of burn. Thermal burns (flame and scald) are the most common type of burns in children, as compared to chemical, electrical or radiation etiologies. Flame burns with coexistent inhalation injury are responsible for the majority of fatalities.[46]
2. In an electrical burn, the extent of injury is often greater than seen externally.
3. A fire in an enclosed space raises the suspicion of smoke inhalation and suggests the need to check carboxyhemoglobin levels and perform bronchosopy. Cyanide toxicity from the byproducts of burned synthetic materials is also a frequent occurrence.
4. Evidence of associated injuries (cervical spine injury, fractures, internal organ injury) should be sought, as well as any pertinent data from the child's medical history.

Physical Examination

1. The physical examination should focus immediately on the airway. With head and neck burns, hoarseness and wheezing may indicate upper airway involvement. The presence of carbonaceous sputum suggests smoke inhalation injury.
2. The extent and depth of the burn should be documented to calculate fluid resuscitation (see Fig. 16-2 to calculate burn percentage).
3. Sites for potential vascular access should be identified.

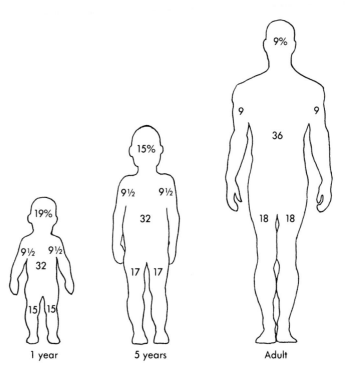

FIG. 16-2. The age of the patient must be considered when calculating the percent of body surface involved in a burn injury. (Adapted from Smith EI: Acute management of thermal burns in children, *Surg Clin North Am* 50:807-814, 1970.)

Securing the Airway

1. All burn patients, especially those with inhalation injuries, are considered hypoxemic and should receive 100% oxygen. Carbon monoxide toxicity is common. Since carboxyhemoglobin is not detected by pulse oximetry, hemoximetry, which fractionates hemoglobin, should be obtained (see Chapter 3, p. 57).
2. If any airway compromise is anticipated, the trachea should be

intubated immediately. Airway edema following a major burn can be extremely rapid, distorting the anatomy.

3. If prolonged endotracheal intubation is anticipated, a nasal tube often is better tolerated.

4 The endotracheal tube must be secured without further compromise to the burned skin.

   a. Tape should be avoided.

   b. Circumferential ties should be observed and readjusted frequently to allow for swelling of the face and neck.

   c. The endotracheal tube may be sutured to the nasal septum or wired to a secure tooth.

   d. A bite block, soft but secure restraints, and adequate sedation are useful in preventing accidental extubation.

5. Nasogastric suction will help to prevent aspiration from post-injury ileus.

Fluid/Electrolyte/Blood Requirements

Fluid requirements are proportional to the extent and depth of the burn.

1. The Parkland formula for initial resuscitation is widely used but may significantly underestimate fluid requirements in small children.

   a. 4 ml/kg/% burn of Ringer's lactate in the first 24 hours.

   b. Half of the above in the first 8 hours (from time of injury).

   c. An additional 100 to 200 ml/kg during the first 24 hours has been recommended for children less than 30 kg.[46,50]

2. Electrolytes, glucose, BUN and creatinine, hematocrit, platelet count, prothrombin time (PT), and partial thromboplastin time (PTT) must be checked frequently.

3. The best estimate of adequate volume replacement is urine output of at least 1.0 ml/kg/hr.

4. Appropriate amounts of blood and blood products must be available before major debridement or grafting procedures.

Anesthetic Management of the Post-burn Patient

PREOPERATIVE ASSESSMENT

Large burn injuries affect nearly every organ system, both in the early phase of injury and during the long recovery process. The pediatric anesthesiologist must be acutely aware of the child's pathophysiology to direct the anesthetic management.

Effects of burn injuries on organ systems[51]

Cardiac	↓ cardiac output initially from hypovolemia ↑ output and hypertension later due to hypermetabolism
Pulmonary	Bronchospasm ↓ FRC ↓ lung and chest wall compliance Pulmonary infection
Renal	↓ glomerular filtration rate (GFR) Tubular dysfunction
Hematopoietic	Initially, ↓ platelets and consumptive coagulopathy Later, tranfusion-related infections
Neurologic	Encephalopathy with ↑ intracranial pressure Seizures
Metabolic	↓ ionized calcium ↑ O_2 consumption

TRANSPORT

1. The child will need adequate sedation and pain control prior to transport to the operating room. Tolerance to both opioids and anxiolytics is common during hospitalization for burn injuries.
2. Fluid boluses may be required during and after administration of opioids or sedatives, depending on the patient's intravascular volume status.
3. Heat loss during transport should be minimized by using warmed blankets and delivering the patient rapidly to a warmed operating room.

INTRAVENOUS ACCESS

Adequate IV access must be established for debridement and grafting procedures. In severely burned children, areas that escaped injury, such as the axilla or web spaces of the digits, may be used. A cutdown may be necessary, or even percutaneous placement of an IV through eschar, though this should be replaced as soon as possible to avoid infection. The surgeon may insert a large-bore cannula into the femoral vein, and transfusions can be given with a bypass pump or rapid infusion device. It is not uncommon for patients to lose 1 to 3 blood volumes during burn excision. Chronic ionized hypocalcemia is common in burn injury patients. Prophylactic replacement of calcium during rapid infusion of titrated blood products is usually required.[47]

MONITORING

1. ECG leads can be wired to the chest wall if the skin is burned, or an esophageal lead can be used.
2. Information from a pulse oximeter is extremely valuable; the probe is attached to the ear, the bridge of the nose, nasal alae,

cheek, or even tongue. It is best to use an oximeter probe that is sterilizable (immersible) and can be applied without tape. Pulse oximeters generally measure the percentage of oxygenated hemoglobin present in the total of oxygenated and deoxygenated hemoglobin. If a large percentage of the total hemoglobin is carboxyhemoglobin, falsely elevated readings will be obtained.[52] Hemoximetry should be used to measure both oxyhemoglobin and carboxyhemoglobin in burn patients with inhalation injuries. Although pulse oximeter probes generally work well over burned tissue, they may malfunction if used in areas with discoloration from silver nitrate. Furthermore, readings may also be inaccurate in patients with methemoglobinemia, which may occur when topical silver nitrate is used in patients with gram-negative sepsis.

3. In major burn injuries an arterial catheter should be placed to facilitate blood pressure monitoring and to obtain laboratory data frequently. End-tidal CO_2 monitoring may be inaccurate with large dead space ventilation and should be verified with blood gas determinations.

4. A central venous catheter is advantageous for monitoring central pressure and for volume administration.

5. Temperature must be monitored carefully, because burned children are extremely vulnerable to heat loss. A warm operating room, a heating blanket, warmed fluids, and warm humidified gases are essential for maintaining the child's temperature and avoiding ventricular dysrhythmias and platelet dysfunction.

ANESTHETIC AGENTS

Choice of anesthetic agents depends upon the underlying condition of the patient, the extent of injury, and the surgery planned.

1. Induction agents
   a. Thiopental is well tolerated in incremental doses if intravascular volume is adequate.
   b. Propofol is likewise well tolerated in the hydrated patient.
   c. Ketamine may be useful for hemodynamic stability, but patients tend to develop tolerance with repeated administration.
   d. High-dose opiate (fentanyl, sufentanil) is useful to block stress response and may provide prolonged analgesia in patients who will remain mechanically ventilated.

2. Nondepolarizing muscle relaxants should be used for induction, to avoid the use of succinylcholine. However, resistance to these relaxants often develops about 1 week postburn, and dosages may need to be increased from 2 to 5 times normal in patients with greater than 20% burn.[47]

3. Succinylcholine administration should be avoided with the burn patient. From 5 days to 6 months following thermal injury, extrajunctional receptors develop on the skeletal muscle,

causing a massive release of potassium when depolarized with succinylcholine.

4. Volatile agents may be used with caution in the postburn period. Cardiac output may be decreased by hypovolemia or myocardial depression from anemia, sepsis, and increased metabolic demands. Further depression from a volatile agent may not be tolerated.

5. Ketamine or propofol may be used for acutely painful dressing changes, but tolerance has been reported.[47] Opiates and benzodiazepines are indicated for analgesia and sedation during the long, painful recovery process, with increasing dosages commonly required.

POISONING AND OVERDOSE[53,54]

- Poisoning in childhood usually involves the accidental ingestion of toxic substances. Overdoses usually occur in adolescence from abuse of alcohol or drugs or from suicide attempts.

- Problems encountered in these patients involve systemic toxicity, need for airway protection, and local skin and mucosal damage from a toxic substance.

- The trachea should be intubated and ventilation assisted as necessary. The level of responsiveness must be ascertained before laryngoscopy, to prevent aspiration.

- Ingestion of a corrosive substance can cause severe burns of the mouth, oropharynx, and esophagus. No attempt should be made to induce vomiting. The airway should be secured if there is any danger of decreased airway reflexes or edema from the mouth or oropharynx. The child may require tracheal intubation for endoscopy to evaluate the extent of the burn.

- A thorough history should be elicited and a urine and serum drug screen performed if appropriate. The poison index or regional poison control center should be consulted to provide specific treatment of the child.

- Systemic toxicity of poisons and drugs may manifest as cardiac, respiratory, neurologic, hepatic, or renal failure. Because of the anesthesiologist's knowledge of physiology and pharmacology, he or she may provide valuable assistance to the pediatrician in the treatment of poisoned and overdosed children.

References

1. Kravitz RM: Congenital malformations of the lung, *Pediatr Clin North Am* 41:453-472, 1994.

2. Hernanz-Schulman M: Cysts and cystlike lesions of the lung, *Radiol Clin North Am* 31:631-649, 1993.

3. Weinstein S, Stolar CJH: Newborn surgical emergencies: congenital diaphragmatic hernia and extracorporeal membrane oxygenation, *Pediatr Clin North Am* 40:1315-1333, 1993.

4. Puri P: Congenital diaphragmatic hernia, *Curr Probl Surg* 10:787-846, 1994.

5. Harrison MR, Adzick S, Estes JM, Howell LJ: A prospective study of the outcome for fetuses with diaphragmatic hernia, *JAMA* 271:382-384, 1994.

6. Vacanti JP, Crone RK, Murphy JD, et al: The pulmonary hemodynamic response to perioperative anesthesia in the treatment of high risk infants with congenital diaphragmatic hernia, *J Pediatr Surg* 19:672-678, 1984.

7. Langer JC, Filler RM, Bohn DJ, et al: Timing of surgery for congenital diaphragmatic hernia: is emergency operation necessary? *J Pediatr Surg* 23:731-734, 1988.

8. West KW, Bengston K, Rescorla FJ, Engle WA, Grosfeld JL: Delayed surgical repair and ECMO improves survival in congenital diaphragmatic hernia, *Ann Surg* 216:454-462, 1992.

9. Breaux CW Jr, Rouse TM, Cain WS, Georgeson KE: Improvement in survival of patients with congenital diaphragmatic hernia utilizing a strategy of delayed repair after medical and/or extracorporeal membrane oxygenation stabilization, *J Pediatr Surg* 26:333-338, 1991.

10. Wilson JM, Lund DP, Lillehei CW, O'Rourke PP, Vacanti JP: Delayed repair and preoperative ECMO does not improve survival in high-risk congenital diaphragmatic hernia, *J Pediatr Surg* 27:368-375, 1992.

11. Kinsella JP, Abman SH: Recent developments in the pathophysiology and treatment of persistent pulmonary hypertension of the newborn, *J Pediatr* 126:853-864, 1995.

12. Morray JP, Krane EJ, Geiduschek JM, O'Rourke PP: Anesthesia for thoracic surgery. In Gregory GA, ed: *Pediatric anesthesia,* ed 3, New York, 1994, Churchill Linvingstone, pp. 421-464.

13. Yaster M: Anesthesia for surgical emergencies in newborns. In Rogers MC, Tinker JH, Covino BG, Longnecker DE, eds: *Prinicples and practice of anesthesiology,* vol 2, St Louis, 1993, Mosby, pp. 2137-2156.

14. Dillon PW, Cilley RE: Newborn surgical emergencies: gastrointestinal anomalies, abdominal wall defects, *Pediatr Clin North Am* 40:1289-1314, 1993.

15. Karrer FM, Hall RJ, Lilly JR: Noncardiac thoracic surgery in children: an overview, *Surg Ann* 25:117-149, 1993.

16. Krasna IH: Is early fascial closure necessary for omphalocele and gastroschisis, *J Pediatr Surg* 30:23-28, 1995.

17. Scherer LR III, Grosfeld JL: Inguinal hernia and umbilical anomalies, *Pediatr Clin North Am* 40:1121-1131, 1993.

18. Yaster M, Buck JR, Dudgeon DL, et al: Hemodynamic effects of primary closure of omphalocele/gastroschisis in human newborns, *Anesthesiology* 69:84-88, 1988.

19. Lacey SR, Carris LA, Beyer AJ III, Azizkhan RG: Bladder pressure monitoring significantly enhances care of infants with abdominal wall defects: a prospective clinical study, *J Pediatr Surg* 28:1370-1375, 1993.

20. Vane DW, Abajian JC, Hong AR: Spinal anesthesia for primary repair of gastroschisis: a new and safe technique for selected patients, *J Pediatr Surg* 29:1234-1235, 1994.

21. Thompson PJ, Greenough A, Dykes E, Nicolaides KH: Impaired respiratory function in infants with anterior abdominal wall defects, *J Pediatr Surg* 28:664-666, 1993.

22. Schafermeyer R: Pediatric trauma, *Emerg Med Clin North Am* 11:187-205, 1993.

23. Yurt RW: Triage, initial assessment, and early treatment of the pediatric trauma patient, *Pediatr Clin North Am* 39:1083-1091, 1992.

24. Jaffe D, Wesson D: Emergency management of blunt trauma in children, *N Eng J Med* 324:1477-1482, 1991.

25. Tepas JJ III, Ramenofsky ML, Molitt DL, Gans BM, DiScala C: The Pediatric Trauma Score as a predictor of injury severity: an objective assessment, *J Trauma* 28:425-429, 1988.

26. Rouse TM, Eichelberger MR: Trends in pediatric trauma management, *Surg Clin North Am* 72:1347-1364, 1992.

27. Elliott WG: Airway management in the injured child, *Int Anesthiol Clin* 32:27-46, 1994.

28. Nakayama DK: Emergency endotracheal intubation in pediatric trauma, *Ann Surg* 211:218-223, 1990.

29. Rasmussen G, Grande CM: Blood, fluids, and electrolytes in the pediatric trauma patient, *Int Anesthiol Clin* 32:79-101, 1994.

30. Bohn D, Armstrong D, Becker L, Humphreys R: Cervical spine injuries in children, *J Trauma* 34:463-469, 1990.

31. Teasdale G, Jennett B: Aspects of coma after severe head injury, *Lancet* 1:878-881, 1972.

32. Rieger A, Berman JM, Striebel HW: Initial resuscitation and vascular access, *Int Anesthiol Clin* 32:47-77, 1994.

33. Stylianos S, Jacir NN, Hoffman MA, Aronovitz MJ, Harris BH: Experimental volume replacement through lower extremity veins, *J Trauma* 35:666-670, 1993.

34. Fleisher G, Templeton J, Delgado-Paredes C: Fluid resuscitation following liver laceration: a comparison of fluid delivery above and below the diaphragm in a pediatric animal model, *Ann Emerg Med* 16:147-152, 1987.

35. Kanter RK, Zimmermen JJ, Strauss RH, Stoeckel KA: Central venous catheter insertion by femoral vein: safety and effectiveness for the pediatric patient, *Pediatrics* 77:842-847, 1986.

36. Guy J, Haley K, Zuspan SJ: Use of intraosseous infusion in the pediatric trauma patient, *J Pediatr Surg* 28:158-161, 1993.

37. Inaba AS, Seward PN: An approach to pediatric trauma, *Emerg Med Clin North Am* 9:523-548, 1991.

38. Fiser DH: Intraosseous infusion, *N Engl J Med* 322:1579-1581, 1990.

39. Freshman SP, Battistella FD, Matteucci M, Wisner DH: Hypertonic saline (7.5%) vs. mannitol: a comparison for treatment of acute head injuries, *J Trauma* 35:344-348, 1993.

40. Battistella FD, Wisner DH: Combined hemorrhagic shock and head injury: effects of hypertonic saline (7.5%) resuscitation, *J Trauma* 31:182-188, 1991.

41. Lanier WL, Stangland KJ, Scheithauer BW, Milde JH, Michenfelder JD: The effects of dextrose infusion and head position on neurologic outcome after complete cerebral ischemia in primates: examination of a model, *Anesthesiology* 66:39-48, 1987.

42. Striker TW: Anesthesia for trauma in the pediatric patient. In Gregory GA, ed: *Pediatric anesthesia,* ed 3, New York, 1994, Churchill Livingstone, pp. 805-812.

43. Brown DL: Anesthetic agents in trauma surgery: are there differences? *Int Anesthiol Clin* 25:75-90, 1987.

44. Brown DI: Trauma management: the anesthesiologist's role, *Int Anesthiol Clin* 25:1-18, 1987.

45. Lloyd TR, Donnerstein RL, Berg RA: Accuracy of central venous pressure measurement from the abdominal inferior vena cava, *Pediatrics* 89:506-508, 1992.

46. Finkelstein JL, Schwartz SB, Madden MR, Marano MA, Goodwin CW: Pediatric burns: an overview, *Pediatr Clin North Am* 39:1145-1163, 1992.

47. Palmisano BW: Anesthesia for plastic surgery. In Gregory GA, ed: *Pediatric anesthesia,* ed 3, New York, 1994, Churchill Livingstone, pp. 699-740.

48. Osgood PG, Szyfelbein SK: Management of burn pain in children, *Pediatr Clin North Am* 36:1001-1013, 1989.

49. Wolfe TM, Rao CC: Anesthesia for selected procedures, *Semin Pediatr Surg* 2:74-80, 1992.

50. O'Neill JA Jr.: Fluid resuscitation in the burned child: a reappraisal, *J Pediatr Surg* 17:604-607, 1982.

51. Szyfelbein SK, Martyn JAJ, Coté CJ: Burn injuries. In Coté CJ, Ryan JF, Todres ID, Goudsouzian NG, eds: *A practice of anesthesia for infants and children,* Philadelphia, 1993, WB Saunders, pp. 357-376.

52. Barker SJ, Tremper KK, Hyatt J: Effects of methemoglobinemia on pulse oximetry and mixed venous oximetry, *Anesthesiology* 70:112-117, 1989.

53. Bond GR: The poisoned child: evolving concepts in care, *Emerg Med Clin North Am* 13:343-355, 1995.

54. Henretig FM: Special considerations in the poisoned patient, *Emerg Med Clin North Am* 12:549-567, 1994.

III

UNIQUE CONCERNS IN PEDIATRIC ANESTHESIA

NEWBORN PHYSIOLOGY AND DEVELOPMENT

17

My brother Jack Jimbo was just born today.
He cries, eats and sleeps in a very strange way.
He has a round face and a small button nose,
and the teeniest, tiniest, littlest nose,
I thought he was cute, so I picked him right up,
and all of a sudden (Oh, yuck!), he threw up!

Caitlin Loeffler, age 10

NEWBORN PHYSIOLOGY

Physiologic characteristics of the newborn

System	Characteristics
Cardiovascular	Decrease in pulmonary vascular resistance (PVR) Closure of patent ductus arteriosus (PDA) Closure of foramen ovale Cardiac output is dependent on heart rate and left ventricular filling pressure (Frank-Starling mechanism)

Respiratory	Increased work of breathing because of:
	    Compliant chest wall
	    Noncompliant lung
	    Fewer Type 1 diaphragmatic muscle fibers
	Prone to hypoxia because of:
	    High O_2 consumption
	    High closing capacity/functional residual capacity (FRC) ratio
	Periodic breathing

Metabolic	Physiologic jaundice
Renal	Decreased glomerular filtration rate (GFR) Poor ability to concentrate or dilute urine Obligatory sodium loss
Temperature	Nonshivering thermogenesis
Neurologic	Immature autonomic nervous system with parasympathetic predominance and poor sympathetic tone Immature central nervous system (CNS) Incomplete myelination

Cardiac Function
FETAL CIRCULATION (FIG. 17-1)

1. Unsaturated blood is carried by the two umbilical arteries to the placenta for oxygenation and then returned to the fetus by the single umbilical vein, with a PO_2 of 30 to 35 mm Hg.
2. The umbilical vein blood primarily enters the inferior vena cava from the ductus venosus and mixes with desaturated blood from the lower extremities. A small amount of umbilical vein blood enters the liver from the portal vein.
3. Blood enters the right atrium from the inferior and superior venae cavae and is shunted across the patent foramen ovale into the left atrium. Blood from the pulmonary artery is shunted across the ductus arteriosus to the aorta.
4. Blood is shunted away from the nonfunctioning lungs by high pulmonary vascular resistance (PVR) caused by:
   a. The relatively hypoxic environment
   b. Compression of vessels by fluid-filled alveoli
5. Oxygenated blood goes from the left atrium into the left ventricle, exiting the heart by the ascending aorta to the coronary, carotid, and subclavian arteries. Carotid artery blood has a PO_2 of 23 to 25 mm Hg.
6. About half the blood in the descending aorta (PO_2 = 23 to 25 mm Hg) perfuses the abdomen and lower extremities, and the rest is returned to the placenta.

CIRCULATORY CHANGES AT BIRTH (FIG. 17-2)

1. Expansion of the lungs, increased PO_2 to 60 mm Hg, and release of vasoactive substances and arachidonic acid metabolites lead to an 80% decrease in the PVR.[1] As a result, both pulmonary circulation and oxygenation increase dramatically. A further decrease in PVR occurs over the next eight weeks.
2. The ductus arteriosus is composed of tissue that is uniquely sensitive to oxygen, prostaglandins, and pH. It will constrict in 90% of term neonates in the first three days of life as PO_2 increases, pH becomes less acidotic, and the placental contribution of prostaglandin (PGE_2) ceases.[2] Permanent closure by endothelial destruction and connective tissue formation may take 2 to 3 weeks.[3]
3. The increase in pulmonary blood flow will result in increased blood volume in the left atrium and subsequent closure of the flap of the foramen ovale as left atrial pressures rise above right atrial pressures. A small left-to-right shunt may persist for several weeks because of incomplete closure, and probe patency persists in 25% to 35% of the adult population.[4]

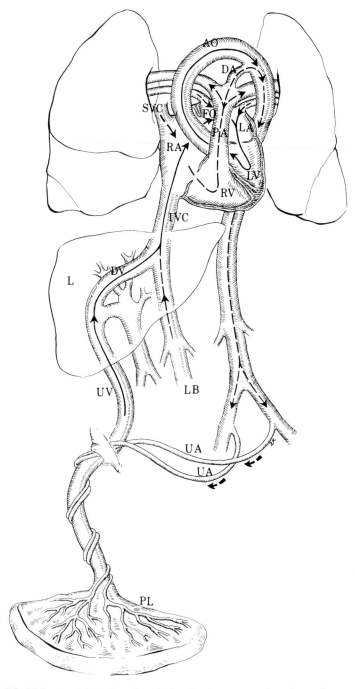

FIG. 17-1. Fetal circulation. The unbroken line demonstrates the pathway of oxygenated blood from the placenta. Desaturated blood returns to the placenta through the umbilical arteries via the broken line. (*PL,* Placenta; *UV,* umbilical vein; *DV,* ductus venosus; *LB,* lower body; *IVC,* inferior vena cava; *SVC,* superior vena cava; *RA,* right atrium, *FO,* foramen ovale; *RV,* right ventricle; *PA,* pulmonary artery; *DA,* ductus arteriosus; *LA,* left atrium; *LV,* left ventricle; *AO,* aorta; *UA,* umbilical artery; *L,* liver.)

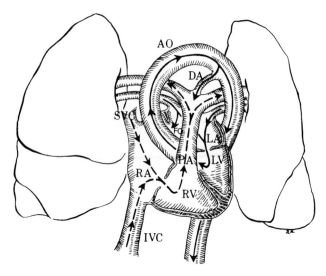

FIG. 17-2. Circulatory changes at birth. Decreased pulmonary vascular resistance at birth results in increased pulmonary blood flow and subsequent flow to the left atrium and ventricle. Increased Po_2 and left-sided pressures typically result in closure of the ductus arteriosus and foramen ovale. A left-to-right shunt will be present if patency persists in either structure. (*IVC,* Inferior vena cava; *SVC,* superior vena cava; *RA,* right atrium; *RV,* right ventricle; *PA,* pulmonary artery; *FO,* foramen ovale; *DA,* ductus arteriosus; *LA,* left atrium; *LV,* left ventricle; *AO,* aorta.)

NEONATAL MYOCARDIAL FUNCTION[5]

The cardiac output of the neonate is dependent upon heart rate and left ventricular filling pressure (Frank-Starling mechanism). In the fetus, augmentation of cardiac output is limited because myocardial performance is near maximum under normal conditions.[6] In contrast, the neonate can achieve twice the cardiac output of the fetus with volume loading and heart rate increase.

1. Thyroid hormone, present in high levels late in fetal gestation, may cause an increase in myocardial contractility.[7]
2. Over the first months of life, the resting cardiac output decreases, with a resultant increase in cardiac reserve. This may be due to the transition from fetal to adult hemoglobin, wherein less cardiac output is needed to provide tissues with an adequate amount of oxygen.[8]
3. The parasympathetic supply to the heart is completely developed at birth, whereas sympathetic innervation continues during the first 6 weeks of life.[9] The neonate is therefore predisposed to bradycardia with minimal chronotropic and inotropic counterbalance.

Respiratory Function
CONVERSION TO AEROBIC LIFE

At birth, the lungs undergo the transition from a fluid-filled organ to an air-filled organ for gaseous exchange. Most of the fluid is expelled from the lungs by compression of the fetal chest during vaginal delivery, with the remainder removed by the lymphatic system over the next 24 hours. In order to overcome surface active forces and fully expand the lungs, the neonate must generate negative intrathoracic pressures of up to 70 cm H_2O. The same pressures are needed for the first few breaths during newborn resuscitation to expand the alveoli.[10]

COMPLIANCE AND WORK OF BREATHING

1. The increased compliance of the chest wall (because of pliable and cartilaginous ribs) and the decreased compliance of the lungs require increased work of breathing for the infant to maintain adequate functional residual capacity (FRC).
2. Respiratory movement is generated mostly by diaphragmatic and abdominal muscles. The diaphragmatic and intercostal muscles of a newborn have a smaller proportion of Type I fibers, the high-oxidative fibers used for repetitive movement.[10]
3. During periods of partial airway obstruction or increased respiratory demands (sepsis, pneumonia) the neonate is more susceptible to respiratory failure from fatigue.

PULMONARY VOLUMES

Tidal volume (V_T) is the same for neonates and adults (7 to 10 ml/kg). However, because neonatal oxygen consumption ($\dot{V}O_2$) is two to three times that of the adult, alveolar ventilation must be increased proportionally.[10]

1. The high minute ventilation/FRC ratio may result in rapid desaturation in the neonate during periods of apnea or airway obstruction. Furthermore, the time required for inhalation induction of anesthesia in neonates is shortened by the higher ratio of minute ventilation to FRC.
2. Neonatal closing volumes are higher than for adults. The high closing capacity/FRC ratio increases the potential for intrapulmonary shunting as exemplified by the rapid desaturation that occurs with airway obstruction.

VENTILATORY DRIVE

In infants less than 3 weeks of age, hypoxia initially stimulates ventilation, followed by a decrease in ventilation. After 3 weeks, hypoxia causes sustained hyperventilation.[10]

1. Chemoreceptors are functional in the full-term infant so that an increase in PCO_2 will stimulate ventilation.
2. Periodic breathing with intermittent apneic spells of less

than 10 seconds is common in neonates up to 3 months of age. Hypoxia, anesthesia, and sepsis may accentuate periodic breathing and apnea in the newborn.

Neonatal Hematology[11]

Blood volume in the newborn is about 90 ml/kg. Hemoglobin content is about 19 g/100 ml, of which 80% is fetal hemoglobin (Hgb F). Hgb F has a higher affinity for oxygen, causing a shift to the left of the oxyhemoglobin dissociation curve. This shift to the left is compensated for by an increased hematocrit (45% to 55%). The level of Hgb F will fall as it is replaced by adult hemoglobin (Hgb A; see Chapter 13, p. 232). Fetal hematopoiesis occurs mainly in the liver and shifts completely to the bone marrow by the sixth week of life.

Hepatic Metabolism and Physiologic Jaundice[12]

Phase I hepatic reactions (degradative), including oxidation, reduction, and hydrolysis, appear to be fully functional at birth. In contrast, Phase II reactions (synthetic) are found in the cytochrome P_{450} microsomal enzyme fraction and are not fully developed in the neonate.

A reduced amount of UDP-glucuronyl transferase results in deficient glucuronide conjugation, which does not reach normal levels until age 2 months. This enzyme is necessary for bilirubin to be rendered water soluble for excretion in bile or renal filtration. The

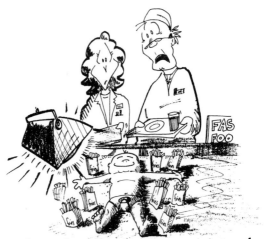

Looks like they are low on Infrared lamps over in Neonatology...

normal newborn produces bilirubin at twice the per kilogram rate of an adult, 75% of which is from red blood cell destruction. Much larger quantities of unconjugated bilirubin are reabsorbed by the enterohepatic circulation in the neonate than the adult. In normal newborns, the median bilirubin is 6 mg/dl 48 hours after birth, with a range from 1 to 12 mg/dl. Other causes of jaundice are to be considered (ABO incompatibility, infection, spherocytosis, etc.) if the bilirubin concentration exceeds 12 mg/dl in a full-term infant or 15 mg/dl in a premature infant. Phototherapy is usually instituted at bilirubin levels of 8 mg/dl in infants between 1500 and 2000 g and at levels greater than 12 mg/dl in neonates of normal birth weight. Exchange transfusion may be necessary when the bilirubin approaches 20 mg/dl.

Renal Function[13]

GLOMERULAR FILTRATION RATE (GFR)

Because fetal waste is removed by the placenta, the fetal kidney produces a minimal amount of urine, which is excreted into the amniotic sac. At birth, renal vascular resistance decreases and both renal blood flow and GFR increase. Although the term newborn has the same number of nephrons as an adult, they are smaller so that the GFR is considerably lower. The GFR at birth is 30% of an adult's, with a rapid increase in function over the first weeks of life. GFR approaches adult levels by the end of the first year. The newborn has a low normal plasma creatinine (0.4 mg/dl) because of small muscle mass/body weight ratio and high anabolic rate.

CONCENTRATING ABILITY

Because renal tubular development and function will not reach adult capacity for 2 to 3 years, the newborn kidney has limited ability to concentrate and dilute urine. The maximal urine concentration of a premature infant is 600 mOsm/L, for a full-term infant 700 mOsm/L, and an adult 1200 mOsm/L.

SODIUM HOMEOSTASIS AND ACID/BASE BALANCE

The newborn kidney is an obligate sodium loser and will continue to excrete sodium even during a severe sodium deficit. Antidiuretic hormone (ADH) synthesis and secretion appear to be intact in the neonate, as does the production of renin, angiotensin, and aldosterone. However, there may be an inability of immature tubular cells to respond to aldosterone. The renal threshold for bicarbonate is low, about 20 mmol/L, making the normal plasma pH for the neonate about 7.34.

Temperature Regulation

Large surface area, poor insulation, a small mass from which heat is generated, and inability to shiver place the newborn at a disadvantage when regulating temperature. Catecholamine-stimulated nonshivering thermogenesis by brown fat is the major source of heat production in the cold-stressed neonate. Complications of increased catecholamine release include elevated pulmonary and systemic vascular resistance and higher O_2 consumption with resultant stress on the newborn heart.

The newborn infant should be maintained in a "neutral thermal environment," the ambient temperature at which an infant can maintain core body temperature with minimal metabolic activity (see box below). The use of radiant heat lamps, warming blankets, hats, and limb wrapping, the delivery of warmed and humidified gases, and the infusion of warmed intravenous fluids in the operating room will help to maintain a neutral thermal environment.

Thermoregulation in infants[14]

Age	Neutral temp*	Critical temp†
Preterm	34° C	28° C
Full term	32° C	23° C
Adult	28° C	1° C

*Neutral temperature is the ambient room temperature that results in minimal oxygen consumption.
†Critical temperature is the temperature below which an unclothed unanesthetized person cannot maintain a normal core temperature.

Central Nervous System (CNS)[15,16]

The CNS of a newborn infant is immature and will undergo major growth and myelination in the first 3 to 4 years of life. The presence of primitive reflexes at birth, such as the rooting reflex, Moro response, and grasp reflex, are indicative of normal fetal CNS development. Normal CNS maturation is reflected in the appearance of developmental milestones at the appropriate ages.

Pediatric neurologic signs

Response	Age of appearance	Age of disappearance
Moro reflex	Birth	1-3 months
Babinski response	Birth	Variable
Horizontal following vision	4-6 weeks	—
Rooting response—awake	Birth	3-4 months
Handedness	2-3 years	—

NORMAL PATTERNS OF GROWTH AND DEVELOPMENT

Gestational Age

Immaturity of most organ systems in the preterm infant necessitates anesthetic considerations different from those for a full-term infant. Postconceptional age (PCA) has been widely used by many investigators as the most important factor for determining increased anesthetic risk in preterm infants. The age at which the infant is at increased risk for postoperative apnea and respiratory complications varies from 44 weeks to 60 weeks PCA depending upon the study cited (see Chapter 1, p. 6). Other preoperative factors such as the presence of respiratory distress syndrome (RDS), history of patent ductus arteriosus (PDA), or preoperative apnea may ultimately be more important than PCA alone in predicting postoperative complications.[17]

Birth Weight/Size

1. The *low birth weight* (LBW) infant (less than 2500 g) has a much higher risk of a complicated postnatal course requiring respiratory and nutritional support. Low birth weights are usually the result of poor prenatal care, smoking, drugs, alcohol, maternal malnutrition, toxemia, or placental insufficiency. A *very low birth weight* (VLBW) infant weighs less than 1500 g.

2. The infant with weight below the 10th percentile is *small for gestational age* (SGA), and intrauterine infection (cytomegalovirus, rubella), congenital malformation, or chromosomal abnormality must be suspected. Many SGA infants are also the result of toxemia or placental insufficiency.

3. The *large for gestational age* (LGA) infant has weight above the 90th percentile, a condition commonly associated with maternal diabetes. These infants should be observed for hypoglycemia.

4. An *appropriate for gestational age* (AGA) infant's weight is between the 10th and 90th percentiles.

COMMON PROBLEMS OF PREMATURITY

Pulmonary

RESPIRATORY DISTRESS SYNDROME (RDS)

Description. Absence or deficiency of surfactant; characterized by hypercarbia and hypoxia with resultant acidosis; may be complicated by pneumothorax, pneumomediastinum, and pulmonary interstitial emphysema

Treatment. Endobronchial surfactant, oxygen therapy, often with some form of positive-pressure ventilation (CPAP, PEEP) and supportive care[18-20]

MECONIUM ASPIRATION SYNDROME

Description.   Perinatal aspiration of meconium; characterized by respiratory insufficiency, pneumonia, and asphyxia

Treatment.   Oxygen, positive-pressure ventilation, and supportive care

APNEA

Description.   Absence of breathing for 15 to 30 seconds, often accompanied by bradycardia and cyanosis

Differential diagnosis.   Hypoxemia, respiratory depression from metabolic disorders (hypoglycemia, hypocalcemia, electrolyte disorders, sepsis), intracranial hemorrhage, airway obstruction, and hyperthermia or hypothermia

Treatment.   Theophylline, caffeine, mechanical ventilation, and supportive care

BRONCHOPULMONARY DYSPLASIA (BPD)

Description.   Chronic obstructive lung disease of neonates exposed to barotrauma and high inspired oxygen concentration; characterized by persistent respiratory difficulty and radiographic evidence of diffuse linear densities and radiolucent areas

Treatment.   Oxygen, bronchodilators, diuretics, mechanical ventilation

PERSISTENT PULMONARY HYPERTENSION

Description.   Pulmonary hypertension and vascular hyperreactivity with resultant right-to-left shunting and cyanosis; associated with cardiac anomalies, respiratory distress syndrome, meconium aspiration syndrome, diaphragmatic hernia, and group B streptococcal sepsis

Treatment.   Oxygen, mechanical ventilation, high-frequency oscillatory ventilation, vasodilator drugs such as tolazoline (nonselective pulmonary and systemic effects), nitric oxide (selective pulmonary effects),[21-23] and extracorporeal membrane oxygenation (ECMO)[24,25]

Cardiac

PATENT DUCTUS ARTERIOSUS (PDA)

(SEE p. 141)

Description.   Left-to-right shunt from the aorta to the pulmonary artery through the ductal remnant of fetal circulation; commonly found in premature infants or infants with RDS; the shunt can result in congestive heart failure and apnea

Treatment.   Indomethacin therapy, surgical ligation of the ductus

CONGENITAL HEART DISEASE
(SEE CHAPTER 7)

Description. Characterized by congestive heart failure or cyanosis unresponsive to oxygen therapy

Treatment. Palliative shunt and complete repair

Gastrointestinal
NECROTIZING ENTEROCOLITIS (NEC)
(SEE p. 249)

Description. Ischemic injury to intestinal mucosa, often complicated by bowel necrosis and perforation, causing abdominal distention, bloody diarrhea, apnea, acidosis, and septic shock

Treatment. Intravenous hydration, antibiotics, discontinuation of feeding, surgical exploration, and resection of damaged intestine

GASTROESOPHAGEAL REFLUX
(SEE p. 245)

Description. Involuntary movement of stomach contents into the esophagus. Physiologic reflux is found in all newborns; pathologic reflux can result in failure to thrive, recurrent respiratory problems (aspiration, bronchospasm, and apnea),[26] irritability, esophagitis, ulceration and gastrointestinal bleeding.

Treatment: Head elevation, small and frequent feedings, H_2 blockers, sucralfate, omeprazole, and surgery (fundoplication)[27,28]

Hematologic
JAUNDICE (SEE p. 256)

Description. Hyperbilirubinemia from increased bilirubin load and poor hepatic conjugation (unconjugated, physiologic) or abnormalities of bilirubin production, metabolism, or excretion (nonphysiologic)

Treatment. Phototherapy, exchange transfusion, and treatment of underlying medical disorder

ANEMIA (SEE p. 281)

Description. Low hematocrit as a result of decreased erythropoiesis (physiologic), blood loss, hemolysis

Treatment. Elimination of causes, transfusion

Metabolic
HYPOGLYCEMIA

Description. Blood sugar less than 40 mg/100 ml, characterized by lethargy, hypotonia, tremors, apnea, and seizures

Treatment. Oral or intravenous glucose

HYPOCALCEMIA

Description. Total serum calcium concentration less than 7 mg/100 ml or ionized calcium less than 3.0 to 3.5 mg/dl; characterized by irritability, jitteriness, hypotonia, and seizures

Treatment. Administration of oral or intravenous calcium

Infectious

CONGENITAL INFECTIONS

Description. Characteristic syndromes caused by congenital bacterial or viral infections. The most common infections are described by the acronym STORCH (syphilis, toxoplasmosis, rubella, cytomegalovirus, herpes).

Treatment. Supportive care

GROUP B STREPTOCOCCAL INFECTION

Description. Characterized by pneumonia, sepsis, and meningitis syndromes

Treatment. Antibiotics and supportive care

Central Nervous System

INTRAVENTRICULAR HEMORRHAGE (IVH)

Description. Periventricular-intraventricular hemorrhage associated with immaturity and hypoxemia. Characterized by bradycardia, respiratory irregularity, apnea, seizures, and hypotonia.

Treatment. Shunting and supportive care

NEONATAL SEIZURES

Description. Convulsion with infectious, metabolic, or traumatic etiology

Treatment. Anticonvulsants and supportive care

Ophthalmologic

RETINOPATHY OF PREMATURITY (ROP)

Description. ROP is a vasoproliferative retinopathy seen in premature infants exposed to high concentrations of oxygen for prolonged periods.

Treatment. Cryotherapy or laser therapy to the avascular retina

References

1. Teitel DF, Iwamoto HS, Rudolph AM: Effects of birth-related events on central blood flow patterns, *Pediatr Res* 22:557-566, 1987.
2. Alenick DS, Holzman IR, Ritter SB: The neonatal transitional circulation: a combined noninvasive assessment, *Echocardiography* 9:29-36, 1992.
3. Clyman RI: Ductus arteriosus: current theories of prenatal and postnatal regulation, *Semin Perinatol* 11:64-71, 1987.
4. Hagen PT, Scholz DG, Edwards WD: Incidence and size of patent

foramen ovale during the first "10" decades: an autopsy study of 965 normal hearts, *Mayo Clin Proc* 59:17-20, 1984.

5. Friedman AH, Fahey JT: The transition from fetal to neonatal circulation: normal responses and implications for infants with heart disease, *Semin Perinatol* 17:106-121, 1993.

6. Teitel DF, Sidi D, Chin T, Brett C, Heymann MA: Developmental changes in myocardial contractile reserve in the lamb, *Pediatr Res* 19:948-955, 1985.

7. Breall JA, Rudolph AM, Heymann MA: Role of thyroid hormone in postnatal circulatory and metabolic adjustments, *J Clin Invest* 73:1418-1424, 1984.

8. Teitel D, Rudolph AM: Perinatal oxygen delivery and cardiac function, *Adv Pediatr* 32:321-347, 1985.

9. Lake CL: Neonatal myocardial and circulatory function. In Lake CL, ed: *Pediatric cardiac anesthesia,* ed 2, Norwalk, Conn, 1993, Appleton & Lange, pp 33-48.

10. Motoyama EK: Respiratory physiology in infants and children. In Motoyama EK, Davis PJ, eds: *Smith's anesthesia for infants and children,* St Louis, 1990, Mosby, pp 11-76.

11. Oski FA: The erythrocyte and its disorders. In Nathan DG, Oski FA, eds: *Hematology of infancy and childhood,* Philadelphia, 1993, WB Saunders, pp 18-43.

12. Cashore WJ: Neonatal hyperbilirubinemia. In Oski FA et al, eds: *Principles and practice of pediatrics,* ed 2, Philadelphia, 1994, JB Lippincott, pp 446-455.

13. Arant BS Jr: Renal and genitourinary diseases. In Oski FA et al, eds: *Principles and practice of pediatrics,* ed 2, Philadelphia, 1994, JB Lippincott, pp 455-465.

14. Krishna G, Haselby KA, Rao CC, Wolfe TM, McNiece WL: The pediatric patient. In Stoelting RK, Dierdorf SF, eds: *Anesthesia and coexisting disease,* ed 3, New York, 1993, Churchill Livingstone, pp 741-810.

15. Ment LR, Fishman MA: Disease of the newborn. In Oski FA et al, eds: *Principles and practice of pediatrics,* ed 2, Philadelphia, 1994, JB Lippincott, pp 342-366.

16. Swaiman KF: Neurologic examination after the newborn period until 2 years of age. In Swaiman KF, ed: *Pediatric neurology: principles and practice,* St Louis, Mosby, 1994, pp 43-52.

17. Gollin G, Bell C, Dubose R, et al: Predictors of postoperative respiratory complications in premature infants after inguinal herniorrhaphy, *J Pediatr Surg* 28:244-247, 1993.

18. Dechant KL, Faulds D: Colfosceril palmitate: a review of the therapeutic efficacy and clinical tolerability of a synthetic surfactant preparation (Exosurf[R] Neonatal[TM]) in neonatal respiratory distress syndrome, *Drugs* 42:877-894, 1991.

19. Corbet A: Clinical trials of synthetic surfactant in the respiratory distress syndrome of premature infants, *Clin Perinatol* 20:737-760, 1993.

20. Verder H, Robertson B, Greisen G, Ebbesen F, Albertsen P, Lundstrom K, Jacobsen T: Surfactant therapy and nasal continuous positive airway pressure for newborns with respiratory distress syndrome, *N Engl J Med* 331:1051-1055, 1994.

21. Kinsella JP, Neish SR, Shaffer E, Abman SH: Low-dose inhalational nitric oxide in persistent pulmonary hypertension of the newborn, *Lancet* 340:819-820, 1992.

22. Kinsella JP, Abman SH: Efficacy of inhalational nitric oxide therapy in the clinical management of persistent pulmonary hypertension of the newborn, *Chest* 105:92S-94S, 1994.

23. Zapol WM, Falke KJ, Hurford WE, Roberts JD Jr.: Inhaling nitric oxide: a selective pulmonary vasodilator and bronchodilator, *Chest* 105:87S-91S, 1994.

24. Ortiz RM, Cilley RE, Bartlett RH: Extracorporeal membrane oxygenation in pediatric respiratory failure, *Pediatr Clin North Am* 34:39-46, 1987.

25. Zapol WM, Snider MT, Hill JD, et al: Extracorporeal membrane oxygenation in severe acute respiratory failure: a randomized prospective study, *JAMA* 242:2193-2196, 1979.

26. Bernard F, Dupont C, Viala P: Gastroesophageal reflux and upper airway diseases, *Clin Rev Allergy* 8:403-425, 1990.

27. Heacock HJ, Jeffery HE, Baker JL, Page M: Influence of breast versus formula milk on physiological gastroesophageal reflux in healthy, newborn infants, *J Pediatr Gastroenterol Nutr* 14:41-46, 1992.

28. Vandenplas Y: Reflux esophagitis in infants and children: a report from the working group on gastro-oesophageal reflux disease of the European Society of Paediatric Gastroenterology and Nutrition, *J Pediatr Gastroenterol Nutr* 18:413-422, 1994.

DELIVERY ROOM RESUSCITATION

18

fly away angel
fly away far
come back angel
let earth embrace your star

Adrienne Coleman

FETAL MONITORING

Knowledge of fetal monitoring techniques allows the physician to anticipate resuscitation and helps to predict treatment and outcome.

Monitors for Uterine Activity

Noninvasive. Tocodynamometry is a technique that uses a pressure-sensitive device to give a qualitative tracing of uterine contraction.

Invasive. A catheter is inserted transvaginally to measure uterine pressure during labor.

1. The transducer should be at the level of parturient's xiphoid process.
2. Normal baseline pressure:
   - Latent phase: < 5 mm Hg
   - Active phase: 10 to 12 mm Hg
3. Normal peak pressure:
   - Early stage 1: 20 to 30 mm Hg above baseline
   - Early stage 2: up to 100 mm Hg

Fetal Heart Rate Monitors

Noninvasive. An external transabdominal Doppler probe monitors fetal heart rate.

1. A poor trace may be present in the obese parturient.
2. The signal is easily lost during maternal or fetal motion.
3. False beat-to-beat variability may be seen, and this technique can be unreliable in a parturient with multiple gestations.

Invasive. More precise measurement of rate and beat-to-beat variability is obtained with a fetal scalp electrode.

Normal fetal heart rate	
Rate	120-150 beats per minute
Pattern	Short-term (±10 beats per minute) rate changes from beat to beat
	Long-term cyclic changes (two to five times each minute)

Abnormal fetal heart rate tracings

Type	Description	Etiology
Early decelerations	10-30 beats/min decrease from baseline U-shaped curve Deceleration ends at or before end of contraction	Compression of fetal head, causing vagal tone
Baseline bradycardia	Rate <120; variability indicates a well-compensated fetus	Common in infants of >42 weeks' gestation Potential etiologies: β-blockade, hypothermia, decreased uterine blood flow, atrioventricular block, congenital cytomegalovirus infection
Baseline tachycardia	>160 beats/min	Maternal causes: amnionitis, infection with fever, thyrotoxicosis, use of atropine or ritodrine Fetal causes: arrhythmias, fetal compromise
Variable decelerations	Alternate rise and fall in fetal heart rate Fetal HR<70 beats/min for more than 60 sec is considered severe	Caused by compression of umbilical cord Often occurs in presence of short or long umbilical cord, or when cord is around neck of the fetus

Ominous fetal heart rate tracings

Type	Description	Etiology
Loss of baseline variability (only reliable when assessed by internal monitors)	≤ 5 beats/min deviation from the baseline FHR tracing Indicative of severe fetal compromise Can occur in presence of CNS depressant drugs	Associated with fetal or maternal acidemia or with significant fetal hypoxemia
Late decelerations	Symmetrical decrease in FHR beginning at or after the peak of contraction; return to baseline occurs only after contraction Changes in FHR are gradual and smooth	Occurs if fetal hypoxia is present prior to stress of contractions Earliest indication in FHR tracing of uteroplacental hypoxia
Prolonged decelerations	Isolated decelerations lasting >60 to 90 sec and <15 min	Multiple causes include cervical examination, uterine hyperactivity, maternal supine hypotension, epidural/spinal analgesia, placental insufficiency or abruption Usually temporary and followed by fetal recovery

Fetal Acid-Base Monitoring

Scalp pH should be obtained in the presence of a worrisome fetal heart tracing to document the degree of fetal distress. A pH value of less than 7.20 usually indicates the need for immediate delivery (cesarean section) if not improved within 15 minutes. Levels of pH are classified as follows:

Normal	7.25 to 7.35
Preacidotic	7.20 to 7.25
Acidotic	<7.20

Treatment of fetal compromise

1. O_2 to mother
2. Left uterine displacement
3. Maternal volume expansion (without dextrose)
4. Discontinuation of oxytocin

GOALS OF NEWBORN RESUSCITATION

Normal physiologic changes at birth are directed toward converting the newborn from dependence on the placenta and fetal circulation to self-sufficient gas exchange.

The *goals of resuscitation* are directed at aiding the infant in completing the above transition to independent life by:
1. Assuring airway patency
2. Maintaining ventilation/oxygenation
3. Maintaining cardiac output
4. Reducing metabolic requirements

Airway

The airway may be obstructed by secretions, flaccid musculature, or dysmorphic anatomy. As a result of a relatively low functional residual capacity and high closing capacity, the PaO_2 of a newborn can fall rapidly in seconds during acute airway obstruction. Successful resuscitation depends on rapid assessment and treatment.

LIGHT SUCTION

This technique recognizes neonatal susceptibility to reflex bradycardia.
1. Thumb control is necessary to prevent applying prolonged, uncontrolled suction to the airway.
2. Intermittent suction allows a period for ventilation (>5 seconds may cause hypoxia). Suction bulbs cause fewer bradyarrhythmias but are less efficient.
3. A trap should be present in the suction circuit for examining aspirated material (e.g., blood, meconium).
4. Traumatic suction to bronchi, trachea, or carina may cause bleeding or edema and worsen airway patency.

AIRWAY PATENCY

1. Congenital anomalies such as choanal atresia, paralyzed vocal cords, laryngeal webs, or the ptotic tongue of infants with Pierre Robin sequence may obstruct the airway. Often a nasal trumpet can bypass oral lesions. As neonates are obligate nose breathers, an oral airway may precipitate bradycardia or laryngospasm and may not improve ventilation.
2. Given that bag-and-mask ventilation of the newborn can be difficult, the use of the laryngeal mask airway (LMA) is being explored. Several case reports have been published demonstrating the efficacy of the LMA in neonatal resuscitation, especially when positive-pressure ventilation cannot be accomplished with bag-and-mask or tracheal intubation.

3. The ultimate assurance of airway patency is the oral endotracheal tube (ETT). The ETT should be advanced under direct vision only 1 to 1.5 cm past the cords, to prevent endobronchial intubation.
4. Complications of intubation in vigorous infants include stridor and a hoarse cry.

POSITIONING

1. When the neonate is supine, the retropharynx and glossopalatine channel can become sealed by soft tissue.
2. Hyperextension of the neck may worsen obstruction and actually cause tracheal collapse. Chin lifts and mandibular extension are more useful for opening the airway. CPAP with bag-mask ventilation is also useful to open the retropharynx.
3. Placing a rolled towel under the shoulders will improve airway patency and make bag mask ventilation easier. If tracheal intubation is necessary, the towel may need to be removed and a better "sniff" position obtained (see Fig. 18-1).

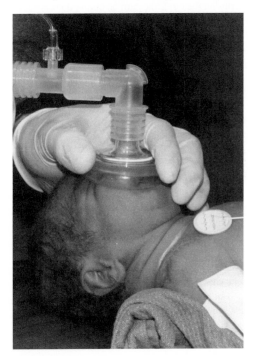

FIG. 18-1. Position for neonatal assisted ventilation.

Ventilation/Oxygenation

After 3 to 4 minutes of apnea, acidosis will cause a drop in cardiac output. In addition, PaO_2 may be too low to measure after 5 minutes of total asphyxia. Treatment of neonatal asphyxia includes basic resuscitative techniques (see table on p. 422).

Cardiac Output

The cardiac output of the neonate is largely rate and preload dependent. The normal heart rate is greater than 120 beats per minute and is best palpated at the umbilicus, where it can be appreciated as a brief forceful (often bounding) pulse.

1. A heart rate of 100 beats per minute may be sufficient if adequate oxygenation and ventilation are maintained.
2. A heart rate of 80 to 100 beats per minute demands assisted ventilation with 100% oxygen.
3. A heart rate between 60 and 80 beats per minute may be acceptable for the first 30 seconds, but chest compressions should begin if there is no improvement with adequate oxygenation.
4. A heart rate of less than 60 beats per minute necessitates immediate chest compressions.
5. Chest compressions should continue until the heart rate is greater than 100 beats per minute.
6. A newborn who requires chest compressions should be tracheally intubated. If the cardiac output does not improve with oxygenation and volume expansion, resuscitative drugs should be used (see table on p. 424).
7. Inadequate cardiac output (low perfusion) with an adequate heart rate may indicate hypovolemia; if volume loss is suspected (as may occur with placental/uterine catastrophe or delayed cord clamping), 10 ml/kg of normal saline or Ringer's lactate can be administered repeatedly as necessary.
8. Other causes of electromechanical dissociation should be considered: hypoxia, hypercapnia, acidosis, pneumothorax, or pneumomediastinum.

Metabolic Requirements

Heat is produced in the newborn by metabolism of brown fat (nonshivering thermogenesis). Oxygen consumption ($\dot{V}O_2$) doubles at a skin-to-air temperature gradient of 10°C and triples at 15°C.

Hypothermia causes hypoxia, hypercapnia, acidosis, and hypoglycemia. These factors increase pulmonary vascular resistance and right-to-left shunting. Normally, 10% of cardiac output goes to brown fat. During hypothermia, 75% of cardiac output is diverted to brown fat. Treatment and prevention are aimed at reducing all forms of heat loss.

BASIC RESUSCITATION IN THE DELIVERY ROOM

Apgar scores (see table on p. 421) are useful in defining the level of neonatal depression. The resuscitator, however, should not stop to calculate the score if therapy will be delayed. A gross impression of neonatal status (vigorous, mildly depressed, depressed, morbid) can be made after delivery to a prewarmed resuscitation area, quick drying with a warm towel, and suctioning of the mouth and nose. Generally the signs appear in the following order: color, respiration, tone, reflex irritability, and heart rate. Regression of signs (i.e., improvement) is generally in the reverse order. It is also unnecessary to delay definitive action in order to count out the heart rate; an impression of normal (>120 beats per minute), slow (80 to 100 beats per minute), or morbid (<80 beats per minute) heart rate is sufficient to initiate therapy. Documentation of the 1-, 5-, and 10-minute Apgar scores is important and can be done by a second observer, or calculated after resuscitation is completed.

Apgar scores

Score	0	1	2
Heart rate (beats/min)	Absent	<100	>100
Respiratory effort	Absent	Slow, regular	Good crying
Muscle tone	Limp	Some flexion of extremities	Active motion
Reflex irritability	No response (nasal catheter)	Grimace	Cough or sneeze
Color	Blue/pale	Extremities blue	Completely pink

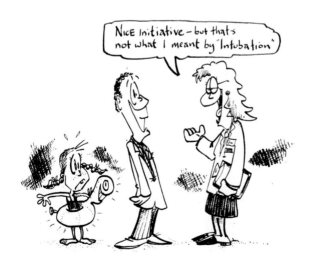

Resuscitation of neonates by Apgar score*

Score	Physical condition	Resuscitation
8-10, vigorous	Heart rate > 100 Good respiratory effort Good motion Grimace or cough Pink or acrocyanotic	1. Suction 2. Dry blankets/radiant warmer 3. Stimulate to cry (rub back, flick feet) 4. Light percussion with mask on back to clear fluid
5-7, mildly depressed	Heart rate > 100 Poor respiratory effort and weak cry Decreased tone No grimace to suction Pale or acrocyanosis	1. Vigorous drying and stimulation/radiant warmer 2. "Blow-by" O_2 3. Bag-mask ventilation if heart rate < 80 4. Naloxone 0.1 mg/kg if received intrauterine opiates 5. Observe in intensive care nursery if continued depression or response to naloxone
3-4, depressed	Heart rate > or < 100 Apneic or gasping Floppy No response to tactile stimulation Blue or pale	1. Immediate bag-mask ventilation (rate 40-60/min, 100% O_2, PIP < 30) 2. Simultaneous vigorous drying and stimulating 3. Intubate if no improvement at one minute 4. If heart rate < 80 after 1 min of positive-pressure ventilation, begin cardiac compressions (rate 120/min, compression: vent 3:1), and treat as morbid
0-2, morbid	Heart rate < 100 beats/min Rare gasp or apneic Limp No response to stimulation Pale, blue or "black" color	1. Brief bag-mask ventilation while drying 2. Immediate intubation if no improvement (within 30 sec) 3. Cardiac compressions immediately if HR < 60 beats/min or any time HR < 80 beats/min after adequate ventilation established 4. If depressed HR and cardiac output, epinephrine 0.1 ml/kg of 1:10,000 (1 mg epi in 10 ml diluent) 5. Volume: 10 ml/kg normal saline or Ringer's lactate 6. Dextrose 0.1-1.0 g/kg 7. Naloxone 0.1 mg/kg 8. Transport to nursery with 100% O_2, warm blankets and warmer

Adapted from Chameides L, Hazinski F, eds: *Textbook of pediatric advanced life support*, American Heart Association, 1994.
*If prematurity or suspicion of intrauterine asphyxia, respiratory distress can occur 5 min to 12 hours after successful resuscitation. Any sign of nasal flaring, retractions, or grunting on reassessment dictates intensive care nursery observation. Prolonged acrocyanosis is normal.

Fetal effects of maternally administered anesthetics

Drug	Placental transfer	Effect on neonate
Thiopental	Rapidly crosses placenta Most removed by fetal liver Diluted in fetal inferior vena cava	Little depression seen in doses < 4 mg/kg
Ketamine	Rapidly crosses placenta	No depression seen in doses <1 mg/kg
Succinylcholine	Limited transfer, because of highly ionized molecule	Motor weakness only seen in neonate homozygous for pseudocholinesterase deficiency
Nondepolarizing muscle relaxants	Limited transfer, because of large, bulky, rigid molecule with steroid nucleus and high ionization	Minimal effect
Nitrous oxide	Rapidly transferred	Exposure should be limited to less than 20 min, for minimal neonatal depression
Halogenated agents	Transfer relative to uptake and distribution of agent	Can depress cardiovascular system if fetus is acidotic—effects rarely seen at levels of halothane 0.5%, enflurane 1%, isoflurane 0.75%
Opioids	Easily transferred	May cause depression reversed by naloxone
Local anesthetics	Transfer dependent on degree of protein binding; fetal acidosis increases accumulation in fetus	
• Chloroprocaine	Eliminated by cholinesterases and does not cross placenta	No effect
• Bupivacaine	Limited transfer, because of high protein binding	Little effect
• Lidocaine	Moderate transfer, because of less protein binding	May see transient neurobehavioral changes

Drugs used in neonatal resuscitation

Drug	Standard concentration	Dose (per kg)	Dose (ml/kg)	Endotracheal route*
Epinephrine	0.1 mg/ml	0.01 mg	0.1 ml	Yes (0.1 mg/kg)
Atropine[†]	0.1 mg/ml	0.01-0.03 mg	0.1-0.3	Yes (0.02-0.06 mg/kg)
Bicarbonate	8.4% = 1 mEq/ml	1 mEq[‡]	1 ml	No
Calcium chloride	100 mg/ml	20 mg	0.2 ml	No
Glucose	$D_{10}W$ (100 mg/ml)	0.5-1 g	5-10 ml	No
Naloxone	0.4 mg/ml	0.1 mg	0.25 ml	Yes (0.1 mg/kg)
PGE_1[§]	0.05 μg/kg/min continuous infusion x 30 min, then titrate according to PaO_2			

*Should be diluted in 3-5 ml normal saline.
†Minimum dose of 0.1 mg.
‡Should be diluted 1:1 with normal saline or Ringer's lactate.
§Side effects of PGE infusion include: apnea, systemic hypotension, CNS irritability (hyperthermia, seizure-like activity), and cardiac arrhythmias.

TRANSPORTATION OF THE CRITICALLY ILL NEWBORN

The problem of stabilization and transportation of the critically ill newborn may be encountered by the anesthesiologist working in a hospital without pediatric or neonatal intensive care capability. The general practitioner, pediatrician, or obstetrician who rarely encounters a critically ill child may consult an anesthesiologist regarding airway management, intravenous access, pharmacotherapy, or general stabilization before transporting the infant to a tertiary care center.

The Receiving Team

Transportation of a critical child generally is performed by a specialized team from the accepting facility. The transport team usually is activated by telephone contact with the on-duty transport coordinator, usually a staff physician from the accepting intensive care unit, who also may advise on management. The coordinator also chooses the mode of transportation. In general, medicolegal responsibility is transferred to the accepting hospital when the transport team arrives at the bedside, and not with acceptance of transportation by telephone. In cases of interstate transportation, most states allow the transport team to function under the "Good Samaritan Act." Conversely, until the transport team arrives at the bed side, medicolegal responsibility falls on the referring physician.

Pretransport Treatment

In addition to treatment already instituted at the referring hospital, the transport coordinator at the accepting hospital may make suggestions to be instituted before arrival of the transport vehicle. Many procedures are difficult to initiate in a moving vehicle and are better applied prior to transport, even if only prophylactically.

1. Maternal and newborn blood clots are obtained along with signed consent for transport.
2. Children with an unstable airway, or whose (presumptive) diagnosis may later threaten the airway, may need elective endotracheal intubation and muscle relaxation.
3. Hyperventilation ($PaCO_2$ of 25 to 30 mm Hg) may be necessary in the child suspected of having increased intracranial pressure.
4. Chest tubes may be needed when even a small pneumothorax is diagnosed.
5. Ideally, two sites of intravenous access should be available through either umbilical or peripheral vessels.
6. A nasogastric tube is usually inserted for bowel obstruction or in patients at risk for aspiration (e.g., tracheoesophageal fistula).
7. Oral feedings should be withheld before transport.
8. Omphalocele, gastroschisis, meningomyelocele, bladder exstrophy are covered with saline-soaked sterile gauze and plastic wrap.
9. If the child is to be transported by air, transfusion may be necessary to raise the hematocrit and increase oxygen-carrying capacity.
10. Blood, urine, and CSF should be cultured before beginning antibiotic administration, which usually is started before transfer.
11. Checking the stool for occult blood helps in diagnosing necrotizing enterocolitis in the newborn.
12. A continuous infusion of PGE_1 is a common therapeutic maneuver for patients with cyanotic congenital heart disease to maintain a patent ductus arteriosus (see table on p. 424).
13. Dopamine may be used for renal perfusion or inotropic support.
14. Sodium nitroprusside is a peripheral and pulmonary vasodilator that can be useful for the treatment of persistent fetal circulation.
15. With the use of anticonvulsants, equipment for controlling the airway (i.e., endotracheal intubation) must be available.
16. Patients with a history of hypoglycemia should be transported with a continuous infusion of $D_{10}W$.

Delivery room stabilization of neonatal emergencies

Clinical manifestation	Treatment	Comments
Respiratory emergencies		
Congenital diaphragmatic hernia (CDH) Respiratory distress with cyanosis Scaphoid abdomen Heart sounds displaced to right Bowel sounds present over thorax CXR shows bowel in thorax	Nasogastric tube for decompression Intubation and ventilation with small tidal volumes and PIP < 30 cm H_2O	Occurs on left in 90% of cases Results in hypoplasia of lungs Prone to pneumothorax on nonherniated side and to pulmonary hypertension
Tracheoesophageal fistula Excessive secretions Coughing, choking, and cyanosis; especially with feeding Inability to pass nasogastric tube	Head-up, prone or lateral positioning Placement of esophageal pouch suction tube	90% with blind upper pouch and fistula between trachea and lower esophagus One third have other anomalies (e.g., VATER association) Aspiration is common with resultant atelectasis and pneumonia
Cystic hygroma Neck mass Stridor Feeding difficulties	If respiratory distress, awake intubation while maintaining spontaneous ventilation	May result in total airway obstruction Mass usually recurs after excision; tracheostomy placement often required during operation
Vascular ring Stridor may be present at birth, but usually develops over first day to weeks	Awake intubation if airway obstruction occurs	Anatomic variations include: • Double aortic arch • Right arch with ligamentum arteriosum • Pulmonary artery sling
Laryngeal/bronchial cysts Stridor	Intubation and ventilatory support as needed Needle aspiration of cyst if its size prevents passage of ETT	Stridor does not respond to medical management
Congenital lobar emphysema Respiratory distress CXR shows hyperlucent lung field with mediastinal shift	Respiratory support as needed	Usually affects left upper lobe Ball-valve mechanism causes air trapping in alveoli

Delivery room stabilization of neonatal emergencies—cont'd

Clinical manifestation	Treatment	Comments
Respiratory emergencies—cont'd		
Choanal atresia Cyanosis at rest or with feeding Unable to pass nasal catheter	Placement of oral airway If bilateral, may need intubation	May be accompanied by other anomalies (e.g., CHARGE association)
Laryngeal web (at level of true vocal cords) Stridor if incomplete Visualization with laryngoscope	Intubation with forcible rupture of web if possible Needle cricothyrotomy followed by tracheostomy	May result in infant's demise if not immediately recognized
Tracheomalacia Inspiratory stridor resulting from pliable airway tissues	Respiratory support as needed	Stridor usually worsens with cry Usually improves with growth
Congenital subglottic stenosis Stridor	Respiratory support or intubation as needed	Stridor does not respond to medical management Usually improves with growth
Cyanotic congenital heart disease (see also Chapter 7)		
Transposition of great vessels Cyanosis May have loud S_2 and a murmur Right axis deviation	Intubation as needed	Balloon septostomy used for immediate palliation
Tetralogy of Fallot Varying degrees of cyanosis Heart murmur Significant right ventricular hypertrophy	Increase FiO_2 to decrease pulmonary vascular resistance Knee-chest positioning	15% with other major extracardiac malformation
Pulmonary stenosis or atresia *Tricuspid atresia* *Truncus arteriosus* *Single or hypoplastic ventricle* *Total anomalous pulmonary venous return* Cyanosis Deterioration or worsened cyanosis with crying or ductus closure	PGE_1 to keep ductus patent Correction of acidosis Inotropic support, emergent septostomy, valvotomy, or shunt if not improving	Diagnosed by echocardiogram

Continued.

Delivery room stabilization of neonatal emergencies—cont'd

Clinical manifestation	Treatment	Comments
Gastrointestinal emergencies		
Omphalocele Midline defect Bowel covered by membrane Within umbilical cord	Nasogastric tube for decompression Saline-soaked gauze or plastic covering of herniated organs	Failure of midgut to return to abdominal cavity Associated with cardiac, urologic, and metabolic abnormalities
Gastroschisis Periumbilical defect Bowel and viscus exposed	Treat as above	Result of omphalomesenteric artery occlusion during gestation Usually not associated with other malformations

Neurologic emergencies

Meningomyelocele Posterior midline defect	Saline-soaked gauze covering defect Keep infant in prone or lateral position	Use of latex-free equipment advised

Nonsurgical neonatal emergencies

Early (first minutes)		
Meconium aspiration Meconium staining Respiratory distress May have low Apgar score	Oropharyngeal suctioning before delivery of shoulders and body Laryngoscopy/intubation if infant depressed Suction via ETT; extubate when aspirate clear and stomach emptied	May develop persistent fetal circulation
Maternal drugs: narcotics, magnesium, anesthetic agents History of recent drug administration Low Apgar score Depression despite resuscitation	Respiratory support as needed Naloxone 0.1 mg/kg/dose IM, IV, ETT Calcium chloride (for hypermagnesemia) 20 mg/kg IV slowly	See table on p. 423

Late (>30 min postpartum)
(sepsis may be etiology for any of these conditions)

Apnea Respiratory pause > 20 sec More severe if accompanied by bradycardia	Stimulation Intubation and ventilation if persistent Evaluation for underlying problem	Often indicative of underlying problems such as acidosis, hypoxia, hypoglycemia, anemia, sepsis, narcotics, CNS trauma, and pulmonary disease Often seen in premature infants (not seen until 2-5 days of age)
Respiratory distress syndrome (RDS) Respiratory distress developing in first hours of life (grunting, flexing, retractions) Low Apgar score CXR with diffuse atelectasis with air bronchograms	Respiratory support as needed PIP 20-25 cm H_2O PEEP 4-5 cm H_2O Maintain Pao_2 40-75 Surfactant therapy Culture and treat for sepsis	Associated with prematurity, maternal diabetes, and perinatal asphyxia May be indistinguishable from neonatal pneumonia
Meconium aspiration syndrome (MAS) Respiratory distress Overdistended chest Coarse breath sounds	Respiratory support as needed May require high peak inspiratory pressure	Pneumothorax common as a result of hyperinflation May develop persistent pulmonary hypertension
Transient tachypnea of the newborn (TTN) Tachypnea Mild retractions	Respiratory support as needed	Self-limited with resolution in 24-48 hours Usually seen in full term infants Associated with cesarean delivery
Pneumothorax Acute unexplained deterioration in respiratory status Decreased breath sounds	Needle aspiration if symptomatic Chest tube thoracostomy	May be due to resuscitation efforts Associated with MAS and RDS
Persistent pulmonary hypertension (PPH) Progressive cyanosis and tachypnea Absence of heart disease Right ventricular hypertrophy	Hyperventilation to achieve $Paco_2$ of 20-25 mm Hg and respiratory alkalosis Consider sedation and muscle relaxation Fluid and inotropic support Vasodilatory support (e.g., tolazoline, nitric oxide after consultation) ECMO	Usually seen in full-term or postdates infant May be history of asphyxia or meconium aspiration Associated with congenital heart disease, MAS, group B streptococcus sepsis

Continued.

Delivery room stabilization of neonatal emergencies—cont'd

Clinical manifestation	Treatment	Comments
Seizures Tonic-clonic movements May present as eye fluttering, sucking, and drooling, tonic posturing, or apnea	Consider immediately treatable etiologies: sepsis, hypoxia, acidosis, hypoglycemia, hypokalemia, maternal drug addiction (withdrawal) Establish adequate airway Phenobarbital 20 mg/kg q30min up to 40 mg/kg to stop seizure Maintenance: 5 mg/kg/24 h divided q12h Phenytoin 20 mg/kg dose × 2 doses q12h Maintenance: 5 mg/kg/24 h divided q12h	May result from central nervous system, metabolic, or infectious etiologies
Sepsis Irritability, lethargy Respiratory distress or apnea Hypothermia Jaundice Abdominal distension	Respiratory support as needed Fluids and blood products administration IV ampicillin 25 mg/kg q12h (≤2.0 kg); 25 mg/kg q8h (>2.0 kg) IV gentamicin 2.5 mg/kg q12h	Consider if history of maternal illness or prolonged rupture of membranes Culture blood, urine and spinal fluid Usual organisms: group B streptococcus, *E. coli, S. aureus, L. monocytogenes*
Hypoglycemia May be asymptomatic Non-specific symptoms include tremors, apnea, poor feeding, seizures, lethargy	If stable: oral glucose If unstable: $D_{10}W$ 2 ml/kg IV then titration of infusion to maintain normoglycemia	Usually seen in infants of diabetic mothers, premature infants, and infants small for gestational age
Opioid withdrawal Nonspecific symptoms include irritability, jitteriness, apnea, poor feeding, seizures	Phenobarbital	Consider if history of maternal substance abuse Taper medicine as tolerated

References

Avery GB, Fletcher MA, MacDonald MG, eds: *Neonatology: pathophysiology and management of the newborn,* Philadelphia, 1994, JB Lippincott.

Chameides L, Hazinski MF, eds: *Textbook of pediatric advanced life support,* American Heart Association, 1994.

Cunningham FG et al, eds: *Williams obstetrics,* East Norwalk, Conn, 1993, Appleton & Lange.

Falciglia HS: Failure to prevent meconium aspiration syndrome, *Obstet Gynecol* 71:349-353, 1988.

Frankel LR: The evaluation, stabilization, and transport of the critically ill child, *Int Anesthesiol Clin* 25:77-103, 1987.

Linder N, Aranda JV: Need for endotracheal intubation and suction in meconium stained neonates, *J Pediatr* 112:613-615, 1988.

Paterson SJ, Byrne PJ, Molesky MG, Seal RF, Finucane BT: Neonatal resuscitation using the laryngeal mask airway, *Anesthesiology* 80:1248-1253, 1994.

Peter G, ed: *Report of the committee on infectious diseases,* ed 23, Elk Grove Village, Ill, 1994, American Academy of Pediatrics.

ANESTHESIA AND SEDATION AWAY FROM THE OPERATING ROOM

19

Leo, master of the "whys"
made the doctors and nurses sigh
didn't the chart say "sedated at four"?
post script note: "he might need MORE!"

Adrienne Coleman

Anesthesia care outside the operating room represents at least 10% of total sedation cases,[1] a number that will no doubt rise as technology becomes increasingly more complex.

Procedures commonly requiring sedation and/or analgesia for infants and children

Diagnostic radiology
  Computed tomography (CT)
  Magnetic resonance imaging (MRI)
  Ultrasound (including echocardiography)
  Fluoroscopy
Interventional radiology
  Angiography/angioplasty/embolizations
  Percutaneous renal and hepatobiliary procedures
  Myelography
Cardiac catheterization laboratory
  Diagnostic catheterizations
  Interventions (angioplasty, valvuloplasty, balloon dilatations, stenting of stenoses, transcatheter closures of septal defects or patent ductus)
Emergency department
  Repair of lacerations
  Closed reductions of fractures
Clinic areas
  Endoscopy/bronchoscopy
  Lumbar puncture
  Bone marrow aspiration
  Biopsies
  Laser treatment
Radiation therapy
  Therapy for neoplastic disease
  Ablation for bone marrow transplant

Many procedures that formerly required a surgical incision can now be accomplished transdermally or percutaneously (e.g., angiographic embolization, lithotripsy, and umbrella occlusion). Equipment necessary for these procedures and for new diagnostic studies cannot be moved to an operating room (e.g., magnetic resonance imaging [MRI] and computed tomographic [CT] scans). Many of these procedures or studies need little or no analgesia, but require prolonged patient cooperation and absence of movement, which make their success nearly impossible in the awake infant or child.

Therefore, it is now common for many pediatric anesthesiologists to administer deep sedation and anesthesia in remote locations of the hospital where equipment is unfamiliar or unavailable and there are no colleagues to assist in an emergency. Similarly, as radiology suites, MRI centers, CT scanners, and fluoroscopy rooms are all built to optimize imaging, they may not be constructed for the needs of an anesthetized patient. Flexibility, resourcefulness, and creativity are required of the anesthesia team.

Safe, effective, and efficient sedation and/or anesthetic practice in infants and children demand special clinical skill, appropriate levels of monitoring and vigilance, and immediate availability of airway and resuscitation equipment tailored to the age and size of the patient.[2,3] For those children scheduled as outpatients, the anesthesiologist may well accept primary patient responsibility during the hospital visit, especially if the procedure is accomplished by technicians and the referring physician is offsite.

PLANNING THE ANESTHETIC

Because of the issues mentioned above, administering anesthesia or sedation to children in locations remote to the operating rooms requires careful preprocedure planning and organization on the part of the anesthetic team. The factors listed in the box at right should be considered well in advance of the scheduled procedure.

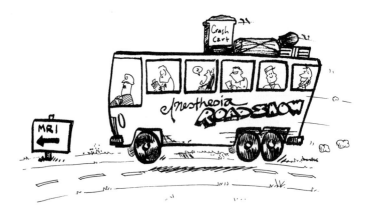

Preprocedure considerations for remote locations:
a checklist

Patient factors

Chronologic and developmental age
Baseline level of sensorium, ability to cooperate, and anxiety
Concomitant illnesses or injuries
Medications and drug allergies
Evaluation of the airway and focused physical exam (risks of loss of
    protective reflexes, airway obstruction, cardiopulmonary dysfunc-
    tion, or neurologic decompensation, particularly increased intracra-
    nial pressure or seizures)
Postprocedure disposition (home, recovery, admission, intensive care
    unit)
Accompanying adult for outpatients

Operator factors

Level of training of anesthesia team for both procedure and anesthetic
Level of training for those performing procedure (technician, nurses,
    physicians)
Availability of personnel for transport, delivery of care, monitoring,
    resuscitation, and recovery
Identification of primary physician (referring doctor, proceduralist,
    anesthesiologist)
Readiness for unexpected complications and/or admission
Availability of anesthesiologists to provide spontaneous support dur-
    ing failed sedation attempts by nonanesthesiologists

Procedure factors

Location (hazards, fixed equipment)
Procedure duration
Anticipated pain or stimulation
Patient positioning
Potential complications
Duration of recovery

The Patient

Proper patient selection is crucial to ensure safe and satisfactory
outcomes for outpatient pediatric patients having "off-floor" procedures with sedation or anesthesia. A preanesthetic visit with the
parent and child (perhaps to follow a scheduled clinic appointment)
is used in many institutions to obtain historical information and a
focused physical examination and to procure information from primary physicians or referring physicians. If this is not practical, a
telephone conversation with a parent and the referring physician is
also helpful to organize information in advance of the procedure.[4]

Many children scheduled for procedures in remote locations
have had or will have other medical procedures. When a child is
scheduled for a series of procedures, the success of the first anesthetic increases both the chances of future successes and parent/
patient satisfaction. Involving the parent and the (verbal) child in

the decision-making process during the preprocedure interview may greatly increase overall cooperation and satisfaction.

1. Often the physician performing the procedure is a consultant not acquainted with the patient. It is important to identify the patient's primary physician and request a preanesthetic history and physical examination. Usually, a repeat history and physical is not required before each procedure when a series of procedures is scheduled.

2. Data from routine laboratory tests and from any special tests pertinent to the condition of the patient should be obtained.

3. Any contraindications to the administration of sedatives, including altered mental status, increased intracranial pressure (ICP), the presence of a difficult airway, compromised respiratory function, hemodynamic instability, or "full stomach," should be noted.

4. For outpatients, it is best to speak with the parent or guardian before the procedure about anesthetic procedures, risks, and plans, by telephone or during a preoperative visit. Fasting schedules should be outlined and critical medications should be continued. Plans for recovery, discharge, and at-home care should be detailed as well.

5. Additionally, patients who may need admission or rescheduling can be identified during the anesthesia preoperative consultation.

The Staff

The rapid evolution of diagnostic and nonsurgical interventional techniques makes it difficult for the anesthesiologist to know or anticipate all of the intricacies for a given procedure. Advance communication with the procedure team is essential to identify each team's needs as well as potential conflicts or difficulties. The procedure team needs to be aware of the basic components and sequence of an anesthetic for a pediatric patient and the amount of time required for equipment set-up, preoperative interview, intravenous access, monitoring, emergence, and recovery.

Typically, scheduling changes are needed to accomodate the anesthetic time, which may seem best accomplished by tacking on anesthetic procedures at the end of the day, where delays will not affect other scheduled patients. Unfortunately, this practice is not in the best interest of the fasting child, nor does it necessarily allow sufficient time for recovery. It is usually best to schedule procedures as early in the day as possible.

It is also important to clarify which members of the procedure team will be present during the procedure. Some diagnostic procedures only require the presence of a technician; neither a nurse nor a physician is available onsite, and the primary referring physician will be even more remote. A two-person anesthesia team is recommended to ensure smooth induction, emergence, and transport to recovery areas. This team must function self-sufficiently in the event of an emergency. Furthermore, back-up anesthetists in the operating room should be identified for emergent support should further help be required.

The Procedure

The following points should be clarified in advance of the procedure and considered when determining the anesthetic goals and plan.

1. What is the specific *technique?* Is the procedure painful or stimulating? Will heparinization for catheter placement be necessary (limiting regional anesthetic choices)? What parts of the body will be accessible to the anesthesia team?

2. Will the procedure involve *radiation exposure* or the use of radiopaque dye (intravenous contrast)? Will ionic or non-ionic compounds be chosen?

3. What is the anticipated *duration* of the procedure? What is the anticipated recovery time after the procedure? Will the patient be hospitalized or discharged?

4. What *position(s)* will the patient be in? Will he or she need to be moved during the procedure? Will he or she need to be transported for part of the procedure to another location while anesthetized? Will the patient be accessible to the anesthesiologist? Must the patient be absolutely motionless (e.g., cerebral angiographic embolization), or can some movement be tolerated (e.g., bone marrow aspiration)?

5. What are the anticipated *complications* and sequelae? Pain? Bleeding? Nausea or vomiting? Hemodynamic compromise?

Special Problems[5]

1. Physical plant: Availability of wall-source oxygen, suction, the appropriate number and type of electrical outlets, and space for an anesthesia machine, ventilator, supply cart, and monitors need to be assessed by the anesthesiologist before beginning the planned procedure in any remote location. Sometimes the physical plant must be modified to accomodate the anesthetic needs and meet standards mandated by medical societies, hospitals, and state law.[6]

   a. *Wall oxygen* should be accessible, or an adequate supply of full cylinders must be available. A separate source of oxygen may be necessary to power a free-standing ventilator.

   b. *Wall suction* is ideal both for patient care and to scavenge gases if inhalation agents will be used. Portable suction is sufficient for patient care but cannot be used to scavenge gases. Suction machines designated for procedure use may not be available to the anesthesiologist during the procedure.

c. *Isolated electrical outlets* usually are not available. Electrical converters or adapters may be needed to power monitoring equipment. Extension cords should be available. Adequate battery supply should be present for transport equipment.

2. Limited access to the patient: A crowded work space, fixed equipment, hazards, and nonmovable tables may make it nearly impossible to position the anesthesiologist or anesthetic equipment close to the patient. Intravenous tubing and breathing circuits may need extensions to prevent disconnections as the patient or table is moved. An emergency plan should be delineated with the person performing the procedure in the event the procedure must be interrupted to treat the patient.

3. Dim lighting: In most radiology suites, overhead lights are dimmed or nonexistent to improve imaging. Task lighting for anesthetic procedures or record keeping should be available.

4. Unpadded tables: With the exception of the emergency department, most locations will utilize fixed hard tables, which cannot be placed in Trendelenburg position if hypotension or vomiting occur. Pressure points require extra padding.

5. Cold rooms: Many radiology sites are kept cold to accomodate superconductors used for imaging. Warming blankets cannot be used on radiology tables, as they interfere with imaging. Warmed fluids, humidified inhalational agents, and radiant warmers may be helpful to maintain normothermia. The radio frequency used in the MRI suite causes body heating equivalent to short wave diathermy, so additional heating devices are not usually required in this location.[7]

6. Radiation exposure: The anesthesia team should take all precautions to protect against excessive radiation exposure, including wearing a lead apron, thyroid shield, and leaded glasses when appropriate. A radiation badge measuring cumulative exposure may be useful for those with frequent exposure. If possible, the anesthesiologist should leave the immediate area during periods of high radiation and observe the patient and monitors from behind a leaded glass shield. With most contemporary shielded and coned equipment, radiation exposure is negligible at a distance of approximately 6 feet.

    When hazards demand that the anesthesiologist leave the patient (e.g., radiation therapy), closed-circuit videography and microphone amplification assist in the maintenance of vigilance. Radio stethoscopes are also available for listening to heart and breath sounds outside of the room.

    The patient should also be protected from the hazards of radiation. Lead shielding should be used for the most radiosensitive areas (eyes, thyroid, testes, ovaries).

Use of Radiopaque Dye

1. Ionic contrast media (sodium meglumine, salts of iodinated acids, or their combinations) commonly are used for IV imaging.

2. The hyperosmolarity of these ionic compounds can cause a typical (*nonallergic*) reaction, characterized by flushing, tachycardia, and nausea, probably caused by endothelial disruption and the subsequent nonimmunologic release of vasoactive substances from mast cells.

3. A small percentage of patients will exhibit true *allergy* to the iodine moiety. Although a history of iodine or shellfish allergy, asthma, or drug allergies may suggest which patients are susceptible, anaphylaxis can occur without significant previous exposure or history.

4. Pretreatment with corticosteroids is most effective in ameliorating allergic reactions. H_2 blockers and dyphenhydramine are useful as adjuvant premedicants.

5. If ionic dyes are used for procedures in children, concentrations of 30% to 60% are preferred to reduce osmolality.

6. Volume contraction, high osmolality, and neuropathy can be anticipated after using ionic contrast because of the hyperosmolarity and high iodine and sodium concentrations. Fluid balance and hemodynamic parameters should be closely monitored.

7. Nonionic compounds are significantly less osmolar than their ionic counterparts and are associated with a decreased incidence of dye reactions. Their use is preferred in children, although they are substantially more expensive.[8]

Treatment for allergic reactions to intravenous contrast

Drug	Dose	Administration
Prophylaxis		
Methylprednisolone	0.5 mg/kg PO	Two doses: 12 hours preprocedure 2 hours preprocedure
Diphenhydramine	0.5-1.0 mg/kg PO/IV	1-2 hours preprocedure
Treatment of anaphylaxis		
Epinephrine	Bolus, 10 µg/kg IV Infusion, 0.1-1.0 µg/kg/min IV	Can be given by intra-osseous infusion or peripheral vessel until central access is established

Properties of intravenous contrast

Compound	Iodine (mg/ml)	Osmolarity (mOsm/L)	Sodium content	Recommended dose in children*
Ionic				
Hypaque Conray Renograffin	~300	1000-2000	May be significant	2 ml/kg of 30% or 60% (maximum dose, 5 ml/kg)
Nonionic				
Hexabrix Iopamidol Iohexal	~300	700-900	Insignificant	2 ml/kg (maximum dose < 4 ml/kg)

*The dose is excreted over time, and doses may be repeated during lengthy procedures with careful attention to hydration.

EQUIPMENT AND MONITORING

Although it is technically feasible to have monitoring systems identical to those in operating rooms, some modification is usually required because of space constraints or physical limitations. Many commercial portable transport monitors are now available with sufficient fields for complete noninvasive and invasive monitoring.

Equipment for general anesthesia in remote locations: a checklist

Suction	If no wall suction is available, a portable suction machine should be placed at the site for the sole use of the anesthesia team. Portable suction is not adequate to scavenge inhaled gases.
Oxygen	Ideally, central oxygen lines are available for patient delivery and the anesthesia machine/ventilator. Full oxygen cylinders with checked circuit are necessary for backup and transport.
Monitors	All monitors needed to fulfill ASA standards should be available and usable (ECG, oximetry, capnography, noninvasive blood pressure, O_2 analyzer, temperature). Electrical adapters and extension cords may be needed. Portable monitors should be adequately charged.
Machines	A portable anesthesia machine/ventilator with appropriate alarms is useful if space and facilities allow. Alternatively, total intravenous general anesthesia obviates the need for an anesthesia machine (electronic infusion devices may be useful).
Cart	A stocked supply cart on casters can be taken to the site with full complement of anesthetic and resuscitative drugs (including naloxone and flumazenil), intravenous and airway equipment (masks, airways, laryngoscopes, endotracheal tubes, stylets), extra circuits, and probes. Intraosseous needles may be needed for emergent IV access.
Defibrillator	All patient areas must have access to a functioning defibrillator. Pediatric settings and paddles should be checked during the preprocedure site visit.

In the United States, equipment and monitors for patients receiving general anesthesia in remote locations must meet the same ASA standards as described for patients in the operating room.[6] In addition, some institutions or states have mandated additional requirements (capnography is required in the state of New York). However, the American Academy of Pediatrics has published separate guidelines for conscious and deep sedation, which are not as stringent as ASA standards.[2] Both standards are listed below.

	American Society of Anesthesiologists standards for basic intraoperative monitoring*	American Academy of Pediatrics standards for sedation
Standard I	Qualified anesthesia personnel continuously[†] present (If a known hazard to personnel exists [e.g., radiation] provisions for remote monitoring must be made)	**Conscious sedation** a. Practitioner knowledgeable in drugs, techniques, monitoring and able to manage complications (minimum: pediatric basic life support) b. Support personnel to monitor physiologic parameters and assist supportive or resuscitative measures **Deep sedation** a. Same b. One person must be available whose *sole* responsibility is monitoring vital signs, adequacy of ventilation and drug administration (either a or b must be able to provide pediatric basic life support; advanced life support recommended)
Standard II	Oxygenation, ventilation, circulation, and temperature shall be continually[†] evaluated	Continuous quantitative monitoring of oxygen saturation (pulse oximetry) and heart rate; intermittent respiratory rate and blood pressure
	Oxygenation a. O$_2$ analyzer* b. Pulse oximetry* c. Patient observation*	a. Not applicable b. Pulse oximetry c. Patient observation

Continued.

	American Society of Anesthesiologists standards for basic intraoperative monitoring*	**American Academy of Pediatrics standards for sedation**
Standard II (cont'd)	**Ventilation** a. Patient observation and auscultation b. $ETCO_2$ analysis with tracheal intubation* c. Disconnect alarm for mechanical ventilation	a. Patient observation (auscultation encouraged for deep sedation) b. Capnography encouraged for deep sedation c. Not applicable
	Circulation a. Electrocardiography* b. Blood pressure and heart rate every 5 minutes* c. Circulatory evaluation by: palpation or pulse auscultation of heart sounds monitoring intraarterial pressure trace ultrasound monitoring of pulse plethysmography oximetry	Available intermittent recording of blood pressure and heart rate (every 5 min for deep sedation)
	Temperature Continuous measurement	

Data from American Academy of Pediatrics Committee on Drugs: Guidelines for monitoring and management of pediatric patients during and after sedation for diagnostic and therapeutic procedures, *Pediatrics* 89: 1110-1115, 1992; American Society of Anesthesiologists: Standards for basic intraoperative monitoring, American Society of Anesthesiologists 1996 Directory of Members, ed 61.

*Under extenuating circumstances, the responsible anesthesiologist may waive the requirements marked with an asterisk(*); it is recommended that when this is done, it should be so stated (including the reasons) in a note in the patient's medical record.

†Continual/Continuous: Note that "continual" is defined as "repeated regularly and frequently in steady rapid succession" whereas "continuous" means prolonged without any interruption at any time.

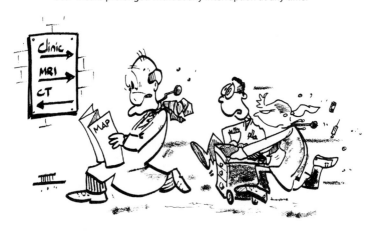

Monitoring for Sedation

The American Academy of Pediatrics has coined the following terms:[2]

Conscious sedation

A medically controlled state of depressed consciousness that:

1. allows protective reflexes to be maintained
2. retains the patient's ability to maintain a patent airway independently and continuously
3. permits appropriate response by the patient to physical stimulation or verbal command.

Deep sedation

A medically controlled state of depressed consciousness or unconsciousness from which the patient is not easily aroused. It may be accompanied by a partial or complete loss of protective reflexes, and includes the inability to maintain a patent airway independently and respond purposefully to physical stimulation or verbal command.

Usually, the anesthesiologist is consulted because the referring physician does *not* want the child to respond appropriately to physical stimulation, by definition necessitating at least deep sedation. The sedation of a child occurs at a continuum between planes of consciousness and deep sedation, with the line to general anesthesia easily crossed. Loss of the airway and cardiorespiratory decompensation may easily and frequently occur, so that early recognition of change by continuous vigilance and monitoring becomes essential to prevent unintentional progression of sedation. All of the equipment and monitoring devices listed in the table on p. 441 are advocated for sedation procedures, with the exception of the anesthesia machine and related alarms.

1. The continuous presence of qualified personnel is required for all sedation procedures. Ideally, the *monitor* is a different person from the *proceduralist.* This distinction becomes mandatory for deep sedation or anesthesia. The monitoring person is responsible for patient observation, recording vital signs, and administering carefully titrated drugs. This person must also be certified in basic pediatric life support and be familiar with the resuscitation cart and equipment.

2. Pulse oximetry is the only monitor recommended by the American Academy of Pediatrics and the American Medical Association for conscious sedation.[9] Unfortunately, oximetry is a late monitor of adequacy of *ventilation;* severe and prolonged hypercapnia and acidosis can occur without changes in oxygen saturation. The following monitoring parameters are recommended for children receiving sedation:

    a. *Adequacy of respiration:* airway patency; rate, depth,

and pattern of respiration; pulse oximetry; capnography (optional with deep sedation per American Academy of Pediatrics published guidelines)

b. *Hemodynamic stability:* heart rate and rhythm (ECG, plethysmography), noninvasive blood pressure

c. *Level of consciousness/responsiveness:* arousable to command, physical stimulation; intact protective reflexes

d. *Temperature:* By thermistor or liquid-crystal adhesive strips

3. No specific monitoring or recording intervals are mandated for vital signs in children receiving conscious sedation. For deep sedation, assessment and recording of vital signs is recommended every 5 minutes and continued until discharge criteria are met. Intravenous access is also recommended (see guidelines, p. 441).

4. Postprocedure observation in a recovery room–type setting that includes trained personnel, vigilance, and appropriate monitors is recommended until the patient meets institutional discharge criteria (see also Chapter 5). The child should return to baseline verbal and motor function, be "awake" with intact protective reflexes, and have stable cardiorespiratory function and adequate hydration. Objective discharge criteria (see p. 103) are particularly useful in areas of the hospital that do not usually recover children from sedation. Final discharge orders and instructions to the parents should be given by the anesthesiologist or responsible physician. It is usually suggested that the parents first contact their primary provider for any postprocedure problems, with appropriate referral information to the anesthesiologist or proceduralist as well.

Equipment and Monitoring in the MRI Suite[7,10,11]

The MRI suite has proved to be one of the most challenging non–operating room locations requiring anesthetic equipment and monitoring. Although the speed of the actual scan has increased tremendously since its inception, sufficient time is still required that most children (and many claustrophobic adults) cannot hold perfectly still for the duration. Three types of energy hazards that affect routine monitoring exist within the suite: a static magnetic field of 1.5 Tesla (1.0 Tesla = 10,000 gauss; the earth's surface is < 1 gauss); radiofrequency (RF); and a time-varied magnetic field. Any equipment used in the scanner suite must pose no danger to the patient or the scanner, must function normally during the scan, and must not affect the quality of the scan obtained. Besides these energy hazards, patients are not easily visualized within the bore of the magnet, and the RF produces accoustic noise of 90 dB (equivalent to light road work), making auscultation difficult if not impossible.

Previously, converting current ferromagnetic equipment into nonferromagnetic for use in the scanner suite required a great deal of creativity. However, newer shielded scanners allow a rapid drop in the magnetic field a short distance from the bore of the magnet. The biomedical engineer associated with the scanner should determine the gauss line—the point in the room at which the magnetic field drops to 30 to 50 gauss. At this distance, many pieces of equipment with nonexchangeable ferromagnetic parts (e.g., intravenous infusion pumps) can be used safely and reliably.

Even with nonferromagnetic monitors, electric cables and cords can act as antennae for the RF present in the suite, causing degradation of the MR image. These monitors can be electronically shielded or positioned outside of the scanner suite. Copper or brass wave guides in the wall of the suite serve as a pass-through for lines and cords without affecting the RF shielding of the suite. Also, many companies now make equipment that is nonferromagnetic and RF-shielded specifically for use within the suite. All equipment, whether converted, maintained at a distance, or purchased specifically for the MR suite, should be checked by an MR-trained biomedical engineer before being used on patients within the MR unit.

Finally, patients and staff must be carefully screened for the presence of ferromagnetic foreign bodies, prostheses, surgical clips, or items on clothing or in hair. Temperature elevations have been noted in the presence of the strong magnetic field; this may be particularly problematic around metallic prosthetic implants. Pacemaker microcircuitry is exquisitely sensitive and may cease to function in a magnetic field of 5 gauss or greater.

PHARMACOLOGY AND ANESTHETIC TECHNIQUES

Principles

Sound decision making for pediatric procedures incorporates all of the preceding information regarding the patient, staff, and procedure, and then utilizes knowledge of the pharmacokinetics and pharmacodynamics of available drugs to design a tailored approach for the individual patient. Ultimately, which drug(s) to use will be based on the physician's experience and expertise, institutional policy and guidelines, and patient and procedural requirements.

1. Titration to effect is the guiding principle for sedation techniques. Beginning with an initial low dose of a single drug and increasing the dose as needed will often achieve the desired result with fewest complications.
2. Adding a second or third drug often precipitates more complications without increasing efficacy than increasing the

dose of a single agent.[12,13] This principle does not preclude the use of EMLA cream or local anesthesia for painful procedures, which can decrease sedative requirements.[14]

3. General anesthesia with endotracheal intubation is usually reserved for lengthy or painful procedures that require absolute immobility, when the airway is compromised ("full stomach," facial anomalies, previous apnea), or when airway access is limited by the procedure or equipment.

4. Cognitive and behavioral therapies can reduce pain and psychological stress. These techniques include guided imagery, music, relaxation, parental presence, or even just swaddling and rocking the infant.[15]

5. For urgent or emergent procedures in nonfasted children, the use of drugs to promote gastric emptying, increase lower esophageal tone, and reduce gastric acidity and volume is advised (see Chapter 2, Premedication, p. 31). Endotracheal intubation is recommended for procedures requiring unconsciousness in patients at risk for aspiration.

6. If the child is to be sedated by oral, rectal, or intramuscular routes, sufficient time should be allowed for drug administration before the onset of the procedure (may require 1 to 2 hours).

7. Children's procedures should be scheduled as the first case in the morning to promote a safe and comfortable fasting interval and allow adequate time for recovery for same-day discharge when appropriate.

8. The essential components and sequence of the sedation or anesthetic plan should be understood by those performing the procedure (i.e., induction and IV access, airway management, maintenance, emergence and recovery). All staff members should realize the importance of communicating with the anesthesia team before moving the patient and before conducting different phases of the procedure that may require changes in anesthetic depth or technique.

9. The anesthetic plan should be agreeable to the parents and the child.

Parameters for selecting sedation pharmacology

Therapeutic goal (sedation, anesthesia, anxiolysis, analgesia, amnesia, immobility)
Experience of those using the technique or medication
Child's age
Preexisting medical conditions of the patient
Procedural requirements
Equipment availability (anesthesia machine?)
Length of procedure
Anticipation of postprocedure pain
Route of drug delivery
Plans for recovery and discharge

Drug Pharmacology

Most of the commonly used medications for sedation and anesthesia in remote locations are listed below. Inhalation anesthesia is not discussed, as its use does not differ for procedures outside of the operating room. The reader is referred to several articles for more complete discussions of sedative pharmacology.[3,16,17]

Routes of drug administration	
IM	Intramuscular
IN	Intranasal
IV	Intravascular
PO	Per os/oral
PR	Per rectum
SL	Sublingual

Chloral hydrate[18,19] is the most commonly used hypnotic for monitored conscious sedation by nonanesthesiologists, probably because it is easily administered orally or rectally and has few cardiorespiratory effects in therapeutic doses. It is indicated for non-painful procedures of moderate duration (30 to 90 min) and is most effective in young children (< 2 yr). It offers no analgesia and may produce prolonged sedation or paradoxical excitation. Mucosal irritation (vomiting or diarrhea) is also common.

Dosage/administration:

Infants and children: 50-100 mg/kg PO (maximum single
  dose = 2.0 g) (onset: 20-40 min; peak blood levels in 30-60 min)

Barbiturates produce sleep by depression of central nervous system (CNS) activity with minimal cardiovascular effects at sedative doses. Although their popularity has been substantially reduced by the benzodiazapines, they still possess an ease of administration by multiple routes and offer cerebral protection to patients with CNS lesions.[20]

Disadvantages include respiratory depression (especially thiopental and methohexital), irritation of rectal mucosa with rectal administration, and slow onset with oral administration. Paradoxical excitation is not uncommon, particularly when barbiturates are used for painful procedures. Pentobarbital in particular is known to offer cerebral radiation protection; it is most predictable when given intravenously. These qualities suggest the barbiturates might be most useful for a young child with an indwelling central venous catheter receiving radiation therapy. Tolerance is commonly seen with barbiturates if daily sedation is needed.

Although drug combinations are not usually advocated for simple sedation procedures, the following scenario might present a notable exception. If sleep does not occur 10 minutes after an initial dose of pentobarbital (2 to 3 mg/kg intravenously), the addition of thiopental 1mg/kg will produce rapid sleep and redistribute quickly with little additional sedation. The initial dose of pentobarbital is usually sufficient to maintain sedation for the duration of the procedure. A second dose of pentobarbital would likely produce prolonged sedation.

Dosage/administration:
Pentobarbital:
    IV: 2-3 mg/kg initial dose (onset 10 min); 1 mg/kg additional doses
    IM: 4-6 mg/kg (onset 40-60 min)
Secobarbital[21]: 5-7 mg/kg PR (onset 10-15 min)

    Ultrashort acting (rapid respiratory depression should be anticipated):
Methohexital: 30 mg/kg PR (onset 6-8 min)
Thiopental[22]: 5-8 mg/kg bolus followed by infusion of 6-8 mg/kg/hr (onset in seconds)

Benzodiazepines[23-25] provide sedation, hypnosis, and anxiolysis by direct action on the CNS. Although they do not provide analgesia, they are antiemetic and provide anterograde and retrograde amnesia. Hemodynamic stability with minimal respiratory depression can be anticipated at therapeutic doses.

Midazolam is very popular for the pediatric population because of the qualities listed above and its timely and predictable results regardless of the route of administration (IV, PO, PR, IM, SL, IN). In the cooperative child, oral midazolam is easily administered if mixed with flavored drink mix or syrup. Older children and adolescents without IV access will have a rapid onset of anxiolysis if the drug is administered sublingually with the end of the syringe dipped in crystalline sugar to increase palatability. A duration of 30 to 45 minutes can be anticipated (may be shortened with IV administration).

Midazolam alone has a very wide therapeutic range, although it does not offer immobility. The practice of combining midazolam with opioids to deepen sedation markedly increases the risk for cardiorespiratory depression and should not be considered conscious sedation.[13] Full monitoring and resuscitative capabilities are required when this technique is used.

Diazepam and lorazepam have also been used for sedation. Both drugs offer slower onset and longer duration. Older children and adolescents having repeated procedures (particularly oncologic) may prefer these benzodiazepines, as they can be taken orally at home so that a therapeutic effect is achieved before reaching the hospital or clinic. These drugs also offer antiemetic and amnestic properties. Lorazepam may have a long duration of action (4 to 6 hours) and a delayed onset. It is best used as an oral preparation in adolescents who are scheduled for prolonged procedures (e.g., chemotherapy, plasmapheresis).[26] Lorazepam is known to cause hallucinations in young children.

Dosage/administration:

Midazolam:

    IV: 0.05-0.10 mg/kg (onset 1-3 min)

    PO: 0.5 mg/kg (onset 15-30 min)

    PR: 1.0 mg/kg (onset 5-15 min)

    IN/SL: 0.2-0.4 mg/kg (onset 10-15 min)

Diazepam: 0.5 mg/kg PO (onset 30-60 min)

Lorazepam: 2-4 mg PO (adolescents) (onset 20-40 min)

Fentanyl is a rapid-onset opioid best reserved for procedures requiring analgesia. Although it offers hemodynamic stability and minimal histamine release, it also produces significant respiratory depression and bradycardia. Prolonged clearance and increased effects are seen in neonates and amplified in preterm infants. Analgesia will be intensified by combination with local anesthesia without increasing respiratory depression.

Respiratory depression can be reversed with naloxone, although hypertension, pulmonary edema, and cardiac arrest have been reported, even with conservative doses. When opioid antagonism is required, incremental doses of 10 to 20 µg should be administered until a satisfactory respiratory rate is achieved.[27]

Dosage/administration:

Fentanyl:

    IV: 0.5-1.0 µg/kg incrementally q5-10 min to a maximum of

        4-5 µg/kg (rapid onset)

    Transmucosal: 15-20 µg/kg over 15-20 min (Oralet) (onset

        10 min)

Ketamine[28] has been termed a "dissociative" anesthetic. It induces rapid unconsciousness by either the IV or IM route and is therefore not recommended for sedation. Spontaneous respiration is usually preserved, and heart rate, blood pressure, and intracranial pressure are usually increased. Copious oral secretions are often noted, which can cause coughing or laryngospasm because of intact airway reflexes. Ketamine has a half-life of about 2 hours and is well known for emergence delirium in older children.

A single intramuscular injection of ketamine will predictably induce anesthesia in the combative or uncooperative older child without the use of an anesthesia machine. An antisialagogue to decrease secretions and a benzodiazepine to reduce emergence phenomena (midazolam 0.03 to 0.1 mg/kg) may be added to the same syringe. Ketamine has also been given orally with effective results.

Dosage/administration:

Ketamine:

    IV: 1-2 mg/kg (onset 1-2 min)

    IM: 5-6 mg/kg (onset 5-10 min)

    PO: 6 mg/kg (onset 30 min)[29]

Propofol[30-34] is a lipid-soluble intravenous anesthetic that provides complete anesthesia outside of the operating room without having to transport an anesthesia machine. The depth of anesthesia can be titrated, usually with preservation of spontaneous ventilation, by either bolus or infusion techniques. It offers rapid onset and rapid emergence with little prolonged sedation, so that patients can be discharged sooner and appear more alert. Less postoperative nausea and vomiting are reported than with other general anesthetics. Propofol does cause significant cardiovascular depression, seen in healthy children as decreased blood pressure. It also causes pain at the injection site, particularly in smaller veins, that is somewhat attenuated by adding lidocaine (0.1 mg/kg) to the syringe.

Dosage/administration:
Propofol:
IV: Bolus 0.5-3.0 mg/kg
Infusion 25-300 µg/kg/min IV

The **lytic cocktail** (or **DPT**),[35] consisting of meperidine (Demerol, 2 mg/kg), promethazine (phenergan, 1 mg/kg), and chlorpromazine (Thorazine, 1 mg/kg), was traditionally used for pediatric sedation, particularly for painful procedures. However, the long duration, low efficacy, and high morbidity and mortality associated with this combination have made it an unacceptable choice in contemporary practice.[36] Excessive and prolonged respiratory depression, central nervous system depression, systemic hypotension, and bradycardia may last for 8 to 10 hours. Since this medication is given as a single intramuscular injection, titration to effect is not possible. Multiple deaths have also been reported.

References

1. Dunbar BS: Remote site survey: initial findings, *Society of Pediatric Anesthesia Newsletter,* vol 11, 1993.
2. American Academy of Pediatrics, Committee on Drugs: Guidelines for monitoring and management of pediatric patients during and after sedation for diagnostic and therapeutic procedures, *Pediatrics* 89:1110-1115, 1992.
3. Coté CJ: Sedation for the pediatric patient, *Pediatr Clin North Am,* 41:31-58, 1994.
4. Patel RI, Hannallah RS: Preoperative screening for pediatric ambulatory surgery: evaluation of a telephone questionnaire method, *Anesth Analg* 75:258-261, 1992.
5. Hughes CW, Bell C: Anesthesia equipment in remote locations. In Ehrenwerth J, Eisenkraft, JB, eds: *Anesthesia equipment, principles and applications,* St. Louis, 1992, Mosby.
6. American Society of Anesthesiologists: Standards for Basic Intraoperative Monitoring, American Society of Anesthesiologists 1996 Directory of Members, ed 61.

7. Gangarosa RE, Minnis JE, Nobbe J, Praschan D, Genberg RW: Operational safety issues in MRI, *Magn Reson Imag* 5:287-292, 1987.

8. Harding MB, Davidson CJ, Pieper KS, et al: Comparison of cardiovascular and renal toxicity after cardiac catheterization using a nonionic versus ionic radiographic contrast agent, *Am J Cardiol* 68: 1117-1119, 1991.

9. Council on Scientific Affairs, American Medical Association: The use of pulse oximetry during conscious sedation, *JAMA* 270: 1463-1468, 1993.

10. Karlik SJ, Heatherley T, Pavan F, et al: Patient anesthesia and monitoring at a 1.5-T MRI installation, *Magnetic Resonance in Medicine* 7:210-221, 1988.

11. Holshouser BA, Hinshaw DB Jr, Shellock FG: Sedation, anesthesia, and physiologic monitoring during MR imaging: evaluation of procedures and equipment, *J Magn Reson Imaging* 3:553-558, 1993.

12. Beebe DS, Belani KG, Chang PN, et al: Effectiveness of preoperative sedation with rectal midazolam, ketamine, or their combination in young children, *Anesth Analg* 75:880-884, 1992.

13. Yaster M, Nichols DG, Deshpande JK, Wetzel RC: Midazolam-fentanyl intravenous sedation in children: case report of respiratory arrest, *Pediatrics* 86:463-467, 1990.

14. Woolf CJ, Chong MS: Preemptive analgesia: treating postoperative pain by preventing the establishment of central sensitization, *Anesth Analg* 77:362-379, 1993.

15. Smith MS, Womack WM: Stress management techniques in childhood and adolescence, *Clin Pediatr* 26:581-585, 1987.

16. Sacchetti A, Schafermeyer R, Gerardi M, et al: Pediatric analgesia and sedation, *Ann Emerg Med* 23: 237-250, 1994.

17. Bell C: Outpatient anesthesia in nonoperating room settings. In McGoldrick K, ed: *Ambulatory anesthesiology: a problem-oriented approach,* Baltimore, 1995, Williams & Wilkins.

18. American Academy of Pediatrics Committee on Drugs and Committee on Environmental Health: Use of chloral hydrate for sedation in children, *Pediatrics* 92(3):471-473, 1993.

19. Greenberg SB, Faerber EN, Aspinall CL, Adams RC: High-dose chloral hydrate sedation for children undergoing MR imaging: safety and efficacy in relation to age, *AJR* 161:639-641, 1993.

20. Olson JJ, Friedman R, Orr K, Delaney T, Oldfield EH: Cerebral radioprotection by pentobarbital: dose-response characteristics and association with GABA agonist activity, *J Neurosurg* 72:749-758, 1990.

21. Montecinos S: Sedation for children undergoing diagnostic procedures, *Anesth Analg* 77:198, 1993.

22. Manache L, Eifel PJ, Kennamer DI, Belli JA: Twice-daily anesthesia in infants receiving hyperfractionated irradiation, *I J Radiation Oncology Biology Physics* 18:625-629, 1990.

23. Weldon BC, Watcha MF, White PF: Oral midazolam in children: effect of time and adjunctive therapy, *Anesth Analg* 75:51-55, 1992.

24. Theroux MC, West DW, Corddry DH, et al: Efficacy of intranasal midazolam in facilitating suturing of lacerations in preschool children in the emergency department, *Pediatrics* 91:624-627, 1993.

25. Sievers TD, Yee JK, Foley ME, Blanding PJ, Berde CB: Midazolam for conscious sedation during pediatric oncology procedures: safety and recovery parameters, *Pediatrics* 88: 1172-1179, 1991.

26. Finder RL, Moore PA: Benzodiazepines for intravenous conscious sedation: agonists and antagonists, *Compendium* 14:972, 974, 976-980, 982, 984, 1993.

27. Neal JM, Owens BD: Hazards of antagonizing narcotic sedation with naloxone (letter), *Ann Emerg Med* 22:145-146, 1993.

28. Reich DL, Silvay G: Ketamine: an update on the first twenty-five years of clinical experience, *Can J Anaesth* 36:186-197, 1989.

29. Bragg CL, Miller BR: Oral ketamine facilitates induction in a combative mentally retarded patient, *J Clin Anesth* 2:121-122, 1990.

30. Blouin RT, Seifert HA, Babenco HD, Conard PF, Gross JB: Propofol depresses the hypoxic ventilatory response during conscious sedation and isohypercapnia, *Anesthesiology* 79:1177-1182, 1993.

31. Westrin P: The induction of propofol in infants 1-6 months of age and in children 10-16 years of age, *Anesthesiology* 74:455-458, 1991.

32. Martin LD, Pasternak LR, Pudimat MA: Total intravenous anesthesia with propofol in pediatric patients outside the operating room, *Anesth Analg* 74:609-612, 1992.

33. Hannallah RS, Baker SB, Casey W, et al: Propofol: effective dose and induction characteristics in unpremedicated children, *Anesthesiology* 74:217-219, 1991.

34. Wetchler BV, Alexander D, Kondragunta RD: Recovery from the use of propofol for maintenance of anesthesia during short ambulatory procedures, *Semin Anesthesia* 11:20-23, 1992.

35. Mitchell AA, Louik C, Lacouture P, Slone D, Goldman P, Shapiro S: Risks to children from computed tomographic scan premedication, *JAMA* 247: 2385-2388, 1982.

36. Nahata MC, Clotz MA, Krogg EA: Adverse effects of meperidine, promethazine, and chlorpromazine for sedation in pediatric patients, *Clin Pediatr* 24:558-560, 1985.

ACUTE PEDIATRIC PAIN MANAGEMENT

20

The sun is out, it's time to play
But something's gone awry
There's so much pain each time I move
I almost want to die.

It hurts to talk, it hurts to walk
Please—don't let me fall!
Don't ask me if it's dull or sharp
It hurts a lot, that's all!

Oh pain, pain, go away
Go ruin someone else's day!

Rivian Bell

Anesthesiologists have become leaders in the field of pain management for children. Consultation may be requested in the perioperative period, in the acute care setting, such as the emergency room or pediatric floor, or in the chronic care setting, which might include the terminally ill child.

The perioperative management of pain begins with the preoperative visit. At that time, analgesic interventions that will be incorporated into the anesthetic plan should be shared with the family, including single-dose regional techniques, placement of epidural catheters, or patient-controlled analgesia.

PAIN ASSESSMENT

The perception of pain is primarily subjective, influenced by sensory and emotional input. What is perceived as pain by one individual is not necessarily perceived to the same degree, or even at all, by another, although nociceptive reception may be the same for both.

Perception and communication of a child's pain closely parallel his or her intellectual and social development. The abilities to understand, quantitate, and communicate are key factors in the expression of pain. A preverbal child cannot articulate analgesic requirements.

When pain in children is evaluated, methods to adequately quantify the degree of pain are essential in determining when to initiate treatment, type of treatment, and effectiveness of treatment. Three types of assessment techniques are available: self-reporting scales, behavioral observation scores, and physiologic monitoring. The assessment scales should be chosen appropriately for the child's developmental stage.

Self-Reporting Measures[1-3]

Self-reporting scales require that a child have sufficient cognitive ability to indicate degree of pain on a relative scale. Adult scales have been modified and converted to a format children can understand. Comparison of scores before and after initiation of treatment helps to determine any necessary adjustments in the treatment protocol. Three types of self-reporting scales are used.

1. *Visual analog scale (VAS)*

   No Pain [————————————————] Worst Pain

   The child is asked to mark the line at a point that corresponds to his or her pain. The VAS is easy to understand and may be useful in children over 7 years of age.

2. *Verbal numerical rating score*

   The child is asked to choose the number that corresponds to the intensity of his or her pain. The child is instructed that 0 corresponds to no pain and 10 corresponds to the worst pain imaginable. This scale is useful for school-age children.

3. *Graphic rating scales*

   • These scales employ a series of cartoon faces or photographs of children depicting a range of facial expressions from a sad or crying face to one that is happy or smiling. The child is asked to select the face that best describes his or her pain.[4]

   • The Oucher scale consists of photographic progression of facial expressions on a number scale, with 0 representing no pain and 100 representing the worst pain (screaming child).[5]

   • These scales are appropriate for use in 3- to 7-year-old children.

Observational Measures

In children under 3 to 7 years of age, observational behavior scales should be employed. These scales can also be used in the older child in whom the verbal or visual analog pain scoring is not effective.

   • OPS: Observation Pain Scale. A standardized scale developed at the Children's Hospital, University of Washington, for postoperative pain assessment (see table at right).[6,7]

   • CHEOPS: Children's Hospital of Eastern Ontario Pain Scale (see table on p. 456).[8]

- NIPS: Neonatal Infant Pain Scale. Neonates are probably the most difficult group for which to objectively assess pain: a combination of behavioral and psychological scoring systems has been used. The NIPS is an assessment of facial expression, cry, breathing pattern, arm position, leg position, and state of arousal.[9]

Observation pain scale

Score	Observation
1	Laughing, euphoria
2	Happy, contented, smiling, playing
3	Neutral; asleep or calm
4	Mild to moderate pain: expresses or vocalizes pain, wrinkles brow, but can be distracted with toy, food or TV
5	Moderate to severe pain; expresses severe pain, crying, inconsolable, screaming, hysteria, sobbing

From Krane EJ, Jacobson LE, Lynn AM, Parrot C, Tyler DC: Caudal morphine for postoperative analgesia in children: a comparison with caudal bupivacaine and intravenous morphine, *Anesth Analg*; 66:647-653, 1987.

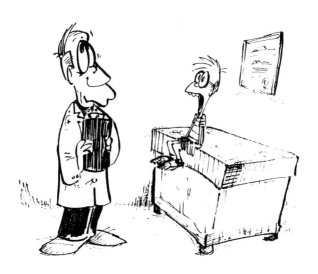

"CAN YOU PROMISE ME I'LL BE NUMBED OUTTA MY MIND?"

Behavioral definitions and scoring of CHEOPS

Item	Behavior	Score	Definition
Cry	No cry	1	Child is not crying
	Moaning	2	Child is moaning or quietly vocalizing; silent cry
	Crying	2	Child is crying, but the cry is gentle or whimpering
	Scream	3	Child is in full-lunged cry; sobbing; may be scored with complaint or without complaint
Facial	Composed	1	Neutral facial expression
	Grimace	2	Score only if definitive negative facial expression
	Smiling	0	Score only if definitive positive facial expression
Child (verbal)	None	1	Child not talking
	Other complaints	1	Child complains, but not about pain; e.g., "I want to see my mommy" or "I am thirsty"
	Pain complaints	2	Child complains about pain
	Both complaints	2	Child complains about pain and about other things; e.g., "It hurts; I want mommy"
	Positive	0	Child makes any positive statement or talks about other things without complaint
Torso	Neutral	1	Body (not limbs) is at rest; torso is inactive
	Shifting	2	Body is in motion in a shifting or serpentine fashion
	Tense	2	Body is arched or rigid
	Shivering	2	Body is shuddering or shaking involuntarily
	Upright	2	Child is in vertical or upright position
	Restrained	2	Body is restrained
Touch	Not touching	1	Child is not touching or grabbing at wound
	Reach	2	Child is reaching for but not touching wound
	Touch	2	Child is gently touching wound or wound area
	Grab	2	Child is grabbing vigorously at wound
	Restrained	2	Child's arms are restrained
Legs	Neutral	1	Legs may be in any position but are relaxed; includes gentle swimming or serpentine-like movements
	Squirming/ kicking	2	Definitive uneasy or restless movements in the legs and/or striking out with foot or feet
	Drawn up/ tensed	2	Legs tensed and/or pulled up tightly to body and kept there
	Standing	2	Standing, crouching, or kneeling
	Restrained	2	Child's legs are being held down

From McGrath PJ, Johnson G, Goodman JT, Schillinger J, Dunn J, Chapman J: The CHEOPS: a behavioral scale to measure postoperative pain in children. In Fields HL, Dubner R, Cervero F, eds: *Advances in pain research and therapy,* New York, 1985, Raven Press, pp. 395-402.

Physiologic Measures

Physiologic monitoring as a technique of pain assessment is based on the principle that the perception of pain initiates a stress response, which in turn triggers cardiorespiratory and hormonal-metabolic changes.

Changes in heart rate, blood pressure, and respiration represent increased sympathetic activity and are presumed to correlate with stress or discomfort. Similarly, increased plasma cortisol, epinephrine, and norepinephrine have been observed with painful procedures and in the postoperative period.[10]

POSTOPERATIVE PAIN MANAGEMENT: DRUG THERAPY

Principles

Analgesic efficacy is improved by the recognition of these basic tenets of pharmacologic management of postoperative pain:

1. Analgesic therapy should be incorporated into the intraoperative anesthetic plan.
2. "PRN" dosing results in a waxing and waning of analgesia with periods of insufficient analgesia alternating with possible oversedation.
3. Patient satisfaction is improved by using the oral, intravenous, or epidural approach rather than intramuscular injections.
4. Common side effects should be anticipated and prophylactic therapy administered when indicated. Alternatively, standing orders should be available to treat anticipated side effects, such as nausea and pruritis.
5. Signs of toxicity and pain scores should be assessed and documented at routine intervals for all patients.
6. The effects of newborn physiology on opioid pharmacokinetics should be considered when determining dosages and intervals for infants.

Infant opioid pharmacokinetics: risk factors for opioid administration

- Increased susceptibility to **apnea** because of a relative imbalance of μ_1 (analgesia) to μ_2 (respiratory depression) receptors[11,12]
- Increased susceptibility to **hypoventilation** because of a decreased ventilatory response to hypoxia/hypercapnia
- Decreased **metabolism** of opioids because of immature liver conjugation (glucuronidation, sulfation, oxidation)
- Decreased **excretion** of drugs and metabolites because of immature renal filtration
- Increased **free drug fraction** because of decreased plasma protein binding (decreased α_1-acid glycoprotein and albumin)
- Higher **drug concentrations** in the brain because of immature blood-brain barrier

Opioid Analgesics

The opioids are used most often for moderate to severe pain. Although initial doses may be chosen by general guidelines, the effective dose must be titrated. Caution must be exercised when using opioids in the neonate or the infant <4 months of age (see box on p. 457).

The route of administration is determined by the needs of the patient as well as the pharmacology of the opioid. Bolus intravenous administration leads to peaks and troughs in analgesic levels, causing breakthrough periods of pain. Continuous intravenous infusions, patient-controlled analgesia, or slow-release oral preparations decrease periods of inadequate analgesia.

The most serious complications of opioid administration are respiratory depression and apnea, appropriately treated by first assisting or controlling ventilation. Intravenous naloxone in incremental boluses of 20 µg (5 to 10 µg/kg for large overdoses) usually reverses ventilatory depression. Repeat doses of naloxone or continuous infusions of 1 to 2 µg/kg/hr may be necessary when long-acting opiates have been used. Large single-bolus doses of naloxone may trigger nausea and vomiting, tachycardia, hypertension, and even pulmonary edema.

More common opioid side effects include pruiritis, which may be treated by diphenhydramine 1 mg/kg PO or IV. Nausea and vomiting, also common, have been reported even after a single dose of morphine.[13] Switching to a different opioid (p. 459) or adding an antiemetic (p. 474) may decrease these symptoms.

Opioid analgesics: continuous intravenous infusions for infants less than 4 months*

Drug	Doses (mg/kg)
Morphine	0.02-0.05 mg/kg bolus, then 0.02-0.05 mg/kg/hr infusion
Fentanyl	1.0-2.0 µg/kg bolus, then 2-4 µg/kg/hr infusion

*Note: Intensive monitoring and nursing observation are strongly recommended for infants receiving opiods (see box on p. 457).

Opioid analgesics: intermittent dosing

Drug	Equianalgesic initial dose (mg/kg)	Interval and route	Comments
Codeine	1.0	q4-6h PO	Dose limited by constipation, nausea, vomiting
Fentanyl	0.001	q1-2h IV	Useful for painful procedures because of rapid onset and short duration
	0.010-0.015	× 1 (transmucosal)	
Hydromorphone (Dilaudid)	0.015-0.02	q3h IV	May cause less itching, nausea, dysphoria
	0.075-0.10	q3-4h PO	Oral preparation is pleasant-tasting liquid
Meperidine (Demerol)	1.0	q3-4h IV	Metabolite (normeperidine) accumulates with chronic use and causes CNS excitation
	2.0-3.0	q3-4h PO	
Methadone	0.1-0.2	q4h (initial) IV	Long acting (12-24 hr)
	0.2-0.4	q8-12h PO	
Morphine	0.1	q2-3h IV	Common side effects include histamine release, nausea, and vomiting
	0.3	q3-4h PO	
Morphine sulfate (MS-Contin)	0.3	q8-12h PO	Useful for chronic pain (slow-release) Smallest tablet is 15 mg Tablet cannot be divided
Oxycodone	0.15	q4h PO	Opioid in Tylox, Percocet, Roxicodone

IV, intravenous; *PO,* orally (per os).

Intravenous regimens for continuous analgesia[14,15]*

Drug/technique	Initial loading dose	Maintenance	Weaning	Comments
Methadone	IV: 0.1 mg/kg in saline over 20 min; may repeat loading dose 2-3 hr SC: 0.2 mg/kg	For IV, sliding scale doses given q4h over 20 min (not prn) unless patient is somnolent or shows signs of toxicity as follows: Mild pain: 0.03 mg/kg Moderate pain: 0.05 mg/kg Severe pain: 0.07 mg/kg	As methadone accumulates, dosing frequency is decreased to q6h and q12h as tolerated In short courses of therapy, drug may be discontinued abruptly and will "self-wean" because of the long half-life	Long half-life (infrequent dosing, self-weaning) Less euphoria and dysphoria than with other narcotics
Continuous-infusion morphine	0.05-0.10 mg/kg IV	0.04-0.06 mg/kg/hr	As for morphine PCA	Patient cooperation and participation not required Easy to titrate to effect
Fentanyl	1-1.5 µg/kg IV	2-4 µg/kg/hr	As for morphine PCA	As for continuous-infusion morphine

	Postoperative pain: 0.05-0.1 mg/kg IV (optional, based on narcotics received intraoperatively)	Postoperative pain: Total hourly dose: 0.05-0.1 mg/kg/hr. Optional background infusion: $\frac{1}{4} - \frac{1}{3}$ of total hourly dose. PCA bolus: remaining hourly dose divided into equal doses at 6-10 min intervals	Discontinue basal infusion after 24-48 hr	Itching can be treated with diphenhydramine or naloxone 0.5-1.0 µg/kg/hr
Morphine/patient-controlled analgesia (PCA)	Sickle cell crisis: 0.10-0.15 mg/kg IV	Sickle cell crisis: Total hourly dose: 0.1-0.2 mg/kg IV. Background infusion: $\frac{1}{2}$ of total hourly dose. PCA bolus: as for postoperative pain	Decrease dose by 20%-30% on first 2 days if patient is improving and then 10%-20% daily	Less respiratory depression. High patient satisfaction. Many patients "self-wean" by decreasing dosage frequency. Include NSAID[†] in sickle cell crisis

*Pain, sedation, scores, and vital signs should be assessed on a regular basis and recorded on the bedside chart.

†NSAID, Nonsteroidal antiinflammatory drug.

Nonopioid Analgesics

Nonopioid analgesics are useful for controlling mild to moderate pain. These drugs exhibit an analgesic ceiling effect.[16] Escalating doses do not provide more analgesia, but will likely increase side effects. It may be helpful to continue administering these drugs when adding opioids, as they have an opioid-sparing effect.[17]

Nonopioid analgesics

Drug	Dose (mg/kg)	Route	Formulation	Comments
Acetaminophen	10-15 q4h	PO PR	Liquid, tablets (chewable), suppository	Maximum 60 mg/kg/day Limited anti-inflammatory effect
Acetylsalicylic acid	10-15 q4h	PO	Tablets (chewable)	Associated with Reye syndrome Antiplatelet effect Gastritis
Choline magnesium trisalicylate	25 q8-12h	PO	Liquid, tablets	Less gastritis Antiplatelet effect
Ibuprofen	5-10 q6-8h	PO	Liquid, tablets	Antiplatelet effect Gastritis Interstitial nephritis Hepatic toxicity with chronic use
Indomethacin	1 q8h	PO, IV PR	Liquid, tablets, suppository	Used in premature infants to close patent ductus arteriosus
Ketorolac	0.5 q6h	IV, IM	Parenteral	Limit to 48-72 hours Only NSAID approved for parenteral analgesia
	10 q6h	PO	Tablets	
Naproxen	5-10 q6-8h	PO	Liquid, tablets	See Ibuprofen
Tolmetin	5-10 q6-8h	PO	Tablets	See Ibuprofen

The nonsteroidal antiinflammatory *ketorolac tromethamine* has recently gained popularity for use in the management of postoperative pain. Its analgesic potency may exceed many of the other NSAIDs and it is available for parenteral administration.[18] It may be administered intramuscularly or intravenously with a loading dose of 0.5 to 1.0 mg/kg followed by a maintenance dose of 0.5 mg/kg every 6 hours.[17,19] When used with morphine, it may exhibit a dramatic opioid-sparing effect.[20] Ketorolac has the disadvantage of prolonging bleeding time because of its effect on platelet aggregation. Clinically, this effect has been shown to increase bleeding during tonsillectomy when ketorolac has been administered before incision.[21]

Adjuvant Drugs

The adjuvant drugs are most commonly used for children with chronic pain. Unfortunately, no comprehensive clinical trials in children are available to guide the use of these drugs. The clinical use of antidepressants[22] and benzodiazepines[23] in adults has recently been reviewed.

Adjuvant drugs useful in pediatric pain management

Drug class	Uses	Drug and dosages	Comments
Tricyclic antidepressants	Decrease pain by central action on pain inhibitory systems Improve sleep cycles Improve mood	Amitriptyline (Elavil): 0.1 mg/kg qhs PO advanced as tolerated to 0.5-2 mg/kg Doxepine: As for amitriptyline (liquid) Imipramine (Tofranil): 1.5 mg/kg/day tid PO	Anticholinergic effect diminished by starting with small doses Contraindicated in patients with cardiac conduction defects Imipramine causes photosensitization, lowers seizure threshold, and has lower metabolism in the presence of methylphenidate (Ritalin)
Stimulants	Increase analgesia and decrease sedation Euphoric effect	Methylphenidate: 0.1-0.3 mg/kg/dose bid PO Dextroamphetamine: 0.1-0.2 mg/kg/dose bid PO	Given in early morning and midday to avoid nighttime insomnia

Continued.

Adjuvant drugs useful in pediatric pain management—cont'd

Drug class	Uses	Drug and dosages	Comments
Anticonvulsants	Neuropathic pain (trigeminal neuralgia) and migraine Alter neuronal excitability	Phenytoin (Dilantin): 5 mg/kg/day PO or IV Carbamazepine (Tegretol): 20-30 mg/kg/day tid PO Clonazepam (Klonopin): 0.01-0.2 mg/kg/day PO	Side effects include sedation, ataxia, dysphoria, GI symptoms, and hepatotoxicity Drug level must be monitored
Corticosteroids	Neuropathic pain (trigeminal neuralgia) and migraine Alter neuronal excitability	Variable, as per patient requirements	Dosage and route determined by patient's medical condition
Benzodiazepines	Anxiolysis Amnesia Antiemetics	Diazepam (Valium): 0.02-0.1 mg/kg q6-8h IV or PO Midazolam (Versed): 0.05-0.1 mg/kg q2-4h IV Lorazepam (Ativan): 0.02-0.05 mg/kg q8-12h IV or PO	Increased respiratory depression when given with opioids Do not provide analgesia Lorazepam causes hallucinations in children under 6 years of age

REGIONAL ANESTHESIA/ANALGESIA

Regional anesthesia is useful when the technique employed will effectively involve the surgical dermatomes or site of injury. It may be used as the sole anesthetic in infants at risk for postoperative apnea undergoing abdominal or lower extremity procedures (most commonly, preterm infants undergoing inguinal herniorrhaphy). Regional procedures in combination with light sedation may be useful in cooperative older children or adolescents in whom general anesthesia is contraindicated or who fear "falling asleep." The former category would include patients with a history (or strong family history) of malignant hyperthermia, or those with severe systemic illness whose conditions might be worsened or complicated by general anesthesia and ventilatory support (for example, patients with cystic fibrosis).

Regional blockade may also be used for analgesia in combination with general anesthesia. When regional blockade is initiated prior to operation, general anesthetic dosing requirements are decreased. Regional blockade may provide postoperative analgesia without the side effects commonly produced by systemic opioids (drowsiness, mood alteration, hypoventilation, nausea and vomiting, etc.). Continuous epidural analgesia is also useful for chronic pain syndromes (sickle cell crisis[24] or malignancy).

Pharmacologic principles of local anesthetics in children[25]

- Because of decreased albumin and α_1-acid glycoprotein serum levels in the infant less than 2 months of age, less bupivacaine will be bound to protein, resulting in higher concentrations of free drug.[26-28]
- Although infants less than 6 months of age have lower levels of plasma cholinesterase, there seems to be little effect of age on the duration of ester anesthetics.[29]
- The effects of incomplete myelination on local anesthetic activity in infants less than 1 year of age are unknown.
- Maximum single doses of lidocaine are identical for infants and adults, possibly because of the infant's increased volume of distribution, balanced by lowered hepatic metabolism.[30]
- Prolonged elimination half-lives ($t\frac{1}{2}$) in children may lead to toxicity when continuous infusions are employed.
- Local anesthetics lower seizure threshold.[27,31]

Contraindications to Regional Anesthesia in Children

ABSOLUTE CONTRAINDICATIONS

- Parental or patient refusal
- Infection (at nerve block site or systemic)
- Uncorrected coagulopathy
- True allergy to local anesthetic

RELATIVE CONTRAINDICATIONS

Practitioner

1. Inadequate technical expertise to properly place or manage the regional technique
2. Lack of in-hospital pain service staffing available to manage any complications of regional blocks (especially if neuraxis opioids are used)

Patient

1. Cannot be properly positioned
2. Poorly controlled seizure disorder
3. Difficult airway
4. Severe hypovolemia

5. Anatomic variation (congenital or acquired) that precludes block placement
6. Actively progressive neurologic disease

Maximum recommended doses of local anesthetics for regional anesthesia [32,33]

Drug	mg/kg (with epinephrine)	Duration (min)
Lidocaine	5 (7)	45-180
Bupivacaine	2.5 (3)	180-600
Tetracaine	1.5	180-600
2-Chloroprocaine	8 (10)	30-60
Procaine	8 (10)	60-90

Note: Never add epinephrine to local anesthetics injected into an area of end-artery distribution (penis, digit).

Spinal

Spinal anesthesia may be used for procedures with surgical dermatomes below T6. It is important to note that the dural sac migrates cephalad during the first year of life.

Anatomy

	Conus medullaris	Dural sac
Neonate	L3	S3
>1 year	L1	S1

POSITION

The sitting position may be especially helpful in neonates to maintain midline needle position and free flow of spinal fluid (see Fig 20-1). The neck and chin must be supported and extended to maintain an unobstructed airway. It may be easier for the novice assistant to hold the infant more securely in the lateral decubitus position. The head should be placed toward the non–needle holding hand (i.e., to the left if the needle is held in the right hand). In the lateral position, the neck is extended to maintain an open airway in small infants.

TECHNIQUE: SPINAL

1. The back is sterilely prepared and draped; a fenestrated adhesive clear plastic drape is useful in small infants.
2. Skin infiltration with local anesthetic should be used for the awake patient.

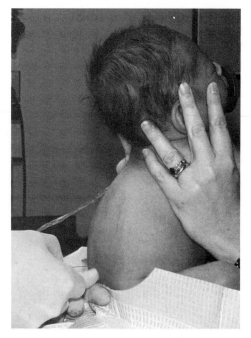

FIG. 20-1. The sitting position is helpful when placing a spinal block in neonates, to maintain midline needle position and free flow of spinal fluid. The neck and chin must be supported and extended to maintain an unintubated airway.

3. A 22 g 1.5 in (4 cm) clear-hubbed spinal needle is placed at the L3-L4 or L4-L5 interspace using the midline approach; a longer or 25 to 27 g spinal needle can be employed in the older child or adolescent.

4. In the small child, the depth is usually 1 to 1.5 cm.

5. After establishing free flow of spinal fluid, local anesthetic is slowly injected using a tuberculin syringe. An additional 0.04 ml of anesthetic is added to the syringe to allow for dead space in the spinal needle.

6. Anesthetic loss through the needle track may be minimized by leaving needle and syringe in place for 5 to 10 sec after injection is complete.

7. Onset of blockade occurs rapidly (tetracaine: 2 min; bupivacaine: 10 min). Elevating the legs after the block is in place (e.g., to place the electrocautery pad) may rapidly extend motor blockade to unacceptable levels.

8. In normovolemic infants, the intravenous catheter may be placed in an anesthetized lower extremity after the block is in place.

9. Hypotension and bradycardia are unusual complications in infants receiving spinal anesthesia.
10. Infants less than 44 to 60 weeks' postconceptional age at risk for apnea are admitted postoperatively for observation (see p. 5).

Doses of local anesthetic for pediatric spinal anesthesia

Local anesthetic	Dose (mg/kg)	Age	Duration (min)
Tetracaine 0.5% in 5% dextrose*[34]	0.8-1.0	Preterm-neonate	80
Tetracaine 0.5% in 5% dextrose*[34] with 20 μg epinephrine	0.8-1.0	Preterm-neonate	120
Bupivacaine 0.5% (isobaric)[35]	0.6-1.0	2-12 mo	70
Bupivacaine 0.75% in 8.25% dextrose [36]	0.3-0.4	0-12 mo	70
Lidocaine 5% in 7.5% dextrose[37]	2	3-10 yr	45

*1% tetracaine combined with equal amounts 10% dextrose.

Epidural Anesthesia and Analgesia
INDICATIONS

1. To reduce general anesthetic requirements for thoracic, abdominal, or pelvic procedures
2. To provide postoperative analgesia for thoracic, lumbar, and sacral dermatomes
3. As part of the management of chronic pain syndromes, including reflex sympathetic dystrophy and neoplasias of the thorax, abdomen, pelvis, and lower extremities
4. To provide anesthesia/analgesia and immobilization of the lower extremities (as for orthopedic procedures)

CONTRAINDICATIONS (also see contraindications for regional anesthesia, p. 465)

1. Treatment of pain above T2 to T4
2. Local or systemic infection
3. Coagulopathy
4. Hemodynamic instability
5. Presence of a neurologic disease that may be exacerbated by conduction blocks (e.g., multiple sclerosis)

Advantages and disadvantages of epidural blockade in children

Advantages	Disadvantages
• Provides continuous analgesia for thoracic, lumbar, and sacral dermatomes • Easily reinforced through an indwelling catheter • Early ambulation • Less respiratory depression than with systemic analgesics • Improved postoperative pulmonary function • Can provide intraoperative muscle relaxation • May improve splanchnic blood flow	• Technically difficult to perform in children because of the shallow epidural space (lumbar and thoracic) • Necessity for concurrent general anesthesia or sedation for placement • Risk of intrathecal block • Risk of air embolism with loss of resistance technique if air used • Risk of spinal cord trauma • Complications of technique (headache, intravascular injection, catheter migration, epidural abscess, or hematoma) • Complications of neuraxial agents (motor blockade, paresthesias, urinary retention, pruritus, respiratory depression)

Caudal Approach (Single-Dose)

In young children, the epidural space can be reached easily by the caudal approach with less risk of dural puncture than with thoracic or lumbar approaches. The technique is simple; blockade can be achieved without using the loss-of-resistance technique or special introducer needles. Further, a standard lumbar epidural continuous-infusion catheter can be placed caudally for blockade of longer duration. Because there is minimal risk of cord injury at the level of the sacrococcygeal ligament, general anesthesia or heavy sedation is not mandatory to prevent the child from making sudden unanticipated movements.

This approach is ideal for analgesia/anesthesia of lumbar and sacral nerve roots. Higher dermatomes can be reached by increasing drug volume or threading a catheter several centimeters into the epidural space.

ANATOMY

The sacral hiatus is bound posteriorly by the sacrococcygeal ligament, superiorly by the sacral cornua and the fused arch of the sacrum. The needle can be misplaced into the bone (bone marrow), subperiostium, sacral ligaments, lateral to the cornua (false hiatus), pelvis (colon or bladder) or the S4 foramen (see Fig. 20-2, next page).

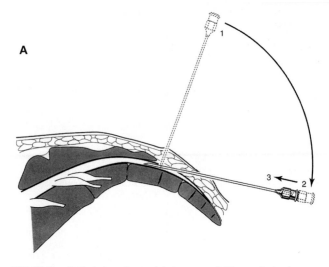

FIG. 20-2. **A,** Technique for caudal placement. *1,* The needle is advanced through the sacral hiatus in the midline between the cornua at a 45-degree angle, bevel facing caudad. *2* and *3,* After the needle pops through the sacrococcygeal ligament, the needle-to-skin angle is reduced so that the needle is advanced 2 to 3 mm into the caudal canal parallel to the spinal axis.

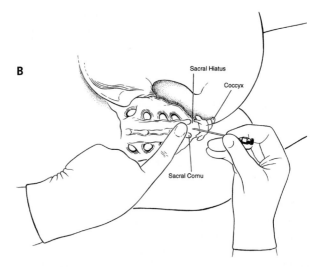

FIG. 20-2, cont'd. **B,** The palpating finger remains over the sacrum during injection (after aspiration for blood and spinal fluid). In this manner, subcutaneous injection can be immediately recognized because a bleb will be raised under the finger.

TECHNIQUE: SINGLE-DOSE CAUDAL BLOCK

1. The block may be placed with the patient in either the prone, lateral decubitus, or knee-chest position.
2. The sacral area is sterilely prepared and draped.
3. The sacral cornu and sacral hiatus are identified by palpation.
4. Local anesthetic is recommended in the awake or mildly sedated patient.
5. A "no-touch" technique can be used, whereby an alcohol wipe is placed under the examiner's finger or thumb at the sacral hiatus.
6. The needle is advanced through the hiatus in the midline between the cornua at a 45-degree angle, bevel facing caudad. Any needle can be employed, although fewer intravascular placements have been noted with short-beveled needles. Short pediatric Touhy needles are useful. Alternatively, an 18 or 20 g IV catheter over a needle can be used.
7. After the needle "pops through" the sacrococcygeal ligament, the needle-to-skin angle is reduced so that the needle is advanced 2 to 3 mm into the caudal canal parallel to the spinal axis (Fig. 20-2, *A*).
8. A test dose of 0.1 ml/kg is injected before the remaining volume.
9. The palpating finger remains over the sacrum during injection (after aspiration for blood and spinal fluid). In this manner, subcutaneous injection can be immediately recognized because a bleb will be raised under the finger (Fig. 20-2, *B*).

SOLUTIONS

Bupivacaine 0.25% with epinephrine 1:200,000 typically provides 3 to 6 hours of analgesia without motor blockade.

DOSING OPTIONS

1. For children over 20 kg in weight and 100 cm in height: 1 ml/10 cm of height. (Use of the lumbar epidural route for larger children reduces the necessary quantity of local anesthetic.)
2. Infants less than 2.5 kg: a more dilute solution is used (0.125%), and volume can be increased to 1.5 ml/kg.
3. *Addition of opioid:* 0.03 to 0.05 mg/kg of preservative-free morphine can be added to the local anesthetic solution. This provides 8 to 24 hours of analgesia. Children receiving a single dose of neuraxal opioids should be admitted to the hospital for monitoring and observation.

Formula to calculate drug volumes for single dose caudal block

Dose (ml/kg)	Local anesthetic	Level
0.06/segment	1% to 1.25% lidocaine + epi 1:200,000[38]	Thoracic
0.056 + (yr × 0.097)	1% lidocaine + epi 1:200,000[39]	Thoracic
ml = C7 to sacral hiatus (in cm) − 13	0.2% to 0.375% bupivacaine[40]	T4-T5
0.5 0.75 1.0	1% to 1.5% lidocaine *or* 0.25%[41] bupivacaine	Sacrolumbar (T11) Lumbothoracic (T10) Midthoracic (T8)

Continuous Lumbar, Thoracic, or Caudal Anesthesia/Analgesia

ANATOMY

Extreme caution should be observed in the placement of thoracic epidural catheters in children, as the spinal cord may be easily injured. The procedure should be reserved for children undergoing major thoracoabdominal procedures, with catheter placement by anesthesiologists with extensive experience in this technique.

POSITION

Catheters are most commonly placed in the lateral decubitus position after induction of general anesthesia. The seated position may be preferred in awake older children or adolescents for lumbar or thoracic placement.

EQUIPMENT

In younger children or infants, the short (2 in) 18 g Touhy needles with 20 g catheters provide safety and ease of insertion. It is difficult to inject through microcatheters (24 g), which kink easily.

TECHNIQUE

1. The *caudal* approach for continuous infusions is identical to the single-dose caudal technique except that an 18 g Touhy needle or an IV catheter over a needle is used. The catheter should be inserted to a predetermined depth as close as possible to the surgical dermatomes to minimize the amount of infusion necessary for analgesia.

2. The *lumbar* or *thoracic* approach is identical to the technique used for adult catheter placement. In the small child, a short 18 g Touhy needle can be used. The ligamentum flavum is very shallow, located only a few millimeters below skin surface in young children.

3. Loss of resistance should be assessed using *normal saline* and *not air,* because of the possibility of air embolus to the paravertebral venous plexus.[42] Children are at increased risk for paradoxical air embolus because of persistent cardiac septal defects.

4. The catheter should be inserted to a premeasured distance to deliver the catheter tip to the middle of the surgical field.

5. The recommended test dose of 0.5 μg/kg epinephrine may be given as 0.1 ml/kg of 1% to 2% lidocaine with 1:200,000 epinephrine. Under halothane or isoflurane anesthesia, the epinephrine test has a high incidence of false-negative results. Therefore, all local anesthetic solutions should be injected slowly and incrementally even if a test dose has been given uneventfully.[43,44]

6. Carefully applied transparent occlusive dressings (Tegaderm) will prevent catheter contamination or change in catheter position with movement. Fecal soiling can easily occur in infants and toddlers with caudal catheters, and the catheter site should be protected by the occlusive dressing.

7. Confirmation of catheter tip placement can be made radiographically when a radiopaque catheter is used or by injecting a small amount of *iohexol (Omnipaque).*

8. Intraoperative anesthesia can be supplemented or analgesia initiated with bupivacaine 0.25% + epinephrine 1:200,000 administered as a bolus with volumes determined by level desired (0.05 ml/kg per segment, not to exceed 1 ml/kg).

9. Infusions of analgesic solution for postoperative pain control can be started during the operative procedure or in the recovery room. Smaller "top-off" boluses of bupivacaine may be needed during the operation if infusions are not begun.

10. The catheter insertion site should be checked twice daily. Typically catheters are removed 72 hours after insertion unless the risks of infection are outweighed by the benefit of continued epidural analgesia. The reported risks of epidural space infection (abscess formation) with placement of epidural catheters for postoperative pain management are extremely low.[45]

Complications of epidural anesthesia/analgesia with local anesthetics and neuroaxis opioids

Complication	Intervention
Cardiovascular collapse	1. Support airway, breathing, and circulation 2. Fluid load 10-20 ml/kg 3. Epinephrine 5-10 µg/kg IV titrated to effect 4. Discontinue infusion; immediately remove catheter after stabilizing patient
Respiratory depression Severe (apnea, obtunded)	1. Support airway; supplemental O_2 2. Naloxone 5-10 µg/kg IV bolus + infusion 5 µg/kg/hr 3. Discontinue infusion and catheter
Mild (slow respiratory rate, sedated)	1. Supplemental O_2 2. Naloxone 0.5 µg/kg IV bolus; repeat as needed 3. Decrease infusion rate 20% to 25% (fentanyl infusions) or stop until patient is alert (morphine or hydromorphone infusions)
Seizure	1. Support airway, breathing, circulation 2. Discontinue infusion and catheter 3. Options for seizure control: Thiopental 2-3 mg/kg IV Midazolam 0.05-0.1 mg/kg/IV Dizepam 0.1-0.3 mg/kg/IV
Motor blockade	1. Decrease concentration of local anesthetic 2. Decrease rate of infusion
Pruritis	1. Diphenhydramine 0.5 mg/kg/dose IV/PO 2. Naloxone 0.5 µg/kg IV ± infusion 0.5-1.0 µg/kg/hr 3. Decrease infusion rate by 10% to 20%; decrease/remove opioid
Nausea/vomiting	1. Metaclopramide 0.1 mg/kg IV/PO q6h 2. Naloxone; see pruritis 3. Ondansetron 0.05-0.15 mg/kg/IV bolus
Urinary retention	1. Warm compresses and gentle massage to bladder 2. Straight catheterization (×1); followed by indwelling catheter 3. Naloxone 0.5 µg/kg IV
Signs of local infection	1. Remove catheter 2. Culture tip 3. Antibiotic therapy if indicated 4. Observe for further signs of local (abscess) or systemic infection

IV, intravenous; *PO,* oral.

Solutions for postoperative continuous epidural analgesia*

Solution	Rate (ml/kg/hr)	Uses
1/16 (0.0625)% bupivacaine + 1 µg/ml fentanyl	0.1-0.2	Neonates, infants <4 mo
1/16 (0.0625)% bupivacaine +2 µg/ml fentanyl	0.2-0.3	Older infants and children; tip at surgical site
1/16 (0.0625)% bupivacaine +10 µg/ml hydromorphone	0.2	Older infants and children; tip distant from surgical site
1/16 (0.0625)% bupivacaine + 0.1 mg/ml morphine	0.1-0.2	Older infants and children; tip distant from surgical site
1-5 µg/ml fentanyl or 10 µg/ml hydromorphone	0.2-0.3	Motor blockade and/or local anesthetic infusion contraindicated

*Maximum bupivacaine dose should not exceed 0.2 mg/kg/hr for neonates and 0.4 mg/kg/hr for older children.

SELECTED COMMON PERIPHERAL NERVE BLCOKS

For a description of the anatomy of various nerve blocks, the reader is referred to any of a number of textbooks of regional anesthesia and nerve blockade.[46,47] The following sections will describe techniques that have selected application to children.

Intercostal Block

Intercostal block provides adequate analgesia to the thorax for 4 to 12 hours. It may be useful for postoperative analgesia after thoracotomy or upper abdominal wall procedures if epidural blockade is not possible or for transient pain relief after multiple rib fractures. In the operative patient, blockade may be placed under direct vision prior to wound closure. A large volume of anesthetic is usually required to effectively block all surgical dermatomes, so that the chance for local anesthetic toxicity with this block is high. Also, placement is difficult in the awake child, as several injections are needed and repeat blockade is usually required every 12 hours.

TECHNIQUE

The patient should be positioned so that the plane of entry is readily exposed. In the semiprone position, the puncture line will be at the midaxillary or posterior axillary line. When the patient is sitting, the posterior axillary line or the paravertebral line just lateral to the sacrospinalis muscle can be used for needle placement. If the paravertebral approach is used, high spinal anesthesia may occur as a result of subarachnoid injection along a nerve root.

A short beveled 25 to 22 g needle is used. The skin is retracted cephalad and infiltrated with local anesthetic. The needle is directed either perpendicular or slightly cephalad at an 80-degree angle to the skin until it encounters the lower border of the rib to be blocked. The retracted skin is relaxed and the needle is carefully walked off the edge of the rib. While the needle is being advanced 1 to 3 mm, a "pop" may be felt. After aspiration for air and blood, the anesthetic solution is injected. Care must be taken to avoid pneumothorax from pleural puncture.

Drugs and Dosing Options

Bupivacaine 0.25% + epinephrine 1:400,000 (maximum total dose 1.0 ml/kg)

Bupivacaine 0.5% + epinephrine 1:400,000 (maximum total dose 0.5 ml/kg)

Axillary Block

This technique can be used for intraoperative anesthesia for upper extremity procedures, as well as postoperative pain relief. Occasionally axillary blockade may be placed for sympathetic blockade. The block has a low incidence of complications, intravascular injection being the most common.

Technique

Few awake children will cooperate with a technique requiring solicitation of paresthesias. In the anesthetized or sedated child, a nerve stimulator is used to localize the injection. A perivascular approach with injection of one-half of the total anesthetic solution volume on either side of the axillary artery is also commonly used, although puncture of the axillary artery may lead to the formation of a local hematoma. A 25 g pinpoint needle may be selected for either technique. As with adults, the intercostal brachial and musculocutaneous nerves must also be blocked by subcutaneous and intramuscular injection.

Drugs and Dosing Options

0.25% to 0.5% bupivacaine + epinephrine 1:200,000 0.5 ml/kg

Fascia Iliaca Compartment Block

This technique blocks the femoral, lateral femoral, cutaneous, and obturator nerves with a single injection using anatomic landmarks and characteristic pops. It is an excellent block for femoral osteotomies and reduction of femoral fractures.

Technique

A line drawn between the anterior superior iliac spine and pubic tubercle will identify the inguinal ligament. A single point that represents the medial two thirds and lateral one third of the inguinal ligament should be noted. 0.5 to 1 cm below (caudad to) this point, a short beveled block needle is advanced until two pops are felt (fascia lata and then fascia iliaca). With injection, there should be a lack of resistance.

DRUGS AND DOSING OPTIONS

A mixture of 1% lidocaine and 0.5% bupivacaine 1:1 with epinephrine 1:200,000 0.7 to 1.0 ml/kg (If bupivacaine is used alone, the block duration may exceed 12 to 18 hours.)

Ilioinguinal and Iliohypogastric Block

This block is useful for orchiopexy or inguinal herniorrhaphy. It allows for a marked reduction in the general anesthetic requirements if placed before incision, as well as providing the patient with postoperative analgesia for several hours. Conversely, it can be placed under direct vision by the surgeon intraoperatively or by either the surgeon or the anesthesiologist after wound closure. Large volumes of local anesthetic at high concentrations have been known to cause prolonged motor blockade of the femoral nerve. This block is inadequate for manipulation or exploration of the spermatic cord or testicle. However, it will block most incisional pain from these procedures.

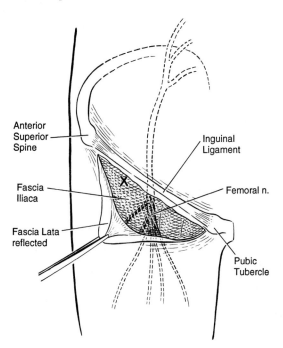

Anterior
Superior
Spine

Inguinal
Ligament

Fascia
Iliaca

Femoral n.

Fascia Lata
reflected

Pubic
Tubercle

FIG. 20-3. Ilioinguinal and iliohypogastric block technique (see description, next page).

TECHNIQUE: ILIOINGUINAL
AND ILIOHYPOGASTRIC BLOCK
(SEE FIG. 20-3, p. 477)

A 22 or 25 g short bevel block needle is placed 1 to 1.5 cm cephalad and 1 to 1.5 cm medial to the anterior superior iliac spine. As the needle passes, two distinct pops—of the external oblique fascia and aponeurosis—are felt. The needle is directed toward the ilium, and half the volume of the anesthetic solution is injected as the needle is withdrawn. The needle is then redirected toward the inguinal ligament, and all but 0.5 to 1 ml is injected. The remaining local anesthetic is injected subcutaneously to block the iliohypogastric nerve.

DRUGS AND DOSING OPTIONS

Bupivacaine 0.25% + epinephrine 1:200,000 0.4 to 0.6 ml/kg

Penile Nerve Block[48]

Most penile nerve blocks are performed by the operating surgeon for circumcision or hypospadias repair. This block will provide surgical anesthesia as well as postoperative pain relief.

TECHNIQUE

The roots from S2-S4 form the penile nerve, located under the symphysis pubis and running along side the dorsal arteries and vein of the penis deep to Buck's fascia. Just to the right and left of the dorsal penile vein, a 25 or 26 g needle is placed at the 10 to 10:30 and 1:30 to 2:00 positions to a depth of 3 to 5 mm until Buck's fascia is pierced. After careful aspiration, the local anesthetic solution is injected. Alternatively, a ring penile block can be performed by circumferentially injecting the base of the penis superficial to Buck's fascia. This avoids injecting volume within the penile fascia with the potential complication of distal ischemia.

DRUGS AND DOSING OPTIONS

All blocks at locations of terminal circulation should avoid epinephrine.
Penile block
Neonates for circumcision: lidocaine 1% 0.8 ml
Older children: bupivacaine 0.25% 1 to 2 ml
Ring block[49]
Bupivacaine 0.25% 2 to 3 ml

Recommended volumes of anesthetic solution (according to patient's weight) for block procedures[50]

Block procedure	Recommended total volume of anesthetic solution according to weight of children (0.25% bupivacaine)			
	Under 20 kg	20-29 kg	30-45 kg	Over 45 kg
Intercostal (total all segments)	1 ml/kg	15-20 ml	20-25 ml	25-30 ml
Axillary	0.3-0.6 ml/kg	10-15 ml	13-18 ml	28-20 ml
FICB* and "3-in-1"	1 ml/kg	20-25 ml	25-30 ml	30-35 ml
Sciatic nerve	0.5 ml/kg	10-12.5 ml	12.5-15 ml	15-17.5 ml
Lumbar plexus	0.7 ml/kg	10-12.5 ml	12.5-15 ml	15-17.5 ml
Penile†	0.1 ml/kg	2-2.5 ml	3-4 ml	5 ml

*FICB, Fascia iliaca compartment block.
†Penile blocks via the subpubic space require two injections (one per each side).

COGNITIVE/BEHAVIORAL TECHNIQUES[51,52]

Preparation

An age-appropriate presentation of the potential postoperative, procedural, or disease-related pain should take place for each child. The child should be given the option of incorporating any support systems into the development of a plan to manage pain or discomfort. This may involve bringing a special stuffed animal, a doll, or any other toys into the operating room or procedure room.

The usefulness of various cognitive and behavioral techniques for pain management in children cannot be underestimated. These techniques can be applied to virtually any pain setting. They can prove invaluable as aids for the completion of painful procedures in children. In addition, they can be used as an adjunct for acute pain management in postoperative, post-traumatic, or disease- and therapy-related pain crises.

Parental Presence[53,54]

Most parents should be encouraged to participate in the pain management of their youngsters. It has become common practice for parents to be present with a child during the entire hospital stay, including nights. They can be very helpful in determining a child's pain level and ability to cooperate and in offering comfort.

Distraction[55-57]

Preschool and early school age children are easily distracted. Techniques which have proven helpful in the management of painful procedures or painful conditions include the use of activity books, party blowers, puppet play, story telling, and various child-oriented videos. Child life therapists and psychologists can design programs of distraction to help children cope with painful situations. Many of the techniques employed for an inhalation induction of anesthesia are examples of distractive techniques, such as pretending the pulse oximeter is a video game.

Guided Imagery/Hypnosis[58-60]

Hypnotic techniques most often require the involvement of a hypnotherapist. Such individuals may be physicians, social workers, nurses, or psychologists. Self-hypnotic techniques can prove quite useful during painful procedures or in coping with the pain of chronic disease. Simple modifications of self-hypnosis involve asking the child to focus on an object in the room while breathing or counting (similar to techniques for management of labor pain) or to concentrate on an image or dream with the eyes closed. Many motivated children can increase relaxation and cooperation for simple procedures if given a few moments to practice focusing techniques in advance. Parents present during procedures may help the child stay focused or guide imagery by gentle suggestions or questions. Having parents and children practice these techniques together before a procedure often increases motivation and cooperation.

TRANSCUTANEOUS ELECTRICAL NERVE STIMULATION (TENS)[61]

Analgesia provided by the transmission of pulse electricity to nerves through electrodes attached to the skin is gaining limited use in pediatrics, particularly with older children and adolescents. This technique has been used successfully after many different surgical procedures as well as for chronic pain syndromes and may significantly diminish opioid requirements.

TENS units are available with three adjustable variables: rate, pulse-width, and amplitude. There are five basic modes of transmission: high rate (conventional); low rate (acupuncture); high rate, high width, and high amplitude (brief intense); pulse train; burst. A beneficial effect can be seen in as little as 15 to 20 minutes.

EMLA (EUTECTIC MIXTURE OF LOCAL ANESTHETICS)[62]

EMLA cream is a topical emulsion containing a mixture of 2.5% lidocaine and 2.5% prilocaine, which is able to penetrate intact skin after application under an occlusive dressing. It must be applied approximately 60 minutes prior to painful stimulation.

Anesthesia reaching 5 mm of depth can be achieved with prolonged application of the mixture. Plasma absorption has remained well below toxic levels in all studies reported.

EMLA has been used and is recommended for venipuncture, venous or arterial cannulation, subcutaneous port access, lumbar puncture, bone marrow aspiration, and skin biopsy. It has also been reported to be beneficial in lithotripsy, circumcision, various otolaryngologic procedures, pulsed-dye laser removal of port-wine stain, post-herpetic neuralgia, and relfex sympathetic dystrophy.

When EMLA is used for intravenous cannulation, it is often helpful to apply the cream to several sites in case difficulty is encountered with cannulation.

References

1. Beyer JE, Aradine CR: Patterns of pediatric pain intensity: a methodological investigation of a self-report scale, *Clnic J Pain* 3:130-141, 1987.
2. Beyer JE, McGrath PJ, Berde CB: Discordance between self-report and behavioral pain measures in children aged 3-7 years after surgery, *J Pain Symptom Manag* 5:350-356, 1990.
3. Manne SL, Jacobsen PB, Redd WH: Assessment of acute pediatric pain: do child self-report, parent ratings, and nurse ratings measure the same phenomenon? *Pain* 48:45-52, 1992.
4. Bieri D, Reeve RA, Champion GD, Addicoat L, Ziegler JB: The Faces Pain Scale for self-assessment of the severity of pain experienced by children: development, initial validation, and preliminary investigation for ratio scale properties, *Pain* 41:139-150, 1990.
5. Beyer JE, Aradine CR: Content validity of an instrument to measure young children's perceptions of the intensity of their pain, *J Pediatr Nursing* 1:386-395, 1986.
6. Krane EJ, Jacobson LE, Lynn AM, Parrot C, Tyler DC: Caudal morphine for postoperative analgesia in children: a comparison with caudal bupivacaine and intravenous morphine, *Anesth Analg* 66:647-653, 1987.
7. Tyler DC, Tu A, Douthit J, Chapman CR: Toward validation of pain measurement tools for children: a pilot study, *Pain* 52:301-309, 1993.
8. McGrath PJ, Johnson G, Goodman JT, Schillinger J, Dunn J, Chapman J: The CHEOPS: a behavioral scale to measure potoperative pain in children. In Fields HL, Dubner R, Cervero F, eds: *Advances in pain research and therapy,* New York 1985, Raven Press, pp 395-402.
9. Lawrence J, Alcock D, McGrath P, Kay J, MacMurray SB, Dulberg C: The development of a tool to assess neonatal pain, *Neonatal Network* 12:59-66, 1993.
10. Anand KJS, Hickey PR: The biology of pain and its effects in the human fetus and neonate, *N Eng J Med* 317:1321-1329, 1987.
11. Zhang AZ, Pasternak GW: Ontogeny of opioid pharmacology and receptors: high and low affinity site differences, *Eur J Pharmacol* 73:29-40, 1981.
12. Pasternak GW, Zhang AZ, Tecott L: Developmental differences between high and low affinity opiate binding sites: their relationship to analgesia and respiratory depression, *Life Sci* 27:1185-1190, 1980.

13. Weinstein MS, Nicolson SC, Schreiner MS: A single dose of morphine sulfate increases the incidence of vomiting after outpatient inguinal surgery in children, *Anesthesiology* 81:572-577, 1994.

14. Berde CB: Pediatric postoperative pain management, *Pediatr Clin North Am* 36:921-940, 1989.

15. Koren G et al: Postoperative morphine infusion in newborn infants: assessment of disposition characteristics and safety, *J Pediatr* 107:963-967, 1985.

16. McCormack K: Non-steroidal anti-inflammatory drugs and spinal nociceptive processing. *Pain* 59:9-43, 1994.

17. Watcha MF, Jones MB, Lagueruela RG, Schweiger C, White PF: Comparison of ketorolac and morphine as adjuvants during pediatric surgery, *Anesthesiology* 76:368-372, 1992.

18. Buckley MMT, Brogden RN: Ketorolac: a review of its pharmacodynamic and pharmacokinetic properties and therapeutic potential, *Drugs* 39:86-109, 1990.

19 Maunuksela EL, Kokki H, Bullingham RE: Comparison of intravenous ketorolac with morphine for postoperative pain in children, *Clin Pharmacol Ther* 52:436-443, 1992.

20. Vetter TR, Heiner EJ: Inravenous ketorolac as an adjuvant to pediatric patient-controlled analgesia with morphine, *J Clin Anesth* 6:110-113, 1994.

21. Rusy LM, Houck CS, Sullivan LJ, Ohlms LA, Jones DT, McGill TJ, Berde CB: A double-blind evaluation of ketorolac tromethamine versus acetaminophen in pediatric tonsillectomy: analgesia and bleeding, *Anesth Analg* 80:226-229, 1995.

22. Watson CP: Antidepressant drugs as adjuvant analgesics, *J Pain Symptom Manag* 9:392-405, 1994.

23. Reddy S, Patt RB: The benzodiazepines as adjuvant analgesics, *J Pain Symptom Manag* 9:510-514, 1994.

24. Yaster M, Tobin JR, Billett C, Casella JF, Dover G: Epidural analgesia in the management of severe vaso-occlusive sickle cell crisis, *Pediatrics* 93:310-315, 1994.

25. Berde CB: Toxicity of local anesthetics in infants and children, *J Pediatr* 122:S14-20, 1993.

26. Wood M: Plasma binding and limitation of drug access to site of action, *Anesthesiology* 75:721-723, 1991.

27. Mazoit JX, Denson DD, Samii K: Pharmacokinetics of bupivacaine following caudal anesthesia in infants, *Anesthesiology* 68:387-391, 1988.

28. Lerman J, Strong HA, LeDez KM, Swartz J, Rieder MJ, Burrows FA: Effects of age on the serum concentration of alpha 1-acid glycoprotein and the binding of lidocaine in pediatric patients, *Clin Pharmacol Ther* 46:219-225, 1989.

29. Zsigmond EK, Downs JR: Plasma cholinesterase activity in newborns and infants, *Can Anaesth Soc J* 18:278-285, 1971.

30. Ecoffey C, Desparmet J, Berdeaux A, Maury M, Giudicelli JF, Saint-Maurice C: Pharmacokinetics of lignocaine in children following caudal anaesthesia, *Br J Anaesth* 56:1399-1402, 1984.

31. Berde CB: Convulsions associated with pediatric regional anesthesia, *Anesth Analg* 75:164-166, 1992.

32. Yaster M, Tobin JR, Maxwell LG: Local anesthetics. In Schecter NL, Berde CB, Yaster CB, eds: *Pain in infants, children and adolescents,* Baltimore, 1993, Williams & Wilkins.

33. Alifimoff JK, Cote CJ: Pediatric regional anesthesia. In Cote CJ, Ryan JF, Todres ID, Goudsouzian NG, eds: *A practice of anesthesia for infants and children,* Philadelphia, 1993, WB Saunders, Co.

34. Abajian JC, Mellish RW, Browne AF, Perkins FM, Lambert DH, Mazuzan JE, Jr: Spinal anesthesia for surgery in the high-risk infant, *Anesth Analg* 63:359-362, 1984.

35. Mahe V, Ecoffey C: Spinal anesthesia with isobaric bupivacaine in infants, *Anesthesiology* 68:601-603, 1988.

36. Blaise GA, Roy WL: Spinal anesthesia in children, *Anesth Analg* 63:1140-1141, 1984.

37. Gouveia MA: [Spinal anesthesia for pediatric patients: our experience in 50 cases]. Raquian estesia para pacientes pediatricas, *Rev Bras Anestesiol* 72:501-511, 1970.

38. Takasaki M, Dohi S, Kawabata Y, Takahashi T: Dosage of lidocaine for caudal anesthesia in infants and children, *Anesthesiology* 47:527-529, 1977.

39. Schulte-Sternberg O, Rahlfs VW: Caudal anaesthesia in children and spread of 1% lignocaine: a statistical study, *Br J Anaesth* 42:1093-1099, 1970.

40. Satoyoshi M, Kamiyama Y: Caudal anesthesia for upper abdominal surgery in infants and children: a simple calculation of the volume of local anesthetic, *Acta Anaesthesia Scand* 28:57-60, 1984.

41. Armitage EN: Regional anesthesia in paediatrics, *Clin Anaesthesiol* 3:553, 1985.

42. Sethna NF, Berde CB: Venous air embolism during identification of the epidural space in children (editorial comment), *Anesth Analg* 76:925-927, 1993.

43. Desparmet JF, Berde CB, Schwartz DC, Lunn RJ, Hershenson MB: Efficacy of adrenaline, lignocaine-adrenaline and isoprenaline as a test dose in halothane-anaesthetized lambs, *Eur J Anaesth* 8:123-128, 1991.

44. Sang CN, Sethna NF, Sullivan L, Berde CB: Evaluation of epinephrine epidural test dose in children under isoflurane anesthesia, *Anesthesiology* 81:A1344, 1994.

45. Strafford MA, Wilder RT, Berde CB: The risk of infection from epidural analgesia in children: a review of 1620 cases, *Anesth Analg* 80:234-238, 1995.

46. Bonica JJ: *The management of pain,* ed 2, Philadelphia, 1990, Lea and Febiger.

47. Cousins MJ, Bridenbaugh PO, eds: *Neural blockade in clinical anesthesia and management of pain,* ed 2, Philadelphia, 1988, JB Lippincott.

48. Dalens B, Vanneuville G, Dechelotte P: Penile block via the subpubic space in 100 children, *Anesth Analg* 69:41-45, 1989.

49. Broadman LM, Hannallah RS, Belman AB, Elder PT, Ruttimann U, Epstein BS: Post-circumcision analgesia: a prospective evaluation of subcutaneous ring block of the penis, *Anesthesiology* 67:399-402, 1987.

50. Dalen SB: Peripheral nerve blockade in the management of postoperative pain in children. In Schecter NL, Berde CB, Yaster M, eds: *Pain in infants, children and adolescents,* Baltimore, 1993, Williams & Wilkins.

51. McGrath PA: *Pain in children: nature, assessment, treatment,* New York, 1990, Guilford Press.

52. Harrison A: Preparing children for venous blood sampling, *Pain* 45:299-306, 1991.

53. Bauchner H, Waring C, Vinci R: Parental presence during procedures in an emergency room: results from 50 observations, *Pediatrics* 87:544-548, 1991.

54. Gonzalez JC, Rough DK, Saab PG, Armstrong FD, Shifman L, Guerra E, Fawcett N: Effects of parent presence on children's reactions to injections: behavioral, physiological and subjective aspects, *J Pediatr Psychol* 14:449-462, 1989.

55. Kuttner L, Bowman M, Teasdale M: Psychological treatment of distress, pain, and anxiety for young children with cancer, *J Dev Behav Pediatr* 9:374-381, 1988.

56. Kuttner L: Management of young children's acute pain and anxiety during invasive medical procedures, *Pediatrician* 16:39-44, 1989.

57. Kuttner L: Helpful strategies in working with preschool children in pediatric practice, *Pediatr Ann* 20:120-122, 124-127, 1991.

58. Hilgard JR, LeBaron S: Relief of anxiety and pain in children and adolescents with cancer: quantitative measures and clinical observations, *Intl J Clin Exp Hypnosis* 4:417-442, 1982.

59. Katz ER, Kellerman J, Siegel SE: Behavioral distress in children with cancer undergoing medical procedures: developmental considerations, *J Consult Clin Psych* 48:356-365, 1980.

60. Zeltzer L, LeBaron S: Hypnosis and nonhypnotic techniques for reduction of pain and anxiety during painful procedures in children and adolescents with cancer, *J Pediatr* 101:1032-1035, 1982.

61. Eland J: The use of TENS with children. In Schechter NL, Berde CB, Yaster M, eds: *Pain in infants, children, and adolescents,* Baltimore, 1993, Williams & Wilkins.

62. Gajraj NM, Pennant JH, Watcha MF: Eutectic mixture of local anesthetics (EMLA) cream, *Anesth Analg* 78:574-583, 1994.

MALIGNANT HYPERTHERMIA

21

monster in my head
scare away the heat
let my muscles go
i'm hot down to my feet

michael buried in the
sand
what he dreamt was not at
hand
no ocean air and no wet
swim
could cool the burning heat
within

Adrienne Coleman

DESCRIPTION

Malignant hyperthermia (MH) is the only clinical entity specifically related to and caused by anesthetic agents. The disorder is an acute hypermetabolic state of skeletal muscle (skeletal muscle is approximately 40% of body weight), resulting in increased oxygen consumption, lactate accumulation, and heat production. The exact cellular mechanism or defect is unknown.

Incidence

The overall incidence of MH reported by various investigators is 1:15,000 anesthetic episodes in children and 1:50,000 anesthetic episodes in adults.[1] The most complete study demonstrating the incidence of MH was conducted in Denmark by Ording with the following results.

Incidence of fulminant malignant hyperthermia[2]

- 1:251,063 total anesthetics
- 1: 84,488 inhalation agents
- 1: 61,961 inhalation agents and succinylcholine

Incidence of suspected malignant hyperthermia[2]

- 1: 16,303 total anesthetics
- 1: 6,167 inhalation agents
- 1: 4,201 inhalation and succinylcholine

MH is of particular concern to the pediatric anesthesiologist because of its increased incidence in children, perhaps because of the prevalence of associated musculoskeletal disorders that are often yet undiagnosed in children. Also, an anesthetic induction with halothane and succinylcholine, a common trigger for masseter spasm and MH, has been used more often with children than adults.

Etiology

MH is an inherited disorder, originally described as having autosomal dominant inheritance. It is now known that MH shows both variable penetrance and expression and that two to three genes are responsible for transmitting the disease.[3]

Genetics of MH

The ryanodine receptor (RYR) is thought to function as a calcium channel. An abnormality of the RYR in the sarcoplasmic reticulum of swine, seen in all MH susceptible pigs, is caused by a single mutation in the receptor gene.[4]

Unfortunately, the human variant is more complicated than the porcine MH syndrome. There appears to be a series of different mutations in humans, and less complete linkage between MH and RYR mutations is observed. The human MH syndrome appears to have a heterogenic basis.[5]

Associated Disorders[6,7]

Two syndromes are uniformly associated with MH: King-Denborough syndrome (short stature, growth retardation and musculoskeletal abnormalities) and central core disease, a myopathy of type I muscle fibers with central degeneration. Other disorders involving the musculoskeletal system have had an inconstant association with MH, with Duchenne's muscular dystrophy being described most commonly and consistently.

Disorders most commonly associated with MH
King-Denborough syndrome
Muscular dystrophy
Myotonia congenita
Central core disease
Schwartz-Jampel syndrome

Triggering Agents

Agents that elicit the clinical manifestations of MH are called triggering agents (see table on p. 487). To date, the halogenated agents and succinylcholine are the anesthetic drugs that are known to trigger MH. The manufacturer of succinylcholine has suggested its relative contraindication in children because of the increased risk of MH and hyperkalemia in children with undiagnosed myopathies (see package insert).

Nonpharmacologic factors that trigger MH include anxiety, stress, and fatigue. Reports of the full syndrome in humans without anesthetic triggers are rare.[8]

Agents that may confuse the clinical diagnosis of MH by causing tachycardia and hyperpyrexia include ketamine, phenothiazines, and anticholinergics.[9] Although caffeine is an agent used in the in vitro contracture test, neither caffeine nor theophylline causes contracture at clinically therapeutic levels.

Anesthetic triggers for MH[9]

Triggering agents	Nontriggering agents
Succinylcholine	Barbiturates
Decamethonium	Opioids
Halothane	Nitrous oxide
Enflurane	Benzodiazepines
Isoflurane	All nondepolarizing muscle relaxants
Desflurane	Etomidate
Sevoflurane	All local anesthetics
	Propofol
	Ketamine
	Anticholinesterases (controversial)

PATHOPHYSIOLOGY

1. The biochemical changes that occur with MH are present only in skeletal muscle and the hematopoietic system. However, the effects of this biochemical error may be seen in multiple organ systems.
2. The precipitating cellular event is a marked increase in intracellular ionized calcium—up to eight times normal resting levels—and blockage of calcium reuptake (see table on p. 488).
3. Increased intracellular calcium combines with troponin, forming the actin-myosin cross-bridges that initiate MH muscle "contracture" (nonpropagated and prolonged, unlike normal contraction). Rigidity may result.
4. Continuous muscle contraction requires constant energy supplied by means of ATP.
   a. Activation of glycogenolysis and phosphorylase kinase produces ATP and heat.
   b. The muscle enters into a hypermetabolic state, which exhausts aerobic metabolism.
   c. Anaerobic metabolism begins with lactate accumulation and hyperpyrexia.

d. Accelerated metabolism results in the following:
- Increased oxygen consumption
- Increased CO_2 production
- Increased heat production

e. Massive muscle edema results in increased membrane permeability and rhabdomyolysis, with the following sequelae:
- Hyperkalemia
- Hypercalcemia
- Myoglobinuria
- Elevated creatinine phosphokinase (CPK)
- Hypernatremia

Effects of elevated calcium in MH

Mechanism		Effect
1. Ionized intracellular Ca^{++} combines with troponin	→	Contractures of skeletal muscle
2. Glycogenolysis and phosphorylase kinase systems are activated to increase ATP production	→	Exhaustion of aerobic metabolism and conversion to anaerobic metabolism
3. Hypermetabolic state	→	Increased: • O_2 consumption • CO_2 production • Heat production
4. Altered muscle membrane permeability and rhabdomyolysis	→	Cellular efflux of: • Potassium • Calcium • Myoglobin • Sodium • CPK

CLINICAL SYNDROME

MH occurs most frequently shortly after induction, particularly if succinylcholine is used. It also commonly occurs at the end of the procedure as the patient emerges from anesthesia. However, the onset of MH has been reported to be delayed for up to 25 hours after the initiation of anesthesia.[10]

Signs and Symptoms

Clinical features of MH	
Cardiovascular	**Body temperature**
Tachycardia	Hyperpyrexia
Arrhythmias	
Hemodynamic instability	**Cutaneous**
	Rash
Respiratory	Diaphoresis
Hypercapnia	
Hypoxia	**Organ system failure**
(Late) Pulmonary edema	Central nervous system
	Renal
Neuromuscular	Hematopoietic
Masseter spasm	
Muscle rigidity	

CARDIOVASCULAR

Tachycardia.   Tachycardia is often one of the earliest signs of MH. Other more common causes of tachycardia should be excluded before the diagnosis of MH is considered, such as light anesthesia, hypercapnia, hypoxemia, hypovolemia, and use of anticholinergic or sympathomimetic agents.

Arrhythmias.   Arrhythmias associated with MH are caused by sympathetic stimulation and increased $PaCO_2$. Premature ventricular contractions (PVCs) and ventricular tachycardia (VT) are common. As hyperkalemia develops, the ECG may show peaked T-waves and widening QRS.

Hemodynamic instability.   Initially there is a rise in blood pressure from sympathetic stimulation. As MH progresses, hypotension may develop secondary to cardiac depression from severe acidosis, conduction abnormalities, and hyperkalemia.

RESPIRATORY

Hypercapnia.   Marked elevations in CO_2 production occur with skeletal muscle hypermetabolism. As a result, tachypnea is one of the earliest signs of MH in spontaneously breathing patients. Patients ventilated mechanically will exhibit a rapid rise in end-tidal CO_2 despite attempts to increase minute ventilation. In a semiclosed circle system, the CO_2 absorber becomes very hot as a result of an accelerated exothermic reaction, and the color indicator will change quickly as the canister becomes exhausted. If hypercapnia is not present, the diagnosis of MH is questionable.

Hypoxia.   Cyanosis may occur from inability to keep up with oxygen requirements or from cardiorespiratory failure and circulatory collapse.

Pulmonary edema.   Pulmonary edema is a late event caused by cardiac decompensation and shifts in intravascular fluids.

NEUROMUSCULAR

Masseter muscle spasm or rigidity (MMR)[11-13]

1. Definition: sustained contracture of jaw muscles after induction of anesthesia, which prevents opening the mouth for laryngoscopy although extremity relaxation is adequate; trismus.
2. Differential diagnosis of masseter muscle spasm[11,14]
   a. Insufficient dose of succinylcholine
   b. Overinterpretation of mild jaw tightness
   c. Normal response to succinylcholine on masseter muscle
   d. Synergistic interaction between succinylcholine and halothane
   e. Underlying myopathy
   f. Malignant hyperthermia

Incidence of masseter muscle spasm

Littleford et al, 1991[11]

   All anesthetics: 16%
   Volatile agent and succinylcholine: 3%

Ording, 1985[2]

   Anesthetics with succinylcholine: 1 in 12,000

Schwartz et al, 1984[12]

   All anesthetics: 12%
   Halothane and succinylcholine: 1%

---

3. Fifty-nine percent of patients referred for muscle biopsy testing were found to be MH susceptible according to the North American Malignant Hyperthermia Group protocol.[15] It is probably best to avoid the use of succinylcholine whenever possible.
4. Suggested treatment of masseter muscle rigidity occurring in a patient undergoing surgery:
   a. Cancel the procedure if elective (conservative approach).
   b. Continue the procedure with nontriggering agents.
   c. Admit all patients postoperatively after an episode of MMR.
   d. Continuously monitor temperature, CPK, myoglobin, and potassium (q4-6h) for 12 to 24 hours.

 e. Maintain adequate hydration and urine output.

 f. Dantrolene sodium therapy need not be given if masseter rigidity resolves promptly without other clinical signs and symptoms (hypercapnia, acidosis, arrhythmias, etc.).

 g. The patient and family should be counseled (see Counseling and Follow-Up), p. 495.

5. CPK levels drawn during an episode of MMR can be difficult to evaluate. Generally, levels below 20,000 IU/L are not considered diagnostic for MH. However, a CPK $\geq$ 20,000 and MMR are 80% reliable predictors of MHS.[15]

Muscle rigidity. Rigidity is frequently observed with MH and simply reflects contractures of the muscles. This finding should not be confused with normal muscle contraction caused by end-plate stimulation with acetylcholine (ACh). Neuromuscular blocking agents will not relieve these contractures.

BODY TEMPERATURE

Hyperpyrexia. Body temperature usually rises in response to the increased metabolic state, not because of a defect in central thermoregulation. Heat production may not be apparent as hyperpyrexia if it does not exceed heat loss mechanisms (cold room, large exposed surgical field, diaphoresis, or use of cardiopulmonary bypass).

CUTANEOUS

Rash. A rash (reddish to mottled purple) is frequently observed about the head, neck, and upper thorax.

Diaphoresis. As the patient's temperature climbs, normal modes of heat loss, such as diaphoresis, take place.

ORGAN SYSTEM FAILURE

Central nervous system (CNS). CNS involvement including cerebral edema, permanent coma, or paralysis has been reported as a late event with MH, usually due to cerebral hypoxia and ischemia.

Renal. Renal failure is usually a consequence of tubular inspissation of myoglobin with inadequate renal perfusion. The osmotic diuresis caused by the mannitol present in dantrolene (150 mg of mannitol per mg dantrolene) will help prevent this sequela.

Hematologic. MH patients have direct involvement of the hematopoietic system both by increased red blood cell fragility and by a change in platelet infrastructure. Disseminated intravascular coagulation is often a late complication of profound rhabdomyolysis or hemolysis or can occur by release of tissue thromboplastin during shock and periods of stasis.

Common laboratory findings in MH

Arterial blood gases	Acidosis—both respiratory and metabolic Hypercapnia Hypoxemia Base deficit
Electrolytes	Hyperkalemia Hypermagnesemia Hypercalcemia (early) Profound hypocalcemia (late) Hypernatremia
Enzymes	Increased CPK—20,000 U/L is diagnostic Increased LDH Increased SGOT
CBC	Decreased hemoglobin Thrombocytopenia
Coagulation profile	Prolonged prothrombin and partial thromboplastin time Decreased fibrinogen Increased fibrin split products

MANAGEMENT OF THE MH SUSCEPTIBLE PATIENT

Population

MH SUSCEPTIBLE CHILD

1. Previous MH episode
2. First-degree relative of individual with a history of MH episode or positive muscle biopsy
3. Previous masseter muscle spasm

HIGH INDEX OF SUSPICION

1. Presence of associated stigmata; history of heat stroke, muscle cramps of large bulky muscles (especially calves), caffeine sensitivity, etc.
2. Presence of associated disorders: strabismus, ptosis, scoliosis, muscular dystrophy, etc.

Preoperative Visit

The MH susceptible child will benefit from a preoperative consultation with the anesthesiologist. If indicated, appropriate laboratory data can be ordered at that time (including CBC, CPK, electrolytes, urinalysis, and ECG). A thorough discussion of the relative risks and proposed anesthetic techniques should be undertaken with the parents.

Premedication

Premedication is advised to reduce stress in the child (see Chapter 2). Benzodiazepines and barbiturates are good choices for premedication. Oral, intranasal, or rectal administration is preferred over intramuscular injections. EMLA (eutetic mixture of local anesthetics) cream may be used 1 hour prior to IV insertion.

Equipment and Monitors for the MH Susceptible Patient

1. Standard monitoring (ECG, blood pressure, temperature, oximetry, capnography, precordial stethoscope); arterial catheter and Foley catheter for repeated sampling in lengthy procedures may be considered
2. Cooling blanket on operating room table
3. Clean anesthesia machine (never exposed to inhalation anesthetics)
4. Previously used (contaminated) anesthesia machine[18]
   a. All vaporizers removed
   b. Accessible plastic and rubber connections changed *(especially fresh gas outlet hose)*
   c. Avoid using contaminated ventilators because of absorption of agents into nonreplaceable rubber parts
   d. CO_2 absorbers changed (absorb inhalation agents minimally)
   e. New circuit and mask
   f. Continuous 10-liter oxygen flow for 10 minutes to reduce the concentration of volatile agents to <1 ppm.[18] MHAUS recommends 10 L/min with 100% O_2 for 20 minutes, or 10 minutes if the fresh gas hose is replaced. Gas analysis by mass spectroscopy or Raman scatter can be used to document presence of detectable levels of inhalation agents after flushing the anesthesia machine.

Pretreatment with Dantrolene Sodium

Controversy exists over the need to pretreat patients. Administration of a nontriggering anesthetic rather than prophylactic dantrolene is believed to be more advantageous in the MH susceptible patient.

1. Carefully monitored patients can be quickly treated with IV dantrolene if necessary.
2. Complications of treatment including nausea, disequilibrium, fatigue, and weakness necessitating ventilatory assistance may outweigh the advantages. These side effects may necessitate hospital admission.
3. Dantrolene sodium 2.5 mg/kg IV administered 2 hours preoperatively will achieve adequate plasma levels for 5 hours.
4. Oral administration of dantrolene is not recommended, as wide variations in plasma concentrations are seen.[19]

Pharmacology of dantrolene sodium

Pharmacokinetics	Onset: 6-20 min Duration (of adequate plasma concentration): 5-6 hr Metabolism: liver Elimination half-life: children 7-10 hr; adult 12 hr Excretion: renal

Actions	**Muscular**
	Inhibits excitation-contraction coupling
	Increases contraction activation threshold voltage
	Decreases intracellular calcium
	Slows calcium release by the sarcoplasmic reticulum
	No effect:
	    Centrally
	    On neuromuscular junction
	    On actin-myosin binding
	    Synergistically with nondepolarizing relaxants
	
	Cardiovascular
	Primary antiarrythmic (increases refractory periods)
	Decreases cardiac contractility and cardiac index
	Increases systemic vascular resistance
	No effect on mean arterial pressure

Toxicity and side effects	Hepatotoxic with prolonged oral use Muscle weakness sufficient to warrant airway protection or prolonged ventilation Decreases LD_{50} of bupivacaine Side effects include drowsiness, dizziness, headache, nausea Synergistic toxicity if given with diltiazem or verapamil, causing hyperkalemia and cardiac arrest

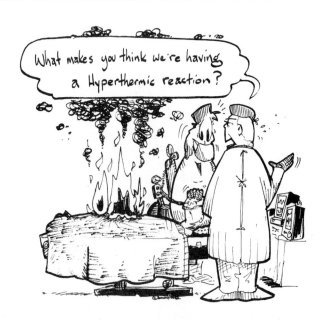

What makes you think we're having a Hyperthermic reaction?

Recommended Anesthetic Techniques for the MH Susceptible Patient

1. Barbiturate induction with balanced technique (nitrous oxide/oxygen, opioid, benzodiazepine, and nondepolarizing relaxant)
2. Propofol infusion
3. Regional anesthesia
4. Local anesthesia with sedation

Postoperative Monitoring

1. Postoperative MH reactions are rare after exposure to nontriggering agents.
2. Postoperatively, inpatients are monitored in the postanesthesia recovery room for 2 to 4 hours, as most MH reactions will occur within the first hour.[20]
3. Confirmed MH susceptible and suspected MH susceptible patients anesthetized with nontriggering agents are acceptable candidates for outpatient surgery. Some children may require readmission if they develop a fever at home.[20]

NEUROLEPTIC MALIGNANT SYNDROME (NMS)

The neuroleptic malignant syndrome (NMS) was first described in 1968 in patients taking major tranquilizers.[21] It is believed that NMS patients may also be MH susceptible, because the clinical features are similar and several NMS patients have had positive muscle biopsies. Although the specific association between the two disorders has not been established, it is probably best to avoid triggering agents in patients with NMS history.

COUNSELING AND FOLLOW-UP

1. A patient who has experienced an acute MH crisis or episode of trismus and his or her family should be counseled at length on the disorder and implications for future anesthetics prior to discharge from the hospital.
   a. This information should be disseminated to first-degree relatives and all second-degree relatives with either a myopathy or elevated CPK activity.
   b. A formal letter describing the event, laboratory documentation, treatment, and future recommendations should be given to the family and mailed to the primary physician.
2. A medical alert bracelet is recommended for the patient and susceptible family members.
3. A muscle biopsy may be performed.
   a. The caffeine-halothane contracture test is now standardized as a result of four conferences held from 1987 to 1991.[22] It

is the only widely accepted test for MH susceptibility. A list of participating test centers may be obtained from MHAUS. However, a "spectrum of susceptibility" has been described, based on variability of test results in susceptible families. Test variability is likely due to heterogeneity in MH susceptibility.[23]

b. The patient must travel to a center where the test is performed, since fresh live muscle tissue is necessary (see Fig. 21-1, p. 497). Dantrolene and droperidol are avoided, as they can normalize a positive response.

c. The recommendation for muscle biopsy is controversial, because susceptible patients are often treated as positive whether or not a biopsy is obtained and because false-negative results have been reported.[24] Therefore, it may be best to perform a muscle biopsy incidentally during other elective surgery. It may be useful for the following reasons:

- To document an acute episode of MH
- To identify modes of genetic transmission
- To give peace of mind to family members
- To resolve concerns about insurance coverage

4. All MH susceptible families should be referred to the Malignant Hyperthermia Association of the United States (MHAUS) for advice and support (Fig. 21-1).

Malignant Hyperthermia Association of the United States (MHAUS)

Address: 32 South Main Street
           Box 1069
           Sherburne, NY 13460

For nonemergency and patient referral calls:
           1-800-98-MHAUS or 607-674-7901

Names of on-call physicians available to consult in MH emergencies 24 hours a day: (209) 634-4917; ask for "Index Zero—Malignant Hyperthermia Consultant List"

Directory

U.S. Malignant Hyperthermia Muscle Biopsy Centers
The following centers are complying with the
standardization protocol for the caffeine-halothane
contracture test that resulted from four conferences
held 11/87, 11/89, 6/90 & 11/91:

Bowman Gray School of Medicine Thomas E. Nelson, Phd
Winston-Salem, NC 27157 (919) 716-4285

Cleveland Clinic Foundation Glenn E. DeBoer, MD/
Cleveland, OH 44106 (216) 444-6331
Hiroshi Mitsumoto, MD/(216) 444-5418

Hahnemann University Henry Rosenberg, MD
Philadelphia, PA 19102 (215) 762-7962

Mayo Clinic Denise Wedel, MD
Rochester, MN 55901 (507) 255-4236

Northwestern University Steven Hall, MD/Silas Glisson, PhD
Chicago, IL 60611 (312) 908-2541

Uniformed Services University Sheila Muldoon, MD
 of the Health Sciences (301) 295-3140
Bethesda, MD 20014

University of California Gerald A. Gronert, MD
Davis, CA 95616 (916) 752-9469

University of California Jordon D. Miller, MD
Los Angeles, CA 90024 (310) 825-7850

University of Massachusetts Barbara E. Waud, MD
Worcester, MA 01605 (508) 856-3160

University of Minnesota Paul A. Iaizzo, PhD
Minneapolis, MN 55455 (612) 624-9990

University of Nebraska Dennis F. Landers, MD, PhD
Omaha, NE 68105-1065 (402) 559-7405

University of South Florida Julius Bowie, MD
Tampa, FL 33612 (813) 251-7438

FIG. 21-1. A listing of Malignant Hyperthermia Muscle Biopsy Centers
in the United States.

TREATMENT PROTOCOL FOR AN ACUTE EPISODE OF MH

Early recognition and aggressive treatment are essential for a successful outcome.

1. *Summon help.*
   - Persons are needed for: resuscitation, line placement, airway management, record keeping, lab delivery.
2. *Discontinue all halogenated volatile agents.*
   - Ideally, an O_2 tank or clean machine and circuit without previous exposure to volatile agents should be brought into the room.
3. *Hyperventilate with 100% O_2 at high gas flows to maintain normocapnia.*
   - Mask ventilation is not usually difficult even in the presence of trismus or rigidity, when intubation may be problematic. Intubation should be performed when clinically feasible to secure the airway.
4. *Inform the surgeon.*
   - The surgical procedure should be terminated as quickly as possible.
5. *Administer dantrolene sodium IV by mixing each 20-mg bottle with 50-60 ml sterile water.*
   - Dantrolene is poorly soluble. The solution may need to be passed through a blood-warming unit or warmed by some other device to ensure it is dissolved thoroughly.
   - INITIAL DOSE: 2.5 mg/kg IV
   - If *ALL* symptoms are not resolved within 45 min, a repeat dose is administered:
     a. 2.5 mg/kg IV every 30 min until all symptoms dissipate
        or
     b. Single repeat bolus of 10 mg/kg IV
   - A typical response (decrease in $ETCO_2$) should be anticipated in 6 min, with normalization of ABG within 20 min.[16]
6. *Establish additional IV access.*
   - Central venous catheter placement should be considered.
7. *Place an intraarterial catheter.*
   - Invasive hemodynamic monitoring and frequent blood sampling will be required.
8. *Send STAT arterial blood gases, electrolytes, and CPK.*
   - Bicarbonate is given intravenously as needed to correct acidosis (1-2 mEq/kg) if ventilation is adequate and $PaCO_2$ is near normal.
   - Supplemental potassium should be avoided (hyperkalemia may occur later).
   - If dangerous hyperkalemia occurs: infuse 10 units regular insulin and 50 ml D_{50} slowly to effect.
9. *Initiate cooling if necessary.*
   - Iced saline 10-15 ml/kg IV every 10 min × 3

- Surface cooling with ice packs, hypothermia units (cooling blanket)
- Iced saline lavage of body cavities (stomach, rectum, peritoneal or thoracic cavities)
- Extracorporeal circulation with cooling if other methods are not successful

10. *Maintain urine output (2 ml/kg/hr) and assess urine myoglobin.*
    - Place foley catheter
    - Mannitol 300 mg/kg IV (*note:* the dantrolene vial contains 150 mg of mannitol/mg dantrolene)
    - Furosemide 0.5-1.0 mg/kg IV
    - Aggressive hydration with central venous pressure monitoring

11. *Give procainamide if arrhythmias are still present after adequate dantrolene therapy.*
    - Presence of arrhythmias may indicate need for additional dantrolene sodium
    - Procainamide loading dose to avoid hypotension:
      a. 1.5 mg/kg IV over 1 min and repeat every 5 min until arrhythmia is controlled or a total dose of 15 mg/kg is given
      or
      b. 15 mg/kg over 30 min
    - Infusion: 0.02-0.08 mg/kg/min
    - Calcium channel blockers should *not* be used, particularly when dantrolene is administered. Verapamil has been shown to cause hyperkalemia and myocardial depression, when used with dantrolene.[17]

12. *Transfer to intensive care unit.*
    - Hemodynamic monitoring should be continued for 24-72 hr after initial episode; recrudescence can occur from 4-36 hr after the event.
    - Laboratory data:
      ABG and electrolytes as dictated by clinical course
      CPK q4-6h × 24 hr
      Urine myoglobin until clear
    - Continue dantrolene administration 1-2.5 mg/kg IV q6h × 24 hr
    - Multi-organ system involvement should be treated as dictated by clinical course.

13. *Counsel patient and family.*
    - A discussion of pretreatment for future anesthetics, possible muscle biopsy for family members, and MHAUS referral should be completed prior to discharge.

References

1. Rosenberg H, Fletcher JE: Malignant hyperthermia. In Barash PG, ed: *ASA Refresher Courses in Anesthesiology,* vol 14, Philadelphia, 1986, JB Lippincott Co., pp. 207-216.
2. Ording H: Incidence of malignant hyperthermia in Denmark, *Anesth Analg* 64:700-704, 1985.
3. Levitt RC: Prospects for the diagnosis of malignant hyperthermia

susceptibility using molecular genetic approaches, *Anesthesiology* 76:1039-1048, 1992.

4. Williams CH, Lasley JH: The mode of inheritance of the fulminant hyperthermia stress syndrome in swine. In Henschel EO, ed: *Malignant hyperthermia: current concepts,* New York, 1977, Appleton-Century-Crofts, p. 141.

5. MacLennon DH, Phillips MS: Malignant hyperthermia, *Science* 25s6:789-794, 1992.

6. Schulman S: Malignant hyperthermia and pediatric anesthesia, *Semin Anesth* 12:54-64, 1993.

7. Heiman-Pattersohn TH, Natter H, Rosenberg H, et al: Malignant hyperthermia susceptibility in x-linked muscle dystrophies, *Pediatr Neurol* 2:356, 1987.

8. Strazis KP, Fox AW: Malignant hyperthermia: a review of published cases, *Anesth Analg* 77:297-304, 1993.

9. *Preventing malignant hyperthermia: an anesthesia protocol,* Malignant Hyperthermia Association of the United States (MHAUS), 1993.

10. Murphy AL, Conlay L, Ryan JF, Roberts JT: Malignant hyperthermia during a prolonged anesthetic for reattachment of a limb, *Anesthesiology* 60:149-150, 1984.

11. Littleford JA, Patel LR, Bose D, Cameron CB, McKillop C: Masseter muscle spasm in children: implications of continuing the triggering anesthetic, *Anesth Analg* 72:151-160, 1991.

12. Schwartz L, Rockoff MA, Koka BV: Masseter spasm with anesthesia: incidence and implications, *Anesthesiology* 61:772-775, 1984.

13. Larach MG, Rosenberg H, Larach DR, Broennle AM: Prediction of malignant hyperthermia susceptibility by clinical signs, *Anesthesiology* 66:547-550, 1987.

14. Hannallah RS, Kaplan RF: Jaw relaxation after a halothane/succinylcholine sequence in children, *Anesthesiology* 81:99-103, 1994.

15. O'Flynn RP, Shutack JG, Rosenberg H, Fletcher JE: Masseter muscle rigidity and malignant hyperthermia susceptibility in pediatric patients: an update on management and diagnosis, *Anesthesiology* 80:1228-1233, 1994.

16. Ryan JF: Malignant hyperthermia: treatment and after care, *Anesth Clin North Am* 4:913-932, 1991.

17. Rubin AS, Zablocki AD: Hyperkalemia, verapamil, and dantrolene, *Anesthesiology* 66:246-249, 1987.

18. Beebe JJ, Sessler DI: Preparation of anesthesia machines for patients susceptible to malignant hyperthermia, *Anesthesiology* 69:395-400, 1988.

19. Harrison GG: Dantrolene: dynamics and kinetics, *Br J Anaesth* 60:279-286, 1988.

20. Yentis SM, Levine MF, Hartley EJ: Should all children with suspected or confirmed malignant hyperthermia susceptibility be admitted after surgery? A 10-year review, *Anesth Analg* 75:345-350, 1992.

21. Guze BH, Baxter LR: Neuroleptic malignant syndrome, *N Engl J Med* 313:163-166, 1985.

22. Larach MG for the North American Malignant Hyperthermia Group: Standardization of the caffeine halothane muscle contracture test, *Anesth Analg* 69:511-515, 1989.

23. Urwyler A, Censier K, Kaufmann MA, Drewe J: Genetic effects on the variability of the halothane and caffeine muscle contracture tests, *Anesthesiology* 80:1287-1295, 1994.

24. Wedel DJ, Nelson TE: Malignant hyperthermia: diagnostic dilemma—false-negative contracture responses with halothane and caffeine alone, *Anesth Analg* 78:787-792, 1994.

PEDIATRIC AMBULATORY SURGERY: UNANTICIPATED ADMISSIONS

22

wait...
i don't have my Batman
pajamas
or my lucky underwear
and mom you know i just can't
sleep
without my Thomas teddy bear.

Adrienne Coleman

The proportion of surgical procedures performed in the ambulatory setting continues to expand at an impressive rate. Children typically are extremely resilient and therefore excellent candidates for outpatient surgery. The advantages of pediatric ambulatory surgery include reduced costs, increased hospital bed capacities for sicker children, minimized separation from parents, and reduction of nosocomial infection.[1]

Prevention of unanticipated postoperative admissions is economically desirable. Even more important, rates of unscheduled hospital admission following "outpatient" surgery are informative measures of outcome in ambulatory surgical care. To date, unexpected admission is a relatively rare event that occurs in approximately 1% of all ambulatory surgery patients,[2] and, interestingly, admission rates have not increased with time despite the growing number of more complicated patients having increasingly complex procedures.[3,4]

INTERPRETING ADMISSION STATISTICS

1. It is widely recognized that hospital-based outpatient surgery units tend to have higher unexpected admission rates compared with freestanding facilities. When evaluating admission rates, therefore, it is essential to compare similar facilities: freestanding ambulatory surgery centers should be compared with other freestanding units, community hospital-based centers with sim-

ilar facilities, and tertiary-care teaching hospitals with comparable institutions. Additionally, patient and procedure mixes must be similar.

2. The extent of care provided by the postanesthesia care unit (PACU) after surgery and the discharge criteria of the PACU provide other variables. For example, some PACUs have considerably longer operating hours than others, thereby preventing possible admissions. Certain PACUs may require intake of oral fluids and micturition prior to discharge, while other units will not insist on these endpoints.

3. When patients cannot be readily admitted to a hospital bed, strict adherence to relatively restrictive patient selection criteria and thoughtful reflection on the proposed surgical procedure become mandatory to minimize the risk of unscheduled postoperative hospitalization and the attendant logistical difficulties. Fatalities reported in the pediatric ambulatory surgery literature[3] underscore the necessity for every surgery center and anesthesiology location to be prepared to manage life-threatening perioperative emergencies.

4. It is important to appreciate that although unexpected admissions are quantifiable endpoints documenting that the procedure did not progress according to plan, the data do not necessarily imply medical, surgical, or anesthetic complications, as patients may be admitted for a variety of social reasons. Monitoring unanticipated admissions helps to:
   a. Identify complications that may require a different anesthetic approach or new therapy.
   b. Target procedures and subgroups of patients that should be excluded from the outpatient arena.

RATES OF AND REASONS FOR PEDIATRIC ADMISSIONS

Published series document unanticipated admission rates ranging from 0.1%[5] to 9.5%.[6] Most large-scale studies report an admission rate slightly above 1%,[3,4,7] and admission rates appear to be comparable for children and adults.[8] Despite the fact that admission rates are similar for children and adults, pediatric patients tend to have very different coexisting diseases and undergo vastly different surgical procedures from their adult counterparts.

Admission rates have remained stable during the past two decades, despite the fact that more people with increasingly complex coexisting medical conditions are undergoing more complicated surgical procedures, possibly because anesthetic and surgical techniques have improved.

1. Endoscopic techniques and other refinements have made surgery less invasive.

2. Anesthetic agents and other pharmaceuticals have been developed and marketed for the outpatient setting to reduce nausea, vomiting, pain, and the duration of recovery.
3. Knowledge of preemptive and multimodal analgesia has grown.

Several problem areas contribute to the overwhelming majority of unanticipated admissions in both the pediatric and adult populations.

1. *Medical problems* are defined as those conditions that are also signs and symptoms of a patient's preexisting disease state, including dysrhythmias, pulmonary edema, and respiratory insufficiency.
2. *Anesthetic problems* are a direct consequence of an anesthesiologist's action or inaction, or are associated side effects or complications of administered drugs (e.g., nausea, vomiting, aspiration, disorientation, postspinal headache, and allergic reactions).
3. *Surgical problems* are those associated with the surgical procedure, such as bleeding, wound care, and intraoperative findings requiring a more extensive procedure or immediate evaluation.
4. *System/social problems* frequently are related to preoperative preparation (perioperative drug administration or lack thereof) and postoperative care (home nursing, appropriate medical and psychological support, etc.).
5. The etiology of some problems may be difficult to differentiate as the result of anesthesia, surgery, preexisting disease, or a combination of these entities. For example, nausea and vomiting can be influenced by the nature of the surgical procedure, preexisting medical conditions and anesthetic and nonanesthetic drugs.

Four comprehensive surveys among patients at pediatric hospitals show postoperative nausea and vomiting, extensive surgery, and respiratory complications (including apnea and croup) as frequent reasons for unanticipated admissions.[3,4,8,9]

Patel and Hannallah[11] compared complications between 10,000 children having outpatient surgery at Children's National Medical Center from 1983 to 1986 and 15,245 children undergoing ambulatory surgery at the same facility from 1988 to 1991. Although the unscheduled admission rate declined impressively by two thirds (from 0.9% to 0.3%), the reasons for admission remained relatively consistent. Vomiting accounted for approximately one third of all admissions in both time segments. In the earlier study period, vomiting was followed in descending order by complicated surgery, croup, parental request, and fever. In the second phase of the study, the most prevalent causes for admission after vomiting were stridor or croup, bleeding, pain, and drowsiness. Complicated surgery accounted for 17% of the earlier admissions but only 9% of the second-phase hospitalizations, leading one to speculate that perhaps procedure selection had improved.

Reasons for admissions to the hospital

Reasons	No. of patients (%) 1983-1986 (N=10,000)	No. of patients (%) 1988-1991 (N=15,245)
Admission rate	**90 (0.9)**	**45 (0.3)**
Protracted vomiting	30 (33)	17 (39)
Complicated surgery	15 (17)	4 (9)
Croup	9(9)	5 (11)
M.D./Parent's request	6 (7)	2 (4)
Fever	6 (7)	0(0)
Bleeding	3 (3)	4(9)
Sleepiness	2 (2)	2 (4)
Others	20 (22)	8 (17)
Pain	0	3 (7)

From Patel RI, Hannallah RS: Complications following pediatric surgery: less of the same? *Anesthesiology* 79(3A):A22, 1993.

PREOPERATIVE PATIENT SELECTION

The first step in controlling unscheduled admissions lies in the selection criteria and process.[10] Not only have selection criteria broadened so that more children are considered at acceptable risk levels for operative procedures, but more increasingly complex surgical procedures have been designated "outpatient" operations by third-party payers. Owing to economic pressures, the days when ambulatory surgery was performed exclusively on healthy individuals undergoing brief, minor procedures have ended. Nevertheless, key elements of a child's medical and social history may increase the risk of postoperative complications to unacceptable levels. These children are unlikely candidates for ambulatory surgery.

Absolute or relative contraindications for pediatric ambulatory surgery

---

Procedure associated with major blood loss or severe postoperative pain

Acute concurrent illness

Severe systemic disease requiring invasive monitoring and intensive postoperative care

Former premature infants <44-60 weeks postconception

Infants with significant bronchopulmonary dysplasia, a history of apnea, or requiring supplemental oxygen

Children <1 year of age with a family history of sudden infant death syndrome

Lack of appropriate social support system, including lack of comprehension of postoperative requirements by family

---

Preoperative screening preparation before the day of surgery can help in cost containment by decreasing last-minute cancellations. The rate of postponed or cancelled surgery among those who could not be screened has been reported as 14.8%, versus 9.7% among patients who were screened.[11]

Objectives of preoperative screening

Evaluate appropriateness of patient and procedure for ambulatory facility

Acquire necessary medical information to assess risk of anesthesia and obtain informed consent

Acquaint patient with ambulatory surgical facility

Evaluate patient's social situation with regard to ambulatory surgery and educate patient's family about preoperative (NPO and medication instructions) and postoperative issues

---

SPECIFIC PROBLEMS NECESSITATING ADMISSION

Emesis

Although in years past, any child vomiting more than four times would have been admitted, now pediatric anesthesiologists are more comfortable discharging children home with current treatment modalities.

1. Adequate parenteral hydration prior to discharge prevents dehydration should vomiting occur.

2. Use of prophylactic antiemetic agents (e.g., propofol and ondansetron) for high-risk patients having certain emetogenic procedures has become more common. While these drugs may prevent vomiting in the hospital, their duration

of action may not be sufficient to prevent vomiting at home.[12,13]

3. Drinking clear fluids prior to discharge is not only unnecessary after ambulatory surgery, but actually increases the incidence of emesis during that period.[14] Liberal hydration (20 ml/kg IV fluid) and offering children clear liquids only if they complain of hunger (which may indicate the return of peristalsis) may be a more reasonable alternative. Liberal IV hydration produces a significantly lower incidence of thirst, drowsiness, and dizziness postoperatively in ambulatory patients.[15]

4. Inadequate pain control can trigger nausea and vomiting and result in postoperative admission. Unfortunately, opiods, especially if given in large doses, may also produce nausea and emesis. A preemptive, multimodal approach to postoperative analgesia, with reliance on local anesthetics, nonsteroidal antiinflammatory drugs (NSAIDs), and limited use of narcotics is often helpful. Ketorolac (0.75 mg/kg IV) can provide analgesia comparable to morphine 0.1 mg/kg IV, with a much lower incidence of nausea and vomiting in the first 24 hours for children recovering from strabismus surgery.[16] However, the clinician must be cognizant of the most recently issued warning from the manufacturer contraindicating the use of ketorolac "intraoperatively when hemostasis is critical." Furthermore, ketorolac (1 mg/kg IV) has been reported to be no more effective as an analgesic for children undergoing tonsillectomy than high-dose (35 mg/kg) rectal acetaminophen and was accompanied by twice the blood loss.[17]

Postextubation Croup

Postextubation croup is characterized—depending on severity—by stridor, a barking, brassy cough, hoarseness, and retractions (suprasternal, intercostal, or subcostal). Typically, these symptoms are caused by mucosal edema in the subglottic region. Postextubation croup is much more common in children (especially those in the 1-4 year old age range) than in adults, probably because anatomically small pediatric airways can be easily compromised by edema, especially in the narrow subglottic area. The incidence in 1977 was reportedly 1%.[18] Knowledge of factors[18,19] that increase susceptibility has decreased this incidence in the past two decades to 0.1% (excluding procedures on the airway).[20] The current standard of practice ensures that an air leak exists around the endotracheal tube, minimizing the incidence of subglottic edema from tight-fitting tubes. More recent studies indicate that 50% to 60% of cases of postextubation croup occur in children with a previous history of infectious or postextubation croup.[20-22]

Factors associated with croup

Age (1-4 years)
Tight-fitting endotracheal tube
Traumatic or repeated intubation
Prolonged intubation
Tissue irritants from endotracheal tube
High-pressure, low-volume cuff
Patient coughing while intubated
Passive head repositioning
History of postextubation or infectious croup

From McGoldrick KE: Otorhinolaryngologic surgery. In McGoldrick KE, ed: *Ambulatory anesthesiology: a problem-oriented approach,* Baltimore, 1995, Williams & Wilkins, pp. 459-506.

CLINICAL COURSE

1. Symptoms of croup usually occur soon after extubation (within 1 hour), with maximum intensity within 4 hours, and complete resolution within 24 hours.

2. Treatment for edema-induced partial airway obstruction is the same whether it occurs at the glottic or subglottic level. Although apparently useful in preventing progression of airway obstruction, steroids do not reliably prevent postextubation edema when administered prophylactically. They may be more useful in reducing symptoms from viral croup (laryngotracheobronchitis), must be given in large doses (dexamethasone 4 to 8 mg IV), and take 4 to 6 hours before maximum effect is achieved. Racemic epinephrine is administered for its vasoconstrictive properties, but, owing to its well-known rebound phenomenon, should be used carefully. Within 2 hours, the clinical efficacy of the drug dissipates, and occasionally the airway obstruction is worse than initially. This potential complication obligates the anesthesiologist to monitor the child for at least 2 or 3 hours, even after only a single dose.

Treatment for postextubation croup

Humidification
Oxygen
Hydration
Nebulized racemic epinephrine (0.5 ml of 2.25% and 2.5 ml saline)
Dexamethasone 4-8 mg IV
Emotional support
Admission as indicated

---

3. Discharge criteria in the outpatient setting should be individualized, depending on a variety of circumstances. The parents

should be given detailed instructions to observe the child frequently throughout the night and to bring the child immediately back to the hospital if there are any signs of respiratory distress. If there is any doubt by either the physician or the parents about the advisability of discharge, the child should be admitted for overnight observation and monitoring.

Factors to consider prior to discharge in patients with postextubation croup[23]

Age
History of prematurity
History of croup or subglottic stenosis
Down syndrome or other germane preexisting conditions
Severity of the child's symptoms
Need for drug therapy
Response to intervention
Parents' comfort level
Distance from the hospital
Availability of supportive measures such as a home humidifier

---

TONSILLECTOMY

During the last decades, tonsillectomy and adenoidectomy (T & A) have been performed increasingly in the outpatient arena, the result in no small part of economic pressures. Although complications following T & A are infrequent, they tend to be serious and have a precipitous onset, which continues to make admission controversial. Hemorrhage and acute airway obstruction are among the potentially life-threatening sequelae. Other postoperative problems include fever, recurrent emesis, pain, and poor oral fluid intake.

Postoperative Sequelae
HEMORRHAGE

Hemorrhage after tonsillectomy may be primary (occurring within the first 24 hours) or secondary (occuring after 24 hours). The documented incidence of hemorrhage ranges from 0.006%[24] to 8.1%[25] when broadly defined (not requiring operative intervention). Multiple studies indicate an incidence of primary hemorrhage requiring reoperation to be between 0.06% and 2.5%, with the greatest majority of incidents occuring within the first 6 hours after surgery.[26-30] A more recent study indicates that primary bleeding occurs most commonly within 75 minutes of arrival in the recovery room.[31] Whereas 6 to 10 hours of postoperative observation was originally advocated for outpatient T & A,[29] these more recent data have supported earlier discharge in otherwise uncomplicated patients.[31]

OBSTRUCTIVE SLEEP APNEA (OSA)

Patients with OSA should be admitted overnight for careful postoperative monitoring,[32] as soft tissue obstruction persists in the immediate postoperative period. Furthermore, these children tend to emerge slowly and exhibit sensitivity to opioids.

CHILDREN LESS THAN 3 YEARS

The safety of outpatient tonsillectomy in young children remains controversial. Patients under age 3 are reportedly at higher risk for immediate postoperative complications, including emesis, fever, airway distress, and poor oral intake, which can lead to dehydration.[27,29] Adenoidectomy alone has less potential for complications than does the combined procedure or tonsillectomy alone.[33] In one series, 60% of children under 3 years of age required more than routine care (necessitating hospitalization), greater than 50% developed airway problems, and 15% of the latter group required ICU admission.[35] Children less than 4 years old reportedly have a lower incidence of postoperative hemorrhage.[27,28]

Challenges encountered with outpatient tonsillectomy

Airway obstruction on induction
Intraoperative hemorrhage
Hypotension
Dysrhythmias
Airway fires
Cervical spine injury secondary to improper head positioning
Compression, obstruction, or dislodgement of endotracheal tube
Laryngospasm
Aspiration
Postoperative apnea or airway obstruction
Nausea and vomiting
Dehydration
Pain
Rebleeding
   Duration of postoperative observation period
   Outpatient status appropriate for age <3 years

From McGoldrick KE: Otorhinolaryngologic surgery. In McGoldrick KE, ed: *Ambulatory anesthesiology: a problem-oriented approach,* Baltimore, 1995, Williams & Wilkins, pp. 459-506.

TECHNIQUES TO DECREASE THE RISK OF UNANTICIPATED ADMISSIONS

Review of the literature reveals that extremely low rates of hospital admission after ambulatory surgery have been achieved and points to those areas in which attention to detail might improve this rate even further. Clearly, however, some factors associated with an increased likelihood of admission, such as the presence of serious coexisting disease or the type and duration of surgery, are beyond our control. Nonetheless, even in the face of multiple confounding variables, patterns do emerge.

1. Postoperative nausea and vomiting are consistently among the most common complications that delay discharge or cause unanticipated admissions.[36]

   a. Patients given propofol for induction and maintenance of anesthesia have less nausea and vomiting and are ready for discharge sooner than control patients who receive thiopental for induction and isoflurane for maintenance.[38] Also, propofol usage may decrease the rate of admission for anesthesia-related reasons.[37]

   b. When given prophylactically, ondansetron appears to be effective in decreasing the incidence of postoperative emesis in children undergoing tonsillectomy[38] and strabismus surgery.[39,40]

   c. Certain nonpharmacologic adjustments, such as not requiring children to drink before discharge, have shown encouraging results in dealing with the challenge of postoperative vomiting.[14]

2. Recent advances in the knowledge of pain mechanisms, as well as preemptive and multimodal analgesia, hold promise for reducing the number of unscheduled hospitalizations for uncontrolled postoperative pain. Many investigators believe there is opportunity for increased use of regional anesthesia[41] and nonsteroidal antiinflammatory drugs[42] in day case surgery.

3. Gentle, skillful airway management, perhaps in combination with increasing use of the laryngeal mask airway where appropriate, may decrease the incidence of postoperative croup.

4. More attention paid to preoperative education might well decrease the incidence of "social" or system admissions.

5. Changes in administrative practices may also improve admission rates. Several studies have suggested that cases started later in the day have an increased likelihood of unplanned admission.[42-44] Perhaps scheduling long procedures early in the day would reduce unexpected admission rates.

6. Preoperative screening[3,37] and extending postanesthesia care unit hours also may improve admission statistics.[37]

7. It is inadvisable to schedule certain interventions, such as tonsillectomy, in a child younger than 3 years of age, as outpatient procedures.

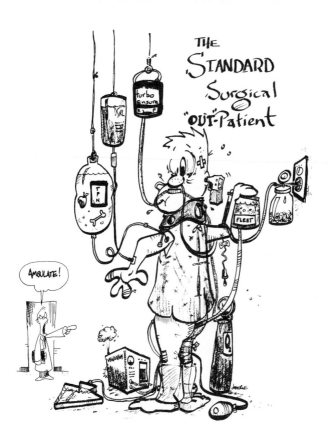

The Standard Surgical "Out"-Patient

AMBULATE!

References

1. Verghese S: Anesthetic management of the ambulatory pediatric surgery patient. In McGoldrick KE, ed: *Ambulatory anesthesiology: a problem-oriented approach,* Baltimore, 1995, Williams & Wilkins, pp. 58-89.

2. Levy ML: Complications: prevention and quality assurance, *Anesthesiol Clin North Am* 5(1):137-166, 1987.

3. Postuma R, Ferguson CC, Stanwick RS, et al: Pediatric day-care surgery: a 30-year hospital experience, *J Pediatr Surg* 22:304-307, 1987.

4. Patel RI, Hannallah RS: Anesthetic complications following pediatric ambulatory surgery: a 3-year study, *Anesthesiology* 69:1009-1012, 1988.

5. Natof HE: Complications associated with ambulatory surgery, *JAMA* 244:1116-1118, 1980.

6. Levin P, Stanziola A, Hand R: Postoperative hospital retention following ambulatory surgery in a hospital-based program, *Am Coll Utilization Rev Phys* 5:90-94, 1990.

7. Gold BS, Kitz DS, Lecky JH, et al: Unanticipated admission to the hospital following ambulatory surgery, *JAMA* 262:3008-3010, 1989.

8. Moir CR, Blair GK, Fraser GC, et al: The emerging pattern of pediatric day-case surgery, *J Ped Surg* 22:743-745, 1987.

9. Patel RI, Hannallah RS: Complications following pediatric ambulatory surgery—less of the same? (abstract) *Anesthesiology* 79(3A):A22, 1993.

10. Feldman M, Pasternak R, Paul S: Morbidity and mortality after ambulatory surgery (correspondence), *JAMA* 271:823, 1994.

11. Patel RI, Hannallah RS: Preoperative screening for pediatric ambulatory surgery: evaluation of a telephone questionnaire method, *Anesth Analg* 75:258-261, 1992.

12. Reimer EJ, Montgomery CJ, Bevan JC, et al: Propofol anaesthesia reduces early postoperative emesis after paediatric strabismus surgery, *Br J Anaesth* 40:927-933, 1993.

13. Rose JB, Martin TM, Corddry DH, Zagnoev M, Kettrick R: Ondansetron reduces the incidence and severity of poststrabismus repair vomiting in children, *Anesth Analg* 79:486-489, 1994.

14. Schreiner MS, Nicolson SC, Martin T, Whitney L: Should children drink before discharge from day surgery? *Anesthesiology* 76:528-533, 1992.

15. Yogendran S, Asokumar B, Cheng DCH, Chung F: A prospective randomized double blind study of the effect of intravenous fluid therapy on adverse outcomes on outpatient surgery, *Anesth Analg* 80:682-686, 1995.

16. Munro HM, Riegger LQ, Reynolds PI, Wilton NCT, Lewis IH: Comparison of the analgesic and emetic properties of ketorolac and morphine for paediatric outpatient strabismus surgery, *Br J Anaesth* 72:624-628, 1994.

17. Rusy LM, Houck CS, Sullivan LJ, et al: Double-blind evaluation of ketorolac tromethamine versus acetaminophen in pediatric tonsillectomy: analgesia and bleeding, *Anesth Analg* 80:226-229, 1995.

18. Koka BV, Jeon IS, Andre JM, Mackay I, Smith RM: Postintubation croup in children, *Anesth Analg* 56:501-505, 1979.

19. Dicarlo JV, Sanders AI, Sweeny MF: Airway complications of endotracheal intubation in pediatric patients (abstract), *Anesthesiology* 69:A775, 1988.

20. Litman RS, Keon TP: Postintubation croup in children (letter), *Anesthesiology* 75:1122-1123, 1991.

21. Neuman GG, Yadlapolli J, Kushins LG: Postintubation croup in children (letter), *J Clin Anesth* 4:346, 1992.

22. Lee KW, Templeton JJ, Dorigal RM: Tracheal tube size and postintubation croup in children (abstract), *Anesthesiology* 53:S325, 1980.

23. Hannallah RS: Postintubation croup, *Soc Amb Anesth Newsletter* 5(2):5, 1990.

24. Chiang TM, Sukis AE, Ross DE: Tonsillectomy performed on an outpatient basis: report of a series of 40,000 cases without a death, *Arch Otolaryngol* 88:307-310, 1968.

25. Kerr AIG, Brodie SW: Guillotine tonsillectomy: anachronism or pragmatism, *J Laryngol Otol* 92(4):317-323, 1978.

26. Allen TH, Steven IM, Sweeney DB: The bleeding tonsil: anesthesia for control of haemorrhage after tonsillectomy, *Anaesth Intensive Care* 1:517-520, 1973.

27. Crysdale WS, Russell D: Complications of tonsillectomy and adenoidectomy in 9409 children observed overnight, *Can Med Assoc J* 135:1139-1142, 1986.

28. Haberman RS, Shattuck TG, Dion NM: Is outpatient suction cautery tonsillectomy safe in a community hospital setting? *Laryngoscope* 100:511-515, 1990.

29. Carithers JS, Gebhart DE, Williams JA: Postoperative risk of pediatric tonsilloadenoidectomy, *Laryngoscope* 97:422-429,1987.

30. Guida RA, Mattucci KF: Tonsillectomy and adenoidectomy: an inpatient or outpatient procedure? *Laryngoscope* 100:491-493, 1990.

31. Nicklaus PJ, Herzon FS, Steinle EW: Short-stay outpatient tonsillectomy, *Arch Otolaryngol Head Neck Surg* 121:521-524, 1995.

32. McColley SA, Apul MM, Carroll JL, et al: Respiratory compromise after adenotonsillectomy in children with obstructive sleep apnea, *Arch Otolaryngol Head Neck Surg* 118:940-943, 1992.

33. Reiner SA, Sawyer WP, Clark KF, et al: Safety of outpatient tonsillectomy and adenoidectomy, *Arch Otolaryngol Head Neck Surg* 102:161-168, 1990.

34. Shott SR, Myer CM, Cotton RT: Efficacy of tonsillectomy and adenoidectomy as an outpatient procedure: a preliminary report, *Int J Pediatr Otorhinolaryngol* 13:157-163, 1987.

35. Tom LWC, DeDio RM, Cohen DE, et al: Is outpatient tonsillectomy appropriate for young children? *Laryngoscope* 102:277-280, 1992.

36. Kapur PA: The big "little" problem (editorial), *Anesth Analg* 73:243-245, 1991.

37. Johnson CD, Jarrett PE: Admission to the hospital after day case surgery, *Ann R Coll Surg Engl* 72:225-228, 1990.

38. Litman RS, Wu CL, Catanzaro FA: Ondansetron prevents vomiting after tonsillectomy in children (abstract), *Anesth Analg* 78:S253, 1994.

39. Lawhorn CD, Brown RE, Huggins DP, et al: Ondansetron dose response curve in pediatric patients (abstract), *Anesth Analg* 78:S240, 1994.

40. Litman RS, Wu CL, Lee A, et al: Prevention of emesis after strabismus repair in children: a prospective, double-blinded, randomized comparison of droperidol versus ondansetron, *J Clin Anesth* 71:58-62, 1995.

41. Parnass SM, McCarthy RJ, Bach BR, et al: Beneficial impact of epidural anesthesia on recovery after outpatient arthroscopy, *Arthroscopy* 9:91-95, 1993.

42. Kong R, Wilson J, Kong KL: Postoperative admissions from a hospital-based day surgery unit, *Ambulatory Surgery* 2:43-48, 1994.

43. Freeman LN, Schachat AP, Manolio TA, et al: Multivariate analysis of risk factors associated with unplanned admission in "outpatient" ophthalmic surgery, *Ophthalmic Surgery* 19(10):719-723, 1988.

44. Fancourt-Smith PF, Hornstein J, Jenkins LC: Hospital admissions from the surgical day care center of Vancouver General Hospital 1977-1987, *Can J Anaesth* 37:699-704, 1990.

PEDIATRIC SYNDROMES AND ANESTHETIC IMPLICATIONS

23

Being new is great
If you're a pencil or a shoe
Your packaging is perfect
And you know just what you're to do.

Being new is different
For a baby boy or girl
Before you can know anything
You're dropped into the world.

And every time you turn around
You find that something's changed
Your head and legs and arms and legs
Keep being rearranged!

Oh, wouldn't it be nice to be
A hammer or a horn,
And know that you are perfect
From the moment that you're born?

Rivian Bell

The pediatric syndromes in this chapter are categorized by type: cardiothoracic, chromosomal, connective tissue, craniofacial, dermatologic, hematologic, immunologic, metabolic/obesity, inborn errors of metabolism, musculoskeletal, and neurologic. Features common to one category are discussed prior to listing individual syndromes. The reader is advised to locate the specifics of the syndrome under its alphabetical listing. To obtain further information, consult the general paragraphs at the beginning of this chapter regarding the pathophysiology and anesthetic implications for that disease. These paragraphs may also refer to other chapters in this book that pertain to the organ systems affected by the particular disease.

CARDIOTHORACIC SYNDROMES (see also Chapter 9)

Congenital cardiac lesions are responsible for more than 90% of all cases of heart disease in children. A thorough understanding of the anatomy and physiology of a specific lesion, by either echocardiography or cardiac catheterization, is essential when developing an anesthetic plan. It is also important to appreciate that the same lesion in two different children may present varying degrees of disability depending on the amount of stenosis, magnitude of shunt, severity of failure, and previous corrective procedures. Children with congenital heart disease (CHD) often have associated noncardiac defects, usually of the genitourinary system. Most children should receive preoperative prophylactic antibiotics (see Appendix F, p. 666).

CHROMOSOMAL SYNDROMES

This category includes a number of specific chromosomal aberrations present in every cell and therefore every organ system. Often the gene has variable penetrance, which affects the severity of the syndrome and the degree of organ involvement. Most of the chromosomal syndromes are associated with mental retardation, which may limit patient cooperation, even in the older child or adolescent. Preoperative ketamine (4 to 5 mg/kg IM) is often useful in the large uncooperative or hyperactive child because of its ease of use, rapid and predictable onset, and preservation of spontaneous ventilation.

CONNECTIVE TISSUE DISORDERS

Patients with these syndromes have defective collagen synthesis and decreased tensile strength properties. Multiple organ systems are usually affected.

These patients are often seen for hernia repair because of increased tissue laxity. Joint hyperflexibility requires extra care in positioning during operative procedures. Involvement of the cervical spine may increase the patient's susceptibility to injury during intubation. Airway management can be affected by arytenoid laxity or dislocation and preexisting tracheomalacia. Generalized alterations of vascular endothelium lead to an increased incidence of accelerated cardiovascular disease. Altered collagen structure may compromise cardiac valvular function.

These patients often have long histories of salicylate, nonsteroidal antiinflammatory drug, and steroid use. Stress dose steroid coverage and a coagulation profile should be considered preoperatively.

CRANIOFACIAL DISORDERS

Children with craniofacial deformities often require corrective operations, with the problem of airway management at issue on each occasion. Preoperative airway assessment becomes more difficult in the nonverbal or preverbal child or if psychomotor retardation is present. Some techniques commonly used for the difficult intubation (awake or fiberoptic intubation) become more difficult in the uncooperative child. Mask induction of anesthesia in spontaneously breathing patients before endotracheal intubation is often a successful option. The endotracheal tube must be adequately secured because it may be present in the operative field and not accessible to the anesthesiologist. Postoperatively, even minimal airway trauma or edema may necessitate prolonged ventilation.

Associated problems in these patients include elevated intracranial pressure, seizure disorders, and congenital heart disease. The extent of neurologic or cardiovascular involvement should be considered when devising anesthetic plans.

DERMATOLOGIC DISORDERS

Children affected by syndromes of primarily dermatologic origin often require repeated surgical intervention. Skin disruption results in increased vulnerability to mechanical trauma and necessitates meticulous care in positioning for surgery. Simple securing of intravenous catheters and endotracheal tubes, placement of ECG pads, and routine eye care should be accomplished without adhesives. Skin injury can be minimized by the use of circumferential gauze bandages, padding under blood pressure cuffs, use of needle electrodes, avoidance of tape, suturing intravenous catheters into place, and wiring endotracheal tubes to teeth.

Disruption of the normal integument causes an inability to maintain body temperature, making temperature monitoring essential and maintenance of normothermia difficult. Standard practices of warming intravenous fluids, warming and humidifying inhaled gases, using warming lights and blankets, and elevation of room temperature should be used.

Intraoperative fluid losses are increased with loss of skin integrity and may be worsened by excessive bleeding from vascular malformations. Fluid and electrolyte balance should be monitored during lengthy procedures.

HEMATOLOGIC DISORDERS

Patients with congenital hematologic disorders often have anemia and decreased oxygen-carrying capacity. The decision to transfuse the patient for elective surgery should be made preoperatively depending on the patient's overall condition. The presence of dyshemoglobins (particularly hemoglobin S [HbS]) may also interfere with the accuracy of pulse oximetry and thereby influence the decision to transfuse perioperatively. Coagulopathy, increased susceptibility to thrombosis, or both may also be present. These patients require specific identification of the clotting defect and delineation of the proposed treatment before the time of operation. Large-bore intravenous catheters and invasive monitoring should be considered if significant volume losses are anticipated.

IMMUNOLOGIC DISORDERS

These syndromes impair the body's defense mechanism by affecting the T cells, B cells, immunoglobins, or other complement cascade. Chronic pulmonary infections often occur, compromising pulmonary function and reserve. These patients require meticulous aseptic technique in the operating room for all invasive procedures, including endotracheal intubation, intravenous (IV) catheter placement, and injection of any drugs into IV tubing.

Also included in this category are syndromes of probable autoimmune etiology involving multiple organ systems (granulomatous disease, systemic lupus). These patients usually require stress dose steroids in the perioperative period.

METABOLIC/OBESITY DISORDERS

Children with these syndromes share the primary clinical manifestations of obesity, whether from a known metabolic derangement or an unknown specific defect. The degree of obesity can be determined from standard growth charts and from calculation of the body mass index (BMI):

$$BMI = \frac{Wt\ (kg)}{Ht^2\ (m)}$$

$$Normal = 20\ to\ 30$$

$$Obese = Over\ 30$$

Multiorgan system dysfunction should be anticipated in the obese pediatric patient, including the cardiovascular, endocrine, musculoskeletal, and autonomic nervous systems. There is an increased incidence of respiratory disease and decreased respiratory reserve.

Specific anesthetic difficulties include airway obstruction from redundant soft tissue, delayed gastric emptying, increased aspiration risk, poor vascular access, and blood pressure lability. A loss of functional residual capacity impairs pulmonary reserve. Decreased sympathetic and parasympathetic function and an increased susceptibility to cardiac failure and pulmonary edema have been described. An increased production of serum fluoride may occur with halothane use.

Preoperative placement of an intravenous catheter and rapid-sequence induction are recommended. Mask induction with spontaneous ventilation often results in acute airway obstruction and rapid oxygen desaturation.

INBORN ERRORS OF METABOLISM

In these diseases, a simple genetically determined biochemical defect results in the blockage of a specific metabolic process. As a result, precursors to the defective reaction accumulate and anticipated products are not made.

Since errors can occur in any biochemical pathway, a broad range of clinical symptoms and pathophysiology should be anticipated. However, most of these diseases produce some common attributes, most notably mental and motor retardation, neurologic abnormalities, and developmental disability. Multisystem involvement is common, particularly hepatorenal dysfunction and cardiomyopathy. Musculoskeletal defects and myotonia may result in respiratory compromise.

Anesthetic management of these patients requires specific delineation of the metabolic defect and thorough evaluation of the organ systems involved and the degree of involvement. Intraoperative and perioperative monitoring of biochemical functions (fluid, electrolyte, and glucose metabolism) is essential. Cardiopulmonary dysfunction and musculoskeletal abnormalities may result in an exaggerated response to inhalation anesthetics, sedatives, opioids, and muscle relaxants. Prolonged drug action and impaired drug elimination may necessitate postoperative ventilation.

MUSCULAR DISORDERS

Progressive weakness is the hallmark of most pediatric syndromes that primarily affect muscle. These myopathies result in atrophy of skeletal muscle and contractures necessitating careful padding and positioning in the operating room. Cardiac muscle involvement may cause cardiomyopathy with arrhythmias, conduction disturbances, or congestive heart failure.

Weakness of respiratory muscles may impair the patient's ability to ventilate. Exaggerated responses to muscle relaxants or sedatives may further decrease ventilatory response. Absent cough or gag may result in recurrent aspiration, with chronic infections and pneumonia. Prolonged airway protection and the need for mechanical ventilation are often necessary in the postoperative period.

SKELETAL DISORDERS

Many congenital disorders of the skeletal system can be categorized under the multiple forms of osteochondrodysplasias (dwarfism). Although symptoms and organ system involvement can vary widely, several features commonly occur.

Short stature, joint laxity or fixed contractures, and brittle bones prone to pathologic fractures necessitate careful padding and positioning in the operating room. Odontoid hypoplasia or atlantoaxial instability may predispose the spinal cord to compression during intubation and positioning. Airway management is further compromised by limited neck mobility or the presence of associated anomalies (micrognathia, cleft palate, tracheal stenosis).

Kyphoscoliosis is a common feature and may result in significant restrictive pulmonary disease and decreased pulmonary reserve. It also increases the problem of positioning, particularly if spinal stenosis with neurologic defects is present.

A significant association exists between many forms of osteochondrodysplasia and congenital cardiac defects, seizure disorders, hydrocephalus, and bone marrow dysfunction (coagulopathy). The full extent of organ system involvement needs to be elucidated during the preoperative evaluation.

NEUROLOGIC DISORDERS

This category encompasses a broad spectrum of clinical problems, the two most commonly encountered being elevation of intracranial pressure (ICP) and seizure disorders. Usual techniques for patients with increased ICP include a barbiturate induction, intraoperative hyperventilation, pharmacologic agents to decrease cerebral edema (osmotic diuretics and steroids), and avoidance of opiate premedications that may raise $PaCO_2$. In general, it is best to avoid ketamine, which elevates ICP.

Barbiturates and benzodiazepines possess antiseizure properties that make them useful agents for patients with seizure disorders. Ketamine can raise seizure threshold. Conversely, enflurane may lower seizure threshold at 2.5 MAC in the presence of hypocapnia.

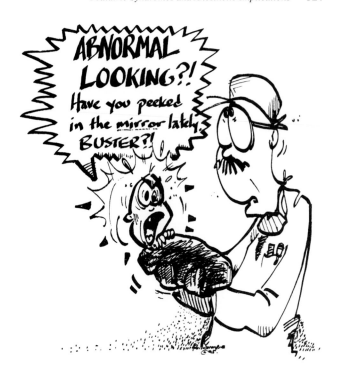

Abbreviations

ANS	Autonomic nervous system
ASD	Atrial septal defect
ATN	Acute tubular necrosis
AVM	Arteriovenous malformation
BUN	Blood urea nitrogen
C-Spine	Cervical spine
CAD	Coronary artery disease
CHD	Congenital heart disease
CHF	Congestive heart failure
CNS	Central nervous system
CPK	Creatinine phosphokinase
CV	Cardiovascular
DDAVP	Desmopressin acetate

Continued.

Abbreviations—cont'd

DIC	Disseminated intravascular coagulation
DTR	Deep tendon reflexes
EACA	Epsilon-aminocaproic acid
ECG	Electrocardiogram
ETT	Endotracheal tube
FFP	Fresh frozen plasma
GE	Gastroesophageal
GH	Growth hormone
GI	Gastrointestinal
Hct	Hematocrit
HTN	Hypertension
ICP	Intracranial pressure
IDDM	Insulin-dependent diabetes mellitus
Ig	Immunoglobulins
INH	Isoniazid
IV	Intravenous
LMA	Laryngeal mask airway
MAC	Minimum alveolar concentration
MH	Malignant hypertension
MVP	Mitral valve prolapse
NSAID	Nonsteroidal antiinflammatory drugs
PAC	Premature atrial contraction
PDA	Patent ductus arteriosus
PS	Pulmonic stenosis
PTH	Parathyroid hormone
SVT	Supraventricular tachycardia
TEF	Tracheoesophageal fistula
TMJ	Temporomandubular joint
TOF	Tetralogy of Fallot
URI	Upper respiratory infection
VF	Ventricular fibrillation
VSD	Ventriculoseptal defect

Pediatric syndromes and anesthetic implications

Disease [category]	Pathophysiology and clinical manifestations	Anesthetic implications
Abetalipoproteinemia (see Bassen-Kornzweig syndrome)		
Acute disseminated histiocytosis (see Letterer-Siwe disease)		
Albers-Schönberg disease (see Osteoporosis)		
Albright-Butler syndrome (primary distal renal tubular acidosis)	Nephrocalcinosis causing interstitial nephritis and renal failure Potassium loss causing weakness and periodic paralysis	Hypokalemia Impaired renal drug excretion Fluid and electrolyte imbalance
[Metabolic]	Anorexia/vomiting Polyuria Dehydration Growth retardation	
Alström syndrome [Metabolic/Obesity]	Diabetes mellitus Blindness Deafness Medullary cystic kidney Obesity	Aspiration precautions required Impaired renal drug excretion Impaired glucose and electrolyte regulation secondary to diabetes

Analbuminemia [Metabolic]	Almost absent albumin (4–100 mg/dl) Altered drug binding and metabolism	Very sensitive to protein-bound drugs including thiopental, curare, coumarin, and bupivacaine
Andersen's disease (Glycogen storage disease—type IV) [Metabolic]	Hepatosplenomegaly Failure to thrive Muscle weakness Cirrhosis Hypoglycemia	Exaggerated response to muscle relaxants Requires maintenance glucose infusion and monitoring of blood glucose Impaired hepatic drug metabolism Liver function tests and coagulation profile may be abnormal
Anderson's syndrome [Craniofacial]	Severe midface hypoplasia Abnormal structure and angle of mandible (triangular facies) Kyphoscoliosis Restrictive lung disease	Potentially difficult airway Decreased pulmonary function
Anhidrotic ectodermal dysplasia (see Christ-Siemens-Touraine syndrome)		
Apert syndrome (acrocephalosyndactyly) [Craniofacial]	Craniosynostosis Hypoplastic midface and prominent mandible Cleft palate Hydrocephalus Exophthalmos Associated CHD Elevated ICP may exist Psychomotor retardation	Potentially difficult airway Preoperative cardiac evaluation required May require prophylactic antibiotics May require anesthetic technique to lower ICP

Continued.

Pediatric syndromes and anesthetic implications—cont'd

Disease [category]	Pathophysiology and clinical manifestations	Anesthetic implications

Arnold-Chiari malformation
 	
[Neurologic]
	Elongation of cerebellar vermis and choroid plexus through foramen magnum with kinking of medulla and upper cervical cord
	Compression causes cranial nerve palsies
	Associated with meningomyelocele and syringomyelia
	Clinical symptoms:
	  Dysphagia
	  Apnea
	  Stridor
	  Opisthotonos
	  Decreased gag reflex
		Aspiration precautions required
		Potentially difficult airway
		Vocal cord paralysis
		Postoperative ventilation or tracheostomy often required
		Consider latex-allergy precautions

Arthrogryposis multiplex congenita [Connective tissue]	Spinal cord involvement causes leg and arm contractures Decreased muscle mass Scoliosis Restrictive pulmonary disease TMJ rigidity Iguinal hernia Cleft palate CHD	Care in positioning required Potentially difficult airway May have exaggerated response to muscle relaxants Pulmonary dysfunction may necessitate postoperative ventilation Preoperative cardiac evaluation required May require prophylactic antibiotics
Arthroopthalmomyopathy (see Stickler syndrome)		

Syndrome	Features	Anesthetic Implications
Asphyxiating thoracic dystrophy (see Jeune syndrome)		
Ataxia telangiectasia (See Louis Bar syndrome) [Immunologic]	Progressive cerebellar ataxia Decreased IgA and IgE Pulmonary infections Bronchiectasis Severe anemia If survival to adolescence, may develop lymphoma	Significant pulmonary dysfunction Preoperative Hct required Careful aseptic technique required
Bardet-Biedl syndrome [Metabolic/Obesity]	Complications of obesity: Delayed gastric emptying Altered ANS response Poor vascular access CHD Renal dysfunction Psychomotor retardation Polydactyly Hypogenitalism	Impaired renal drug excretion Preoperative cardiac evaluation required May require prophylactic antibiotics Aspiration precautions necessary
Bartter syndrome [Metabolic]	Hypokalemic, hypochloremic metabolic alkalosis Hyperaldosteronism with normal blood pressure In infancy: Failure to thrive Polyuria, polydipsia Increased prostaglandins	Fluid and electrolyte imbalance Decreased response to norepinephrine Impaired renal drug excretion

Continued.

Pediatric syndromes and anesthetic implications—cont'd

Disease [category]	Pathophysiology and clinical manifestations	Anesthetic implications
Bassen-Kornzweig syndrome (Abetalipoproteinemia) [Metabolic]	Retinal abnormalities Ptosis; strabismus Spinocerebellar degeneration with ataxia Vitamin A deficiency	Exaggerated response to muscle relaxants
Beckwith-Wiedemann syndrome (infantile gigantism) [Craniofacial]	50% born prematurely; birth weight > 4000 g Macroglossia, exophthalmos Visceromegaly, omphalocele CHD Severe neonatal hypoglycemia secondary to islet cell hyperplasia Medullary renal dysplasia Polycythemia	Potentially difficult airway Requires constant glucose infusion, avoidance of IV glucose boluses, and close monitoring of blood glucose Impaired renal drug excretion Preoperative cardiac evaluation required May require prophylactic antibiotics

Behçet syndrome
 	
[Immunologic]
	Triad:
	  Recurrent uveitis
	  Aphthous stomatitis
	  Genital ulcerations
	Optic atrophy
	CNS signs: spastic paresis, ataxia, seizures
	Pericarditis and vasculitis
	Obstructive pulmonary disease
	Skin lesions
		Oropharyngeal scarring causes potentially difficult airway
		May require stress dose steroids
		Preoperative assessment of cardiopulmonary dysfunction needed

Bird-headed dwarfism (see Seckel syndrome)		
Blackfan-Diamond syndrome [Hematologic/Immunologic]	Congenital idiopathic red cell aplasia Hepatosplenomegaly Thrombocytopenia Recurrent pulmonary infections	May require stress dose steroids Coagulation studies needed Platelet transfusion may be necessary
Bloch-Sulzberger syndrome (incontinentia pigmenti) [Dermatologic]	Skin lesions: erythematous streaks, verrucous lesions, hyperpigmentation CNS involvement: cortical atrophy, spastic paresis, seizures, hydrocephalus, and increased ICP Ocular manifestations: strabismus, cataracts, retinal detachment Skeletal anomalies: spina bifida, cleft lip or palate Impaired thermoregulation	Succinylcholine should be avoided in presence of spastic paresis Teeth are susceptible to injury during laryngoscopy Consider latex precautions if spina bifida present Requires careful temperature monitoring
Bowen syndrome (cerebro-hepatorenal syndrome) [Craniofacial]	Facial dysmorphism Congenital glaucoma Flexion contractures of fingers and toes, equinovarus CHD Psychomotor retardation	Potentially difficult airway Preoperative cardiac evaluation required May require prophylactic antibiotics

Continued.

Pediatric syndromes and anesthetic implications—cont'd

Disease [category]	Pathophysiology and clinical manifestations	Anesthetic implications
Carpenter syndrome (acrocephalopolysyndactyly) [Craniofacial]	Short neck Hypoplastic mandible Omphalocele CHD Hypogenitalism Premature closure of cranial sutures and elevated ICP Psychomotor retardation	Potentially difficult airway Preoperative cardiac evaluation required May require prophylactic antibiotics Management of elevated ICP
Central core disease [Musculoskeletal]	Muscular dystrophy Hypotonia with muscle wasting	Increased sensitivity to respiratory depressants Exaggerated response to muscle relaxants Increased risk of malignant hyperthermia
Cerebral gigantism (see Sotos syndrome)		
Cerebrohepatorenal syndrome (see Zellweger syndrome)		

Charcot-Marie-Tooth disease [Neurologic]	Chronic peripheral neuropathy Distal muscle weakness and wasting Sympathetic postganglionic fibers impair autonomic function, particularly the control of temperature	Autonomic nervous system hypersensitivity Impaired thermoregulation Potential for postoperative respiratory dysfunction May be sensitive to muscle relaxants
Chediak-Higashi syndrome [Hematologic/Immunologic]	Albinism Hepatosplenomegaly Recurrent chest infections Malignant lymphoma Thrombocytopenia Prolonged bleeding time	May require stress dose steroids Abnormal coagulation May have hepatitis and pulmonary dysfunction
Cherubism [Craniofacial]	Intraoral vascular masses Mandibular and maxillary tumors Chronic upper airway obstruction may cause cor pulmonale	Tracheostomy may be necessary for extremely difficult airway May have cardiopulmonary dysfunction

Christ-Siemens-Touraine syndrome (anhidrotic ectodermal dysplasia)
 	
 [Connective tissue]
	Triad:
	  Absence of sweat glands
	  Absence of teeth
	  Hypotrichosis
	 Midfacial hypoplasia
	 Inability to control temperature by sweating
	 Persistent respiratory infections
		Potentially difficult airway
		 Risk of hyperpyrexia
		 Anticholinergics decrease sweat production and may further contribute to hyperthermia

Continued.

Pediatric syndromes and anesthetic implications—cont'd

Disease [category]	Pathophysiology and clinical manifestations	Anesthetic implications
Chronic nonsuppurative panniculitis (see Weber-Christian disease)		
Chromosome 10 qtr deletion syndrome [Chromosomal]	Microcephaly, broad beak-like nose, micrognathia, short neck, hypertelorism CHD: VSD, TOF, PDA Pulmonary hypertension and CHF	Potentially difficult airway Cardiopulmonary dysfunction Preoperative cardiac evaluation required May require prophylactic antibiotics
CHARGE syndrome [Craniofacial]	Nasal discharge and obstruction Coloboma, heart defects, atresia choanae, mental retardation, genital hypoplasia and ear deformations with or without hearing loss	Bilateral choanal atresia may necessitate placement of oral airway Preoperative cardiac evaluation required
Cockayne-Touraine syndrome (dystrophic epidermolysis bullae) [Dermatologic]	Subepidermal bullae primarily on hands, feet, sacral areas and mucous membranes Scarring of skin leading to strictures, especially of oral aperture Recurrent respiratory infections Poor nutritional status and anemia	Potentially difficult airway Friction on skin surfaces (adhesives) disrupt skin integrity Fluid and electrolyte imbalance Impaired thermoregulation
Congenital facial disease (see Möbius syndrome)		

Syndrome	Clinical Findings	Anesthetic Implications
Congenital hypothyroidism (see Cretinism)		
Congenital ichthyosis (see Ichthyosiform erythrodermia)		
Conradi syndrome [Connective tissue]	Chondrodystrophy with contractures Saddle nose CHD Psychomotor retardation Renal dysfunction	Impaired renal drug excretion Preoperative cardiac evaluation required May require prophylactic antibiotics
Cori disease (glycogen storage disease—Type III) [Metabolic]	Glycogen deposition in liver and muscle Hepatosplenomegaly Hypoglycemia, acidosis, and hyperuricemia	Requires glucose infusion, frequent monitoring of blood glucose and acid-base status Exaggerated response to muscle relaxants Abnormal coagulation profile
Cornelia de Lange syndrome [Craniofacial]	Upper airway obstruction Cleft palate Micrognathia Macroglossia Short stature Microcephaly Hand and feet abnormalities CHD Severe developmental delay	Potentially difficult airway Strabismus associated with MH Preoperative cardiac evaluation required May require prophylactic antibiotics

Continued.

Pediatric syndromes and anesthetic implications—cont'd

Disease [category]	Pathophysiology and clinical manifestations	Anesthetic implications
Cranium bifidum (see Encephalocele)		
CREST syndrome [Connective tissue]	Calcinosis Raynaud's phenomenon Esophageal dysmotility Scleroderma, syndactyly Telangiectasias Renal dysfunction Pulmonary hypertension	Restriction of oral aperture and difficult intubation May require stress steroids Cardiopulmonary function may be impaired Extremities must be kept warm to prevent vasoconstriction Impaired renal drug excretion
Cretinism (congenital hypothyroidism) [Metabolic]	Goiter Macroglossia Hypotension with markedly decreased intravascular volume Low cardiac output Cold intolerance Myxedema Delayed gastric emptying Decreased metabolic rate Respiratory depression and impaired ventilatory response to hypoxia and hypercarbia Hypoglycemia Hyponatremia Adrenal insufficiency	Increased sensitivity to cardiovascular and respiratory depressants Prolonged recovery from opioids Exaggerated response to sedation and premedication Fluid and electrolyte imbalance Aspiration precautions Stress dose steroids may be required May need postoperative ventilatory support

Cri-du-chat syndrome [Chromosomal]	Deletion or translocation of chromosome 5 Abnormal larynx leading to a catlike cry Microcephaly; micrognathia CHD Psychomotor retardation	Difficult intubation Stridor caused by laryngomalacia may be worsened by anesthesia Propensity to hypothermia Preoperative cardiac evaluation required May require prophylactic antibiotics
Crouzon syndrome (craniosynostosis) [Craniofacial]	Wide skull Proptosis Maxillary hypoplasia: sagittal and coronal suture synostosis Nystagmus, strabismus High arched palate and cleft palate Elevated ICP	Potentially difficult airway Management of increased ICP Strabismus associated with MH
Cutis laxa [Connective tissue]	Skin hangs in loose pendulous folds due to disorder of elastin synthesis Premature wrinkling Vocal cord laxity Diaphragmatic atony GI tract diverticula Rectal prolapse In severe form: Emphysema Pulmonary artery stenosis Aortic aneurysmal dilation	Cardiopulmonary dysfunction Vascular catheters are difficult to maintain Soft tissue laxity around larynx may lead to airway obstruction

Continued.

Pediatric syndromes and anesthetic implications—cont'd

Disease [category]	Pathophysiology and clinical manifestations	Anesthetic implications
Cystinosis [Metabolic]	Fanconi syndrome Epistaxis Portal hypertension Esophageal varices Hypothyroidism Diabetes Renal dysfunction Anemia and coagulopathy	Requires preoperative evaluation of thyroid and renal function, glucose regulation and hematologic profile Impaired renal drug excretion Nasal intubation should be avoided
Dandy-Walker syndrome [Neurologic]	Hydrocephalus Associated CNS malformations: meningomyelocele Developmental delay	May have elevated ICP if no functioning shunt in place Consider latex precautions
DiGeorge syndrome [Immunologic]	Defect of third and fourth branchial arches PTH deficiency leading to hypocalcemia, tetany, and cardiac failure Thymic hypoplasia; immunodeficiency CHD Micrognathia Tracheomalacia	Potentially difficult airway Requires frequent monitoring of serum calcium Exaggerated response to nondepolarizing muscle relaxants Blood transfusions must be irradiated to prevent graft-versus-host reaction Preoperative cardiac evaluation required May require prophylactic antibiotics

Syndrome [Category]	Features	Anesthetic Implications
Down syndrome (Trisomy 21) [Chromosomal]	Microcephaly; macroglossia Hypotonia CHD: VSD, TOF, PDA Duodenal atresia Atlantoaxial instability Congenital subglottic stenosis Increased neoplastic disease Obstructive sleep apnea Recurrent pulmonary infections Polycythemia in neonates	Potentially difficult airway; select endotracheal tube one size smaller than anticipated Decreased CNS catecholamine stores may decrease MAC Exaggerated response to muscle relaxants Consider obtaining C-spine films prior to neck manipulation Preoperative cardiac evaluation required May require prophylactic antibiotics
Duchenne muscular dystrophy [Musculoskeletal]	Progressive muscle weakness Kyphoscoliosis, lumbar lordosis Restrictive lung disease Pharyngeal weakness, dysphagia, aspiration Cardiac arrhythmias, impaired contractility CPK elevation with myoglobinuria and rhabdomyolysis CHF	Postoperative ventilation may be required Associated with malignant hyperthermia Succinylcholine causes increased serum K^+ and possible cardiac arrest Exaggerated response to respiratory depressants, muscle relaxants, and inhalation agents
Dystrophic epidermolysis bullae (see Cockayne-Touraine)		

Continued.

Pediatric syndromes and anesthetic implications—cont'd

Disease [category]	Pathophysiology and clinical manifestations	Anesthetic implications
Dwarfism (osteochondrodystrophies) 1. Achondrogenesis 2. Thanatophoric dwarfism 3. Short-rib-polydactyly syndromes (type I and type II) 4. Type I osteogenesis imperfecta 5. Camptomelic dwarfism (lethal form) 6. Cerebrocostomandibular syndrome 7. Hypophosphatasia [Musculoskeletal]	Odontoid hypoplasia and/or atlantoaxial instability Micrognathia Cleft palate Tracheal stenosis and malacia Small chest cavity Kyphoscoliosis Restrictive lung disease CHD	Need preoperative C-spine and cardiac evaluation Potentially difficult airway Consider pulmonary function tests Care in OR positioning May require prophylactic antibiotics
Ebstein's anomaly [Cardiothoracic]	Patent foramen ovale Small right ventricle Coexistent tricuspid stenosis and tricuspid insufficiency Cor pulmonale Cardiac arrhythmia, usually paroxysmal atrial tachycardia	Management of CHF, cyanotic heart disease Agents that precipitate tachycardia should be avoided

Edward syndrome (Trisomy 18) [Chromosomal]	CHD Micrognathia Rocker bottom feet Apneic spells and airway obstruction Renal dysfunction	Potentially difficult airway Impaired renal drug excretion May be at risk for postoperative apnea Preoperative cardiac evaluation required May require prophylactic antibiotics
EEC syndrome [Connective tissue]	Ectrodactyly, ectodermal dysplasia, and cleft lip/palate Chronic respiratory tract infections Chronic blepharitis, conjunctivitis, keratitis Malnutrition; anemia Mental retardation Genitourinary problems Hypohidrosis	Difficulty with thermoregulation Need intraoperative eye care Potentially difficult intubation May have chronic pulmonary dysfunction Skin fragility
Ehlers-Danlos syndrome [Connective tissue]	Deficiency of procollagen lysyl hydroxylase Joint hyperextensibility Lens subluxation Retinal detachment Cystic renal involvement GI bleeding Dissecting aortic aneurysm Mitral valve prolapse and conduction defects Kyphoscoliosis Restrictive lung disease Coagulopathy	Increased risk of spontaneous pneumothorax Skin integrity easily disrupted Impaired renal drug excretion Impaired cardiac function Abnormal coagulation profile Impaired pulmonary function

Continued.

Pediatric syndromes and anesthetic implications—cont'd

Disease [category]	Pathophysiology and clinical manifestations	Anesthetic implications
Eisenmenger syndrome [Cardiothoracic]	Pulmonary hypertension and increased pulmonary vascular resistance Right to left shunt at both atrial and ventricular level Cor pulmonale Cyanosis	Abnormal ventricular function Positive-pressure ventilation may increase right-to-left shunt and worsen cyanosis Prolonged postoperative ventilation may be necessary
Encephalocele (cranium bifidum) [Neurologic]	Herniation of cerebral tissue through defect in skull Anterior encephalocele appears as mass in nasopharynx Basal encephalocele may cause feeding difficulties and respiratory obstruction Posterior encephalocele associated with hydrocephalus, epilepsy, paraplegia, and blindness	Potentially difficult airway Difficulty maintaining normothermia Brainstem compromise may precipitate changes in heart rate and blood pressure
Encephalotrigeminal angiomatosis (see Sturge-Weber syndrome)		

Epidermolysis bullosum (Herlitz's syndrome) [Dermatologic]	Spontaneous skin/mucosal blisters Narrow scarred airway and esophagus and restriction of oral aperture Potential for laryngeal involvement Feeding problems and poor nutrition Mitten-hand deformities Anemia Impaired thermoregulation	Often requires fiberoptic intubation Meticulous avoidance of trauma with: Airway manipulation Regional anesthetic IV, ETT securing Pressure point padding Eye care May need stress dose steroids
Erythema multiforme [Dermatologic]	Acute inflammatory diseases with IgM and complement deposition in tissues in response to vascular damage Erythematous plaques, blisters, and target or bull's eye lesions of distal extremities and mucous membranes Associated malignancies	Sulfonamides, salicylates, penicillins, barbiturates, and hydantoin should be avoided Loss of skin integrity

Continued.

Pediatric syndromes and anesthetic implications—cont'd

Disease [category]	Pathophysiology and clinical manifestations	Anesthetic implications
Erythema multiforme major (Stevens-Johnson syndrome) [Dermatologic]	Prodrome: fever, malaise, arthralgia, URI Extensor surface bullae Bullae of visceral pleura may cause pneumotho-races, pleural effusions, and pulmonary infections GI ulceration and hemorrhage Pericarditis Atrial fibrillation Corneal ulcerations, uveitis, and staphylococcal panophthalmitis Anemia Dehydration and poor nutritional status Renal: ATN and nephritis	Avoidance of skin trauma Bullae may compromise upper airway May need stress dose steroids Sulfonamides, salicylates, penicillins, barbiturates, and hydantoin should be avoided Preoperative cardiac evaluation required Fluid and electrolyte imbalance
Eulenburg syndrome (see Paramyotonia congenita)		
Fabry's disease (lysosomal storage disease) [Metabolic]	Galactosidase deficiency Angiokeratomas of skin Corneal opacities Hypertension Myocardial ischemia Progressive azotemia Lipid deposition in blood vessels	Impaired renal drug excretion Preoperative cardiovascular evaluation required

Familial dysautonomia (see Riley-Day syndrome)		
Familial periodic paralysis: Type I—Hypokalemic Type II—Hyperkalemic Type III—Normokalemic [Musculoskeletal]	Severe muscle weakness, may spare respiratory muscles Loss of cough reflex, dysphagia Cardiac dysrhythmias *Type I* Paralysis (lasts 36 hr) exacerbated by high-carbohydrate meals, salt loading, exercise, or cold Treatment: spironolactone, acetazolamide *Type II* Paralysis (lasts 1-2 hr) related to exercise and cold Treatment: calcium, insulin, and glucose *Type III* Weakness may last several days Recurrent respiratory infections	May have exaggerated response to non-depolarizing muscle relaxants Careful monitoring of fluids and electrolytes Avoidance of hypothermia *Type I* IV fluids should be free of sodium and dextrose *Type II* IV fluids should contain dextrose and be free of potassium *Type III* As for type I
Familial xanthomatosis (see Wolman's disease)		

Continued.

Pediatric syndromes and anesthetic implications—cont'd

Disease [category]	Pathophysiology and clinical manifestations	Anesthetic implications
Fanconi syndrome [Metabolic]	Impaired tubular reabsorption of glucose, amino acids, phosphate, bicarbonate, and K^+; slow progression to renal failure Metabolic acidosis Hypokalemia Hypophosphatemia Polyuria, hypercalciuria, glucosuria and aminoaciduria Rickets and osteomalacia	Requires careful preoperative evaluation and frequent intraoperative monitoring of fluids, electrolytes, and acid-base status. Impaired renal drug excretion
Farber's disease [Metabolic]	Deficiency of ceramidase resulting in accumulation of ceramide in the tissues Laryngopharyngeal involvement may occur Triad: subcutaneous nodules, arthritis, and psychomotor retardation Hepatomegaly Cardiomyopathy	Potentially difficult airway Postoperative risk for acute renal and hepatic failure due to ceramide accumulation Tracheal intubation is best avoided in patients presenting with laryngopharyngeal involvement
Favism (G-6-PD deficiency) [Metabolic]	Hemolytic anemia Vitreous hemorrhage Recurrent infections Hepatitis Bacterial pneumonia Mononucleosis Hemolysis occurs with oxidant drugs: salicylates, sulfur, phenacetin, vitamin K, methylene blue, INH, quinidine, antimalarials, nitrofurans	Prilocaine may cause methemoglobinemia Impaired hepatic drug metabolism Liver function and coagulation need preoperative assessment

Syndrome	Features	Anesthetic Implications
Fazio-Londe syndrome [Musculoskeletal]	Anterior horn cell degeneration of bulbar nuclei and cervical and upper thoracic cord Bulbar neuropathy impairs swallowing and gag reflexes	Succinylcholine may cause hyperkalemia May have exaggerated response to muscle relaxants Aspiration precautions needed
Fibrodysplasia ossificans (see Myositis ossificans)		
Focal dermal hypoplasia (see Goltz syndrome)		
Fragile X (Martin–Bell syndrome) [Chromosomal]	Mental retardation Hyperactivity Autistic features Midfacial hypoplasia High arched palate Cardiac abnormalities develop in late childhood (MVP, aortic root dilation)	Potentially difficult airway Consider echocardiography in older children
Freeman-Sheldon syndrome (Whistling face syndrome) [Craniofacial]	Craniocarpotarsal dysplasia Hypertelorism Blepharophimosis Small mouth; pursed lips V-shaped fibrous tissue band at the midchin	Potentially difficult airway

Continued.

Pediatric syndromes and anesthetic implications—cont'd

Disease [category]	Pathophysiology and clinical manifestations	Anesthetic implications
Freidreich's ataxia [Neurologic]	Progressive degeneration throughout CNS, including mental deterioration Scoliosis Restrictive lung disease Myocardial necrosis, muscle degeneration Arrhythmias	Preoperative cardiopulmonary evaluation is required May have exaggerated response to muscle relaxants
G-6-PD deficiency (see Favism)		
Gardner syndrome [Metabolic]	Multiple polyposis Bony tumors and fibromas Sebaceous cysts Anemia from GI bleeding	May have loss of skin integrity Care in positioning required Preoperative blood count required
Gaucher disease [Metabolic]	Defect of glucocerebrosidase Accumulation of lipids in the pulmonary tissue may lead to progressive respiratory failure and cor pulmonale Hypersplenism may lead to pancytopenia Vertebral fractures (osteoporosis) GE reflux Seizures and neurologic deterioration Copious oral secretions	Potentially difficult airway May need careful padding and positioning Preoperative cardiopulmonary evaluation is needed May have impaired hepatic drug metabolism Preoperative Hct and platelet count are required Aspiration precautions are required

Globoid cell leukodystrophy (see Krabbe's disease)		
Glycogen storage disease (see: von Gierke disease—Type I Pompe disease—Type II Cori disease—Type III Andersen's disease—Type IV McArdle disease—V Hers disease—Type VI Tauri disease—Type VII)		
Goldenhar syndrome (oculo-auriculovertebral syndrome) [Craniofacial]	CHD Eye and ear abnormalities Renal abnormalities Maxillary hypoplasia Micrognathia Cleft or high arched palate Hemivertebra or vertebral fusion; may involve upper neck and odontoid elongation Spina bifida Psychomotor retardation	Potentially difficult airway and intubation Requires preoperative assessment of cardiac status and cervical spine May require prophylactic antibiotics

Continued.

Pediatric syndromes and anesthetic implications—cont'd

Disease [category]	Pathophysiology and clinical manifestations	Anesthetic implications
Goltz–Corlin syndrome (focal dermal hypoplasia) [Craniofacial]	Hypoplasia and change in skin pigmentation Papillomas of the mucous membranes and the larynx Strabismus CHD Head asymmetry Incomplete segmentation of cervical and thoracic vertebrae Renal dysfunction	Potentially difficult airway Airway obstruction from laryngeal papillomas Association with strabismus and MH Impaired renal drug excretion Preoperative cardiac evaluation required May require prophylactic antibiotics
Gorlin–Chaudhry–Moss syndrome [Craniofacial]	Craniofacial dysostosis Hypertrichosis Dental and ocular anomalies CHD (PDA common)	Potentially difficult airway Preoperative cardiac evaluation required May require prophylactic antibiotics
Groenblad–Strandberg syndrome (Pseudoxanthoma elasticum) [Connective tissue]	Degenerative multisystem disorder of elastin tissue Premature peripheral, cerebral and coronary vascular disease Decreased visual acuity, retinal detachment GI hemorrhage Renal HTN	Loss of skin integrity Need preoperative evaluation of cardiac and renal function

Syndrome	Features	Anesthetic Implications
Guillain-Barré syndrome [Neurologic]	Acute polyneuropathy Peripheral neuritis involving cranial nerves Bulbar palsy leading to hypoventilation and hypotension Autonomic dysfunction may lead to CV instability	Succinylcholine may cause hyperkalemia Bulbar involvement may necessitate tracheostomy and mechanical ventilation CV instability Drugs potentiating catecholamine release should be avoided
Hallermann-Streiff syndrome (oculomandibulofacial syndrome) [Craniofacial]	Dwarfism TMJ displacement Brittle teeth Hypoplastic nose and deviated septum Normal size tongue in a small mouth Microphthalmia and nystagmus Psychomotor retardation Lordosis, scoliosis, spina bifida	Upper airway obstruction and potentially difficult airway A blind nasal intubation may be difficult Superior displacement of trachea Association with strabismus and MH Evaluation of pulmonary function and reserve is required
Hallervorden-Spatz disease [Neurologic]	Disorder of basal ganglia Dementia Dystonia leading to scoliosis, trismus, torticollis Restrictive lung disease	Succinylcholine should be avoided Potentially difficult airway Inhalation agents may relax torticollis
Hand-Schüller-Christian disease [Hematologic]	Histiocytic granuloma in bones and viscera including larynx, lungs, liver, and spleen Laryngeal fibrosis Hypersplenism may lead to pancytopenia Diabetes insipidus Respiratory failure Cor pulmonale	May need stress dose steroids Coagulation profile may be abnormal Preoperative assessment of pulmonary status is required

Continued.

Pediatric syndromes and anesthetic implications—cont'd

Disease [category]	Pathophysiology and clinical manifestations	Anesthetic implications
Harlequin fetus (see Ichthyosiform erythrodermia)		
Hartnup disease [Metabolic]	Defective intestinal absorption of tryptophan, leading to niacin deficiency (like pellegra) Scaly red skin Cerebellar ataxia	Potential loss of skin integrity Behavioral manifestations may have implications for induction technique
Heart-Hand syndrome (see Holt-Oram syndrome)		
Hemochromatosis	Inherited disorder of iron metabolism with iron deposition in liver, pancreas, skin, heart Hepatic fibrosis and cirrhosis Diabetes mellitus Abnormal skin pigmentation CHF and cardiac arrhythmias	Preoperative cardiac evaluation needed May have abnormal coagulation status Impaired hepatic drug metabolism

Hemolytic uremic syndrome [Hematologic]	Triad: 　Nephropathy 　Thrombocytopenia 　Hemolytic anemia 　Seizures Heart failure caused by HTN, volume overload, se- 　vere anemia, and progressive renal disease Associated metabolic derangements: hyperkalemia, 　metabolic acidosis, hypocalcemia, hyponatremia	Fluid and electrolyte imbalance May have abnomal coagulation profile Cardiac evaluation may be needed Blood count, BUN, creatinine needed 　preoperatively
Henoch-Schönlein purpura [Hematologic]	Vasculitis of small blood vessels Nonthrombocytopenic purpura Nephritis can progress to renal failure Abdominal pain GI hemorrhage	May need stress dose steroids Impaired renal drug excretion May have abnormal coagulation profile
Hepatolenticular degeneration (see Wilson's disease)		

Continued.

Pediatric syndromes and anesthetic implications—cont'd

Disease [category]	Pathophysiology and clinical manifestations	Anesthetic implications
Hereditary angioneurotic edema [Hematologic/Immunologic]	Abnormal levels of C_1 and C_4 esterase inhibitors and accumulation of vasoactive substances which increase vascular permeability Episodic edema of trunk, extremities, face, abdomen, and airway lasting (average) 24-92 hr Mortality about 30%, mostly from laryngeal edema Often induced by vibration or trauma, may have prodromal tingling or tightness	Preoperative complement assay needed Recommended prophylaxis: EACA for 2-3 days and/or FFP 1 day preoperatively Acute attack is treated with epinephrine, antihistamines, and steroids Hoarseness or dysphagia may be present Extreme care should be exercised in airway manipulation because minor trauma may elicit response
Hereditary hemorrhagic telangiectasia (see Osler-Weber-Rendu syndrome)		
Herlitz's syndrome (see Epidermolysis bullosum)		
Hers disease (Type VI glycogen storage disease) [Metabolic]	Hepatomegaly Poor muscle development Hypoglycemia	May have coagulopathy May have exaggerated response to muscle relaxants

Holoprosencephaly [CNS]	Median deformities of face/brain Dextrocardia and VSD Incomplete rotation of colon; biliary stenosis Hepatic malfunction and hypoglycemia Mental retardation and seizures	Difficult endotracheal intubation and use of mask Possible postoperative apnea Preoperative cardiac evaluation is needed Hepatic drug metabolism may be impaired
Holt-Oram syndrome (Heart-hand syndrome) [Chromosomal]	Upper limb anomalies (e.g., radial dysgenesis) CHD: septal defects, dextrocardia, TOF Sudden death secondary to pulmonary embolus or coronary occlusion reported	Preoperative cardiac evaluation is needed May require prophylactic antibiotics
Homocystinuria [Metabolic]	Deficiency of cystathionine synthetase leading to increase plasma and urinary levels of methionine and homocysteine Tall, thin habitus with kyphoscoliosis Hypercoagulability and thromboembolic events Growth retardation and seizures Hypoglycemia and hyperinsulinemia	Increased incidence of cerebral, pulmonary, renal, mesenteric, and coronary thrombosis in the perioperative period Preoperative assessment of pulmonary status and reserve needed Abnormal coagulation profile
Hunter syndrome (Type II mucopolysaccharidosis) [Metabolic]	Retinitis pigmentosa Nodular, ivory-colored skin lesions Dwarfism, stiff joints Hepatosplenomegaly Kyphoscoliosis; restrictive lung disease Valvular heart disease and cardiomyopathy Hydrocephalus and elevated ICP Severe psychomotor retardation	Potentially difficult airway because of abnormal anatomy and progressive tracheomalacia and tracheal collapse Restrictive lung disease and recurrent pulmonary infection Management of increased ICP

Continued.

Pediatric syndromes and anesthetic implications—cont'd

Disease [category]	Pathophysiology and clinical manifestations	Anesthetic implications
Hurler syndrome (Type I mucopolysaccharidosis) [Metabolic]	Accumulation of mucopolysaccharides in the oropharynx, the epiglottis, and tracheal wall Short thick neck Coarse facies Macroglossia; large tonsils and adenoids Odontoid hypoplasia and atlantoaxial subluxation Decreased joint mobility and flexion contractures Thoracic kyphosis Hepatosplenomegaly Severe CAD, valvular disease and cardiomyopathy Psychomotor retardation Hydrocephalus	Potentially difficult airway Coagulation profile may be abnormal Postoperative subglottic edema (croup) common Restrictive lung disease and recurrent pulmonary infection Cardiac and cervical spinal evaluation required
Hutchinson-Gilford syndrome (see Progeria)		
Ichthyosiform erythrodermia (Congenital ichthyosis or harlequin fetus) [Dermatologic]	Contraction and decreased thickness of skin Strangulation of smaller appendages (i.e., ears, lips, nose, and digits) Impaired thermoregulation	Maintenance of normothermia Loss of skin integrity
Immotile cilia syndrome (see Kartagener's syndrome)		

Incontinentia pigmenti (see Bloch-Sulzberger syndrome)		
Infantile gigantism (see Beckwith-Wiedemann syndrome)		
Ivemark syndrome [Cardiothoracic]	Malposition of abdominal viscera Complex cyanotic CHD Splenic agenesis may cause immunocompromise	Aseptic technique required Preoperative cardiac exam required May require prophylactic antibiotics
Jervell and Lange-Nielsen syndrome [Cardiothoracic]	Prolonged QT interval Congenital deafness Syncopal attacks due to paroxysmal ventricular fibrillation Extreme sensitivity to sympathetic stimulation Sudden cardiac death	Halothane, lidocaine, catecholamines, atropine, phenothiazines, and quinidine should be avoided Failure of medical therapy may necessitate left stellate ganglion blockade
Jeune syndrome (asphyxiating thoracic dystrophy) [Musculoskeletal]	Dwarfism Short ribs, prominent rib rosary in midaxillary line Small larynx Pulmonary hypoplasia and cysts Stiff thorax Renal disease with proteinuria, uremia HTN is problematic if child survives infancy	May require surgical intervention to enlarge thorax, with substantial blood loss High incidence of barotrauma, hypoxia, and hypercarbia Small larynx may necessitate a smaller ETT than usual
Juvenile rheumatoid arthritis (see Still's disease)		

Continued.

Pediatric syndromes and anesthetic implications—cont'd

Disease [category]	Pathophysiology and clinical manifestations	Anesthetic implications
Kartagener's syndrome (immotile cilia syndrome) [Cardiothoracic]	Dextrocardia Bronchiectasis Chronic bronchitis Sinusitis Heart block	Nitrous oxide should be avoided with bronchiectasis
Kasabach-Merritt syndrome [Hematologic/Immunologic]	Giant hemangiomas of cavernous type (usually on face and scalp) Thrombocytopenia Hyperfibrinogenemia Chronic consumptive coagulopathy Gastrointestinal bleeding Laryngeal hemangiomas may occur CHF may occur	May need stress dose steroids Surgical excision of hemangiomas can precipitate DIC Invasive monitoring and large bore IVs needed for volume resuscitation Airway difficulties depend on hemangioma location
Kawasaki disease (mucocutaneous lymph node syndrome) [Cardiothoracic]	Acute febrile erythematous disease; vasculitis Desquamative conjunctivitis Nonsuppurative lymphadenitis Myocarditis, coronary artery aneurysms, and ischemia Pyelonephritis and renal failure	Preoperative cardiovascular evaluation is needed; late ischemia and infarction may occur

King-Denborough syndrome [Musculoskeletal]	Low progressive myopathy with contractures Low set ears Malar hypoplasia Micrognathia Pectus carinatum Kyphoscoliosis Growth retardation May be subset of Noonan syndrome	Potentially difficult airway May have exaggerated response to muscle relaxants Uniformly MH susceptible Preoperative evaluation of pulmonary function needed
Klinefelter syndrome (XXY) [Chromosomal]	Tall stature Vertebral collapse due to osteoporosis Microcephaly Prognathism Strabismus, lens dislocation Aggressive behavior	Care in positioning Potentially difficult airway Management of disruptive and uncooperative patient
Klippel-Feil syndrome [Connective tissue]	Scoliosis Congenital heart disease Sprengel deformity Congenital synostosis of cervical vertebrae Renal dysfunction	Care in neck manipulation for intubation Impaired renal drug excretion Assessment of CHD Progressive airway obstruction and difficult intubation may require tracheal intubation

Continued.

Pediatric syndromes and anesthetic implications—cont'd

Disease [category]	Pathophysiology and clinical manifestations	Anesthetic implications
Klippel-Trenaunay syndrome [Neurologic]	Spinal cord hemangiomas Varicose veins Bone and soft tissue hypertrophy Cutaneous hemangiomas Seizures Scoliosis Sensory motor paralysis May be associated with chronic Sturge-Weber syndrome	Possible spinal hemangiomas Scoliosis associated pulmonary and heart disease Risk of coagulopathy and hemorrhage
Köhlmeier-Degos disease (malignant atrophic papulosis) [Dermatologic]	Occlusive vasculitis of unknown etiology Multiple infarcts of skin, GI tract, and CNS Porcelain white papules that form atrophic scars Pericarditis, pericardial and pleural effusions Restrictive pulmonary disease Cerebral edema, increased ICP, and herniation	Preoperative cardiorespiratory evaluation required Management of increased ICP
Krabbe's disease (globoid cell leukodystrophy) [Neurologic]	Blindness Deafness Psychomotor retardation	Supportive care

Syndrome [Category]	Features	Anesthetic Implications
Kugelberg-Welander disease [Musculoskeletal]	Anterior horn cell degeneration Juvenile proximal hereditary muscular atrophy Hypotonia Cardiac arrhythmias and CHF Kyphoscoliosis	Succinylcholine may induce hyper-kalemia May have exaggerated response to muscle relaxants and respiratory depressants Aspiration precautions may be needed
Larsen's syndrome [Connective tissue]	Congenital joint dislocations including the cervical spine Cervical kyphoscoliosis Cartilage weakness in ribs, epiglottis, arytenoids Cleft palate, subglottic stenosis, tracheomalacia CHD Hydroencephalopathy	Potentially difficult airway management C-spine evaluation should be performed Preoperative cardiac evaluation required May require prophylactic antibiotics
Lawrence-Moon-Biedl syndrome [Metabolic/Obesity]	Obesity Retinitis pigmentosa Polydactyly CHD Psychomotor retardation Diabetes insipidus	Aspiration precautions Preoperative cardiac evaluation required May require prophylactic antibiotics
Leber's hereditary optic neuropathy [Neurologic]	Bilateral loss of central vision Cardiac dysrhythmias May have encephalopathy and movement disorders	Inability to metabolize sodium nitroprusside due to rhodanase deficiency leads to severe cyanide toxicity

Continued.

Pediatric syndromes and anesthetic implications—cont'd

Disease [category]	Pathophysiology and clinical manifestations	Anesthetic implications
Leigh's syndrome (subacute necrotizing encephalomyelopathy, SNE) [Neurologic]	Encephalopathy, convulsions, ataxia, peripheral neuropathy External ophthalmoplegia Lactic acidosis Psychomotor retardation Swallowing difficulties	May have impaired ventilatory response Acid-base status needs frequent monitoring
Leopard syndrome [Craniofacial]	Congenital pulmonary stenosis Hypertelorism Cardiac conduction defects Ptosis Kyphosis, pectus carinatum	Potentially difficult airway Preoperative ECG and cardiopulmonary evaluation required
Lesch-Nyhan syndrome [Metabolic]	Absence of hypoxanthine-guanine phosphoribosyl transferase needed for purine metabolism Hyperuricemia, causing: Urolithiasis Urinary obstruction Acute renal failure Self-mutilation Hyperreflexia, clonus Psychomotor retardation and aggressive behavior	Exaggerated response to muscle relaxants Careful hydration needed to maintain alkaline urine Impaired renal drug excretion

Letterer-Siwe disease (acute disseminated histiocytosis) [Hematologic]	Lymphocytic infiltration of liver, spleen, lymph nodes, lung, and bone Mandibular hypoplasia Diabetes insipidus if sella turcica involved Pulmonary fibrosis, respiratory failure, cor pulmonale May have leukocytosis or pancytopenia High serum uric acid leading to renal stones	Potentially difficult airway; may have laryngeal fibrosis Loss of skin integrity May need stress steroids May have had chemotherapeutic agents Preoperative cardiorespiratory evaluation required
Louis Bar syndrome (see Ataxia telangiectasia)		
Lowe syndrome (oculocerebrorenal syndrome) [Musculoskeletal]	Hypotonia Cataracts, glaucoma Osteoporosis and rickets Seizures Psychomotor retardation Renal tubular dysfunction; hyperchloremic metabolic acidosis	Strabismus associated with MH susceptibility Exaggerated response to muscle relaxants Electrolyte and acid-base imbalance
Lyell disease (toxic epidermal necrolysis) [Dermatologic]	Acute bullous eruption of skin and mucous membranes, oropharynx, tongue, tracheobronchial tree Pneumonia GI hemorrhage Septicemia, shock, hypovolemia, DIC	Loss of skin integrity May need stress dose steroids Impaired thermoregulation
Lysosomal storage disease (see Fabry's disease)		

Continued.

Pediatric syndromes and anesthetic implications—cont'd

Disease [category]	Pathophysiology and clinical manifestations	Anesthetic implications
Malignant atrophic papulosis (see Köhlmeier-Degos disease)		
Mandibulofacial dysostosis (see Treacher Collins syndrome)		
Maple syrup urine disease [Metabolic]	Decreased activity of oxoacid dehydrogenase causes increased leucine, isoleucine, valine, and oxoacids In early infancy: 　Poor feeding 　Vomiting 　High-pitched cry 　Seizures, stupor, coma Severe acidosis, hyperammonemia, and hypoglycemia can occur	Frequent monitoring of acid-base status, blood glucose, fluids, and electrolytes is needed
Marble bone disease (see Osteopetrosis)		

Marfan's syndrome
[Connective tissue]
	Atlantoaxial instability
	Dilation of aortic root (aortic aneurysm)
	Aortic valvular insufficiency and mitral valve prolapse
	Cystic medial necrosis leading to coronary disease,
	    valvular disease
	Kyphoscoliosis
	Bullous emphysema
	Lens subluxation
		C-spine evaluation before laryngoscopy
		    is required
		Preoperative cardiovascular evaluation
		    required
		Care in positioning needed
		Increased potential for pneumothorax

Maroteaux-Lamy syndrome (Type VI mucopolysaccharidosis) [Metabolic]	Short stature Odontoid hypoplasia Coarse facies Joint stiffness Hydrocephalus; elevated ICP CHD Kyphosis	Requires care in positioning Potentially difficult airway C-spine evaluation before laryngoscopy is required Preoperative cardiac evaluation required May require prophylactic antibiotics
McArdle disease (Type V glycogen storage disease) [Metabolic]	Deficiency of muscle phosphorylase Muscle cramps Muscle wasting and myoglobinuria	Succinylcholine may cause hyperkalemia IV regional technique (Bier block) may increase chance of muscle ischemia Symptoms may be confused with MH

McCune-Albright syndrome
 	
[Metabolic]
	Classic triad:
	    Café-au-lait spots
	    Fibrous dysplasia
	    Endocrine abnormalities: hyperthyroidism, GH
	        excess, hyperparathyroidism
	Hypophosphatemia and hypercortisolism
		Severity of endocrine derangement
		    should be evaluated

Continued.

Pediatric syndromes and anesthetic implications—cont'd

Disease [category]	Pathophysiology and clinical manifestations	Anesthetic implications
Meckel syndrome [Craniofacial]	Occipital encephalocele Microcephaly; micrognathia Cleft epiglottis, lip, and palate Polycystic kidney CHD Polydactyly Cataracts	Potentially difficult intubation Impaired renal drug excretion Preoperative cardiac evaluation needed May require prophylactic antibiotics

Menkes syndrome
 	
[Metabolic]
	Disorder of copper metabolism
	Growth deficiency
	CNS degeneration
	   Feeding difficulty
	   Seizure disorder
	   Hypothermia
	   Hypotonia
	Usually fatal by age 3
		Potential for difficult airway
		Possible susceptibility to MH

Metaphyseal dysplasia (see Pyle's disease)		
Miller's syndrome [Craniofacial]	Facial features similar to Treacher Collins syndrome Micrognathia, molar hypoplasia, low-set ears, cleft lip/palate Severe limb deformities CHD: VSD, ASD, PDA	Difficult tracheal intubation Consider early tracheostomy Preoperative cardiac evaluation required May require prophylactic antibiotics

Syndrome	Features	Anesthetic Implications
Möbius syndrome [Craniofacial]	Nonprogressive determinations of motor nuclei of CN VI and VII causing facial palsy Limb deformities Micrognathia and upper airway obstruction Recurrent aspiration Muscle weakness of tongue, neck, chest	Potentially difficult airway Exaggerated response to muscle relaxants may occur in distribution of involved nerves Aspiration precautions
Morquio syndrome (Mucopolysaccharidosis—Type IV) [Metabolic]	Defective degradation of keratin sulfate Coarse facies Prominent maxilla Severe skeletal abnormalities Short neck Kyphoscoliosis Odontoid hypoplasia with subluxation Recurrent pulmonary infections	Potentially difficult intubation Preoperative C-spine and pulmonary evaluation is required
Moschkowitz disease (thrombotic thrombocytopenic purpura) [Hematologic]	Hemolytic anemia Thrombocytopenia Neurologic damage Renal disease	May need stress dose steroids Coagulation profile needed Impaired renal drug excretion
Mucocutaneous lymph node syndrome (see Kawasaki disease)		

Continued.

Pediatric syndromes and anesthetic implications—cont'd

Disease [category]	Pathophysiology and clinical manifestations	Anesthetic implications
Mucopolysaccharidoses (see: Hurler syndrome—Type I Hunter syndrome—Type II Sanfilippo syndrome—Type III Morquio syndrome—Type IV Scheie disease—Type V Maroteaux-Lamy syndrome—Type VI)		
Multiple endocrine neoplasia Type I—see Wermer syndrome Type II—see Sipple syndrome		
Myasthenia gravis [Musculoskeletal]	Autoimmune disorder of the neuromuscular junction caused by a decreased number of acetylcholine receptors Weakness and easy fatigability of voluntary muscles Ocular muscles commonly involved (ptosis, diplopia) Dysarthria and dysphagia	Increased sensitivity to nondepolarizing muscle relaxants (use 1/20 of normal dose) May be resistant to effects of succinylcholine for muscle relaxation Hypothermia and hypokalemia may worsen respiratory function Regional techniques may decrease need for postoperative ventilation

Myelomeningocele (spina bifida) [Neurologic]	Failure of fusion of vertebral arches Usually varying degrees of paralysis below level of lesion Thoracic lesions can cause progressive spinal deformity, resulting in restrictive lung disease May have hydrocephalus	Care in positioning required Large blood and fluid losses should be anticipated during repair Lateral position should be used for intubation to avoid trauma to sac May be difficult to maintain normothermia Requires latex allergy precautions
Myositis ossificans (fibrodysplasia ossificans) [Musculoskeletal]	Bony infiltration of tendons, fascia aponeuroses, and muscle Decreased thoracic compliance Recurrent aspiration	Difficulty opening mouth and inability to manipulate neck may hinder intubation Decreased pulmonary reserve
Myotonia congenita (Thomsen's disease) [Musculoskeletal]	Decreased ability to relax muscles after contraction Muscle hypertrophy Absence of cardiac involvement	See Myotonic dystrophy
Myotonic dystrophy [Musculoskeletal]	Myotonia made worse by exercise and cold Weakness primarily of limb muscles, increased CPK Ptosis; cataracts Cardiac conduction defects and arrhythmias Impaired ventilation Dysphagia, aspiration Mental retardation	Succinylcholine and neostigmine can precipitate myotonic crisis Exaggerated response to nondepolarizing muscle relaxants Extreme sensitivity to respiratory depressants Often require prolonged postoperative ventilation

Continued.

Pediatric syndromes and anesthetic implications—cont'd

Disease [category]	Pathophysiology and clinical manifestations	Anesthetic implications

Neonatal ectopia cordis
 	
[Cardiothoracic]
	Craniofacial deformities:
	  Microcephaly
	  Hydrocephalus
	  Omphalocele
	Intracardiac anomalies
	Usually fatal in infancy
		Controlled hyperventilation for respiratory acidosis
		Extensive intraoperative monitoring is required

Neurofibromatosis (von Recklinghausen syndrome) [Neurologic]	CNS neurofibromas Cafe-au-lait spots Increased incidence of pheochromocytoma Kyphoscoliosis Honeycomb cystic lung changes Renal artery dysplasia and HTN Tumors may involve larynx and right ventricle outflow tract	Prolonged paralysis with depolarizing muscle relaxants Difficult airway management if tumor involvement Preoperative screening for pheochromocytoma and pulmonary function needed
Niemann-Pick disease [Metabolic]	Deficiency of sphingomyelinase leading to tissue (cerebral) deposition of sphingomyelin Hepatosplenomegaly Epilepsy Psychomotor retardation Thrombocytopenia and anemia	May have abnormal coagulation profile Management of seizure disorder
Noack syndrome [Metabolic/Obesity]	Craniosynostosis Obesity Digital anomalies	Potential elevation of ICP Aspiration precautions needed Preoperative pulmonary evaluation needed Difficult vascular access

Noonan syndrome (male Turner) [Chromosomal]	"Shield-shaped" chest, kyphoscoliosis, short stature Webbed neck Micrognathia, hypertelorism, ptosis CHD: ASD, PS Hydronephrosis or hypoplastic kidneys Mild mental retardation	Potentially difficult airway Preoperative cardiorespiratory evaluation needed May require prophylactic antibiotics Impaired renal drug excretion C-spine x-ray is advisable to exclude atlantoaxial instability
Oculoauriculovertebral syndrome (see Goldenhar syndrome)		
Oculocerebrorenal syndrome (see Lowe syndrome)		
Oculomandibulofacial syndrome (see Hallermann-Streiff syndrome)		
Oro-facial-digital syndrome [Craniofacial]	Cleft lip and palate Lobed tongue Hypoplasia of mandible and maxilla Hydrocephalus, elevated ICP Polycystic kidney Digital abnormalities	Potentially difficult airway Management of elevated ICP Renal dysfunction

Continued.

Pediatric syndromes and anesthetic implications—cont'd

Disease [category]	Pathophysiology and clinical manifestations	Anesthetic implications
Osler-Weber-Rendu syndrome (hereditary hemorrhagic telangiectasia) [Hematologic]	Ectatic vascular lesions in skin, mucosa, viscera Pulmonary AV fistulas Normal clotting factors, but bleeding may be difficult to control and cause severe anemia Recurrent chest infections, dyspnea, and cyanosis	Traumatic intubation may cause severe bleeding from oral mucosal lesions Nasal intubation is contraindicated Large AVM's can cause significant shunts (Qs/Qt) Large-bore intravenous catheters may be needed for volume replacement
Osteochondrodystrophies (see Dwarfism)		
Osteogenesis Imperfecta *Type I:* O.I. congenita (newborn, most severe) *Type II:* O.I. tarda gravis (birth-1 year) *Type III* O.I. tarda levis (1 year onward) [Musculoskeletal]	Defect in synthesis of collagen and associated dysfunction of platelet aggregation Classic triad: Blue sclera Multiple fractures Deafness Bleeding diathesis Kyphoscoliosis Cardiac anomalies Increased metabolic rate and hyperpyrexia Severe congenita form: Small mandible Mid-face hypoplasia Short limbs and trunk	Requires careful positioning and padding Difficult intubation and airway management may occur with the severe forms Hyperpyrexia under anesthesia can be confused with MH Tourniquets and blood pressure cuffs may cause fractures Restrictive lung disease Atropine should be used with caution as it may exacerbate the pyrexia Severe metabolic acidosis may occur under anesthesia

Osteopetrosis (Albers-Schönberg disease, or marble bone disease) [Musculoskeletal]	Generalized skeletal density on x-ray with disturbed mineralization at the growth plates; high incidence of pathologic fractures Optic atrophy and abnormal eye movements Hepatosplenomegaly Anemia, neutropenia, thrombocytopenia Hypocalcemia with propensity for cardiac arrhythmias and seizures	Requires care in positioning and padding May have exaggerated response to non-depolarizing muscle relaxants Need coagulation profile
Paramyotonia congenita (Eulenberg syndrome) [Musculoskeletal]	Myotonia on exposure to cold and stress Paroxysmal weakness Serum K^+ fluctuations	Succinylcholine may induce hyperkalemia Nondepolarizers do *not* relax myotonia Halothane can cause shivering and induce myotonia Extreme sensitivity to respiratory depressants
Patau syndrome (Trisomy 13) [Chromosomal]	Microcephaly Micrognathia Dextrocardia and CHD Cleft lip and/or palate Psychomotor retardation Fatal by age 3	Potentially difficult airway Preoperative cardiac evaluation needed May require prophylactic antibiotics
Pfeiffer syndrome (acro-cephalopolysyndactyly) [Craniofacial]	Craniosynostosis Hypoplastic maxilla and nasal bridge Hypertelorism Proptosis Cleft palate Congenital deafness	Management of difficult airway Association of strabismus with MH

Continued.

Pediatric syndromes and anesthetic implications—cont'd

Disease [category]	Pathophysiology and clinical manifestations	Anesthetic implications
Phenylketonuria (PKU) [Metabolic]	Deficiency of phenylalanine hydroxylase Progressive mental retardation, hyperactivity Seizures	Loss of skin integrity Tendency to hypoglycemia Sensitive to respiratory depressants
Pierre Robin sequence [Craniofacial]	Micrognathia Glossoptosis Cleft palate CHD Chronic upper airway obstruction may cause hypoventilation, pulmonary HTN, and cor pulmonale	Difficult intubation Preoperative cardiac evaluation required May require prophylactic antibiotics In supine position the tongue may cause total airway occlusion, which may require nasal airway, tongue suture, or tracheostomy; LMA may be useful (see p. 47)
Poikiloderma atrophicans vasculare (see Rothmund-Thomson syndrome)		
Pompe disease (Type II glycogen storage disease) [Metabolic]	Absence of acid maltase Hypotonia Hepatomegaly Cardiomegaly and CHF Macroglossia Glossoptosis Airway obstruction Recurrent pneumonia	Potentially difficult airway Cardiac and pulmonary depressants should be avoided May have exaggerated response to muscle relaxants Coagulation profile may be abnormal

Porphyria [Metabolic]	Inherited disorder of increased σ-aminolevulinic acid synthetase and decreased uroporphyrinogen synthetase activity resulting in increased porphobilinogen Demyelination of peripheral nerves and axonal degeneration Flaccid paralysis and skeletal muscle weakness Autonomic nervous system imbalance leading to HTN and tachycardia Diabetes mellitus Severe abdominal pain	Drugs that induce liver enzymes precipitating an attack include: Barbiturates Steroids Etomidate Enflurane Ketamine Safe anesthetics include: opiates, local anesthetics, N_2O, isoflurane, halothane, atropine Exaggerated response to muscle relaxants
Prader-Willi syndrome [Metabolic]	Neonate: Hypotonia Poor feeding Dolichocephaly, small mouth, narrow face Older child: Polyphagia, obesity Hypogonadism Hyperactivity Mental retardation Diabetes, hypoglycemia Aberrations in chromosome 15	Propensity to cardiopulmonary failure requiring postoperative ventilation May have prolonged response to muscle relaxants Aspiration precautions needed
Primary distal renal tubular acidosis (see Albright-Butler syndrome)		

Continued.

Pediatric syndromes and anesthetic implications—cont'd

Disease [category]	Pathophysiology and clinical manifestations	Anesthetic implications
Progeria (Hutchinson-Gilford syndrome) [Cardiothoracic]	Premature aging (start 6 mo-3 yr) Cardiac disease: HTN, ischemia, cardiomegaly Alopecia Micrognathia Joint stiffness Small stature	Careful padding and positioning Potentially difficult airway May need monitoring and treatment of cardiac ischemia
Progressive infantile spinal muscle atrophy (see Werdnig-Hoffman disease)		
Prune belly syndrome (urethral obstruction malformation complex) [Metabolic]	Deficiency of abdominal wall musculature Renal dysplasia Pulmonary hypoplasia Colonic malrotation Ineffective cough from lack of abdominal wall musculature, recurrent respiratory infections	Preoperative pulmonary evaluation required Impaired renal drug excretion
Pyle's disease (metaphyseal dysplasia) [Craniofacial]	Enlarged mandible Cranial nerve palsies Skeletal anomalies	Potentially difficult airway

Refsum syndrome [Metabolic]	Deficiency of phytanic acid alpha-hydroxylase Polyneuropathy, ataxia Cardiac arrhythmias and heart block Deafness Ichthyosis Anosmia	Loss of skin integrity Requires care in positioning Preoperative cardiac evaluation required
Rieger syndrome [Musculoskeletal]	Subset of myotonic dystrophy Hypoplastic maxilla Imperforate anus Hypertelorism Psychomotor retardation	Succinylcholine may cause hyperkalemia Difficult airway management Sensitivity to respiratory depressants and nondepolarizing muscle relaxants
Riley-Day syndrome (familial dysautonomia) [Neurologic]	Focal demyelination of posterior columns of spinal cord and degeneration of dorsal root ganglia Deficiency of dopamine β-hydroxylase leads to hypo- and hypertensive attacks Hypotonia Deficient tear production Absent corneal reflex and DTR's Insensitivity to pain Recurrent aspiration and pneumonia Respiratory insensitivity to CO_2	Lack of compensatory cardiovascular re- flexes, especially in presence of po- tent cardiovascular depressants Difficult to assess anesthetic depth be- cause of pain insensitivity and auto- nomic lability Phenothiazines and β-blockers recom- mended for adrenergic blockade Exaggerated response to muscle relaxants Impaired thermoregulation

Continued.

Pediatric syndromes and anesthetic implications—cont'd

Disease [category]	Pathophysiology and clinical manifestations	Anesthetic implications
Ritter disease Staphylococcal scalded skin syndrome [Dermatologic]	Staphylococcal sepsis secondary to exotoxin Epidermolysis and intraepidermal desquamation	Fluid and electrolyte imbalance Strict aseptic technique required Impaired thermoregulation
Romano-Ward syndrome [Cardiothoracic]	Prolongation of the QT interval Ventricular tachyarrhythmia Syncopal attacks secondary to paroxysmal VF following emotional or physical stress	Halothane, lidocaine, procaine, quinidine, and phenothiazines may adversely affect cardiac conduction Sympathetic stimulation may stimulate ventricular tachydysrhythmia
Rothmund-Thomson syndrome (poikiloderma atrophicans vasculare) [Dermatologic]	Atrophic telangiectatic dermatosis Cataracts Defective dentition Hypogenitalism Congenital bone defects including pathologic fractures	Poor dentition requires caution with dentition laryngoscopy Loss of skin integrity Care in positioning and padding required
Rubinstein-Taybi syndrome [Cardiothoracic]	CHD: ASD, PS Microcephaly Dysphagia, aspiration Psychomotor retardation Recurrent pulmonary infections	Preoperative cardiac evaluation needed May require prophylactic antibiotics Aspiration precautions

Russell-Silver syndrome
 	
[Musculoskeletal]
	Dwarfism
	Dysmorphic facial features, midline facial hypoplasia
	Limb asymmetry
	Endocrine abnormalities
	    hypoglycemia
	    hypogonadism
		Hypothermia
		Potentially difficult intubation
		Underdosing of anesthetics may occur
		    because surface area–to–weight ratio
		    is increased

Saethre-Chotzen syndrome (acrocephalopolysyndactyly) [Craniofacial]	Craniosynostosis Strabismus Prominent mandible High arched palate Renal dysfunction	Potentially difficult airway Association of strabismus with MH Impaired renal drug function
Sanfilippo syndrome (Type III mucopolysaccharidosis) [Metabolic]	Coarse facial features Joint stiffness Severe psychomotor retardation Usually fatal by second decade	Induction technique should be appro- priate for uncooperative child

Scheie disease (Type V
mucopolysaccharidosis)
 	
[Metabolic]
	Deposition of mucopolysaccharides in connective
	    tissue
	Corneal clouding
	Joint stiffness, especially in hands and feet
	Cardiac valvular disease
		Requires care in positioning
		Preoperative cardiac evaluation is
		    required

Schwartz-Jampel syndrome [Musculoskeletal]	Dwarfism Skeletal abnormalities Muscle stiffness and abnormal contractions Progressive myotonic dystrophy	Elevated temperature with anesthesia; MH susceptibility Requires careful positioning

Continued.

Pediatric syndromes and anesthetic implications—cont'd

Disease [category]	Pathophysiology and clinical manifestations	Anesthetic implications
Scleroderma [Connective tissue]	Autoimmune process causing deposition of fibrous tissue in skin and internal organs Inflammatory polyarthritis Diffuse pulmonary fibrosis and cor pulmonale Cardiac conduction defects Esophageal dysmotility increased GE reflux, and strictures Telangiectasias may cause anemia Renal dysfunction	Restriction of oral aperture causes difficult intubation May need stress steroids Aspiration precautions needed Preoperative cardiopulmonary evaluation is required
Senior-Loken syndrome [Metabolic]	End-stage renal disease Leber's amaurosis	Anesthetic considerations of renal failure (see p. 320) Unable to metabolize sodium nitroprusside
Seip-Lawrence syndrome [Dermatologic]	Generalized lipodystrophy Generalized loss of subcutaneous fat Skin pigmentation Hepatomegaly; cirrhosis Impaired thermoregulation Development of IDDM Glomerulonephritis	Requires care in positioning and padding Renal and hepatic drug excretion may be impaired May have coagulopathy

Syndrome	Features	Anesthetic Implications
Shone syndrome [Cardiothoracic]	Mitral stenosis (parachute mitral valve) Associated aortic stenosis and mitral regurgitation Coarctation of aorta Increased susceptibility to pulmonary infections	Need preoperative cardiopulmonary evaluation
Shy-Drager syndrome [Neurologic]	Diffuse CNS degeneration and autonomic dysfunction Defective baroreceptor response causes blood pressure and heart rate lability Orthostatic hypotension Decreased sweating	Neosynephrine used to treat hypotension Anticholinergics that decrease sweating should be avoided
Sipple syndrome (Multiple endocrine neoplasia—Type II) [Metabolic]	Pheochromocytoma Medullary carcinoma of thyroid Parathyroid adenoma CNS tumors Cushing disease	See anesthetic management of pheochromocytoma (p. 332) Preoperative thyroid functions tests needed Frequent monitoring of electrolytes
Smith-Lemli-Opitz syndrome [Craniofacial]	Microcephaly; micrognathia Strabismus Hypotonia Pyloric stenosis Syndactyly Increased susceptibility to recurrent infections Psychomotor retardation	Potentially difficult airway Association of strabismus with MH May have exaggerated response to muscle relaxants

Continued.

Pediatric syndromes and anesthetic implications—cont'd

Disease [category]	Pathophysiology and clinical manifestations	Anesthetic implications
Sotos syndrome (cerebral gigantism) [Skeletal]	Accelerated growth Scoliosis Acromegalic features (large mandible and maxilla) Mental retardation Normal ICP but dilated ventricles	Potentially difficult airway
Spina bifida (see Myelomeningocele)		
Staphylococcal scalded skin syndrome (see Ritter disease)		
Stevens-Johnson syndrome (see Erythema multiforme major)		
Stickler syndrome [Musculoskeletal]	Joint laxity and arthritis Cleft palate Micrognathia Kyphoscoliosis Cataracts, retinal detachment, glaucoma	Potentially difficult airway

Syndrome	Features	Anesthetic Implications
Still's disease [Connective tissue]	Cervical spine arthritis; atlantoaxial subluxation TMJ involvement and decreased oral aperture Mandibular hypoplasia Cricoarytenoid arthritis Myocarditis and conduction abnormalities Anemia Renal dysfunction	Potentially difficult airway; may require fiberoptic intubation (easier via nasal route) May need stress dose steroids Chronic NSAID therapy may cause coagulopathy Cricoarytenoid arthritis may lead to airway obstruction
Sturge-Weber syndrome (encephalotrigeminal angiomatosis) [Neurologic]	Vascular malformations and hemangiomas (along CN V) Intracranial calcifications cause seizure disorder and hemiparesis Congenital glaucoma Developmental delay	Significant intraoperative blood loss should be anticipated with hemangioma resection Preoperative evaluation of seizure disorder
Sydenham's chorea [Neurologic]	Antistreptococcal antibodies to neurons of the subthalamic and caudate nuclei Involuntary choreoathetoid movements Persistent dopaminergic sensitivity	Central stimulants and neuroleptics should be avoided
Syringomyelia [Neurologic]	Associated with Arnold-Chiari malformation Skeletal muscle wasting Scoliosis Bulbar involvement, dysphagia, aspiration Defect in intermedullary blood supply to cord Impaired thermoregulation	See Arnold-Chiari malformation Exaggerated response to muscle relaxants Succinylcholine-induced hyperkalemia

Continued.

Pediatric syndromes and anesthetic implications—cont'd

Disease [category]	Pathophysiology and clinical manifestations	Anesthetic implications
Systemic lupus erythematosus [Immunologic]	Immune complex vasculitis with inflammatory involvement of connective tissue Nephritis Hypertension Arthritis Dermatitis (malar butterfly rash) CNS involvement, seizures, chorea Pericarditis; pleuritis Hepatosplenomegaly Anemia	Impaired renal drug excretion and hepatic drug metabolism ASA, NSAID may impair coagulation May need stress dose steroids
Tangier disease (lipoproteinemia) [Metabolic]	Orange tonsils and rectal mucosa Splenomegaly Peripheral neuropathy Premature coronary artery disease Anemia, thrombocytopenia	May have exaggerated response to muscle relaxants Preoperative cardiac evaluation required May require prophylactic antibiotics May have coagulopathy
TAR syndrome (Thrombocytopenia and absent radius) [Hematologic]	Profound thrombocytopenia (<15,000) Bilateral radial aplasia High incidence of intracranial hemorrhage CHD	Preoperative cardiac evaluation needed May require prophylactic antibiotics Elective surgery should be avoided in first year of life Platelet transfusions may be required

Syndrome	Features	Anesthetic Implications
Tauri disease (glycogen storage disease—type VII) [Metabolic]	Muscle cramps Myoglobinuria Altered liver function	May be confused with MH May have abnormal coagulation profile
Tay-Sachs disease [Metabolic]	Motor weakness causing dysphagia Ganglioside storage disease Cherry red spot on macula Deafness Blindness Seizures Recurrent respiratory infections Usually fatal in first few years of life	Aspiration precautions needed Preoperative evaluation of seizure disorder May have decreased pulmonary reserve
Thomsen's disease (see Myotonia congenita)		
Thrombocytopenia and absent radius (see TAR syndrome)		
Thrombotic thrombocytopenic purpura (see Moschkowitz disease)		
Toxic epidermal necrolysis (see Lyell disease)		
Treacher Collins syndrome (mandibulofacial dysostosis) [Craniofacial]	Facial and pharyngeal hypoplasia; aplastic zygomatic arches Micrognathia Microstomia Choanal atresia CHD	Marked narrowing of airway above larynx Extremely difficult intubation, LMA may be useful Antibiotic prophylaxis and preoperative cardiac evaluation if CHD exists

Continued.

Pediatric syndromes and anesthetic implications—cont'd

Disease [category]	Pathophysiology and clinical manifestations	Anesthetic implications
Trisomy 13 (see Patau syndrome)		
Trisomy 18 (see Edward syndrome)		
Trisomy 21 (see Down syndrome)		

Tuberous sclerosis
 	
[Neurologic]
	Triad:
	    Adenoma sebaceum
	    Seizures
	    mental retardation
	Hamartomas in lungs, kidney, heart, brain, and elsewhere
	Cardiac arrhythmias
	Polycystic renal disease
		Avoid agents which may lower the seizure threshold; for example, enflurane, ketamine and etomidate
		Patients with ECG abnormalities should have echocardiographic evaluation

Turner's syndrome (XO) [Chromosomal]	Short stature Micrognathia Web neck Dissecting aortic aneurysm Aortic coarctation Pulmonary stenosis Renal dysfunction	Potentially difficult airway Preoperative cardiac evaluation required Impaired renal drug excretion

Urbach-Wiethe disease [Immunologic]	Histiocytosis Cutaneous and mucosal hyalinosis Hyaline deposits in larynx and pharynx cause hoarseness and aphonia	Potentially difficult airway
Urethral obstruction malformation complex (see Prune belly syndrome)		
VATER syndrome [Cardiothoracic]	Vertebral segmentation Imperforate anus Tracheo-esophageal fistula Absent radius CHD (VSD) Renal dysfunction Recurrent pulmonary infections	See management of TEF on p. 374 Preoperative cardiac evaluation is required May require prophylactic antibiotics Impaired renal drug excretion
Velocardiofacial syndrome [Craniofacial]	Characteristic facies: malar hypoplasia, long face, long prominent nose, square nasal bridge CHD: VSD, TOF, pulmonary atresia Episodic bronchospasm	Preoperative cardiac evaluation is required May require prophylactic antibiotics

Continued.

Pediatric syndromes and anesthetic implications—cont'd

Disease [category]	Pathophysiology and clinical manifestations	Anesthetic implications
von Gierke's disease (Glycogen storage disease—Type I) [Metabolic]	Deficiency of G-6-phosphatase Glycogen accumulation leading to massive hepatomegaly Fanconi-like syndrome: Acidosis Aminoaciduria Glycosuria Phosphaturia Hyperuricemia Poor muscle development Hyperlipidemia Severe hypoglycemia Short stature Increased bleeding time and platelet dysfunction	Preoperative coagulation profile needed Impaired hepatic drug metabolism and renal drug excretion May have exaggerated response to muscle relaxants Increased intraabdominal pressure from hepatomegaly
Von Hippel—Lindau syndrome [Neurologic]	Retinal or CNS hemangioblastomas (posterior fossa or spinal cord) Renal, pancreatic, and hepatic cysts Neurologic changes resulting from compression or hemorrhage	Associated with pheochromocytoma Possible impaired hepatic drug metabolism and renal drug excretion
Von Recklinghausen syndrome (see Neurofibromatosis)		

Von Willebrand's disease [Hematologic]	Decreased factor VIII activity causing defective platelet adhesiveness	Salicylates should be avoided May need cryoprecipitate or DDAVP preoperatively (see p. 293)
Weber-Christian disease (chronic nonsuppurative panniculitis) [Cardiothoracic]	Necrosis of fat, including pericardial (restrictive pericarditis) and meningeal Retroperitoneal involvement may cause acute or chronic adrenal insufficiency Seizures	Heat, cold, and pressure may increase fat necrosis May need stress steroids
Wegener's granulomatosis [Immunologic]	Necrotizing granulomatous arteritis Recurrent pulmonary infections Upper respiratory bleeding and hemoptysis Glomerulonephritis	May need stress dose steroids Potentially difficult airway May have impaired renal drug excretion
Werdnig-Hoffman disease (progressive infantile spinal muscle atrophy) [Musculoskeletal]	Degenerative disease of anterior horn cells and cranial nerve motor nuclei Generalized muscle weakness Bulbar involvement leads to recurrent aspiration and pneumonia Kyphoscoliosis	Succinylcholine may cause hyperkalemia Increased sensitivity to nondepolarizing muscle relaxants Restrictive lung disease
Werner syndrome [Cardiothoracic]	Premature aging Coronary artery disease Scleroderma-like changes Alopecia Hypogonadism Psychomotor retardation Diabetes mellitus	Cardiovascular concerns of the elderly Management of diabetes mellitus (see p. 324) Careful positioning and padding required

Continued.

Pediatric syndromes and anesthetic implications—cont'd

Disease [category]	Pathophysiology and clinical manifestations	Anesthetic implications
Whistling face syndrome (see Freeman-Sheldon syndrome)		
Williams syndrome [Cardiothoracic]	Elfin facies Hypercalcemia in infancy Supravalvular aortic stenosis Joint contractures Psychomotor retardation	Careful positioning and padding required Left ventricular failure and fixed cardiac output
Wilson-Mikity syndrome [Cardiothoracic]	Prematurity; <1,500 g birth weight Pulmonary fibrosis and cystic areas; severe chronic lung disease Recurrent pulmonary infections and aspiration Cor pulmonale	Decreased pulmonary reserve May need stress dose steroids Cardiac depressants should be avoided Aspiration precautions needed
Wilson's disease (hepatolenticular degeneration) [Metabolic]	Decreased plasma ceruloplasmin causing abnormal copper deposition in liver and CNS Kayser-Fleischer rings on cornea Malabsorption syndrome Cirrhosis and jaundice Renal tubular acidosis and aminoaciduria	Decreased pseudocholinesterase Abnormal coagulation profile Impaired renal and hepatic drug clearance

Syndrome	Features	Anesthetic Implications
Wiskott-Aldrich syndrome [Immunologic]	X-linked recessive immunodeficiency (T cell and IgM) Severe recurrent bacterial and opportunistic infections Intracranial hemorrhage Thrombocytopenia Propensity for hypothermia Progressive renal dysfunction	Absolute aseptic technique required May need preoperative transfusions of red cells and platelets (irradiated to prevent graft-versus-host disease) Antibiotic prophylaxis preoperatively
Wolff-Parkinson-White syndrome [Cardiothoracic]	Reentry pathway: accessory bundle of Kent Arrhythmias; SVT Associated CHF, most commonly with Ebstein anomaly Digoxin often used to control arrhythmias, rarely causes VF in children	Sympathetic stimulation or atropine may trigger tachyarrhythmias Halothane may predispose to PACs and trigger reentry pathway Countershock should be used for SVT Consider antibiotic prophylaxis if associated CHD
Wolman's disease (familial xanthomatosis) [Metabolic]	Foam cell infiltration of tissue including myocardium Adrenal calcification Hepatomegaly Death by 6 months of age	May have abnormal coagulation profile and platelet function Multisystem failure
Xeroderma pigmentosum [Dermatologic]	Disorder of pyrimidine metabolism Excessive erythema and blistering following minimal sun exposure Keratosis and skin cancer develop at an early age	Loss of skin integrity
Zellweger syndrome (Cerebrohepatorenal syndrome)	Similar to Bowen syndrome with craniofacial dysmorphism, glaucoma Also has peroxisomal abnormalities of kidney and liver	Exaggerated response to muscle relaxants Electrolyte imbalance Impaired renal drug excretion Abnormal coagulation Possible difficult intubation

Bibliography and Suggested Readings

General

Berry FA, Steward DJ: *Pediatrics for the anesthesiologist,* New York, 1993, Churchill Livingstone.

Gibson J, Potparic O: *A dictionary of medical and surgical syndromes,* Park Ridge, Ill, 1992, Parthenon Publishing Group.

Katz J, Steward DJ: *Anesthesia and uncommon pediatric diseases,* Philadelphia, 1987, W.B. Saunders.

Magalini SI, Magaline SC, de Francisci G: *Dictionary of medical syndromes,* Philadelphia, 1990, J.B. Lippincott.

Oski FA, DeAngelis CD, Feigin RD, Warshaw JB: *Principles and practice of pediatrics,* Philadelphia, 1990, J.B. Lippincott.

Steward DJ: *Manual of pediatric anesthesia,* ed 4, New York, 1995, Churchill Livingstone.

Cardiothoracic Syndromes

Adu-Gyamfi Y, Said A, Abomelha A: Anaesthetic-induced ventricular tachy-arrhythmia in Jervell and Lange-Nielsen syndrome, *Can J Anaesth* 38:345-346, 1991.

Diaz JH: Perioperative management of neonatal ectopia cordis: report of three cases, *Anesth Analg* 75:833-837, 1992.

Gersony WM: Diagnosis and management of Kawasaki disease, *JAMA* 265:2699-2700, 1991.

Holland JJ: Cardiac arrest under anesthesia in a child with previously undiagnosed Jervell and Lange-Nielsen syndrome, *Anaesthesia* 48:149-151, 1993.

Kaplan P, Kirschner M, Watters G, Costa MT: Contractures in patients with Williams syndrome, *Pediatrics* 84:895-899, 1989.

Yanagida H, Kemi C, Suwa K: The effects of stellate ganglion block on the idiopathic prolongation of the Q-T interval with cardiac arrhythmia (the Romano-Ward syndrome), *Anesth Analg* 55:782-787, 1976.

Chromosomal Syndromes

Amitai Y, Gillis D, Wasserman D, et al: Henoch-Schonlein purpura in infants, *Pediatrics* 92:865-867, 1993.

Basson CT, Cowley GS, Solomon SD, et al: The clinical and genetic spectrum of the Hold-Oram syndrome (Heart-Hand syndrome), *N Engl J Med* 330:885-891, 1994.

Bhimji S. What is fragile X syndrome? *Resident and Staff Physician,* pp. 63-68, August 1992.

Crabbe LS, Bensky AS, Hornstein L, Schwartz DC: Cardiovascular abnormalities in children with fragile X syndrome, *Pediatrics* 91:714-715, 1993.

Committee on Sports Medicine and Fitness: Atlantoaxial instability in Down syndrome: subject review, *Pediatrics* 96:151-154, 1995.

Enjoiras O, Riche MC, Merland JJ, Escande JP: Management of alarming hemangiomas in infancy: a review of 25 cases, *Pediatrics* 85:491-498, 1990.

Kobel M, Steward DJ: Anesthetic considerations in Down's syndrome: experience with 100 patients and a review of the literature, *Anaesth Soc J* 29:593-599, 1982.

Marcus CL, Keens TG, Bautista DB, von Pechman WS, Ward SL: Obstructive sleep apnea in children with Down syndrome, *Pediatrics* 88:132-139, 1991.

Pueschel SM, Scola FH, Pezzullo C: A longitudinal study of atlanto-dens relationships in asymptomatic individuals with Down syndrome, *Pediatrics* 89:1194-1198, 1992.

Schwartz N, Eisenkraft JB: Anesthetic management of a child with Noonan's syndrome and idiopathic hypertrophic subaortic stenosis, *Anesth Analg* 74:464-466, 1992.

Connective Tissue Disorders

Goldhagen JL: Cricoarytenoiditis as a cause of acute airway obstruction in children, *Ann Emerg Med* 17:532-533, 1988.

Mizushima A, Satoyoshi M: Anaesthetic problems in a child with ectrodactyly, ectodermal dysplasia and cleft lip/palate: the EEC syndrome, *Anaesthesia* 47:137-140, 1992.

Smith BL: Anaesthesia and Still's disease (letter), *Anesthesia* 40:209, 1985.

Stevenson GW, Hall SC, Palmieri J: Anesthetic considerations for patients with Larsen's syndrome, *Anesthesiology* 75:142-144, 1991.

Craniofacial Disorders

Billette de Villemeur T, Bijaoui G, Beauvais P, Richardet JM: Bowen syndrome: congenital glaucoma, flexion, contracture of fingers and facial dysmorphism without peroxisomal abnormalities, *Eur J Pediatr* 151:146-147, 1992.

Chadd GD, Crane DL, Phillips RM, Tunell WP: Extubation and reintubation guided by the laryngeal mask airway in a child with the Pierre-Robin syndrome, *Anesthesiology* 76:640-641, 1992.

Davis ST, Ducey JP, Fincher CW, Hosking MP: The anesthetic management of a patient with chromosome 10qter deletion syndrome, *J Clin Anesth* 6:512-514, 1994.

Duggar RG, DeMars PD, Bolton VE: Whistling face syndrome: general anesthesia and early postoperative caudal analgesia, *Anesthesiology* 70:545-547, 1989.

Ebata T, Nishiki S, Masuda A, Amaha K: Anaesthesia for Treacher Collins syndrome using a laryngeal mask airway, *Can J Anaesth* 38:1043-1045, 1991.

Gurkowski MA, Rasch DK: Anesthetic considerations for Beckwith-Wiedemann syndrome, *Anesthesiology* 70:711-712, 1989.

Jedele KB, Michels VV, Puga FJ, Feldt RH: Velo-cardio-facial syndrome associated with ventricular septal defect, pulmonary atresia, and hypoplastic pulmonary arteries, *Pediatrics* 89:915-919, 1992.

Jones R, Dolcourt JL: Muscle rigidity following halothane anesthesia in two patients with Freeman-Sheldon syndrome, *Anesthesiology* 77:599-600, 1992.

Langer RA, Yook I, Capan LM: Anesthetic considerations in McCune-Albright syndrome: case report with literature review, *Anesth Analg* 80:1236-1239, 1995.

Lynch M, Underwood S: Pulmonary oedema following relief of upper airway obstruction in the Pierre-Robin syndrome: a consequence of early palatal repair? *Br J Anaesth* 66:391-393, 1991.

Madan R, Trikha A, Venkataraman R, Batra R, Kalia P: Goldenhar's syndrome: an analysis of anaesthetic management: a retrospective study of seventeen cases, *Anaesthesia* 45:49-52, 1990.

Ravindran R, Stoops CM: Anesthetic management of a patient with Hallermann-Streiff syndrome, *Anesth Analg* 58:254-255, 1979.

Rothman G, Wood RA, Naclerio RM: Unilateral choanal atresia masquerading as chronic sinusitis, *Pediatrics* 94:941-944, 1994.

Scheller JG, Schulman SR: Fiber-optic bronchoscopic guidance for intubating a neonate with Pierre-Robin syndrome, *J Clin Anesth* 3:45-47, 1991.

Sklar GS, King BD: Endotracheal intubation and Treacher-Collins syndrome, *Anesthesiology* 44:247-249, 1976.

Stevenson GW, Hall SC, Bauer BS, Viacari FA, Seleny FL: Anaesthetic management of Miller's syndrome, *Can J Anaesth* 38:1046-1049, 1991.

Tobias JD, Lowe S, Holcomb GW: Anesthetic considerations of an infant with Beckwith-Wiedemann syndrome, *J Clin Anesth* 4:484-486, 1992.

Dermatologic Disorders

Lyos AT, Levy ML, Malpica A, Sulek M: Laryngeal involvement in epidermolysis bullosa, *Ann Otol Rhino Laryngol* 103:542-546, 1994.

Touloukian RJ, Schonholz SM, Gryboski JD, Oh T, McGuire J: Perioperative considerations in esophageal replacement for epidermolyis bullosa: report of two cases successfully treated by colon interposition, *Am J Gastroenterol* 83:857-861, 1988.

Hematologic/Immunologic Disorders

Amitai Y, Gillis D, Wasserman D, Kochman RH: Henoch-Schönlein purpura in infants, *Pediatrics* 92:865-867, 1993.

Enjoiras O, Riche MC, Merland JJ, Escande JP: Management of alarming hemangiomas in infancy: a review of 25 cases, *Pediatrics* 85:491-498, 1990.

Metabolic Disorders

Asada A, Tatekawa S, Terai T, et al: The anesthetic implications of a patient with Farber's lipogranulomatosis, *Anesthesiology* 80:206-209, 1994.

Birkinshaw, KJ: Anaesthesia in a patient with an unstable neck: Morquio's syndrome, *Anaesthesia* 30:46-49, 1975.

Christensen E, Brandt NJ, Rosenberg T, Bömers K, Jakobs C: The segregation of glutaryl-CoA dehydrogenase deficiency and Refsum syndrome in a family, *J Inher Metab Dis* 17:287-290, 1994.

Holm VA, Cassidy SB, Butler MG, et al: Prader-Willi syndrome: consensus diagnostic criteria, *Pediatrics* 91:398-402, 1993.

Jones AEP, Croley TF: Morquio syndrome and anesthesia, *Anesthesiology* 51:261-262, 1979.

Kazim, R, Weisberg, R, Sun LS: Upper airway obstruction and Menkes syndrome, *Anesth Analg* 77:856-857, 1993.

King DH, Jones RM, Barnett MD: Anaesthetic considerations in the mucopolysaccharidoses, *Anaesthesia* 39:126-131, 1984.

Lowe S, Johnson DA, Tobias JD: Anesthetic implications of the child with homocystinuria, *J Clin Anesth* 6:142-144, 1994.

Nicolson SC, Black AE, Kraras CM: Management of a difficult airway in a patient with Hurler-Scheie syndrome during cardiac surgery, *Anesth Analg* 75:830-832, 1992.

Scriver CR, Mahon B, Levy HL, et al: The Hartnup phenotype: mendelian transport disorder, multifactorial disease, *Am J Hum Genet* 40:401-412, 1987.

Shapiro LR: The McCune-Albright syndrome: the whys and wherefores of abnormal signal transduction, *N Engl J Med* 325:1738-1740, 1991.

Sloan TB, Kaye CI: Rumination risk of aspiration of gastric contents in the Prader-Willi syndrome, *Anesth Analg* 73:492-495, 1991.

Tobias JD, Atwood R, Lowe S, Holcomb GW: Anesthetic considerations in the child with Gaucher disease, *J Clin Anesth* 5:150-153, 1993.

Warady BA, Cibis G, Alon U, Blowley D, Hellerstein S: Senior-Loken syndrome: revisited, *Pediatrics* 94:111-112, 1993.

Musculoskeletal Disorders

Dinner M, Goldin EZ, Ward R, Levy J: Russell-Silver syndrome: anesthetic implications, *Anesth Analg* 78:1197-1199, 1994.

Hall RMO, Henning RD, Brown TCK, Cole WG: Anaesthesia for children with osteogenesis imperfecta: a review covering 30 years, and 266 anaesthetics, *Peadiatr Anaesth* 2:115-121, 1992.

Jones D, Doughty L, Brown K: Anaesthesia for a child with Sotos' syndrome (letter), *Anaesthesia and Intensive Care* 19:298-299, 1991.

Ravindran R, Stoops CM: Anesthetic management of a patient with Hallermann-Streiff syndrome, *Anesth Analg* 58:254-255, 1979.

Suresh D: Posterior spinal fusion in Sotos' syndrome, *Br J Anaesth* 66:728-732, 1991.

Neurologic Disorders

de Leon-Casasola OA, Lema MJ: Anesthesia for patients with Sturge-Weber disease and Klippel-Trenaunay syndrome, *J Clin Anesth* 3:409-413, 1991.

Gaiser RR, Cheek TG, Gutsche BB: Major conduction anesthesia in a patient with Klippel-Trenaunay syndrome, *J Clin Anesth* 7:316-319, 1995.

Greenberg RS, Parker SD: Anesthetic management for the child with Charcot-Marie-Tooth disease, *Anesth Analg* 74:305-307, 1992.

Katende RS, Herlich A: Anesthetic considerations in holoprosencephaly, *Anesth Analg* 66:908-910, 1987.

Lee JJ, Imrie M, Taylor V: Anaesthesia and tuberous sclerosis, *Br J Anaesth* 73:421-425, 1994.

Moorman CM, Elston JS, Matthews P: Leber's hereditary optic neuropathy as a cause of severe visual loss in childhood, *Pediatrics* 91:988-989, 1992.

Pincus JH: Subacute necrotizing encephalomyelopathy (Leigh's disease): a consideration of clinical features and etiology, *Develop Med Child Neurol* 14:87-101, 1972.

Schweiger JW, Schwartz RE, Stayer SA: The anaesthetic management of the patient with tuberous sclerosis complex, *Paediatr Anaesth* 4:339-342, 1994.

Ward DS: Anesthesia for a child with Leigh's syndrome, *Anesthesiology* 35:80-81, 1981.

APPENDIXES

DRUG LIST

A

CONTENTS

ANTIDYSRHYTHMIC/INOTROPE

ANTIEMETIC

ANTIHISTAMINES

ANTIHYPERTENSIVES

ANTITHYROID PREPARATIONS

BARBITURATES

BENZODIAZEPINES

BENZODIAZEPINE ANTAGONIST

LIST OF ABBREVIATIONS

α	Alpha
AVB	Atrioventricular blockade
ACT	Activated clotting time
AF	Atrial fibrillation
β	Beta
BBB	Blood-brain barrier
CBC	Complete blood count
CHF	Congestive heart failure
CV	Cardiovascular
E	Elimination route (unchanged drug or metabolites)
ED	Effective dose
ETT	Endotracheal tube
g	Gram
GI	Gastrointestinal
GU	Genitourinary
hr	Hour
HSV	Herpes simplex virus
IM	Intramuscular
IN	Intranasal
IV	Intravenous
K^+	Potassium
kg	Kilogram
M	Metabolism
MAO	Monoamine oxidase
μg	Microgram
mEq	Milliequivalent
mg	Milligram
min	Minute
msec	Millisecond
Na^+	Sodium
NSS	Normal saline solution
PABA	Para-aminobenzoic acid
PCN	Penicillin
PIT	Partial thromboplastin time
PO	Per os (orally)
PR	Per rectum
PRN	As needed
q	Every
SA	Sinoatrial
SC	Subcutaneous
SL	Sublingual
SLE	Systemic lupus erythematosus
SVR	Systemic vascular resistance
SVT	Supraventricular tachycardia
TB	Tuberculosis
$T_{1/2}\beta$	Elimination half-life
VF	Ventricular fibrillation
VT	Ventricular tachycardia
WPW	Wolff-Parkinson-White
yr	Years
>	Greater than
<	Less than

Drug	Class	Dose	Pharmacokinetics	Comments
Acetaminophen (Tylenol, Panadol)	Analgesic	0-3 mo: 40 mg/dose PO 4-11 mo: 80 mg/dose PO 12-24 mo: 120 mg/dose PO 2-3 yr: 160 mg/dose PO 4-5 yr: 240 mg/dose PO 6-8 yr: 320 mg/dose PO 9-10 yr: 400 mg/dose PO 11-12 yr: 480 mg/dose PO or 5-10 mg/kg q6h PO	Onset: 30-60 min Duration: 3-4 hr M = liver E = kidney $t_{1/2}\beta$ = 1-3 hr	A metabolite of phenacetin but low risk of methemoglobinemia or hemolytic anemia Hepatotoxicity occurs at doses >140 mg/kg. Treatment with N-Acetylcysteine is most effective if begun within 10 hr of ingestion
Acetazolamide (Diamox)	Diuretic	*Diuretic:* PO/IV: 5 mg/kg qd or qod *Glaucoma:* IV: 20-40 mg/kg/day divided q6h IM: 20-40 mg/kg/day divided q6h PO: 8-30 mg/kg/day divided q6-8h	E = kidney IV onset: 2 min Duration: 4-5 hr PO onset: 1-1.5 hr Duration: 8-12 hr	Carbonic anhydrase inhibitor Side effects: hypokalemia, acidosis, alkaline urine, paresthesias, vomiting, and diarrhea
Acyclovir	Antiviral	*Herpes simplex virus:* Neonate: IV: 30 mg/kg/day divided q8h Child: <12 yr IV: 750 mg/m²/day divided q8h	E = kidney $t_{1/2}\beta$ = 2.5 hr	Can cause renal dysfunction (if rapidly infused), thrombophlebitis, headache, rash Encephalopathy can occur with IV use Widely distributed to all tissue and body fluids (including CSF)

Drug	Class	Dose	Pharmacokinetics	Comments
Adenosine (Adenocard)	Antiarrhythmic	*SVT:* 0.1 mg/kg rapid IV push; may increase dose by 0.05 increase dose by 0.05 mg/kg q2min to max of 0.25 mg/kg (or 12 mg)	M: plasma adenylate cyclase $t_{1/2}\beta$: <10 sec	Not effective for AF, VT Do not use in 2° AVB, 3° AVB, or sick sinus syndrome unless paced
Albuterol (Proventil, Ventolin)	Bronchodilator	*Enteral:* 2-5 yrs: 0.1 mg/kg/day divided q8h PO May increase to 12 mg/day 6-11 yr: 2 mg PO tid May increase to 24 mg/day >12 yr: 2-4 mg PO tid or qid *Inhaler:* 1-2 puffs q4-6h *Nebulizer:* 0.01-0.03 ml/kg in 2 ml NSS tid-qid (Concentration = 5 mg/ml with 1 ml maximum dose)	Peak Effect: 30-60 min after inhalation Duration: 4-6 hr	Selective β_2 agonist Tachyphylaxis with long-term use Side effects: tachycardia, nausea, vomiting, nervousness, and hypokalemia
Alprostadil (Prostin VR)	Prostaglandin E_1	IV = 0.05 µg/kg/min continuous infusion Increase incrementally up to 0.4 µg/kg/min *Maintenance:* Increase until acceptable Po_2, then immediately decrease to lowest effective dose	M = lungs (70%) E = kidney	Aids in maintaining a patent ductus arteriosus in ductus-dependent cyanotic heart defects Side effects include apnea, seizures, bradycardia, hypotension, hyperpyrexia, and bronchoconstriction

Continued.

Drug	Class	Dose	Pharmacokinetics	Comments
Alfentanil (Alfenta)	Opioid	*Load:* 30-50 μg/kg IV *Maintenance:* 10-15 μg/kg IV single boluses or infusion of 0.5-1.5 μg/kg/min	Onset: 1-2 min M = liver E = kidney	Slow elimination in patients with liver disease Hypotension potential when used with diazepam May cause truncal rigidity
Amantadine (Symmetrel)	Antiviral	*Child:* 1-9 yr: PO: 4-8 mg/kg/day divided q8-12h 9-12 yr: PO: 200 mg/kg divided q12h	E = kidney $t_{1/2}\beta$ = 15-20 hr (prolonged with renal dysfunction)	Side effects include depression, nausea, seizures, CHF and orthostatic hypotension Give for 90 days after influenza exposure for prophylaxis if vaccine contraindicated Adjust dose in renal failure
Amikacin (Amikin)	Antibiotic Aminoglycoside	*Neonate:* <7 days and <1000 gm IV/IM: 7.5 mg/kg q24h <7 days and 1000-2000 gm IV/IM: 7.5 mg/kg q12h <7 days and >2000 gm IV/IM: 10 mg/kg q12h >7 days IV/IM: 7.5-10 mg/kg q8h *Child:* IV/IM: 15 mg/kg/day divided q8h	E = kidney $t_{1/2}\beta$ = 2-3 hr (prolonged with renal dysfunction, neonates)	Excellent gram negative coverage especially *Pseudomonas* Side effects include ototoxicity, nephrotoxicity and potentiation of neuromuscular blockade Infuse slowly IV Therapeutic levels: Peak = 25-30 mg/L Trough = 5-8 mg/L

Drug	Class	Dose	Pharmacokinetics	Comments
Aminophylline	Bronchodila- tor	*Load:* 6 mg/kg IV over 20-30 min *Maintenance:* IV infusion: Neonate 0.2 mg/kg/hr <1 yr 0.2-0.9 mg/kg/hr 1-9 yr 1 mg/kg/hr	Onset: IV rapid M = liver E = kidney $t_{1/2}\beta$ = 3-10 hr (children); 15-58 hr (neonates)	Indicated for relief of bron- chospasm and treatment of neonatal apnea Side effects include tachycardia, dysrhythmias, nervousness, nausea, and vomiting Metabolism slowed with CHF, cimetidine administration and β-blockers Therapeutic levels Asthma: 10-20 mg/L Apnea: 6-13 mg/L
Amoxicillin (Amoxil)	Antibiotic Penicillin	PO: 20-40 mg/kg/day divided q8h	E = kidney	Achieves serum levels twice those of ampicillin Less GI effects than ampicillin
Amphotericin B (Fungizone)	Antifungal	*Test dose:* IV: 0.1 mg/kg infants, up to 0.5 mg in children *Initial dose:* IV: 0.25 mg/kg/day, increase daily by 0.125-0.25 mg/kg in- crements to a maximum total dose of 1.5 mg/kg/day	E = kidney $t_{1/2}\beta$ = 15 days	Does not penetrate CNS Premedicate with diphenhy- dramine and acetaminophen Side effects include renal dysfunc- tion, shaking chills, anemia, thrombocytopenia, allergic re- actions, hypokalemia, hypo- magnesemia, and seizures

Continued.

Drug	Class	Dose	Pharmacokinetics	Comments
Ampicillin (Omnipen, Polycillin)	Antibiotic Penicillin	*Neonate:* IV or IM* 0-7 days: 50-100 mg/kg q12h >7 days: 75-100 mg/kg q8h *Child:* Mild-moderate infection: IV/IM/PO: 50-100 mg/kg/day divided q6h Maximum dose = 2-4 g/day Severe infection: IV/IM: 200-400 mg/kg/day divided q4-6h Maximum dose = 12 g/day	M = liver (about 50%) E = kidney, liver $t_{1/2}\beta$ = 2-4 hr (age dependent)	Has gram negative activity, including enterococcus Higher doses are for treatment of *H. flu* meningitis in conjunction with chloramphenicol After 5-10 days: Delayed skin rash is common and may not indicate hypersensitivity May cause interstitial nephritis
Amrinone (Inocor)	Inotrope	*Load:* IV: 0.75 mg/kg over 2-3 min may repeat in 30 min if needed *Infusion:* IV: 5-10 µg/kg/min	Onset: 2-5 min Duration: 0.5-2 hr (depending on dose) M = liver E = kidney $t_{1/2}\beta$ = 3.6 hr (adults)	Inotropic agent that acts via inhibition of phosphodiesterase May act as a negative inotrope in infants Has direct relaxant effect on vascular smooth muscle to decrease preload and afterload Do *not* dilute with dextrose solutions or mix with furosemide Side effects include thrombocytopenia, hepatotoxicity, hypotension, and arrhythmias Avoid in patients sensitive to bisulfites

*Doses increase for meningitis.

Drug	Class	Dose	Pharmacokinetics	Comments
Atracurium (Tracrium)	Nondepolarizing muscle relaxant	*Intubation:* IV: 0.5-0.5 mg/kg *Maintenance:* IV: 0.25 mg/kg Infusion: 6 µg/kg/hr	Onset: 1-2 min Duration: 20-30 min M = Hoffman elimination Ester hydrolysis	Lacks cumulative effects Laudanosine metabolite can cause CNS stimulation Significant histamine release only occurs at $3 \times ED_{95}$
Atropine	Anticholinergic	IV: 10-20 µg/kg IM: 20 µg/kg Maximum dose for resuscitation = 1 mg IV	Onset: IV = rapid; IM = 2-5 min Duration: 4 hr M = liver E = kidney $t_{1/2}\beta$ = 2 hr	Indicated to prevent reflex bradycardia with suction, intubation, etc. and to treat symptomatic bradydysrhythmias Side effects include hyperpyrexia, urinary retention, dry mouth, confusion, and rash
Bretylium (Bretylol)	Antiarrhythmic	*Initial:* IV: 5-10 mg/kg over 10-30 min may repeat in 20-30 min × 1 *Maintenance:* IV bolus: 5-10 mg/kg q6h over 10 min IV infusion: 1-2 mg/min	Onset: 2 min-2 hr Duration: 6-24 hr M = minimal E = kidney $t_{1/2}\beta$ = 5-10 hr	Indicated for management of recurrent life-threatening ventricular dysrhythmias Causes initial catecholamine release followed by sympathectomy-like state manifested by orthostatic hypotension
Bupivacaine (Marcaine)	Local amide anesthetic	Maximal safe dose: 2.5 mg/kg With epinephrine: 3 mg/kg	Duration: 240-480 min M = liver E = kidney $t_{1/2}\beta$ = 2-6 hr	Slow onset and long duration agent with high in vivo toxic potential Severe cardiotoxicity has limited use of 0.75% solution Toxic levels = 1.5 µg/ml

Continued.

Drug	Class	Dose	Pharmacokinetics	Comments
Calcium chloride	Inotrope	IV bolus: 10 mg/kg, may repeat	Onset: rapid	Should be given centrally to avoid phlebitis Do not mix with bicarbonate Once injected, calcium is bound to protein and incorporated into muscle, bone, and other tissues
Calcium gluconate*	Inotrope	IV bolus: 100 mg/kg, may repeat IV infusion: 200-500 mg/kg/day	Onset: rapid	May produce arrhythmias in digitalized patients Do not mix with bicarbonate Formulation of choice for peripheral IV administration Can cause tissue necrosis if extravasation occurs Protein binding and incorporation into tissue occurs as with calcium chloride
Captopril (Capoten)	Antihypertensive	*Neonate:* PO: 0.1-0.4 mg/kg q6-24h *Infant:* PO: 0.5-0.6 mg/kg/day divided q6-12h *Child:* PO: 25 mg/day divided q12h	Onset: 30 min-2 hr M = liver E = kidney	Indicated in renovascular hypertension and in the management of congestive heart failure Competitively inhibits angiotensin converting enzyme Side effects include hyperkalemia, elevated creatinine, neutropenia, proteinuria, cough, and acute hypotension after first dose

*See p. 664 for infusion preparation.

Drug	Class	Dose	Pharmacokinetics	Comments
Carbamazepine (Tegretol)	Anticonvul-sant	*>6 years:* PO: 10 mg/kg/day divided q12-24h initially Maximum dose = 20 mg/kg/day *6-12 years:* PO: 10 mg/kg/day divided qd or bid initially Maintenance = 20-30 mg/kg/day divided q6-8h Maximum dose = 1000 mg/day *Adolescent:* PO: 200 mg bid initially Maintenance: 600-1200 mg/day divided q6-8h Maximum dose = 1000 mg/day	Onset: 2-6 hr Duration: 6-8 hr M = 98% liver $t_{1/2}\beta$ = 13-17 hr	Indicated for trigeminal/glos-sopharyngeal neuralgias, and psychomotor epilepsy Obtain pretreatment CBC Side effects include: sedation, diplopia, vertigo, nausea, vomiting, and ataxia *Life threatening:* aplastic anemia, thrombocytopenia, oliguria, hypertension, acute heart failure and hepatic dysfunction Therapeutic drug levels 4-12 mg/L
Carbenicillin (Geopen)	Antibiotic Penicillin	*Neonate:* IV or IM 0-7 days: 50-75 mg/kg q6h *Children:* IV or IM UTI: 50-200 mg/kg/day divided q4-6h Severe infection: 400-500 mg/kg/day divided q4-6h Maximum dose = 3 g/day	M = liver E = kidney $t_{1/2}\beta$ = 1-4 hr, age dependent	Indicated for *Pseudomonas* and *Proteus* resistant to ampicillin Interferes with normal platelet aggregation such that bleeding time is prolonged 1 gram contains 4-7 mEq Na^+ May lead to urinary K^+ loss and cardiac failure

Continued.

Drug	Class	Dose	Pharmacokinetics	Comments
Cefazolin (Ancef/Kefzol)	Antibiotic cephalosporin—first generation	*Infant/child:* IV or IM 25-100 mg/kg/day divided q6-8h	M = minimal E = kidney $t_{1/2}\beta$ = 2 hr	Reduce dose in renal failure Use caution in penicillin-allergic patients Active against *Staphylococcus, E. coli* and *Klebsiella*
Cefamandole (Mandol)	Antibiotic cephalosporin—second generation	*Child:* IV/IM: 50-150 mg/kg/day divided q4-8h	M = minimal E = kidney $t_{1/2}\beta$ = 30-60 min	1 gm = 3.3 mEq Na^+ Not recommended in children <1 mo Can produce hypoprothrombinemia Greater gram negative and less gram positive coverage than 1st generation drugs
Cefoperazone (Cefobid)	Antibiotic cephalosporin—third generation	*Infant/child:* IV/IM: 25-100 mg/kg/day divided q12h	M = minimal E = bile $t_{1/2}\beta$ = 2 hr (neonate 6-12 hr)	Penetrates into CNS when meninges are inflamed Dose reduction not necessary in renal insufficiency Can produce hypoprothrombinemia Less gram positive coverage than 1st generation drugs but has excellent *Pseudomonas* coverage

Drug	Class	Dose	Pharmacokinetics	Comments
Cefotaxime (Claforan)	Antibiotic cephalo-sporin—third generation	*Neonate:* IV/IM <7 days: 50-100 mg/kg/day divided q12h 7-30 days: 75-150 mg/kg/day divided q8h *Infant/child:* (<50 kg) IV/IM: 50-180 mg/kg/day divided q4-6h	M = liver (50%) E = kidney $t_{1/2}\beta$ = 1-1.5 hr	Broad gram negative coverage, especially against *Serratia* Little dose adjustment in renal insufficiency Good CNS penetration
Cefotetan (Cefotan)	Antibiotic cephalo-sporin—second generation	IV: 40-60 mg/kg divided q12h	M = minimal E = kidney, bile $t_{1/2}\beta$ = 3-5 hr	Special role in clinical use is against *B. fragilis*
Cefoxitin (Mefoxin)	Antibiotic cephalo-sporin—second generation	*Infant/child:* IV/IM: 80-160 mg/kg/day divided q4-6h	M = minimal E = kidney $t_{1/2}\beta$ = 45-60 min	Special role in clinical use is against *B. fragilis*
Ceftazidime (Fortaz)	Antibiotic cephalo-sporin—third generation	*Neonate:* IV: 60 mg/kg/day divided q12h *Infant/child:* IV: 75-150 mg/kg/day divided q8h	M = none E = kidney $t_{1/2}\beta$ = 2-4 hr	Active against gram positive, gram negative and anaerobes, but not *B. fragilis* Not active against most enterococci
Ceftizoxime (Cefizox)	Antibiotic cephalo-sporin—third generation	*Infant/child:* IV/IM: 150-200 mg/kg/day divided q6-8h	M = none E = kidney $t_{1/2}\beta$ = 1.3-1.6 hr	Active against gram positive, gram negative and anaerobic organisms, including *B. fragilis* Inactive against most enterococci

Continued.

Drug	Class	Dose	Pharmacokinetics	Comments
Ceftriaxone (Rocephin)	Antibiotic cephalosporin—third generation	*Infant/child:* IV/IM: 50 mg/kg/day qd *Meningitis:* IV: 75 mg/kg × 1 dose then 100 mg/kg/day divided q12h	M = none E = kidney $t_{1/2}\beta$ = 4-8 hr	Good CNS penetration Active against gram positive, gram negative and anaerobes Inactive against most enterococci
Cefuroxime (Zinacef)	Antibiotic cephalosporin—second generation	*Neonates:* IV/IM: 10 mg/kg/day divided q12h *Infant/child:* IV/IM: 50-100 mg/kg/day divided q6-8h *Meningitis:* IV: 200-240 mg/kg/day divided q6-8h	M = none E = kidney $t_{1/2}\beta$ = 1-4 hr, age dependent	Broad gram positive coverage, except enterococci Good gram negative coverage except *Pseudomonas*, most strains of *Serratia* and *Proteus vulgaris*
Cephalothin (Keflin)	Antibiotic cephalosporin—first generation	*Neonate:* IV or IM 0-7 days: 40 mg/kg/day divided q12h >7 days: 60 mg/kg/day divided q8h *Child:* 80-160 mg/kg/day divided q4-6h	M = liver (50%) E = kidney $t_{1/2}\beta$ = 0.5-1 hr	See cefazolin For treatment of staphycoccal infections
Cephapirin (Cefadyl)	Antibiotic cephalosporin—first generation	40-80 mg/kg/day divided q6h IV, IM	M = liver (50%) E = kidney $T_{1/2}\beta$ = 0.5-1 hr	Similar to Cephalothin

Drug	Class	Dose	Pharmacokinetics	Comments
Cephradine (Velosef)	Antibiotic cephalosporin—first generation	*Children:* IV: 50-100 mg/kg/day divided q6h IM: 50-100 mg/kg/day divided q6h PO: 25-100 mg/kg/day divided q6-12h	M = minimal E = kidney $T_{1/2}\beta$ = 0.7-2 hr	For treatment of gram positive infections as well as *E. coli, Proteus mirabilis,* and *Klebsiella*
Chloral hydrate (Noctec)	Sedative/ hypnotic	PO/PR: 50-100 mg/kg Up to 1.0 g	Onset: PO/PR: 13-60 min Duration: PO/PR: 4-8 hr M = liver and RBC to active trichloroethanol E = kidney (some liver)	Useful for preoperative sedation Excellent PO/PR absorption, but has a bitter taste Side effects include gastric irritation, myocardial depression (in cardiac diseases), and potentiation of oral anticoagulants Contraindicated in marked hepatic or renal dysfunction
Chloramphenicol (Chloromycetin)	Antibiotic	Loading dose (all ages) IV/PO: 20 mg/kg *Neonates:* IV <7 days: 10 mg/kg/day divided q12-24h, initiate 24 hr after load 7-21 days: 20 mg/kg/day divided q8-12h >21 days: 30 mg/kg/day divided q6-12h *Children:* IV/PO: 50-100 mg/kg/day divided q6-8h	M = liver E = kidney $T_{1/2}\beta$ = 1.5-3.5 hr	Few indications for use exist but indicated for typhoid fever and ampicillin-resistant *H. flu* meningitis Must monitor drug levels (15-20 mg/L) May cause aplastic anemia Inhibits hepatic microsomal enzymes

Continued.

Drug	Class	Dose	Pharmacokinetics	Comments
Chlorpromazine (Thorazine)	Phenothiazine	PO: 0.5 mg/kg q4-6h IV/IM: 2 mg/kg/day divided q6-8h *Maximum daily doses:* <5 yrs: 40 mg 5-12 yrs: 75 mg	Onset: IV: rapid IM: 30 min PO: 30-60 min Duration: IM: 3-4 hr PO: 4-6 hr M = liver E = liver, kidney $T_{1/2}\beta$ = 10-20 hr	A neuroleptic Also useful as an antiemetic, major tranquilizer Side effects include sedation, orthostatic hypotension (α-blockade), extrapyramidal reactions, cholestatic jaundice and leukopenia Not recommended in children <6 mo or in those with suspected Reye's syndrome
Cimetidine (Tagamet)	H$_2$ receptor antagonist	*Neonate:* PO/IV: 10-20 mg/kg/day divided q4-6h *Child:* PO/IV: 20-40 mg/kg/day divided q6h	Onset: 45-90 min PO Duration: IV/IM/PO: 4-5 hr M = liver E = kidney $T_{1/2}\beta$ = 2 hr	Side effects include drowsiness, dizziness, gynecomastia, and neutropenia May cause increased levels of active propranolol, benzodiazepines, phenytoin, theophylline by inhibiting hepatic microsomal enzymes
Clindamycin (Cleocin)	Antibiotic	IV/IM: 15-40 mg/kg/day divided q6-8h PO: 8-25 mg/kg/day divided q6-8h	E = kidney $T_{1/2}\beta$ = 2-4 hr	Use with caution in nenonates, infants and in hepatic and renal insufficiency Gram positive and anaerobic activity Associated with pseudomembranous colitis

Drug	Class	Dose	Pharmacokinetics	Comments
Clonazepam (Klonopin)	Benzodi- azepine	Children up to 10 yrs, 30 kg: PO: 0.01-0.03 mg/kg/day divided q8h May be increased to maximum 0.1-0.2 mg/kg/day divided q8h	M = liver E = kidney $T_{1/2}\beta$ = 24-48 hr	Side effects include depression, drowsiness, ataxia, behavioral changes and increased bronchial secretions May cause GI, CV, GU, renal and hematopoietic toxicity
Cloxacillin (Cloxapen)	Antibiotic Penicillin	<20 kg: 50-100 mg/kg/day divided q6h PO >20 kg: 1-2 gm/day divided q6h PO Maximum dose = 4 g/day	M = liver (50%) E = kidney and liver $T_{1/2}\beta$ = 6 hr	Rapid, but incomplete PO absorption Better PO absorption achieved with dicloxacillin Antistaphylococcal activity
Cocaine	Ester local anesthetic	*Topical:* 4% solution (1 drop = 2 mg) Maximum safe dose = 3 mg/kg (1.5 mg/kg if used with a volatile anesthetic)	M = liver, plasma esterases E = kidney $T_{1/2}\beta$ = 1 hr	Sympathomimetic which blocks reuptake or norepinephrine May cause tremors, seizures, tachycardia, and hyperpyrexia
Codeine	Opioid	*Analgesic:* IV: 0.5-1.0 mg/kg q4-6h PO: 0.5-1.0 mg/kg q4-6h *Antitussive:* PO: 0.25-0.5 mg/kg q4h Maximum dose = 30 mg/day	M = liver E = kidney $T_{1/2}\beta$ = 3-3.5 hr	Semisynthetic opioid Best used in combination with ac- etaminophen for analgesia Side effects include sedation, nau- sea, and vomiting

Continued.

Drug	Class	Dose	Pharmacokinetics	Comments
Corticotropin (ACTH)	Hormone	*Aqueous:* IV/IM/SC: 1.6 unit/kg/day divided q6-8h *Gel:* IV/IM/SC: 0.8 unit/kg/day divided q12-24h	Onset: rapid by any route Duration: 2 hr	Used diagnostically to evaluate suspected primary adrenal insufficiency Side effects include sodium retention and hypokalemic metabolic alkalosis Contraindicated in Cushing's disease, peptic ulcer disease, psychosis, TB, fungal disease and pork sensitivity
Co-trimoxazole (Bactrim, Septra)	Antibiotic Sulfonamide	*Moderate infections:* PO: 8 mg/kg/day trimethoprim *plus* 40 mg/kg/day sulfamethoxazole divided q12h *Severe infections or pneumocystis:* PO/IV: 20 mg/kg/day trimethoprim *plus* 100 mg/kg/day sulfamethoxazole divided q6h *Prophylaxis* in immunocompromised patients: PO: 5 mg/kg/day trimethoprim *plus* 25 mg sulfamethoxazole divided q12h	M = liver E = kidney $T_{1/2}\beta$ = 10 hr	Side effects include rash, glossitis, stomatitis May cause jaundice or worsen renal dysfunction In folate-deficient patients, anemia, leukopenia and thrombocytopenia can occur

Drug	Class	Dose	Pharmacokinetics	Comments
d-tubocurarine	Nondepolariz-ing muscle relaxant	*Intubation:* Premature = 0.125 mg/kg IV 0-2 mo = 0.25 mg/kg IV >2 mo = 0.3-0.6 mg/kg IV Supplemental doses, ½ initial dose	Onset: 3-5 min Duration: 30 min M = liver (minimal) E = kidney $T_{1/2}\beta$ = 1-3 hr	Neonates and infants are more sensitive to drug effects Causes significant histamine re-lease resulting in hypotension in the usual dose range
Desmopressin acetate (DDAVP)	Pituitary hor-mone	In: (solution = 100 μg/ml) 3 mo-12 yr = 5-30 μg/kg/day di-vided q12-24 hr (endocrine replacement) IV: 0.3 μg/kg over 30 min (hematologic dose)	Duration: 6-20 hr	Drug of choice for central dia-betes insipidus, *not* useful for nephrogenic diabetes insipidus Side effects include nausea, hy-pertension, water retention, and hypotension (especially with rapid administration) Will stimulate release of von Willebrand's factor (VIII$_A$)
Dexamethasone (Decadron)	Corticosteroid	*Increased intracranial pressure:* Initial: 0.5-1.5 mg/kg IV/IM Maintenance: 0.2-0.5 mg/kg/day divided q6h IV/IM *Croup/airway edema:* IV: 0.25-0.5 mg/kg q6h PRN (begin 24 hr prior to planned extubation then re-peat × 4-6 doses)	Duration: 36-54 hr M = liver E = kidney $T_{1/2}\beta$ = 2-4 hr	Glucocorticoid activity 40 times hydrocortisone Little mineralocorticoid activity

Continued.

Drug	Class	Dose	Pharmacokinetics	Comments
Diazepam (Valium)	Benzodiazepine	*Premedicant:* IM: 0.3-0.4 mg/kg PO: 0.1-0.2 mg/kg *Status epilepticus:* 1 mo-5 yr: 0.2-0.5 mg/kg IV q10-30 min to effect, then repeat q2-4h Maximum dose = 5 mg >5 yr: 1 mg IV q15-30 min to effect then repeat q2-4h Maximum dose = 10 mg	Onset: IV: rapid IM: 15-30 min M = liver (Active metabolites-oxazepam + desmethyl diazepam) E = kidney $T_{1/2}\beta$ = 7-20 hr (Metabolites 5-20 hr)	Indicated for sedation, treatment of status epilepticus Avoid in children <1 yr due to prolonged drug action IM route may cause pain on injection, poor absorption, and aseptic necrosis
Diazoxide (Hyperstat)	Antihypertensive	*Hypertensive crisis:* IV: 1-3 mg/kg slow bolus, may repeat q15-30min then q6-8h PRN *Refractory hypoglycemia:* (insulin producing tumors) Newborn/infant: 8-15 mg/kg/day divided q8-12h PO/IV Child: 3-8 mg/kg/day divided q8-12h PO/IV	Onset: 1-2 min IV Duration: 2-12 hr M = liver E = kidney	Primary site of action is arteriolar resistance vessels Chemically related to thiazide diuretics Side effects include sodium and water retention, hyperglycemia, hypotension, and reflex tachycardia

Drug	Class	Dose	Pharmacokinetics	Comments
Digoxin (Doses given are for treatment of CHF)	Antidysrhythmic, inotrope	*Total digitalizing dose (TDD):* Premature: 20 µg/kg IM or IV Full term: 30 µg/kg IM or IV <2 yr: 30-50 µg/kg IM or IV 35-60 µg/kg PO 2-10 yr: 15-30 µg/kg, IM or IV, 20-40 µg/kg PO > 10 yr: 10-15 µg/kg IV or PO *Maintenance:* PO Premature: 5 µg/kg Full term: 8-10 µg/kg <2 yr: 10-12 µg/kg 2-10 yr: 8-10 µg/kg >10 yr: 2-5 µg/kg	Onset: IV: 5-30 min IM: 30 min PO: 1-2 hr M = Minimal E = kidney $T_{1/2}\beta$ = 42 hr	TDD given as ½ dose stat then ¼ TDD q6h × 2 followed by maintenance Maintenance dose divided bid in children <10 yr IV/IM doses are 75% of PO dose except IV = PO in children >10 yr Side effects of toxicity include anorexia, nausea, vomiting, disorientation, and AVB Toxicity potentiated by hypokalemia, hypomagnesemia, and hypercalcemia Therapeutic level = 0.8-2.0 µg/L
Diphenhydramine (Benadryl)	Antihistamine	*Sedation:* IV/IM/PO = 5 mg/kg/day divided q6h *Anaphylaxis/phenothiazine overdose:* IV: 1-2 mg/kg slowly	Onset: IV: rapid IM/PO: 15-30 min M = liver E = kidney $T_{1/2}\beta$ = 3-7 hr	Indicated for sedation, treatment of allergic/anaphylactic reactions/extrapyramidal reactions or as an antiemetic Side effects include dry mouth, tachycardia, hypotension, and respiratory depression
Dobutamine* (Dobutrex)	Inotrope	IV: 1-10 µg/kg/min continuous infusion Maximum recommended dose = 40 µg/kg/min	Onset: 2 min IV Duration: 10 min IV M = liver E = kidney, liver $T_{1/2}\beta$ = 2 min	Synthetic catecholamine with primarily β₁ stimulation properties Increases cardiac output with minimal effect on heart rate or peripheral resistance

*See p. 664 for infusion preparation.

Continued.

Drug	Class	Dose	Pharmacokinetics	Comments
Dopamine* (Intropin)	Inotrope	IV: 1-20 µg/kg/min continuous infusion	Onset: 5 min IV Duration: 10 min IV M = kidney, liver, nerve endings E = kidney $T_{1/2}\beta$ = 2 min	Natural catecholamine with effects on dopaminergic, β-, and α-adrenergic receptors Indicated in low output states associated with hypotension Side effects include tachycardia, tachydysrhythmias, hyperglycemia and intense vasoconstriction with skin sloughing if accidental extravasation occurs
Droperidol (Inapsine)	Antiemetic	IM/IV: 10-70 µg/kg PRN	Onset: 5-8 min IV/IM Duration: 3-6 hr M = liver E = kidney $T_{1/2}\beta$ = 100 min	Inhibits dopamine receptors in chemoreceptor trigger zone of medulla to decrease nausea and vomiting Side effects include extrapyramidal reactions and hypotension (α blockade) May cause dysphoria
Edrophonium (Tensilon)	Cholinesterase inhibitor	IV: 0.5-1 mg/kg	Onset: 1-5 min Duration: 60 min M = liver (30%) E = kidney (70%) $T_{1/2}\beta$ = 1.8 hr	Less muscarinic side effects than longer acting cholinesterase inhibitors Duration of action similar to neostigmine but less than pyridostigmine

*See p. 664 for infusion preparation.

Drug	Class	Dose	Pharmacokinetics	Comments
Epinephrine (Adrenalin)*	Inotrope	IV: 0.1-1 µg/kg/min continuous infusion or 10 µg/kg IV bolus PRN *Cardiac arrest:* 50 µg/kg IV of 1:10,000 solution (100 µg/ml)	Onset: rapid IV Duration: 10 min IV M = liver, nerve terminals E = kidney, liver	Natural catecholamine with α_1, β_1, β_2 adrenergic activity Side effects include dysrhythmias, hypertension, tachycardia, nausea, vomiting, and necrosis at site of repeated injection May be given via endotracheal tube Pediatric infusion dose is ten times usual adult infusion
Erythromycin (numerous)	Antibiotic	*Children:* IV: 10-20 mg/kg/day divided q6h (slow infusion) PO: 30-50 mg/kg/day divided q6-8h *Rheumatic Fever Prophylaxis:* PO: 500 mg/day divided q12h	M = liver E = kidney $T_{1/2}\beta$ = 1.4 hr	Effective against *Legionella, Mycoplasma, Streptococci* and *Neisseria gonorrhea* GI side effects common Avoid IM (pain/necrosis) Use with caution in liver disease (cholestatic hepatitis) May increase digoxin, theophylline, and carbamazepine levels Indicated for penicillin allergic patients
Esmolol (Brevibloc)	Beta blocker	*Load* (extrapolated from adult doses): IV: 500 µg/kg over 1 min, may repeat after infusion started if response inadequate *Infusion:* IV: 50-200 µg/kg/min	Onset: rapid IV M = blood esterases E = kidney $T_{1/2}\beta$ = 9 min	β_1 selective β-blocker Drug must be diluted to a concentration of <10 mg/ml to avoid venous irritation Side effects include bradycardia, hypotention and *rarely* sedation, confusion and bronchospasm

*See p. 665 for infusion preparation.

Continued.

Drug	Class	Dose	Pharmacokinetics	Comments
Etidocaine (Duranest)	Local amide anesthetic	Infiltration: 4 mg/kg	Onset: slow Duration: 2-4 hr (infiltration) M = liver E = kidney $T_{1/2}\beta$ = 6 hr	Resembles lidocaine but is 50× more lipid soluble and lasts 2-3× longer Toxic levels = 2 μg/ml Indicated for local infiltration, peripheral nerve block and epidural anesthesia
Etomidate (Amidate)	Nonbarbiturate induction agent	*Induction of anesthesia:* IV: 0.3 mg/kg (children >10 yr)	Onset: 30 sec Duration: 3-12 min M = liver E = kidney $T_{1/2}\beta$ = 2.5 hr	Awakening more rapid than with thiopental Causes less hemodynamic depression than barbiturates Side effects include pain on injection, myoclonus, and adrenocortical suppression
Fentanyl (Sublimaze)	Opioid	*Analgesia:* IV: 1-2 μg/kg initial dose *As the sole agent for cardiovascular surgery:* IV: 50-75 μg/kg	Onset: 1-2 min Peak: 10 min Duration: 20-30 min M = hepatic (85%) E = kidney $T_{1/2}\beta$ = 2-4 hr	Synthetic opioid that is 75-125 times more potent than morphine Side effects include bradycardia, respiratory depression and truncal rigidity
Flumazenil (Romazicon)	Benzodiazepine antagonist	8-15 μg/kg titrated to desired effect	M = liver E = liver $T_{1/2}\beta$ = 41-79 min onset: <2 min	Half-life may be shorter than half-life of benzodiazepine being reversed

Drug	Class	Dose	Pharmacokinetics	Comments
Furosemide (Lasix)	Diuretic	PO: 2 mg/kg q6-8h IV: 1 mg/kg q12h IM: 1 mg/kg q12h May increase dose by 1 mg/kg with maximum single dose 6 mg/kg	Onset: IV: 2-10 min IM: 5-30 min PO: 30-60 min Duration: IV: 2 hr PO: 6-8 hr M = minimal E = kidney $T_{1/2}\beta$ = 1 hr	Side effects include ototoxicity, hypokalemia, alkalosis, increased urinary calcium excretion, and volume depletion
Gentamicin	Antibiotic Aminoglycoside	*Neonate:* under 2000 g <30 wk: 2.5 mg/kg/day divided q24h IV/IM 30-34 wks: 2.5 mg/kg/day divided q18h IV/IM >34 wks: 2.5 mg/kg/day divided q12h IV/IM over 2000 gm <7 days: 2.5 mg/kg/day divided q12h IV/IM >7 days: 2.5 mg/kg/day divided q8h IV/IM *Children:* IV/IM: 5-7 mg/kg/day divided q8h	M = liver (40%) E = kidney $T_{1/2}\beta$ = 2-3 hr (nonneonates)	See amikacin Therapeutic levels peak = 6-10 mg/L trough = <2 mg/L Adjust dose with renal dysfunction Give intrathecally for CNS infections

Continued.

Drug	Class	Dose	Pharmacokinetics	Comments
Glycopyrrolate (Robinul)	Anticholinergic	IV: 5-10 µg/kg IM: 10 µg/kg	Onset: Rapid IV M = minimal E = probably kidney	Primarily indicated as an antisialagogue and in conjunction with neostigmine and pyridostigmine for reversal of neuromuscular blockade Poorly lipid-soluble and doesn't cross BBB well
Heparin sodium	Anticoagulant	IV: 50 units/kg bolus For cardiac bypass: 300-400 units/kg (3-4 mg/kg) *Maintenance:* IV: 10-25 units/kg/hr as continuous infusion or 100 units/kg q4h	Onset: immediate Duration: 2-6 hr M = liver E = kidney $T_{1/2}\beta$ = 1-2 hr	Potency of commercial preparations range from 140-190 units/mg Acts by accelerating Antithrombin III neutralization of activated clotting factors Follow drug effect with PTT and/or ACT Contraindicated in patients with known bleeding tendencies or who are to undergo intraocular or intracranial procedures Side effects include hemorrhage, thrombocytopenia, allergic reactions, and altered protein binding (displacement of basic drugs)

Drug	Class	Dose	Pharmacokinetics	Comments
Hydralazine (Apresoline)	Antihypertensive	*Hypertensive crisis:* IV/IM: 0.1-0.5 mg/kg q4-6h *Chronic hypertension:* PO = 0.75-3 mg/kg/day divided q6-12h	Onset: IV: 2.5-20 min IM: 10-30 min PO: 20-30 min M = liver E = kidney $T_{1/2}\beta$ = 2-4 hr	Acts by direct smooth muscle dilatation (arterioles > venules) May cause SLE and arthritis-like syndrome May cause enhanced defluorination of enflurane Reflex tachycardia is common
Hydrochlorothiazide (HydroDIURIL)	Diuretic	PO: 2-3 mg/kg/day divided q12h	E = kidney	Side effects include hyperbilirubinemia, hypokalemia, alkalosis, hyperuricemia, hyperglycemia, and hyponatremia
Hydrocortisone (Solu-Cortef)	Corticosteroid	*Physiologic replacement:* 10-14 mg/m²/day IM/IV *Stress dose:* 4-8 mg/kg/day in 3 divided doses or 2-4 × physiologic replacement IV *Acute adrenal insufficiency* 1-2 mg/kg/dose bolus, then 25-200 mg/day in divided doses IV *Status asthmaticus:* Load: 4-8 mg/kg IV Maintenance: 8 mg/kg/day divided q6h IV	Duration: 4-6 hr M = liver E = kidney $T_{1/2}\beta$ = 1-2 hr	Side effects include psychosis, GI ulceration, impaired wound healing, adrenal suppression, hyperglycemia, water retention, hypernatremia, hypokalemia, and myopathy Appropriate for sole replacement in adrenocortical insufficiency

Continued.

Drug	Class	Dose	Pharmacokinetics	Comments
Hydroxyzine (Atarax/Vistaril)	Antihistamine	IM: 0.5-1 mg/kg q4-6h PO: 2 mg/kg/day divided q6h	Onset: 15-20 min PO Duration: 4-6 hr PO M = liver E = kidney, liver $T_{1/2}\beta$ = 3 hr	Same indications as for diphenhydramine Minimal cardiorespiratory depression IV injection can cause thrombosis, hemolysis; arterial injection can cause necrosis
Ibuprofen (Motrin)	Analgesic	10 mg/kg PO max: 40 mg/kg/day	M = liver E = renal $T_{1/2}\beta$ = 3.5-7 hr	Used with caution in asthmatics and those with aspirin allergy or nasal polyps
Insulin—regular	Insulin	Diabetic ketoacidosis: Load: 0.1 unit/kg IV bolus to saturate insulin receptors Infusion: 0.1 unit/kg/hr	Onset: 30-60 min Peak: 2-5 hr Duration: 5-8 hr	Rapid onset and short duration
Insulin— semi-lente	Insulin	As indicated SC, never IV	Onset: 30-90 min Peak: 5-10 hr Duration: 12-16 hr	Rapid onset and short duration
Insulin—lente	Insulin	As indicated SC, never IV	Onset: 1-2.5 hr Peak: 7-15 hr Duration: 24 hr	30% semi-lente + 70% ultralente Intermediate onset and duration
Insulin—NPH	Insulin	As indicated SC, never IV	Onset: 1-2 hr Peak: 6-12 hr Duration: 18-24 hr	Intermediate onset and intermediate duration Human NPH may be more potent and shorter acting than pork-derived NPH

Drug	Class	Dose	Pharmacokinetics	Comments
Insulin—protamine zinc (PZI)	Insulin	As indicated SC, never IV	Onset: 4-8 hr Peak: 14-24 hr Duration: 36 hr	Delayed onset, long duration
Insulin—ultra-lente	Insulin	As indicated SC, never IV	Onset: 4-8 hr Peak: 10-30 hr Duration: 36+ hr	Delayed onset and long duration
Isoetharine (Bronkosol)	Bronchodilator	*Inhaler:* 1-2 puffs q3-4h *Nebulizer:* 0.25-0.5 ml 1% solution diluted to 2 ml with NSS q4h	Peak effect: 15-60 min Duration: 2-4 hr	See albuterol
Isoproterenol (Isuprel)*	Bronchodilator/inotrope	*Inhaler:* 1-2 puffs q3-4h *Nebulizer:* 0.01 ml/kg diluted to 2 ml with NSS q4h Maximum dose = 0.05 ml/dose *Inotrope/Chronotrope/Severe Bronchospasm:* IV: 0.1-1 µg/kg/min continuous infusion	Onset: IV: rapid Inhaled: 2-5 min Duration: IV:1-2 min Inhaled: 1-3 hr M = liver, nerve endings E = kidney, liver	Synthetic catecholamine that is the most potent activator of β_1 and β_2 adrenergic receptors Indicated as an inhaler to produce bronchodilation, to increase the heart rate in complete heart block and to decrease pulmonary resistance IV infusion for severe refractory bronchospasm or circulatory support Side effects include dysrhythmias and hypertension (especially with epinephrine) Tachyphylaxis is common

*See p. 665 for infusion preparation.

Continued.

Drug	Class	Dose	Pharmacokinetics	Comments
Kanamycin (Kantrex)	Antibiotic Aminoglycoside	*Neonate:* under 2000 gm <7 days: 15 mg/kg/day divided q12h IV/IM >7 days: 20 mg/kg/day divided q12h IV/IM over 2000 gm <7 days: 20 mg/kg/day divided q12h IV/IM >7 days: 30 mg/kg/day divided q8h IV/IM *Infant/child:* IV/IM: 15-30 mg/kg/day divided q8-12h *Suppression of bacterial flora* PO = 50-100 mg/kg/day divided q6h	E = kidney $T_{1/2}\beta$ = 2-3 hr	See amikacin Used to suppress intestinal flora prior to GI surgery Therapeutic levels: peak = 15-30 mg/L trough = 5-10 mg/L
Ketamine (Ketalar)	Nonbarbiturate induction agent	*Induction:* IV: 1-3 mg/kg IM: 5-10 mg/kg PO: 6 mg/kg *Analgesia:* IV: 0.2-0.5 mg/kg	Onset: IV: 30-60 sec IM: 3-5 min PO: 30 min Duration: IV: 5-10 min IM: 10-20 min M = liver E = kidneys, liver $T_{1/2}\beta$ = 2.5 hr	Produces a "dissociative" state as well as profound analgesia, bronchodilation Side effects include tachycardia, hypertension, salivation, elevated intracranial pressure, prolongation of non-depolarizing muscle relaxants, and emergence delirium Emergence delirium is diminished by prior administration of barbiturates and benzodiazepines, not by recovery in a quiet room

Drug	Class	Dose	Pharmacokinetics	Comments
Ketorolac (Toradol)	Analgesic	0.5 mg/kg IV; max 4 mg/kg/day	M = liver E = renal $T_{1/2}\beta$ = 3.5-6.5 hr	Used with caution in asthmatics and those with aspirin allergy or nasal polyps
Levothyroxine (Synthroid)	Thyroid preparation	*Neonates:* PO: 25-50 μg/day IV: 20-40 μg/day *<1 year:* PO: 50-75 μg/day IV: 40 μg/day *Children:* PO: 3-5 μg/kg/day IV: 75% PO dose	M = liver	Levothyroxine 100 mg = thyroid 65 mg Titrate dose to serum free T_4 and thyroid stimulating hormone levels Increases catabolism of vitamin K-dependent factors
Lidocaine (Xylocaine)*	Amide local anesthetic	*Local anesthesia:* Maximal safe dose: 5 mg/kg With epinephrine: 7 mg/kg	M = liver E = kidney Duration: 60-120 min	Extensive metabolism results in plasma clearance being proportional to hepatic blood flow Monoethylglycinexylide metabolite has 80% of parent drug's activity against arrhythmias
	Antiarrhythmic	*Ventricular dysrrhythmias:* Bolus = 1 mg/kg IV, may repeat q5-10 min to maximum dose of 3-5 mg/kg Infusion = 30-50 μg/kg/min	Onset: immediate M = liver E = kidney (10% unchanged) $T_{1/2}\beta$ = 1.5 hr	Indicated for ventricular dysrhythmias Contraindicated in WPW syndrome, amide-type drug hypersensitivity, and severe SA, AV, or intraventricular block in the absence of a pacemaker Therapeutic levels 1-5 μg/ml Toxicity occurs at levels >7 μg/ml

*See p. 665 for infusion preparation.

Continued.

Drug	Class	Dose	Pharmacokinetics	Comments
Lorazepam (Ativan)	Benzodi-azepine	*Sedation:* IV = 0.03-0.05 mg/kg q6h PRN PO = .05 mg/kg > age 6	Onset: IV: 5-20 min Duration: IV: 10 hr M = liver E = kidney $T_{1/2}\beta$ = 10-20 hr	Long $t_{1/2}\beta$ makes it less attractive than other benzodiazepines for preoperative sedation May cause mild respiratory depression and paradoxical excitation Has some antiemetic properties Hallucinations reported in children <6 yr
Meperidine (Demerol)	Opioid	*Premedication:* IM: 1-2 mg/kg *Analgesia:* IV/IM/PO/SC: 1-1.5 mg/kg q3-4h	Onset: IV: 5 min IM/SC: 10 min PO: 15 min Duration: 2-4 hr M = liver 95% E = kidney $T_{1/2}\beta$ = 1.5-4 hr	Synthetic opioid with $\frac{1}{10}$ the activity of morphine Major metabolite normeperidine is active and has an elimination half-life of 15-40 hr (CNS stimulant) Side effects include orthostatic hypotension, negative inotropy, seizures, and respiratory depression Tachycardia and mydriasis reflect atropine-like activity
Mepivacaine (Carbocaine)	Amide local anesthetic	Maximal dose: 5-6 mg/kg	M = liver E = kidney $T_{1/2}\beta$ = 2 hr Duration: 90-180 min	Similar to lidocaine but lacks vasodilator activity and is a better choice when addition of epinephrine is undesirable Toxic levels = >5 mg/ml

Drug	Class	Dose	Pharmacokinetics	Comments
Metaproterenol (Alupent)	Bronchodilator	*Inhaler:* 1-2 puffs q3-4h *Nebulizer:* 0.2-0.3 ml of 5% solution in 2-5 ml NSS q4-6h	Peak Effect: 30-60 min Duration: 3-4 hr	See albuterol May repeat q1h for severe bronchospasm with careful monitoring
Methicillin (Staphcillin)	Antibiotic Penicillin	*Neonate:* 0-7 days 50-100 mg/kg/day divided q12h IV/IM >7 days 100-200 mg/kg/day divided q6-8h IV/IM *Child:* IV/IM = 100-400 mg/kg/day divided q4-6h	E = kidney	Contains 2.5 mEq Na$^+$/gram Very effective against *S. aureus* Poor PO absorption
Methimazole (Tapazole)	Antithyroid preparation	*Child:* Initial dose: 0.4-0.7 mg/kg/day divided q8h *Maintenance:* 50% initial daily dose divided q8h once euthyroid	Onset: days to weeks Duration: 8-12 hr E = kidney $T_{1/2}\beta$ = 6-13 hr	Inhibits iodine incorporation into thyroglobin Only available as PO form Improvement usually seen in 1-2 days Side effects include urticarial rash, pruritis, and granulocytopenia
Methohexital (Brevital)	Barbiturate	*Induction:* PR: 20-30 mg/kg of 10% solution IM: 10 mg/kg of 5% solution IV: 1-2 mg/kg of 1% solution	Onset: IV: Rapid PR: 5-10 min M = liver E = kidney $T_{1/2}\beta$ = 1-2 hr	Psychomotor recovery is more rapid than thiopental after repeated doses due to greater hepatic clearance Side effects include involuntary muscle movements, hiccoughs, mild cardiovascular depression Intraarterial injection can cause necrosis Avoid in porphyria

Continued.

Drug	Class	Dose	Pharmacokinetics	Comments
Methyldopa (Aldomet)	Antihypertensive	PO = 10 mg/kg/day divided q6-12h Maximum dose = the lesser of 65 mg/kg or 3 mg/day *Hypertensive Crisis:* IV: 20-40 mg/kg/day divided q6h	Onset: IV: 1-2 hr PO: 4-6 hr M = liver E = kidney $T_{1/2}\beta$ = 2 hr	Converted to α-methylnorepinephrine which inhibits central α-adrenergic receptors Side effects include sedation, liver dysfunction, positive direct Coomb's test, and rebound hypertension
Methylprednisolone (Solu-Medrol)	Corticosteroid	*Immunosuppression:* PO = 0.4-1.6 mg/kg/day divided q6-12h *Status asthmaticus:* Load: 1-2 mg/kg IV *Maintenance:* 1.6 mg/kg/day divided q6h IV	Duration: 12-36 hr $T_{1/2}\beta$ = 2-4 hr	Preferred over prednisone in liver disease or methylation may be impaired Glucocorticoid activity 5 × hydrocortisone but little mineralocorticoid activity
Metoclopramide (Reglan)	Gastric motility stimulant	*Gastric Dysmotility:* 1-6 yr: 0.1 mg/kg q6h PO/IV 6-12 hr: 3-9 mg q6h PO/IV *Antiemetic:* IV: 1-2 mg/kg q2-6h	Onset: peak PO levels in 40-120 min M = liver E = kidney $T_{1/2}\beta$ = 2-4 hr	Dopamine antagonist; increases esophageal sphincter tone, stimulates small bowel motility, acts as an anti-emetic Contraindicated in pheochromocytoma, GI obstruction, and in patients with extrapyramidal symptoms or those receiving phenothiazines, butyrophenones, MAO inhibitors or tricyclic antidepressants Side effects include sedation, dry mouth, dysphoria, and extrapyramidal reactions Decrease dose in renal failure

Drug	Class	Dose	Pharmacokinetics	Comments
Mezlocillin (Mezlin)	Antibiotic Penicillin	Moderate infection: IV, IM: 50-100 mg/kg/day divided q6h Severe infection: IV, IM: 200-300 mg/kg/day divided q6h	E = kidney $T_{1/2}\beta$ = 1.5 hr	Contains approximately 2 mEq Na^+ per gram Active against *Klebsiella* and *Pseudomonas*
Metronidazole (Flagyl)	Antibiotic	*Initial dose:* Neonate = 15 mg/kg IV Child = 15 mg/kg IV *Maintenance:* Neonate: <7 days = 7.5 mg/kg divided q12h IV >7 days = 7.5 mg/kg divided q8h IV Children = 7.5 mg/kg divided q6h IV	M = liver E = kidney	Effective against anaerobic organisms Potentiates anticoagulants and causes disulfuram-type reaction with alcohol Side effects include nausea, diarrhea, leukopenia and vertigo Infuse over 1 hr Good CNS penetration
Midazolam (Versed)	Benzodi-azepine	*Sedation:* IM = 0.07-0.08 mg/kg IV = 0.03 mg/kg IN = 0.2 mg/kg *Induction of anesthesia:* IV = 0.2-0.3 mg/kg	Onset: IV: 3-5 min IM: 15-30 min IN: 5-10 min Duration: IV: <2 hr IM: 2 hr M = liver E = kidney $T_{1/2}\beta$ = 1-4 hr	Water soluble so less pain on IM injection 2-3 times more potent than diazepam

Continued.

Drug	Class	Dose	Pharmacokinetics	Comments
Mivacurium (Mivacron)	Nondepolarizing muscle relaxant	*Intubating:* 0.2 mg/kg over 5-15 sec *Continuous infusion:* 10-14 µ/kg/min	M = plasma cholinesterase E = renal $T_{1/2}\beta$ = 2 min	Continuous infusion requires titration to effect with neuromuscular twitch monitor Dose requirements are higher in the pediatric population
Morphine sulfate	Opioid	*Premedication:* IM: 0.1-0.2 mg/kg *Analgesia:* IV/IM/SC: 0.1-0.2 mg/kg q2-4h	Onset: IV: 5-10 min IM: 30-60 min SC: 30-90 min Duration: 4-6 hr M = liver E = kidney $T_{1/2}\beta$ = 2-4 hr	Side effects include orthostatic hypotension due to histamine release, bradycardia, respiratory depression, miosis, nausea, vomiting, and biliary spasm Useful in treatment of cyanotic spells in tetralogy of Fallot
Nafcillin (Unipen)	Antibiotic Penicillin	*Neonate:* 0-7 days: 40 mg/kg/day divided q12h IV/IM >7 days: 60 mg/kg/day divided q6-8h IV/IM *Child:* IV: 100-200 mg/kg/day divided q4h IM: 100-200 mg/kg/day divided q12h PO: 50-100 mg/kg/day divided q6h	M = liver (90%) E = kidney	See Methicillin Poor PO absorption Causes more vein irritation than oxacillin

Drug	Class	Dose	Pharmacokinetics	Comments
Neomycin	Antibiotic Aminoglyco-side	*Neonate:* PO: 50 mg/kg/day divided q6h *Infant/child:* PO: 50-100 mg/kg/day divided q6h *Hepatic encephalopathy:* Acute: 2.5-7 g/m^2/day divided q6h × 5-7 days PO Chronic: 2.5 g/m^2/day divided q6h PO *Bowel prep:* PO: 90 mg/kg/day divided q4h × 3 days	E = GI tract (PO drug does not undergo systemic absorption)	Indicated to decrease intestinal flora prior to intestinal surgery and to manage hepatic encephalopathy
Naloxone (Narcan)	Narcotic antagonist	IV/IM: 5-10 μg/kg, repeat q3-5min PRN	Onset: IV: 1-2 min IM: 2-5 min Duration: IV: 60 min IM: 1-4 hr M = liver E = kidney $t_{1/2}\beta$ = 1-1.5 hr (adult); 3 hr (neonate)	Side effects include nausea, vomiting, tachycardia, hypertension, and pulmonary edema May need 100-200 μg/kg for large narcotic overdoses followed by a continuous infusion of 1-2 μg/kg/hr, especially if long acting narcotic was given

Continued.

Drug	Class	Dose	Pharmacokinetics	Comments
Neostigmine (Prostigmine)	Cholinesterase inhibitor	IV: 0.05–0.07 mg/kg	Onset: 1–5 min Duration: 60 min M = liver (50%) E = kidney (50%) $t_{1/2}\beta$ = 1.3 hr	Duration more similar to glycopyrrolate than atropine
Nifedipine (Procardia)	Calcium channel blocker	PO: 0.25–0.5 mg/kg q6–8h SL: 0.25–0.5 mg/kg q6–8h	Onset: 15–30 min PO M = liver E = liver/kidney $t_{1/2}\beta$ = 4–5 hr	Side effects include hypotension, tachycardia, and syncope Little effect on automaticity
Nitroglycerin	Vasodilator	IV: 0.5–20 µg/kg/min continuous infusion	Onset: 1–2 min IV Duration: 10 min IV M = smooth muscle, liver $t_{1/2}\beta$ = 2 min	Acts primarily on venous capacitance vessels but at higher doses has effects on systemic resistance vessels Side effects include headache, flushing, hypotension, reflex tachycardia and methemoglobinemia
Norepinephrine (Levophed)	Inotrope	IV: 0.1–1.0 µg/kg/min continuous infusion, increase as required	Onset: rapid IV Duration: 1–2 min IV M = liver, nerve terminals E = kidneys (minimal)	Natural catecholamine with primarily α activity (some β_1) Indicated for hypotension due to low SVR states (septic shock) Side effects include hypertension, reflex bradycardia and skin sloughing after extravasation

Drug	Class	Dose	Pharmacokinetics	Comments
Oxacillin (Prostaphlin)	Antibiotic Penicillin	*Neonate:* IV or IM >7 days: 100-200 mg/kg/day divided q8h *Child:* PO PO: 50-100 mg/kg/day divided q6h	E = kidney, liver $t_{1/2}\beta$ = 1 hour	Good staphlococcal coverage Hepatitis can occur with high doses Well-absorbed PO
Pancuronium (Pavulon)	Nondepolarizing muscle relaxant	*Intubation:* IV: 0.07-0.1 mg/kg *Maintenance:* IV: 0.05 mg/kg	Onset: 1-3 min Duration: 35-55 min M = liver (minimal) E = kidney 80% liver 20% $t_{1/2}\beta$ = 1-2 hr	Neonates and infants are more sensitive to drug effects Tachycardia occurs and is due to blockade of cardiac muscurinic receptors and vagolysis
Penicillin G	Antibiotic Penicillin	*Neonate:* IV or IM 0-7 days: 50-100,000 unit/kg/day divided q12h >7 days: 100-250,000 unit/kg/day divided q8h *Child:* IV/IM: 25-500,000 unit/kg/day divided q4-6h PO: 40-80,000 unit/kg/day divided q6h (125 mg = 200,000 u for all PCN)	E = kidney $t_{1/2}\beta$ = 1 hr	Na^+ salt: 1 million units contains 1.68 mEq Na^+ K^+ salt: 1 million units contains 1.68 mEq K^+ Side effects include skin rash, anaphylaxis, and serum sickness

Continued.

Drug	Class	Dose	Pharmacokinetics	Comments
Pentobarbital (Nembutal)	Barbiturate	*Premedication:* IM/PO: 3-5 mg/kg, maximum 100 mg	Onset: IM: 10-30 min PO: 30-60 min M = liver E = kidney $t_{1/2}\beta$ = 20-50 hr	Paradoxical excitation may occur in presence of pain IM injection painful Avoid in porphyria
Phenobarbital (Luminal)	Barbiturate	*Sedation:* IM: 2-3 mg/kg divided q8h PO: 2-3 mg/kg divded q8h *Status epilepticus:* IV: 15-25 mg/kg no faster than 30 mg/min *Maintenance:* PO: 4-6 mg/kg/day divided q12h	Onset: 2-3 hr PO M = liver microsomes E = kidney $t_{1/2}\beta$ = 96 hr	Indicated for grand mal and focal epilepsy as well as for prophylaxis against the recurrence of febrile seizures Paradoxical reaction may occur in children resulting in agitation and hyperactivity Contraindicated in porphyria Stimulates hepatic microsomes Therapeutic levels 10-20 µg/ml
Phenylephrine (Neosynephrine)	Vasoconstrictor	IV = 0.1-1 µg/kg/min continuous infusion or 10 µg/kg IV bolus PRN	Onset: rapid IV Duration: IV: 5-20 min M = liver, intestine	Synthetic catecholamine that acts primarily on α_1 receptors to increase SVR May cause carotid reflex-mediated bradycardia Useful in treatment of cyanotic spells in tetralogy of Fallot

Drug	Class	Dose	Pharmacokinetics	Comments
Phenytoin (Dilantin)	Anticonvulsant	*Status epilepticus:* IV: 15-25 mg/kg no faster than 50 mg/min *Maintenance:* 4-7 mg/kg/day divided q12-24h IV/PO *Antiarrhythmic:* IV: 2-4 mg/kg over 5 min PO: 2-5 mg/kg/day	Onset: IV: 3-5 min PO: slow M = 98% liver (metabolites inactive) E = kidney $t_{1/2}\beta$ = 7-42 hr	Indicated for control of all types of seizure disorders (except petit mal) as well as ventricular and digitalis-induced dysrhythmias Side effects include nystagmus, ataxia, diplopia, vertigo, allergic reactions, peripheral neuropathy, and gingival hyperplasia Therapeutic drug levels 10-20 µg/ml Above plasma levels of 10 µg/ml elimination follows zero-order kinetics 90% protein bound; increased free level in patients with low albumin
Potassium iodide	Antithyroid preparation	*Thyrotoxicosis:* Child: 200-300 mg/day PO divided q8-12h	E = kidney	Indicated for preoperative preparation before thyroidectomy for hyperthyroidism as well as in treatment of thyrotoxicosis Inhibits thyroid hormone formation and release Effects can be seen in 24 hr Side effects include angioedema, laryngeal edema, nausea, vomiting, rash, rhinitis SSKI contains 1 gm of KI in 1 ml

Continued.

Drug	Class	Dose	Pharmacokinetics	Comments
Prednisone	Corticosteroid	*Physiologic replacement:* PO = 4-5 mg/m²/day divided q12h *Stress dose:* 2-4 x physiologic replacement *Asthma:* Acute: 0.5-1.0 mg/kg/day PO up 20-40 mg/day × 3-5 days *Antiinflammatory:* 0.5-2 mg/kg/day PO divided q6-12h	Duration = 18-36 hr $t_{1/2}\beta$ = 1-1.5 hr	Glucocorticoid activity 4 × hydrocortisone; slightly less mineralocorticoid activity than hydrocortisone Appropriate for sole replacement in adrenal insufficiency
Procainamide (Pronestyl)	Antiarrhythmic	*Loading dose:* IV: 2-5 mg/kg over 30 min *Maintenance:* IV: 20-80 µg/kg/min continuous infusion Maximum dose = 50-60 mg/kg/day	Onset: IV: <5 min M = liver, plasma E = kidney $t_{1/2}\beta$ = 2.5-5 hr (active metabolites 6 hr)	Indicated for ventricular and atrial dysrhythmias Contraindicated in myasthenia gravis and complete heart block Hepatic acetylation yields NAPA, an active metabolite that is renally excreted Side effects include hypotension, lupus-like syndrome, asystole and thrombocytopenia Therapeutic levels 4-12 µg/ml and likelihood of toxicity increases at >8 µg/ml and is indicated by QRS >0.2 msec

Drug	Class	Dose	Pharmacokinetics	Comments
Prochlorperazine (Compazine)	Phenothiazine	PO: 0.4 mg/kg/day divided q6-8h PR: 0.4 mg/kg/day divided q6-8h IM: 0.2 mg/kg/day divided q6-8h	Onset: PO: 30-40 min IM: 10-20 min PR: 60 min Duration: IM/PR: 3-4 hr M = liver E = kidney $t_{1/2}\beta$ = 10-20 hr	Indicated for postoperative nausea and vomiting Side effects and cautions regarding use are similar to chlorpromazine Do not use in children <10 kg or under 2 yr
Promethazine (Phenergan)	Antihistamine	*Sedation:* IM: 0.5-1 mg/kg q6h PRN *Antiemetic:* IM/PO/PR/ 0.25-0.5 mg/kg q4-6h PRN *Antihistamine:* PO = 0.1 mg/kg q6h	Onset: IV: 3-5 min IM/PO: 20 min M = liver E = kidney, liver $t_{1/2}\beta$ = 4.4-7 hr	Same indications as for diphenhydramine Low incidence of extrapyramidal reactions

Continued.

Drug	Class	Dose	Pharmacokinetics	Comments
Propranolol (Inderal)	Beta blocker	*Arrhythmias:* IV: 0.01-0.1 mg/kg slow IV push; may repeat q5-10 min PRN *Maintenance:* PO: 0.5-4 mg/kg/day divided q6-8h Maximum daily dose 60 mg *Hypertension:* PO: 0.5-1.0 mg/kg/day divided q6-12h Maximum daily dose 2 mg/kg/day *Tetralogy spells:* IV: 0.15-0.25 mg/kg slowly; may repeat × 1 after 15 min PO: 1-2 mg/kg divided q6h	Onset: IV: 2 min PO: 20 min M = liver E = kidney $t_{1/2}\beta$ = 2-6 hr	Non-selective β-blocker Contraindicted in asthma and advanced heart block Use cautiously in CHF, diabetes mellitus and with hepatic and renal disease Extensive hepatic first pass effect 4-OH propranolol metabolite is active
Propofol (Diprivan)	Nonbarbiturate induction agent	*Induction:* 2.5-3.5 mg/kg *Continuous infusion:* 50-200 µg/kg/min	$t_{1/2}\alpha$ = 7-9 min $t_{1/2}\beta$ = 250-400 min	Requires strict aseptic technique Pharmacokinetics are *not* altered by chronic cirrhosis/renal failure

Drug	Class	Dose	Pharmacokinetics	Comments
Propylthiouracil (PTU)	Antithyroid preparation	*Child:* 0-10 yr: 50-150 mg/day PO divided q8h >10 yr: 150-300 mg/day PO divided q8h Maintenance: 30-50% initial daily dose divided q8h	Onset: days to weeks Duration: 2-3 hr E = kidney $t_{1/2}\beta = 2$ hr	Blocks thyroid hormone synthesis as well as peripheral conversion of T_4 to T_3 100 mg PTU = 10 mg methimazole *Not available in parenteral form* Side effects rare and include rash and granulocytopenia
Protamine sulfate	Heparin antagonist	IV = According to heparin dose-response curve or give 1-1.3 mg for every 100 units of heparin given in previous 2 hr	Onset: 5 min Duration: 2 hr	Binds with heparin to form an inactive complex Can cause myocardial depression and peripheral vasodilation with resultant sudden hypotension or bradycardia Allergic reactions are more common in patients with fish allergy and those on protamine zinc insulin
Pyridostigmine (Regonal, Mestinon)	Cholinesterase inhibitor	IV: 0.25 mg/kg	Onset: 2-5 min Duration: 90 min M = liver (30%) E = kidney (70%) $t_{1/2}\beta = 1.9$ hr	See neostigmine

Continued.

Drug	Class	Dose	Pharmacokinetics	Comments
Ranitidine (Zantac)	H₂ receptor antagonist	PO: 2-4 mg/kg/day divided q12h IV: 1-2 mg/kg/day divided q6-8h	Onset: PO: 30-60 min Duration: IV/PO: 8-12 hr M = liver E = kidney (50% unchanged) $t_{1/2}\beta$ = 2-3 hr	Fewer androgenic effects than cimetidine
Ribavirin (Virazole)	Antiviral	*Aerosol:* Dilute 6 g vial in 300 ml (20 mg/ml) Administer by aerosol 12-18 hr/day × 3-7 days		Treatment for severe lower respiratory RSV (respiratory syncytial virus) infection Particles may obstruct ventilator
Scopolamine	Anticholinergic	IV: 5-10 µg/kg IM: 10 µg/kg	Onset: Rapid IV E = kidney	Indicated for preoperative sedation and antisialagogue activity Crosses BBB
Secobarbital (Seconal)	Barbiturate	*Premedication:* IM/PO: 3-5 mg/kg	Onset: IM: 7-10 min PO: 15-30 min M = liver E = kidney $t_{1/2}\beta$ = 20-28 hr	See pentobarbital

Drug	Class	Dose	Pharmacokinetics	Comments
Sodium nitroprus-side (Nipride)*	Vasodilator	IV: 0.5-10 µg/kg/min continuous infusion	Onset: rapid IV Duration: 1-10 min IV M = RBC and liver (thiocyanate) E = kidney	Smooth muscle dilator affecting primarily resistance vessels Absolutely contraindicated in Leber's hereditary optic atrophy and tobacco amblyopia, avoid with B$_{12}$ deficiency and severe liver or renal disease Side effects include hypotension, reflex tachycardia, and cyanide toxicty
Spironolactone (Aldactone)	Diuretic	PO: 1-3 mg/kg/day divided q6-12h	E = kidney	Competitive aldosterone antagonist May potentiate ganglionic blocking agents and other antihypertensives Side effects include hyperkalemia, nausea and vomiting
Streptomycin	Antibiotic Aminoglycosides	*Neonate:* IM: 20-30 mg/kg/day divided q12h × up to 10 days *Child:* IM: 20-40 mg/kg/day divided q8h × up to 10 days *Tuberculosis:* IM: 20-50 mg/kg × 1 dose (use higher dose for TB meningitis)	M = liver E = kidney $t_{1/2}\beta$ = 2-3 hr	See amikacin Need to follow with auditory tests Commonly used with other antibiotics for synergistic action against bacterial endocarditis, tularemia, and plague Rarely causes nephrotoxicity

*See p. 664 for infusion preparation.

Continued.

Drug	Class	Dose	Pharmacokinetics	Comments
Succinylcholine (Anectine)	Depolarizing muscle relaxant	IV: 1-2 mg/kg IM: 4-5 mg/kg	Onset: IV: 30-60 sec IM: 2-3 min Duration: IV: 10-15 min IM: 10-30 min M= plasma pseudo-cholinesterase E = kidney	Use upper dose limit in infants Fasciculations rare in children less than 3 yr old Pretreat with atropine 0.01 mg/kg IV or 0.02 mg/kg IM to prevent vagally mediated bradycardia Prolonged action with severe liver disease, hypothermia, treatment with antibiotics (aminoglycosides), hypothermia, hyperkalemia, and pseudo-cholinesterase deficiency
Terbutaline (Brethine)	Bronchodilator	PO: <12 yr: 0.05 mg/kg q8h up to 0.3 mg/kg/day >12 yr: 2.5 mg q8h up to 5 mg q8h SC: <12 yr: 0.005-0.01 mg/kg q15-20 min × 2 maximum dose of 0.25 mg >12 yr: 0.25 mg q15-30 min; do not exceed 0.5 mg/4 hr	Peak effect: PO: 60 min SC: 15-30 min Duration: PO: 8 hr SC: 4-6 hr	See albuterol Less β_2 selectivity with SC administration

Drug	Class	Dose	Pharmacokinetics	Comments
Tetracaine (Pontocaine)	Ester local anesthetic	Maximum safe dose: 1.5 mg/kg	M = plasma cholinesterase E = kidney Duration: 60-180 min	PABA metabolite may be an antigen resonsible for future allergic reactions
Tetracycline	Antibiotic	*Child:* PO: 25-50 mg/kg/day divided q6h IM: 15-25 mg/kg/day divided q8-12h (not to exceed 250 mg/dose)	M = liver E = biliary, kidney $t_{1/2}\beta$ = 6-9 hr	IV administration scleroses veins Broad spectrum of activity against gram positive and negative organisms Not recommended in children <8 yr due to tooth staining and impaired bone growth May cause nausea and vomiting May cause increased ICP in infants Outdated drug has been associated with a form of Fanconi's anemia
Thiopental sodium (Pentothal)	Barbiturate	*Induction:* IV: 3-5 mg/kg PR: 20-30 mg/kg	Onset: rapid IV M = liver E = kidney $t_{1/2}\beta$ = 5-10 hr	Intraarterial injection can cause necrosis Avoid in porphyria Side effects include anaphylactic/anaphylactoid reactions and histamine release
Ticarcillin (Ticar)	Antibiotic Penicillin	Moderate infection: IV/IM 50-100 mg/kg/day divided q6h Severe infection: IV/IM: 200-300 mg/kg/day divided q6h	E = kidney $t_{1/2}\beta$ = 1.5 hr	Contains >5 mEq Na$^+$ per gram Effective against *Pseudomonas*

Continued.

Drug	Class	Dose	Pharmacokinetics	Comments
Tobramycin (Nebcin)	Antibiotic Aminoglyco-side	*Neonate:* See gentamycin *Children:* IV/IM: 7.5 mg/kg/day divided q8h	M = liver (40%) E = kidney $t_{1/2}\beta$ = 2-3 hr	See amikacin
Valproic acid (Depakene, Depakote)	Anticonvulsant	PO = 10-15 mg/kg/day divided q12h Increase by 5-10 mg/kg/day q week Maximum dose = 60 mg/kg/day	Onset: peak PO levels in 1-4 hr M = 70% liver (inactive metabolites) $t_{1/2}\beta$ = 12 hr	Indicated in petit mal epilepsy Side effects include impairment of platelet aggregation, false-positive urine ketone test, hepatotoxicity, nausea and vomiting Results in increased plasma levels of phenytoin, diazepam, and phenobarbital Therapeutic levels 50-100 mg/L

Drug	Class	Dose	Pharmacokinetics	Comments
Vancomycin (Vancocin)	Antibiotic	*Neonate:* Under 1000 g: <7 days: 10 mg/kg q24h IV >7 days: 10 mg/kg q18h IV 1000-2000 g: <7 days: 10 mg/kg q18h IV >7 days: 10 mg/kg q12h IV Greater than 2000 g: <7 days: 10 mg/kg q12h IV >7 days: 10 mg/kg q8h IV *Infant/child:* IV: 30 mg/kg/day q8h (45 mg/kg for CNS infections)	E = kidney (90%) $t_{1/2}\beta$ = 6 hr	Side effects include ototoxicity and nephrotoxicity Therapeutic levels: 10-25 mg/L Drug induced rashes and hypotension caused by histamine release; must be given slowly over 1 hour Must adjust dose in renal insufficiency
Vasopressin (Pitressin)	Pituitary hormone	*Aqueous:* 0.5-3 ml/day divided q8h SC (ampule contains 20 u/ml) *Tannate in oil:* 0.25 ml Q 1-3 day IM/SC PRN (ampule contains 5 u/ml) *Nose drops:* 1-2 drops in each nostril, q4-6h PRN	Duration: Tannate: 48-96 hr SC/IM Aqueous: 2-8 hr SC/IM M = liver/kidney E = kidney $t_{1/2}\beta$ = 10-20 min	Indicated for treatment of central diabetes insipidus Side effects include nausea, vomiting, abdominal pain, tremor, sweating, urticaria, and anaphylaxis Physiologic half-life does not correlate with $t_{1/2}\beta$

Continued.

Drug	Class	Dose	Pharmacokinetics	Comments
Vecuronium (Norcuron)	Nondepolarizing muscle relaxant	*Intubation:* IV: 0.05–0.1 mg/kg	Onset: Infant—1.5 min Child—2.4 min Duration: Infant—73 min Child—35 min M = liver (80%) E = kidney (20%)	$t_{1/2}\beta$ is prolonged by liver failure when dose exceeds 0.2 mg/kg Devoid of circulatory effects except when given with high-dose narcotics, when bradycardia is sometimes seen Less renal excretion than pancuronium
Verapamil (Isoptin/Calan)	Calcium channel blocker	IV: 0.1–0.3 mg/kg not to exceed 5 mg	Onset: IV: 1–10 min PO: 15–30 min Duration: 6 hr M = liver E = liver/kidney $t_{1/2}\beta$ = 5–7 hr	Indicated for treatment of SVT Contraindicated in 2nd or 3rd degree heart block, CHF, hypotension, and right-to-left shunt Use in infants <1 yr can result in apnea, bradycardia, and hypotension
Vidarabine (Ara-A)	Antiviral	*HSV encephalitis/neonatal HSV infection:* IV: 15 mg/kg/day over 12 hr × 10 days	E = kidney	Poorly soluble in water so must be diluted in large volumes

PEDIATRIC RESUSCITATION ALGORITHMS

B

BRADYCARDIA DECISION ALGORITHM

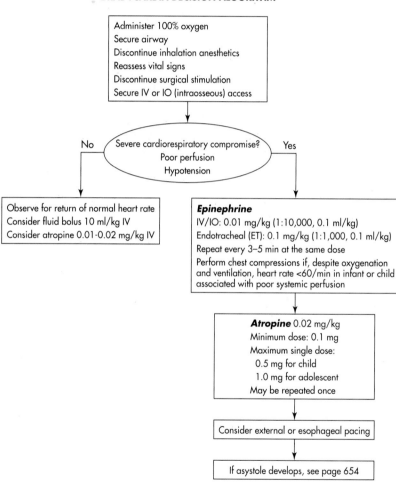

FIG. B-1. Bradycardia decision algorithm (Data from Cardiac rhythm disturbances. In Chameides L, Hazinski MF, eds: *Textbook of pediatric advanced life support,* Dallas, 1994, American Heart Association.)

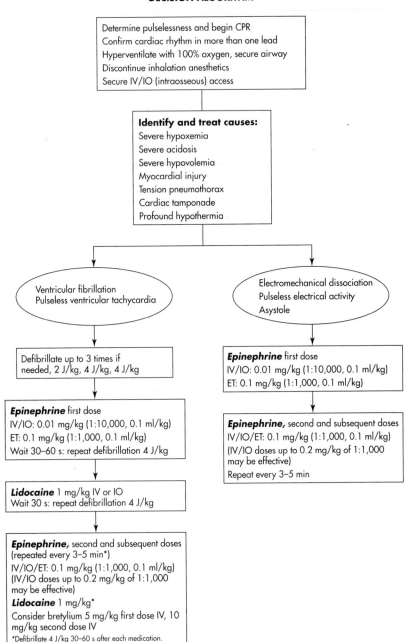

FIG. B-2. Asystole and pulseless arrest decision algorithm (Data from Cardiac rhythm disturbances. In Chameides L, Hazinski MF, eds: *Textbook of pediatric advanced life support,* Dallas, 1994, American Heart Association.)

VASCULAR ACCESS

The preferred site of vascular access remains the largest vein that can be accessed rapidly without interfering with CPR.

Vascular access

	Site	Complications	Comments

Peripheral	Upper extremity
	  Cephalic
	  Basilic
	  Median
	    cubital
	  Dorsal venous
	    arch
	Lower extremity
	  Saphenous
	  Median
	    marginal
	  Dorsal venous
	    arch
	  Scalp
		Thrombosis
		Hematoma
		Cellulitis
		Phlebitis
		Infiltration
		Compartment
		  syndrome
		Air embolus
		Catheter embolus
			Complications
			  infrequent
			Difficult to locate in
			  well-nourished
			  children or those
			  in shock, trauma,
			  or arrest
			Scalp veins are frag-
			  ile and prone to
			  infiltration

Intraosseous	Tibia
	  (anteromedial)
		Tibial fracture
		Compartment
		  syndrome
		Osteomyelitis
		Skin necrosis
		Bone embolus
		Fat embolus
			Emboli are not usu-
			  ally clinically
			  significant
			Not indicated in the
			  presence of pelvic
			  fracture or proxi-
			  mal extremity
			  fracture.
			Onset of drug effect
			  comparable to in-
			  travascular site.

Central	Femoral
	External jugular
	Subclavian
	Internal jugular
		Thrombosis
		Cellulitis
		  hematoma
		Phlebitis
		Infiltration
		Compartment
		  syndrome
		Air embolus
		Catheter embolus
		Arterial
		  cannulation
		Hemothorax
		Hydrothorax
		Pneumothorax
		Cardiac
		  tamponade
		Dysrhythmia
			Femoral vein is most
			  predictable in lo-
			  cation and course.
			Central access of
			  head and neck
			  often requires in-
			  terruption of CPR
			Hemo-, hydro-,
			  pneumo-, and
			  chylothorax more
			  common on left
			  side because of
			  higher left lung
			  apex
			Central cannulation
			  complications
			  more common
			  than in adults

EMERGENCY VASCULAR ACCESS ALGORITHM

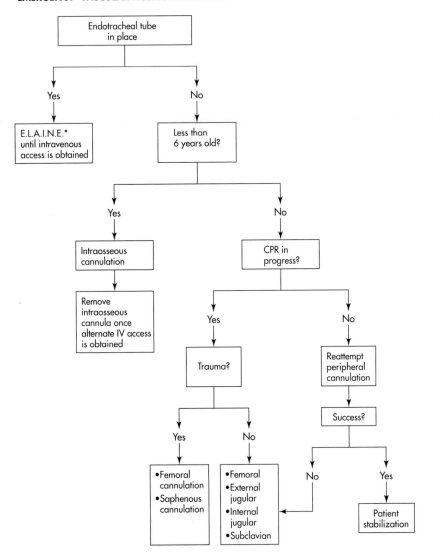

*E.L.A.I.N.E.—Epinephrine, **L**idocaine, **A**tropine, **I**soproterenol, **N**aloxone.
Resuscitative medications effective through the endotracheal tube.

FIG. C-1. Emergency vascular access algorithm. Ultimately, the order of attempted cannulation will vary with a practitioner's familiarity and expertise with a given technique. (Adapted from Vascular access. In Chameides L, Hazinski MF, eds: *Textbook of pediatric advanced life support.* Dallas, 1994, American Heart Association.)

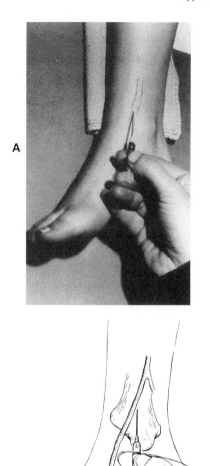

FIG. C-2.   Peripheral. Intravenous access may be secured even when the vein is not visualized, by knowing venous anatomy. The saphenous vein can almost always be cannulated 0.5 to 1.0 cm superior and anterior to the medial malleolus running parallel to the tibia (**A** and **B**).

Continued.

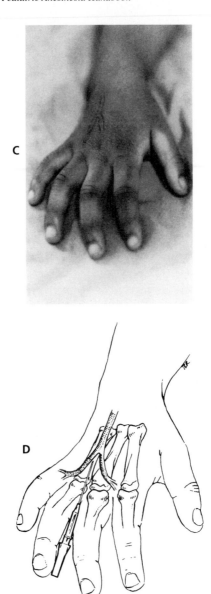

FIG. C-2, cont'd. A vein is also usually found on the middorsum of the hand between the middle and ring metacarpals (**C** and **D**).

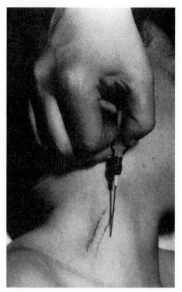

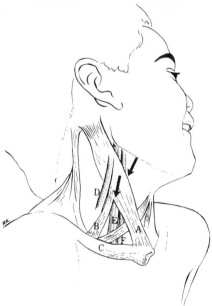

FIG. C-3. Jugular. The internal jugular vein can be cannulated by inserting a needle at the apex of the triangle of the two heads of the sternocleidomastoid (*SCM*) and aiming for the ipsilateral nipple (*lower arrow and photograph*). The vein can also be located by inserting the needle anteriorly to the SCM at a point halfway between the mastoid process and sternal notch, aiming at the ipsilateral nipple (*higher arrow*). *A,* medial head of the SCM; *B,* lateral head of the SCM; *C,* clavicle; *D,* external jugular vein; *E,* internal jugular vein; *F,* carotid artery.)

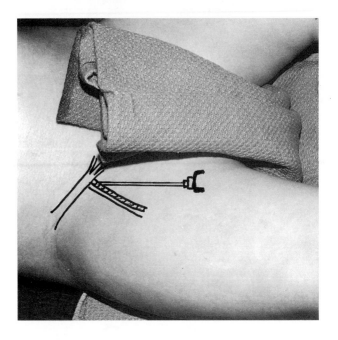

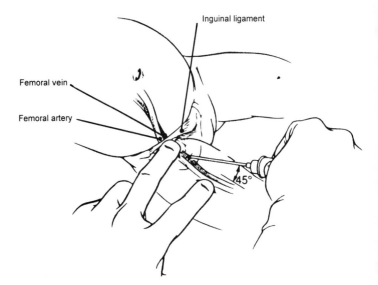

FIG. C-4. Femoral access. The femoral artery is located inferior to the inguinal ligament at the midpoint between the superior iliac spine and symphysis pubis. The femoral vein is medial to the artery and is best accessed approximately 1 finger's breadth below the inguinal ligament, with the needle directed toward the umbilicus at a 45° angle. (Adapted from Vascular access. In Chameides L, Hazinski MF, eds: *Textbook of advanced pediatric life support,* Dallas, 1994, American Heart Association.)

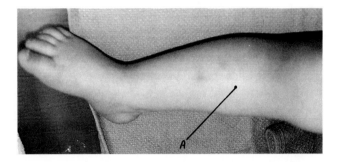

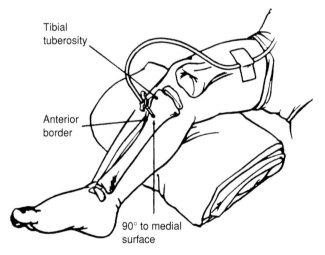

FIG. C-5. Intraosseous access. The site of cannulation (*A*) is approximately one finger's width below and just medial to the tibial tuberosity. At this site the tibia is just under the skin surface. A sudden decrease in resistance to forward motion of the needle indicates entrance into the bone marrow cavity. (Adapted from Vascular access. In Chameides L, Hazinski MF, eds: *Textbook of Advanced pediatric life support,* Dallas, 1994, American Heart Association.)

PEDIATRIC RESUSCITATION DRUG DOSAGES

D

Drug	Dose (mg/kg)	Stock solution	Preparation
*†Atropine	0.01-0.02	Many, commonly: 0.4 mg/ml, 0.5 mg/ml	*Undiluted:* **0.4 mg/ml stock solution:** 0.025 ml/kg = 0.01 mg/kg 0.05 ml/kg = 0.02 mg/kg **0.5 mg/ml stock solution:** .02 ml/kg = 0.01 mg/kg .04 ml/kg = 0.01 mg/kg Minimum dose = 0.1 mg Maximum dose = 1.0 mg
†Calcium chloride	10-30	10% solution (100 mg/ml)	*Undiluted:* 0.1 ml/kg = 10 mg/kg
Calcium gluconate	100	10% solution (100 mg/ml)	*Undiluted:* 1 ml/kg = 100 mg/kg
*†Epinephrine	0.01 (0.05 for cardiac arrest)	1:10000 (1 mg/ml)	*Diluted* 1:10 gives: 1:10,000 solution = 0.1 mg/ml 0.1 ml/kg = 0.01 mg/kg
*†Lidocaine	1	4% solution (40 mg/ml)	*Diluted:* 2 ml of 4% lidocaine + 6 ml diluent = 1% solution (10 mg/ml) 0.1 ml/kg = 1 mg/kg

Drug	Dose (mg/kg)	Stock solution	Preparation
*Naloxone	0.01-0.02	0.4 mg/ml Neonatal = 0.02 mg/ml	*Undiluted* (neonatal): 0.5-1.0 ml/kg = 0.01-0.02 mg/kg 0.4 mg/ml DILUTED 1:4 gives 0.1 mg/ml, then .01 ml/mg = .01 mg/kg
†Phenylephrine	0.01	1% solution (10 mg/ml)	*Diluted* 1:10 twice to a 0.01% solution (0.1 mg/ml) 0.1 ml/kg = 0.01 mg/kg
Sodium bicarbonate	1 mEq/kg	1 mEq/ml	*Undiluted:* 1 ml/kg = 1 mEq/kg Dilute: 1:1 OR 1:2 for infants and neonates
Tolazoline (Priscoline)	1 followed by infusion	25 mg/ml	*Diluted:* 1:10 gives: 2.5 mg/ml 0.4 ml/kg = 1 mg/kg

*Drugs can be given via endotracheal tube.

†Because of small volumes these drugs should be administered with a Tb syringe in infants < 10 kg.

E

DRUG INFUSIONS FOR PEDIATRIC RESUSCITATION

Drug	Dose (μg/kg/min)	Undiluted concentration (mg/ml)	Preparation (mg in diluent to equal 100 ml total volume)	Infusion rate
Calcium gluconate	200-500 mg/kg/day	100 mg/ml	—	Dilute total dose in desired volume and infuse over 24 hr
Dopamine	1-15	40	A: (wt in kg) × 6 or B: 30 mg or C: Alternative: 150 mg (3.75 ml) in 250 ml	A: 1 ml/hr= 1 μg/kg/min B: 1 ml/kg/hr = 5 μg/kg min or wt in kg = ml/hr = 5 μg/kg/min C: 1 ml/kg/hr = 10 μg/kg/min or wt in kg = ml/hr = 10 μg/kg min
Dobutamine	1-15	50	Same as dopamine A	Same as dopamine A
Sodium nitroprusside	1-10	25	Same as dopamine A	Same as dopamine A (do not mix with saline)

Drug	Dose (μg/kg/min)	Undiluted concentration (mg/ml)	Preparation (mg in diluent to equal 100 ml total volume)	Infusion rate
Amrinone	5-10 μg/kg/min	5 mg/ml	Same as dopamine A	Same as dopamine A
Epinephrine	0.1-1	1	(wt in kg) × 0.6	1 ml/hr = 0.1 μg/kg/min
Isoproterenol	0.1-1	0.2	Same as epinephrine	Same as epinephrine
Lidocaine	20 (10-50)	40	120 (3 ml)	1 ml/kg/hr = 20 μg/kg/min
Tolazoline	1	25	100 (4 ml)	1 ml/kg/hr = 1 mg/kg/hr (begin after 1 mg/kg IV loading dose)
Trimethaphan (Arfonad)	10-200	50	60 mg	1 ml/kg/hr = 10 μg/kg/min
PGE-1	0.01-1	0.5	0.06 (0.12 ml)	1 ml/kg/hr = 0.01 μg/kg/min

ANTIBIOTIC PROPHYLAXIS AGAINST BACTERIAL ENDOCARDITIS

F

CARDIAC CONDITIONS FOR WHICH PROPHYLAXIS IS RECOMMENDED:

Prosthetic heart valves (including bioprosthetics)
Previous history of endocarditis
Most congenital heart disease
Idiopathic hypertrophic subaortic stenosis
Surgically constructed systemic-pulmonary shunts
Mitral valve prolapse with mitral insuficiency
Permanent endocardial pacemaker electrode
Rheumatic and other valvular dysfunction

PROCEDURES FOR WHICH PROPHYLAXIS IS INDICATED:

All dental procedures likely to induce gingival bleeding
Tonsillectomy and/or adenoidectomy
Surgical procedure involving respiratory mucosa
Bronchoscopy
Incision and drainage of infected tissue
Most GI and GU procedures especially in high risk, except
- Percutaneous liver biopsy
- Upper GI endoscopy *without* biopsy
- Proctosigmoidscopy *without* biopsy
- Straight catheterization of bladder

In high-risk patients or if infection is suspected, give prophylactic antibiotics even in these lower-risk procedures

CARDIAC CONDITIONS FOR WHICH PROPHYLAXIS IS NOT RECOMMENDED:

Isolated secundum atrial septal defect (ASD)
Secundum ASD repaired WITHOUT a patch more than 6 months earlier
Patent ductus arteriosus ligated and divided more than 6 months earlier
Permanent epicardial pacemaker electrode

DRUG REGIMENS FOR CARDIAC PROPHYLAXIS:

Dental/respiratory tract procedures

1. *Standard regimen*
   Amoxicillin 50 mg/kg (maximum 3.0 g) PO 1 hr before procedure, then 25 mg/kg (maximum 1.5 g) 6 hours after initial dose
2. *Unable to take oral medication*
   Ampicillin 50 mg/kg (maximum 2.0 g) IM/IV 30-60 min before procedure, and 25 mg/kg (maximum 1.0 g) 6 hours after initial dose or amoxicillin 25 mg/kg (maximum 1.5 g) PO 6 hours after initial dose
   OR
   Amoxicillin/Ampicillin/Penicillin allergic
   Clindamycin 10 mg/kg (maximum 300 mg) IV 1 hour before procedure and 5 mg/kg (maximum 150 mg) IV (or PO) 6 hours after initial dose
3. *Amoxicillin/Ampicillin/Penicillin allergic*
   Erythromycin 20 mg/kg (maximum 1.0 g) PO 1 hour before procedure, then 10 mg/kg (maximum 500 mg) 6 hours after initial dose
   OR
   Clindamycin 10 mg/kg (maximum 300 mg) PO 1 hour before procedure and 5 mg/kg (maximum 150 mg) PO 6 hours after initial dose
4. *Maximum protection*
   Ampicillin 50 mg/kg (maximum 2.0 g) IM/IV plus
   Gentamicin 1.5 mg/kg IM/IV (maximum 80 mg) 30 min before procedure followed by amoxicillin 25 mg/kg (maximum 1.5 g) PO 6 hours after initial dose or repeat the parenteral regimen 8 hours after the initial dose
   OR
   Amoxicillin/Ampicillin/Penicillin allergic
   Vancomycin 20 mg/kg (maximum 1.0 g) IV slowly over 1 hour before procedure (only 1 dose necessary)

Gastrointestinal or genitourinary procedures

1. *Standard regimen*
   Ampicillin 50 mg/kg (maximum 2.0 g) IV/IM plus gentamicin 1.5 mg/kg (maximum 80 mg) IV/IM 30-60 min before procedure followed by amoxicillin 25 mg/kg (maximum 1.5 g) PO 6 hours after initial dose or may repeat entire regimen 8 hours after initial dose
2. *Minor or repetitive procedures in low risk patients*
   Amoxicillin 50 mg/kg (maximum 3.0 g) PO 1 hour before procedure and 25 mg/kg (maximum 1.5 g) PO 6 hours after initial dose
3. *Amoxicillin/Ampicillin/Penicillin allergic*
   Vancomycin 20 mg/kg (maximum 1.0 g) IV slowly over 1 hour plus gentamicin 1.5 mg/kg (maximum 80 mg) IM/IV 1 hour before procedure
   May repeat entire regimen once 8 hours after initial dose

APPENDIX
BIBLIOGRAPHY

American Hospital Formulary Service: *American Hospital Formulary,* Bethesda, MD, 1989, American Society of Hospital Pharmacists.

Behrman RE, Vaughan VC III: *Nelson textbook of pediatrics,* ed 13, Boston, 1987, Little, Brown.

Benitz WE, Tatro DS: *The pediatric drug handbook,* ed 2, Chicago, 1988, Year Book Medical Publishers, Inc.

Drug facts and comparisons, Philadelphia, 1988, JB Lippincott Co.

Gilman A et al: *The pharmacological basis of therapeutics,* ed 8, New York, 1990, Pergamon Press.

Greene MG, ed: *The Harriet Lane handbook,* ed 12, Chicago, 1990, Mosby.

Physicians' desk reference, ed 44, Oradell, NJ, 1990, Medical Economics Co.

Prevention of bacterial endocarditis: recommendations by the American Heart Association by the Committee on Rheumatic Fever, Endocarditis, and Kawaski Disease, *JAMA* 1990; 264:2919-2922.

Stoelting RK: *Pharmacology and physiology in anesthetic practice,* Philadelphia, 1987, JB Lippincott.

Ziai M: *Pediatrics,* ed 3, Boston, 1984, Little, Brown.

INDEX

Page numbers in italics indicate illustrations.